D0556230

Child and adolescent mental health services: strategy, planning, delivery, and evaluation

Edited by

Richard Williams
Professor of Mental Health Strategy
Welsh Institute for Health and Social Care
School of Care Sciences
University of Glamorgan
Glamorgan, UK
and Consultant Child and Adolescent Psychiatrist
Gwent Healthcare NHS Trust
Newport, UK

and

Michael Kerfoot
Professor of Child and Adolescent Policy and Research
School of Psychiatry and Behavioural Sciences
University of Manchester
Manchester, UK

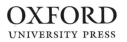

OXFORD
UNIVERSITY PRESS

OXFORD

UNIVERSITY PRESS

Great Clarendon Street, Oxford OX2 6DP

Oxford University Press is a department of the University of Oxford.
It furthers the University's objective of excellence in research, scholarship,
and education by publishing worldwide in

Oxford New York

Auckland Cape Town Dar es Salaam Hong Kong Karachi
Kuala Lumpur Madrid Melbourne Mexico City Nairobi
New Delhi Shanghai Taipei Toronto

With offices in

Argentina Austria Brazil Chile Czech Republic France Greece
Guatemala Hungary Italy Japan South Korea Poland Portugal
Singapore Switzerland Thailand Turkey Ukraine Vietnam

Oxford is a registered trade mark of Oxford University Press
in the UK and in certain other countries

Published in the United States
by Oxford University Press Inc., New York

© Oxford University Press, 2005

The moral rights of the author have been asserted

Database right Oxford University Press (maker)

First published 2005

All rights reserved. No part of this publication may be reproduced,
stored in a retrieval system, or transmitted, in any form or by any means,
without the prior permission in writing of Oxford University Press,
or as expressly permitted by law, or under terms agreed with the appropriate
reprographics rights organization. Enquiries concerning reproduction
outside the scope of the above should be sent to the Rights Department,
Oxford University Press, at the address above

You must not circulate this book in any other binding or cover
and you must impose this same condition on any acquirer

A catalogue record for this title is available from the British Library

ISBN 0 19 850844 1 (Pbk)

10 9 8 7 6 5 4 3 2 1

Typeset by Cepha Imaging Pvt. Ltd., Bangalore, India
Printed in Great Britain
on acid-free paper by
Biddles Ltd., King's Lynn

Foreword

We know that some 450 million people in our world live with a mental disorder.

We know that 1 in 3 of us will be affected directly or indirectly in our lifetime.

We know that 1 million people in our world commit suicide - 10 million try each year, including far too many children and young people.

We know that 121 million of us have depression - 3 in every 100 of us.

We know that neuropsychiatric disorders are responsible for one third of disabilities, 15% of in-patient costs, nearly a quarter of drugs costs and half the caseload of our social workers.

We also know that mental health, especially in the young, is rarely given the attention and priority it needs and deserves.

We are also aware that eating disorders and behavioural problems are the visible, if often misunderstood, tip of an adolescent iceberg.

We are to some extent aware of the pressures of lifestyle, school, college, and early careers can lead to stress and depression.

We are perhaps less aware of the impact, physical, and psychological, on young minds of decisions taken and events occurring before or at birth and in the early years.

A few years ago, as Health and Social Services Minister, I remember presenting to a not very expectant world the Messages from Research about child welfare and intervention, and the need to focus on those families and children apparently or probably finding it difficult to cope.

In 1995 I also launched with Richard Williams the HAS publication *Together we stand,* the thematic review which fed into the Health of the Nation Handbook on CAMHS. This is a follow up to that, highlighting as it does the advances in policy, strategy, commissioning, delivery, and evaluation over the subsequent nine years.

Child and adolescent mental health is one of the scandals of inadequate provision by health services across the world. It is doubly a scandal when one thinks that so much is preventable and so much is treatable and that failure to provide the services to do so condemns a young person to a life with the cruel burden of stigma added to the burden of the disorder.

Nor should one believe that it is all down to health services, fundamental as they may be. So often a young person loses out because health and social services and education cannot agree to share responsibility – and budgets – for his or her needs.

We have a great deal of expertise and professional excellence in our child and adolescent services; we need to blend it to a greater extent and we need to share best practice and impart these skills to those entering the services. We also need to learn from service users and their families and to help them to understand better what they are experiencing and what is being done to help them through.

Richard Williams and Michael Kerfoot and their team of contributors to this study take us through the history of CAMHS and steer us through the practice and policies, the theories and the settings, with the compass of their seven broad principles or themes and the recurring reminder that policy should determine services and not be dictated by them. Policy itself comes from a synthesis of science and practice, leavened by the needs and preferences of those for whom the services are to be provided. It is a book that is written, not as a textbook, but for a wider readership of practitioners, managers, and policymakers. It should be widely read – and its messages understood and acted upon.

John Bowis OBE MEP
November 2004

John Bowis was UK Health Minister responsible for Mental Health, from 1993 to 1996. From 1997 to 1999 he worked in support of the WHO Global Campaign "Nations for Mental Health". Since 1999 he has been MEP for London and his Party's Health Spokesman.

Child and adolescent mental health services

Oxford University Press makes no representation, express or implied, that the drug dosages in this book are correct. Readers must therefore always check the product information and clinical procedures with the most up to date published product information and data sheets provided by the manufacturers and the most recent codes of conduct and safety regulations. The authors and the publishers do not accept responsibility or legal liability for any errors in the text or for the misuse or misapplication of material in this work.

Preface

The idea that gave rise to this book was not ours alone, it belongs to a number of people. Oxford University Press agreed with the concept and asked us to edit this text. Initially simple, the aim was to write a follow-up to *Together we stand*. However, as we began work, we became aware that we were taking on an ambitious task.

Together we stand, published by Her Majesty's Stationery Office for the NHS Health Advisory Service (HAS) in 1995, is both a report and a manual summarizing a philosophy and a strategic approach to policy for child and adolescent mental health services (CAMHS) in England and Wales, as well as making innovating and creative suggestions for the way forward in commissioning and delivering better services. Hitherto, children's mental health had been a neglected topic in the domains of healthcare, social care, and education policy and investment as our opening chapter shows.

The work that led to *Together we stand* was requested in 1992 by the then Secretary of State for Health in England, Mrs Virginia Bottomley. At that time, the HAS was a non-departmental public body that was responsible for advising and making recommendations to Ministers and the responsible authorities on the state of mental health and eldercare services in England and Wales. One of us, Richard Williams, was its director and a number of the authors of this book, including, particularly, Mike Kerfoot, were involved in the CAMHS thematic review. That thematic review was conducted for the HAS by many talented practitioners, managers, and academics; thereby, it drew on contemporary wisdom. Through its many site visits, the HAS rapidly became aware that CAMHS, as the services became widely known thereafter, were grossly under resourced but being sustained by many committed practitioners though not by policy, commissioning, or strategically-directed investment. In his foreword to this book, John Bowis describes circumstances of that nature as a 'scandal'.

It is clear that a huge amount has changed for the better for CAMHS in the UK since 1995. England and Wales now have overt and widely-supported policies though, as we write, differing scales of proposed investment. Despite a change in the political complexion of the UK government in 1997, CAMHS remain high on the agenda. The practitioners remain committed and are, as ever, the vital positive asset in current services in the UK, but now workforce development is recognized as the most substantial hurdle to cross in moving forward. Interest in getting commissioning right is growing and management of CAMHS is improving. Many of the directions for development that we flagged, commended, or recommended in *Together we stand* have been taken up. The philosophy in that report has stood the test of time and is now adopted universally in the UK and a huge amount of practice, research, and managerial expertise has been brought to bear since 1995. Indeed, we see the philosophy and the expertise underlined in the separate National Service Frameworks for Children, Young People, and Maternity Services launched by the English and Welsh governments in 2004. Gradually, services for children, young people, and their families are improving as a result. The whole scene has become more complex as a result of burgeoning knowledge, skill, and interest and this is why the simple request to write an update to *Together we stand* has proved a challenge.

In this book, we follow the lead provided by *Together we stand* by writing one text for a plural audience; policymakers, strategic and operational managers, and practitioners of all disciplines. This is not, then, a textbook of clinical practice though, in it, we are attempting to bring together and integrate the knowledge, skills, and evidence from clinical experience and research with the tested principles and skills of good strategic leadership and management, operational management, and developmental principles from adult educational theory and practice. These topics are surveyed in Parts I and II. In Part III, we draw on experiences from North America, Australasia, the developing countries, and countries post major conflict to benchmark services in western Europe in the early twenty-first century and to learn lessons for improving policy, practice, and management. We leave readers to extract and integrate those lessons; they are clear and potent. Finally, Part IIII looks more closely at progress made with service commissioning, delivery, and evaluation in the UK since *Together we stand* was published.

The result is 38 chapters written by 54 renowned authors. Although we focus most on the UK, our intention was to edit a book that would have much wider geographical interest and applicability. We think that practitioners, policymakers, and managers worldwide will find the result helpful. At the very least, our authors provide a summary of accumulated wisdom as it was early in 2004.

John Bowis wrote the foreword to *Together we stand* in 1995 and we are extremely grateful to him for writing the foreword to this book.

Richard Williams and Michael Kerfoot
December 2004

Acknowledgement

One other thing stirs me when I look back at my youthful days ... The fact that so many people gave me something or were something to me without knowing it. Such people, with whom I never perhaps exchanged a word, yes, and others about whom I merely heard things by report, had a decisive influence on me; they entered into my life and became powers within me. Much that I should otherwise not have felt so clearly or done so effectively was felt or done as it was, because I stand, as it were, under the sway of these people. Hence I always think that we all live, spiritually, by what others have given us in the significant hours of our life. ... Often, indeed, their significance comes home to us first as we look back, just as the beauty of a piece of music or of a landscape often strikes us first in our recollection of it. ... If we had before us those who have thus been a blessing to us, and could tell them how it came about, they would be amazed to learn what passed over from their life into ours.

Albert Schweitzer (1875-1965)

Sadly, during the time in which we have been editing this book, two of its authors have died. Professor Richard Harrington and Dr David R. (Dan) Offord were both prominent figures on the world stage of child and adolescent mental health. We were privileged to know Richard Harrington very well as both colleague and friend and our lives, and the lives of countless others, were enriched by his brilliant intellect and unceasing good humour. We knew Dan Offord much less well but his work and reputation have also influenced us and the approach and contents of this book. Both were committed clinicians, researchers, and teachers who earned and retained the confidence and interest of colleagues from many different disciplines associated with the needs of troubled children.

Richard Williams and Michael Kerfoot
December 2004

Contents

List of contributors

Susan Bailey
Consultant Adolescent Forensic Psychiatrist
Adolescent Forensic Unit
Mental Health Services of Salford
Bury New Road
Prestwich
Manchester, UK

Wendy Barber
Consultant Child and Adolescent Psychiatrist
and Visiting Fellow University of
Glamorgan
Ty Bryn Child and Adolescent Unit
St Cadoc's Hospital
Lodge Road
Caerleon
Newport, UK

John Benington
Institute of Governance and Public
Management
University of Warwick
Coventry, UK

Peter Bower
National Primary Care Research and
Development Centre
University of Manchester
Williamson Building
Oxford Road
Manchester, UK

Anna Brazier
Clinical Psychologist
Childrens Centre
University Hospital of Wales
Health Park
Cardiff, UK

David Browning
formerly Associate Director
Audit Commission
1st Floor, Millbank Tower
Millbank
London, UK

Sarah Byford
Centre for the Economics of Mental Health
Institute of Psychiatry
De Crespigny Park
Denmark Hill
London, UK

Ted Cole
Senior Research Officer
University of Birmingham
Edgbaston
Birmingham, UK

Colin Coles
Honorary Research Professor
School of Education
King Alfred's College
Winchester, UK

Ilana B. Crome
Academic Director of Psychiatry
Professor of Addiction Psychiatry
Academic Psychiatry Unit
Keele University Medical School
Harplands Hospital
Hilton Road
Stoke-on-Trent, UK

Harry Daniels
Deputy Head of School
School of Education
University of Birmingham
Edgbaston
Birmingham, UK

Owen Davies
Consultant Psychiatrist
Marsburg House
Bowbridge Lane
Stroud, UK

Richard Dean
IT Specialist
Centre for Public Mental Health
Durham University
Elvet Riverside Building
New Elvet
Durham, UK

Kedar Nath Dwivedi
Director
International Institute of CAMH
Consultant Child and Adolescent Psychiatrist
Child, Adolescent, and Family Services
8 Notre Dame Mews
Northampton, UK

Bob Foster
National CAMHS Implementation Lead
LNR Strategic Health Authority
Lakeside House
4 Smith Way
Leicester, UK

William Fraser
146 Wenallt Road
Cardiff, UK

KWM (Bill) Fulford
Department of Philosophy
University of Warwick
Coventry, UK

Fiona Gale
CAMHS Regional Developmental Worker -
East Midlands National CAMHS
Support Service (NCSS)
LNR Strategic Health Authority
Lakeside House
4 Smith Way
Leceister, UK

Richard Gater
Department of Psychiatry
Rawnsley Building
Manchester Royal Infirmary
Oxford Road
Manchester, UK

Eilish Gilvarry
Northern Regional Drug & Alcohol
Services
Plummer Court
Carliol Place
Newcastle upon Tyne, UK

Gyles Glover
Professor of Public Mental Health and
Director, Centre for Public Health
Durham University
Elvet Riverside Building
New Elvet
Durham, UK

Rajesh Gowda
Department of Psychological Medicine
University Hospital of Wales
Heath Park
Cardiff, UK

Richard Harrington*
Professor of Child and Adolescent
Psychiatry
Royal Manchester Children's Hospital
Hospital Road
Pendlebury
Manchester, UK

Claire Hartley
National Child Health Mapping Team
Appleton House
Lanchester Road
Durham, UK

Philip Hazell
Director
Child and Youth Mental Health
Service
Harker Building
Wallsend Hospital
Wallsend
New South Wales, Australia

*It is with regret that we announce that Professor Richard Harrington died during the preparation of this book.

Christopher Heginbotham
Chief Executive
Mental Health Act Commission
Maid Marion House
Hounds Gate
Nottingham, UK

Peter Hill
Department of Psychological Medicine
Great Ormond Street Hospital for Children
Great Ormond Street
London, UK

Peter Hindley
Hightrees Deaf Child and Family Service
61 Glenburnie Road
London, UK

Cathy James
Wellington House
133-155 Waterloo Road
London, UK

Carol Joughin
Honorary Visiting Senior Research Fellow
Child Health Research and Policy Unit
City University
20 Bartholomew Close
London, UK

Michael Kerfoot
Professor of Child and Adolescent Policy
   and Research
School of Psychiatry and Behavioural
   Sciences
University of Manchester
Mathematics Building
Oxford Road
Manchester, UK

Martin Knapp
Professor of Child and Adolescent Policy
   and Research
Centre for the Economics of Mental Health
Institute of Psychiatry
De Crespigny Park
Denmark Hill
London, UK

Zarrina Kurtz
Consultant in Public Health and
   Health Policy
12 Blithfield Street
London, UK

Alison Lagier (née Sparrow)
Director of Operations
Rhondda Cynon Taff Local Health Board
Centre Court
Treforest Industrial Estate
Pontypridd
Glamorgan, UK

Wendy Macdonald
National Primary Care Research and
   Development Centre
University of Manchester
Williamson Building
Oxford Road
Manchester, UK

Barbara Maughan
Social, Genetic and Developmental
   Psychiatry Research Group
Institute of Psychiatry
De Crespigny Park
Denmark Hill
London, UK

Howard Meltzer
Professor
Office for National Statistics
1 Drummond Gate
London, UK

David R. (Dan) Offord*
Offord Centre for Child Studies
McMaster University and Hamilton
   Health Sciences Corporation
1200 Main Street West
Hamilton, Ontario
Canada

Ian Partridge
Prospect House
338 Hollingwood Lane
Bradford, UK

*It is with regret that we announce that Dr Dan Offord died during the preparation of this book.

Dave Pottage
Senior Research Fellow
School of Psychiatry & Behavioural Sciences
University of Manchester
Mathematics Building
Oxford Road
Manchester, UK

Atif Rahman
Consultant in Child and Adolescent
    Psychiatry
Royal Manchester Children's Hospital
Hospital Road
Pendlebury
Manchester, UK

Sarah Rawlinson
Child and Adolescent Mental Health Services
Bristol Royal Hospital for Children
Upper Maudlin Street
Bristol, UK

Greg Richardson
Consultant Child and Adolescent Psychiatrist
Lime Trees Child and Adolescent Family Unit
31 Shipton Road
York, UK

Gill Salmon
Senior Lecturer in Child and Adolescent
    Mental Health
Swansea Child and Family Clinic
Trehafod
Waunarlwydd Road
Cockett
Swansea, UK

Jane Scourfield
Department of Psychological Medicine
University of Wales College of Medicine
Cardiff, UK

Michael Shooter
President of the Royal College of
    Psychiatrists
17 Belgrave Square
London, UK

Anita Thapar
Department of Psychological Medicine
University Hospital of Wales
Heath Park
Cardiff, UK

Margaret Thompson
Senior Lecturer in Child and Adolescent
    Psychiatry
University of Southampton
Child Mental Health Services
Ashurst Hospital
Lyndhurst Road
Ashurst
Southampton, UK

Karen Tingay
Academic Unit
Family Consultation Clinic
Dunstable Health Centre
Priory Gardens
Dunstable, UK

John Visser
Senior Lecturer
School of Education
University of Birmingham
Edgbaston
Birmingham, UK

Panos Vostanis
Professor of Child and Adolescent
    Psychiatry
Division of Child Psychiatry
University of Leicester
Westcotes House
Westcotes Drive
Leicester, UK

Morton Warner
Professor of Health and Social Care
Welsh Institute of Health and Social Care
University of Glamorgan
Glyntaff Campus
Pontypridd
Glamorgan, UK

Richard Williams
Professor of Mental Health Strategy
Ty Bryn Child and Adolescent Unit
St Cadoc's Hospital
Lodge Road
Caerleon
Newport, UK

Miranda Wolpert
Consultant Clinical Psychologist
Family Consultation Clinic
Dunstable Health Centre
Priory Gardens
Dunstable, UK

Part 1

Background issues and concepts

Chapter 1

Setting the scene: perspectives on the history of and policy for child and adolescent mental health services in the UK

Richard Williams and Michael Kerfoot

Introduction

Underpinning our selection of the contents of this book is our assumption that its readers are seeking to develop or, at the least, to better understand child and adolescent mental health services. When doing either, there is a great temptation to get to grips immediately with the front line of provision of services with a view to examining what is happening there and what we would prefer to happen with a view to closing the gap between the two. While we agree that no one should forget that benefits to the public are usually delivered through relationships between them and practitioners, we also believe that the context in which patients, clients, users and their carers relate to staff of services is vital to the success of the whole enterprise. The context frames not only knowledge, skill, and attitudes but, most significantly, can exhort or hold back their acquisition and application, and also shapes the wishes, expectations, and demands of the public. Therefore, we start this text from a position that is about as remote from delivering healthcare as one can get. This is because this book is about the context of practice rather than about that practice itself.

Our book has a clear focus on strategy and its relationship to improving service delivery with the intention of obtaining better harmony between the needs and preferences of children, young people, and their families, and the realities of practice (Children's Commissioner for Wales 2003). In the next three chapters, we examine what is strategy and its role in promoting better mental healthcare for children and young people. But, we believe that it is important to begin with policy, as it should both shape strategy and be responsive to its effects. In this chapter, we propose a model for better connecting policy with practice and show how there should be reciprocal relationships between them. Inevitably, this takes us into exploring the relationships between policy and strategy. Put another way, we set the scene for the chapters that follow by asserting that strategy should be the two-way connecting link between policy and delivery of improved healthcare. In its essence, this chapter explores the relationship sketched by Fig. 1.1.

Plainly, in a text that endeavours to deal with issues of principle, we cannot attempt to present a comprehensive, comparative worldwide review of policy relating to children's mental health. Rather, in order to illustrate policy for child and adolescent mental health (CAMH), we have elected to take two countries' development of child and adolescent mental health services (CAMHS) and the policy that has underpinned them as an example of general principles.

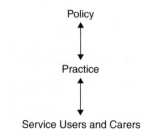

Fig. 1.1 The practice link between service users and policy.

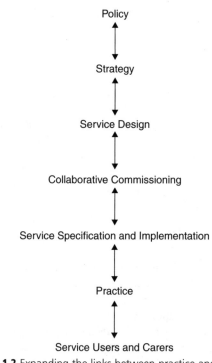

Fig. 1.2 Expanding the links between practice and policy.

While we have elected to present the policies of two jurisdictions in the UK in some detail, our intention is not to limit this chapter and its application to the UK, but to use the UK as an example upon which to build a model that links policy with the experiences of children and young people who use CAMHS, which could have much wider applicability. We look at how modern concepts of evidence-based practice, values-based practice, and clinical governance are related to, and mirrored in, modern concepts of policy development and implementation. The model on which we propose this and the following four chapters is shown in Fig. 1.2.

What is policy?

In everyday language, we tend to use the word 'policy' at two different levels. The first relates to the activities of government and 'politicians' or other large organizations, while the second relates to the detailed procedures by which some more limited enterprise should be put into effect. Thus, the Concise Oxford Dictionary (1990) defines policy as 'a course or principle of action adopted or proposed by a government, party, business or individual, etc.' and as 'prudent conduct; sagacity'. On reflection, a third use of the term, which might appear relevant at actual as well as metaphorical levels, due to modern-day preoccupations of policy with risk-avoidance (Williams 1999), relates to contracts issued for insurance purposes. Significantly, the roots of the word lie in the Greek for citizenship.

In a paper published in 2001, Black distinguishes between *practice* (or operational) *policies* (application of resources by practitioners), *service* (or strategic) *policies* (that determine the pattern of services) and *governance policies* (organizational and financial structures). Here, while very mindful of the implications of these wider meanings, we focus on policy as meaning those statements made by governments to explain the thinking and principles that they intend to guide their actions and investment of public monies to achieve improvements in the health of the nation and people within it.

In this chapter, we offer a summarized historical analysis of how CAMHS have developed in the UK, which shows the paucity of policy until the 1990s and recent rapid developments. Later, we return to examine some modern general conceptions about policy and, in particular, the notions of evidence-based and value-based policy and link them to how policy is formulated and implemented. But, to set the scene, we begin by considering a number of universal themes that impact on healthcare policy and which emerge from retrospective reviews of the twentieth century because they are as applicable to CAMH as all other public sector services.

Healthcare policy in the UK

In essence, our view is that policy should set the broad principles on which are based more detailed strategies to guide design and implementation of the service developments that are required. So, at this point, we take a side step from CAMHS to examine, albeit superficially, some very broad themes that appear to us to have driven, and to be continuing to drive, healthcare policies in the UK. They are not an exhaustive or exclusive list. Although we have drawn these seven themes from our experience in parts of the UK, there are clear parallels for CAMHS in the world more broadly. They are:

universality;

risk reduction and management and promoting resilience;

progressive improvement in capability;

manufactured risk;

limitations of resource;

the dynamics of need, demand and supply; and

the workforce.

Universality of high-quality services

Universality is a core principle that drove the creation of the National Health Service (NHS) in the UK in 1948 and it has been re-examined repeatedly and re-stated in different forms by successive governments. By it is meant the intention to provide the best of healthcare services to all on the basis of individuals' needs rather than on the basis of other determinants such as, for instance, rank, religion, and affluence. Universality sets extreme challenges and every review has shown how far our services can fall from achieving it.

Over the last 65 years in the UK, differing manifestations of this principle have come to the forefront of policy debate. Present concerns centre on: the relationships between adversity, disadvantage, poverty, and social exclusion, and the need for, and access to, services (see, for example, National Assembly for Wales 2000, and National Assembly for Wales Statistical Directorate 2000); the issues raised by cultural diversity and equitable access for all, regardless of culture, to appropriate services; and a particularly challenging issue for mental health services is the ubiquitous matter of stereotyping and stigma. But, underlying these issues are vital questions about whether it is proper and feasible that all components of healthcare can, or should be, provided free of charge at the point of need. If yes, then how should the finance and resources be found and delivered; and, if no, what healthcare functions should be so delivered?

Initially, policies to achieve universality of state-funded healthcare were implemented in an environment in which there was a considerable trust that those who did so would deliver high-quality care. However, increasing democratization has brought with it in the UK a culture of reduced deference to professional people, who are perceived as holding authority. Reduced trust and its consequences (O'Neil 2002, 2004; Pendleton and King 2002; Williams 2002) has been fanned by some highly publicized recent professional and managerial failings in the UK.

The principle of universality of high-quality healthcare has driven a wide range of subsidiary policies that have been designed to achieve equity and non-discrimination of access to services of assured and rising quality. In parallel, trust has been replaced by a culture of risk aversion, much greater scrutiny and regulation. Editorials written by one of us explore this area in more depth (Williams 1997, 1999, 2000, 2002).

Salter (2001) provides an analysis of the compact of relationships between the state (within which, policy-makers set the imperatives for, and directions of, services that are funded from the public purse), the public (who use and pay for all publicly funded services), and the professions (which deliver services to the public) (see Fig. 1.3).

Salter argued for a re-examination of the triad of relationships (i.e. the relationships between: the state and the public; the state and the professions; and the professions and the public) that spring from this triangle of stakeholders. He drew particular attention to his perception of the importance of putting energy into examining the relationship between the public and the professions. The wish of the people who use our services to have their voices heard is continuing to

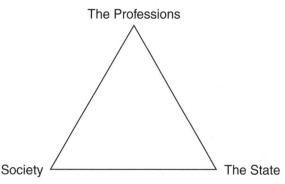

Fig. 1.3 A triangle of relationships representing an implicit compact about publicly funded healthcare.

rise, and associated with this is the rising position of advocacy—particularly for vulnerable people, so that they too may make their full contribution, have their needs met, and have their rights protected.

Salter's analysis sets the scene for debate on health policy. In this chapter, we examine in some detail communications between policymakers and the professions. That relationship is, arguably, mediated by managers and so, in this chapter, we are implicitly looking at another triangle of relationships: that between policymakers, public sector service managers, and the professions.

Reducing and managing risk and promoting resilience

Over the 80 years in which CAMHS have emerged in the UK as separate entities, knowledge of the factors that impact on the risks of contracting disease or other healthcare problems has increased dramatically (Wallace *et al.* 1997). This has contributed to two broad approaches to understanding risk and two approaches to delivering improved health. First, knowledge of the factors that impact on individuals' states of health and their risks of developing particular disorders and diseases has increased profoundly. Similarly, there have been rapid increases in the knowledge of the broad societal and environmental risk factors that impact, not only on the health of individuals but also, on groups and populations of individuals. The dramatic impacts of intervening indirectly with the health of individuals through environmental approaches to populations of people have been evident for some considerable period (for example, a very considerable impact on the health of the nation resulted from improved sanitation and, again, wider-scale fluoridization of the water supply is another, this time current, issue in the UK). The two related approaches to healthcare are those of practice relating to relieving ill health and reducing risk for identified individuals, and public health practice relating to communities and health promotion for groups of people.

In 1974, government policy resulted in simultaneous re-organization of local government and health services in England and Wales. One effect was that local management of the NHS passed from administering hospitals and groups of hospitals to Area Health Authorities (AHAs) which took responsibility for the health of geographically defined populations as well as premises. AHAs took over much (but not all) of the responsibility for public health and community medicine from the local authorities. Previously, responsibilities for the two branches of healthcare depicted in Fig. 1.4 were split, in England and Wales, between the NHS and the local authorities. Thus, policy developments in the early 1970s reflected deliberate re-adjustments to the balance between individual and public approaches to healthcare. Although the changes that occurred in 1974 and thereafter adjusted the allocation of responsibilities between them, they did not resolve the situation as some healthcare functions (e.g. environmental health) remain still in the responsibility of the local authorities (though further adjustments took place in Wales in 2003 with the creation of the National Public Health Service for Wales).

In parallel with increased prominence being given to healthcare approaches that are based on recognition of risk factors and endeavours to reduce them, other approaches have begun to look at improving the resilience of both individuals and populations to developing ill health. Thus, in more recent years, we see increasing concerns about health promotion both at individual (e.g. well-people's clinics and health-promoting schools) and at community and population levels (e.g. the healthy schools initiatives of Lister-Sharp *et al.* 1999).

In effect, these approaches have produced a matrix for policy and service development, which is summarized by the examples in Fig. 1.4.

	Prevention	Intervention
Health and Social Care Approaches to Individual Service Users (Individual Healthcare)	Health in schools programmes Well-adolescent clinics Parenting programmes targeted on families most at risk (e.g. pregnant, young, and unpartnered women) Targeted education programmes to aid young people who are identified as at particular risk to resist substance use and/or misuse or to resist progressing from substance use to misuse	Consultation and advice provided for, and joint working with, staff in Tier 1 provided by staff of Tier 2 Specialist CAMHS Indicated education programmes to aid young people who are already using substances and/or misusing substances Parenting interventions for families whose children already have mental health problems Referral of children and young people to Specialist CAMHS
Health and Social Care Approaches to the Public (Public Healthcare)	Work with the Media Healthy schools programmes Ante-natal and post-natal parenting classes Provision of information and information leaflets on common problems for families Universal education programmes to aid young people to resist substance use and/or misuse	Advice on service policies to the responsible health, education and social services authorities provided by professionals who work in Specialist CAMHS with the aim of reducing the risk of young people developing co-morbid mental disorders Supervision of the work of other agencies and staff when they design and deliver universal parenting classes Training for staff in Tier 1 provided by staff of Tier 2 Specialist CAMHS

Fig. 1.4 Prevention and intervention: individual and public health approaches to child and adolescent mental health.

Inevitably, there have been tensions between public health and individual health approaches and between directing new resources towards health promotion and relief of existing disease and disorder. CAMH has evidently been caught up in this policy and service matrix alongside most other services. Generally, we think that this wide approach is to be greatly welcomed. However, it does also have a less satisfactory impact, which is that many authorities and agencies now have quite different conceptions of what the zone of responsibilities of CAMHS should be within the spectrum of possibilities represented by the matrix. These differences may not be recognized, negotiated, or resolved when they plan or deliver local services.

Progressive improvement in capability

Another theme with which policy for healthcare throughout the world has had to contend, is that of the very rapid increases in capability and the ever-widening array of people who are able to influence the health and/or otherwise of populations and individuals, and they highlight the importance of better co-ordination between agencies (Williams and Salmon 2002).

In retrospect, it seems to us highly likely that the true pace and extent of development of healthcare knowledge, skill, and potential for intervention was not envisaged when the NHS was established in the UK in the 1940s. Ingenuity has driven spectacularly rapid improvements in the potential to deliver healthcare interventions that appear to go well beyond what was anticipated when the concept for the NHS was first developed. This applies fully to mental healthcare. It has led to increasing debate about the role of the NHS and whether the principle of universality can continue to underpin the roles and responsibilities of the state.

Manufactured risk

Similarly, growth of knowledge and potential capability has also driven much greater awareness that the number of disorders and diseases to which humans might fall prey is not static or limited. Instead of a portfolio of a fixed number of risks, which have reduced in degree and impact as the affluence of society has risen and as public health measures have greatly reduced or removed the risks of particular diseases and disorders resulting in improvements to the health of the public, it is now evident that changes have resulted in new risks for ill health and for deviation from what might be broadly considered a state of health. Entirely new disorders have arisen, other disorders have been defined and recognized, and there are now new possibilities for effective intervention with previously intractable conditions and undesirable circumstances. As examples within our field, attention deficit/hyperactivity disorder has arisen as a syndrome that has been defined progressively as the Diagnostic and Statistical Manual of the American Psychiatric Association has developed. Within the last 15 years, its diagnosis and treatment in the UK, as elsewhere, has increased dramatically. Similarly, autism spectrum disorders are much more frequently detected and diagnosed, and the period of our study has been marked by increasing awareness of the frequency of young people deliberately harming themselves and the wide spectrum of their needs.

Some of the new disorders have arisen from evolution of existing risks and others have occurred as a consequence of technological and other innovation (e.g. radiation hazards and diseases relating to antibiotic resistance), or with changing conditions and circumstances in society. Thus, some of the new risks can be termed 'manufactured risks' and all of these developments have broadened the scope, nature, and volume of demand for health services. Plainly, evolutions of all of these kinds operate within the realm of younger people's mental health.

Limitations of resource

Thus, from the core principle of universality of high-quality healthcare has stemmed a rapidly increasing array of potential work for health services that include health promotion and prevention, as well as services to intervene with individuals who have established disorder. Similarly, the task of commissioning and delivering health services now falls to many more

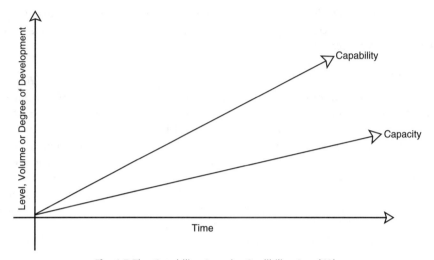

Fig. 1.5 The Capability-Capacity Credibility Gap (C3).

agencies than the NHS. Democratization of knowledge and rapid improvements in communications have played their part in accelerating public expectations of healthcare services. It is fair to say that the public's wishes, expectations, and demands are better aligned to the potential capability of services than they are to the reality, which is that the affluence of society as a whole and its willingness to give priority to healthcare, even less mental healthcare, have not expanded in parallel with the rise of potential capability.

Thus, although increasing volumes of resource have been put into healthcare for the last 70 years, the gap between the ability and/or willingness of the state to fund healthcare services and what could be done continues to increase (see Fig. 1.5).

Need, supply, and demand

Thus, there is a triangle of tension linking demands made by individuals and communities for expanded health and social care interventions, objective measures of benefit that might reasonably be achieved by high-quality services for target populations (that we might consider here as need), and the capacity of society to supply the services that are needed or demanded.

Our view is that this rising gap between public expectation and the potential capability of healthcare services, and their actual and affordable capacity, is one of the most powerful drivers of all health and social care policy. Looking back, we see successive governments in England and Wales endeavouring to balance the tensions between public wishes and expectations for its public sector services, and capacity and capability. We consider that this applies as much to mental healthcare as to all other arenas of health.

This general challenge has lain behind recurrent examinations of the purpose of health and social care in the UK. Each successive government in England and Wales has been faced with the dilemma on taking office. Prior to doing so, all political parties tend to make statements to suggest that public sector services will be safe with them and each suggests how it will manage better the triangle of tensions of Fig. 1.6. But each government, on taking office, has to reconcile

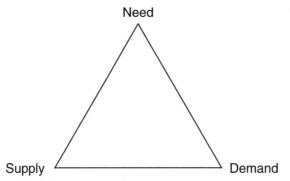

Fig. 1.6 The Triangle of Tension linking Need, Supply and Demand.

	Mode of Governance		
Dominant Mode of Governance	Hierarchies	Markets	Networks
Dominant Nature of Interaction of Government with Service Providers	Commands	Competition on price and quality	Trust and enabling organizations to deliver

Fig. 1.7 Dominant Modes of Governance (after Powell and Glendinning 2002).

itself to not only trying to grapple with the realities of the runaway scenario depicted by Fig. 1.5, but also with endeavouring to keep the promises that it has made prior to election.

How have successive governments responded to the challenge? In their chapter in a recent book on partnerships, Powell and Glendinning (2002, p. 1) cite an argument to the effect that the dominant mode of government in the UK has shifted (see Fig. 1.7) from hierarchies (in which commands are the core feature), through markets (in which the levers are competition on price and quality), to networks (in which governance is effected through trust and enabling organizations to deliver).

Looking back, we argue that, prior to the period of Conservative government from 1979 to 1997, command was indeed the dominant mode of governance of the health and welfare services, though history shows that strong themes of interdependent partnership between the state and the voluntary sector preceded the creation of the modern welfare state in the late 1940s.

Although recent governments (post-1979) have developed and adopted different dominant modes when trying to manage the conundrum set by the need–supply–demand triangle of tension within healthcare, each has also retained other modes. The Conservative Party retained use of command hierarchies alongside the market approach it introduced formally in 1990. Since its election in 1997, the Labour Party has replaced markets with networked quasi-contractual approaches to commissioning healthcare, while also retaining use of command through its National Service Frameworks and Priorities and Planning Frameworks and greater concentration on managing performance that is, often, related to delivery processes rather than outcomes.

As we shall see, these mixtures of governance modes have affected and been reflected in policy for CAMHS.

Workforce issues

Finance is not the only limiting factor that impacts heavily on health and social care, and education possibilities. Throughout the world, the supply of appropriately trained staff for our health and welfare services is now the most significant rate-limiting factor in producing service change.

There are three issues that we identify here. The first relates to the supply of staff who are enabled to keep up to date with a rapidly changing field. The second relates to the environment in which those staff work. The environment of modern social welfare and health services is shifting from one of respect and trust for professionals, with a belief that they will do what is right, to its replacement with a much more heavily regulated scenario. In part, this relates to a democratization of social welfare services and it also picks up on much greater public awareness of particular situations in which professionals have not performed in a way that politicians, the media, and/or the public or their professional peers see as satisfactory.

A third issue relates to the gap between capacity and capability that we have already identified. In such a setting, there is a real possibility of tension between policymakers and practitioners. While it is possible that policymakers and practitioners may see eye-to-eye over the direction of travel for certain aspects of service, it is also possible that they might not. Practitioners are faced with dealing with the public at the point at which they require services, and the professions that provide those practitioners have their own value systems and ethics, which may or may not concur with those of policymakers. Thus, it is conceivable that, in any given situation, there is the real possibility of practitioners experiencing a tension between what they see as right and proper in delivering services for the service users to whom they relate, and their perceptions of what it is that policymakers are asking them to do. From the policymakers' perspective, the tensions may be experienced as them straining to deliver their promises to a public whose expectations they have raised against a background of limitations to the public purse. A contemporary example from the UK is that of the tension between public safety, protection of individuals' freedoms, and user-centred services that has arisen between the governments in England and Wales, on one side, and service users, their carers, and the professions, on the other, over the contents of the draft Mental Health Bill published in 2002. The UK government published the Bill with the intention of improving public safety and patient care, among many other important matters, while a coalition between service users, carers, managers and the professions argues that key provisions in the Bill are non-evidenced, impractical, and unethical.

Ham and Alberti (2002) refer to 'the implicit contract' determining the relationship between the government, the medical profession, and the public. They say that this was based on:

> the government guaranteeing access to care for all citizens and determining the budget for the NHS;

> the medical profession taking responsibility for ensuring clinical standards and delivering care to patients;

> the public accepting from the government its right to healthcare that is delivered to appropriate standards by the profession, and paying taxes to fund the NHS.

Ham and Alberti believe that the implicit contract has weakened progressively since the 1960s with the rate of change accelerating since 1997. They call for a new and explicit contract that balances patients' rights with public responsibilities and greater accountability, provision of enough resources, better partnerships between doctors and their patients, and support for effective care in a setting in which the government exercises open stewardship. Interestingly, Ham and Alberti see increased accountability of professionals as essential to 'preserve appropriate discretion and autonomy and to avoid doctors becoming mere technicians, slavishly following rules and regulations determined by others. Equally the profession has to accept the legitimate role of managers in the NHS while being willing to play their part in steering the system at all levels'.

Managing the gap between capability and capacity of CAMHS

Our seven themes are well exampled by CAMHS. As later chapters will show, there is now documented evidence of rising prevalences of mental disorders affecting children and adolescents, and progressive developments of potential capability. Furthermore, recognition of the mental health problems faced by young people has increased very substantially, and a willingness of families to request and accept CAMHS has improved resulting in greater public expectations. However, the capacity of services to deliver improvements in mental health for individuals and populations, and intervention with established disorders, remains much more limited. Despite undoubted, though often poorly planned and co-ordinated, increases in investment, that gap is continuing to grow (see Fig. 1.5). Unfortunately, while each of the seven policy themes operates in respect of children's mental health, governments in the UK were substantially silent on CAMHS until the 1980s.

A historical perspective on policy for and development of CAMHS in the UK

Now that we have considered some general matters that bear on modern healthcare policy, we trace, in three epochs, the history of those services and policy for them in the UK by way of illustration and to provide a platform of understanding for our analysis of recent and current policy challenges relating to CAMHS.

Developments from 1920 to 1974

Although some practitioners took an interest in children's mental ill health, the psychiatric disorders of children and adolescence do not feature prominently in the early history of psychiatry. While, as Black (1993) says, 'the history of the treatment of children's deviant behaviour goes back to ancient times…', it was not until the late nineteenth century, that 'serious medical interest began to be shown in the emotional and intellectual problems of young people and the importance of a developmental perspective in understanding disorder'. But, 'Increasingly, attention was paid to differences in intellectual ability which allowed psychiatric disordered young people to be distinguished from those with mental handicap'.

As Williams and Skeldon (1992) say:

> Developments in the USA and later in England were strongly influenced by the teaching of Adolf Meyer whose concern with the uniqueness of the individual rather than clinical descriptions of mental disorder was enthusiastically taken up by those struggling to understand troubled young people. His psychobiological approach embraced physical, psychological and environmental influences and enabled a multi-factorial clinical and social-developmental perspective to be taken.

It is fascinating to observe that Meyer might consider his approach compatible with modern CAMHS policy.

The first child-guidance clinic for delinquent children was founded in Boston, USA, in the early 1920s and, according to Black, this 'marked the beginning of the application of "scientific" methods to the study and treatment of deviant children'. Meyer's psychobiological approach helped to fuse the contributions of psychiatrists, psychologists, and social workers leading to child-guidance clinics being set up in England on this model. Black says:

> The first child-guidance clinic in the UK, and indeed in Europe, was founded in the East End of London by the Jewish Health Organization in 1927 and a psychiatrist, Emmanuel Miller, was appointed as honorary director together with a psychiatric social worker who had trained in Boston and a psychologist.

Williams and Skeldon say that thereafter 'development spread rapidly and by 1939 there were 46 out-patient clinics in Great Britain based on the child guidance model of multi-disciplinary work with contributions from psychiatry, psychology, social work and child psychotherapy'. Initially, there was no training for staff specific to children and adolescents. Most services were staffed by recruiting practitioners trained to work with adults who were willing to spend part of their time in clinics working with children and their families.

By 1948, when the National Health Service (NHS) was founded, there were often rudimentary child-guidance services, in most areas (Black 1993). By the 1970s, most towns, boroughs and counties had at least out-patient services. Services often developed in response to the needs of schools and, increasingly, to provide services to the courts, which valued and continue to value advice from experts in making decisions about the needs and welfare of children in trouble. In most instances prior to 1974, these child-guidance clinics were administered and funded by the local authorities with their Medical Officers of Health providing the medical staff input, while other departments of the local authorities provided social workers and psychologists.

Around 50 years ago in the UK, there were only a few hospital-based child psychiatric clinics. But, in parallel with, if slightly later than, the child guidance movement, separate developments took place of mental health departments for children and adolescents in NHS teaching hospitals. Once again, many of the staff developed interests in working with children from their bases in adult psychiatry. Often, these services were associated with existing mental hospitals or with specialist paediatric hospitals. They provided out-patient services and, later, some developed inpatient psychiatric services for children and adolescents.

Williams and Skeldon point out that the result of these largely unco-ordinated parallel streams of development was that, by the 1970s, a situation had been reached in which a number of towns had two services (one substantially hospital-based offered by the NHS and the other offered by the local authority in the community). In some instances, there was overlapping of staff but, in many, a formal mechanism for co-ordination did not exist. Similarly, until the early 1970s in England and Wales, both hospital management committees and local authorities employed social workers and doctors.

At this point, contrasts were beginning to be made in academic and professional circles between the availability of services and research into the prevalence of child psychiatric disorder. For example, Kolvin (1973) found that less than 1% of the child population was receiving help from child-guidance clinics but that between 7 and 20% of children (depending on severity) were identified as suffering from a definite child psychiatric disorder (Rutter *et al.* 1970).

Academic departments of child and adolescent psychiatry were established earlier in the US than in Europe, and the first academic department of psychiatry opened in England in 1972.

Since then, the academic contributions to CAMH have grown dramatically. Most major medical schools in universities now make some level of commitment to child psychiatry and/or related disciplines and to training professionals who work in CAMHS.

As a result, Black identified a number of landmark scientific developments in the last 60 years, and it is salutary to remember that many of the disorders and mental health problems that are in common parlance now have been identified and delineated, and treatment approaches developed, in the interval. In her view: Kanner's definition of the syndrome of infantile autism (1943); Robertson's work on managing children in hospital (1952); Bowlby's seminal ideas on attachment (1969, 1973, 1980); Winnicott's concept of parenting (1965); Robins long-term follow-up of child-guidance clinic patients (1966); Rutter's (Rutter *et al.* 1970; Rutter and Smith 1995) and Graham's (1976) work on the epidemiology of childhood mental disorder; and Kolvin's assessment of treatment approaches (1973); constitute some of these groundbreaking developments between 1940 and 1980. Since then, of course, much more has developed including, particularly, development of more effective intervention techniques and the new molecular genetics which promise so much for the future.

So far, we have traced very briefly the origins in the UK of out-patient mental healthcare for younger people. When doing so, we found that their development was largely due to advocacy by dedicated people rather than the result of deliberate policy. Arguably, prior to 1980, one of the most notable oases in this dessert was the Court Report (1976). The situation has been similar for in-patient services.

In-patient units specifically for children and adolescents began to appear in the nineteenth century, mainly to care for young people who were described as severely mentally retarded. In the USA, units were set up in the 1920s primarily for young people suffering the after effects of encephalitis. Thereafter, growing experience of the positive effects of environments that focus on the needs of young people was reported and excited interest in the UK. In the UK, the first in-patient adolescent units were opened in the late 1940s at St Ebbas in Epsom and at the Bethlem Hospital. The number of units grew very slowly until the mid-1960s.

Concern over the plight of adolescents admitted to adult psychiatric wards was raised in the House of Commons and spurred a brief policy foray into the field when the then Ministry of Health issued Memorandum HM64(4) (1964), which gave guidance to health regions on the number of mental illness beds required specifically for adolescents. This speeded up the previously slow development of adolescent units across the country with a number of new in-patient services being established in the decade to 1974. Although largely provided by health agencies, significant contributions of staff were made to those units by local authority education and social services departments. The history indicates variations in structure, function, and therapeutic model and a good general account of staff roles in and the functioning of the, then, contemporary UK adolescent units is offered by Steinberg (1986).

Developments from 1974 to 1990

Earlier, we referred to the changes of approach to healthcare strategy and its administration consequent on the re-organization of the public sector in England and Wales in 1974. There were two key consequential matters that were important for CAMH. One effect was that the focus of service planners moved from considering the needs of those people who used the services of particular hospitals to include the wider needs of defined populations, whether service users or otherwise. Second, the new AHAs took over much of the responsibility for public health from the local authorities. Responsibility for school medical services passed to the new health authorities as did most of the medical staff who worked in the child-guidance clinics. The employment of all social workers based in the NHS passed in the other direction to local authority social services departments.

At this point, some attention was given by the, then, Department of Health and Social Security (DHSS) in the UK government to getting the AHAs and local authorities to better co-ordinate the child guidance and hospital-based mental health services for children and young people in each area. As Williams and Skeldon say:

> Although these intentions were admirable, resulting in improved services in many places, the new arrangements also sowed the seeds of great difficulties for child and adolescent mental health services. Major problems have sprung from the struggle to produce effective services in circumstances in which staff were employed by and the capital and revenue found by at least two different authorities. Each had its own responsibilities, priorities and planning machinery—one responsible to local government and the other direct to central government. These inherent structural weaknesses were containable throughout the 1970s but, in the 1980s they contributed powerfully to reductions in service and the consequent forced movement away from the child guidance multi-disciplinary model of service when financial pressures on public services began to bite hard.

Thus, it is pertinent to look at, not only what happened to the volume and distribution of services but also to consider, what we know of the effects on the nature and approach of CAMHS.

Cruelly for CAMHS, the enormous opportunities offered by policy-driven re-organization of public sector services in the mid-1970s were accompanied by a down-turn in the economic circumstances of the UK and this slowed up investment in and, therefore, the development of both out-patient and in-patient mental health services for minors, which lasted for much of the next 25 years. Indeed, many dedicated in-patient places and units were closed in this period due, we think, to the absence of effective planning and funding mechanisms at regional and national levels.

Thus, by the mid 1990s, England and Wales had inherited a circumstance in which, although services have continued to develop slowly, and the potential capability of practitioners had grown dramatically in the last 50 years, the ability of the country to afford, and the lack of will-ingness of its policymakers and managers to prioritize, CAMH in practice within what could be afforded had resulted in, overall, a situation in which the estimates are that between 1 and 2% of the child population received treatment, while the incidence and prevalence of disorder have risen. Furthermore, recognition of the mental health problems faced by young people has increased very substantially and a willingness of families to request and be prepared to accept CAMHS has improved, resulting in greater public expectation, which continues to rise, and in growing gaps between the potential capability and the actually capacity of services. However, in the 1980s, even this came under erosion.

In our view, the erosion that appeared to occur from the mid 1980s, took place, not necessarily on the basis of the application of any evidence but from two roots that relate to the different styles and mechanisms of administration of local authority and national health services in the UK: from service pressures that continued to rise irrespective of pressures on the public purse, and from differing ideological and value-based developments within the professions. We do not suggest that these changes or any greater gulf between services provided by local authorities and NHS were in any way orchestrated or managed. Indeed, we have already provided a background picture of the growth of CAMHS in England and Wales that has been driven in a substantially unco-ordinated way. Thus, CAMH was only the focus of prominent policy at intervals until the 1990s. Rather, services have grown in the UK as a result of the advocacy of strong minded, committed, and determined individuals who were often senior practitioners or took their origin from the sapiential authority of academic development. As the NHS Health Advisory Service (HAS) was to show later (1995), management investment in child and adolescent mental healthcare was extremely low until very recently. Also, the attention given to CAMH by policymakers was, arguably, scant until the 1990s and any statements that were made (e.g. in response to the Bridges over Troubled Waters report from the HAS) were not necessarily followed through into implementation.

We have described an opening investment in children's mental healthcare in the UK as founded on psychosocial approaches and multidisciplinary care. But, what happened over approximately a 15-year period, from the mid-1980s through to the end of the last century, was that overt involvement of the local authorities declined in delivering what we would now call Specialist CAMHS. Arguably, this mirrored the very real and increasing pressure on the local authorities for them to deal effectively with rapid increases in our recognition of physical, sexual, and emotional abuse inflicted on young people, and must be set against the scenario of major budgetary pressures that did not reflect the growing demands placed on local authorities.

However, it is also evident that other influences also underpinned this separation, between the NHS and local authority input to Specialist CAMHS which involved growing differences in the ideologies and values adopted by social care and healthcare practitioners and managers. The work of the Dartington Social Research Unit (DSRU) provides a contemporary commentary on the tensions between the major public service sectors (Bullock and Little 1999; Williams and Salmon 2002; Little and Bullock 2004). This situation has been accompanied by and has reflected apparent reductions in emphasis on child development and casework in training social workers.

In parallel, the abilities of educational psychologists (also employed by local authorities) to invest time in working closely with other mental healthcare practitioners and directly with pupils in need also declined during the 1980s. This reflected rising demands from parents and schools, and challenges that can be traced to the otherwise laudable Education Act of 1980 and its successor legislation dealing with special educational need. It brought an extremely important improvement in approach to children's educational, emotional, and behavioural needs by endeavouring to remove a categorical approach in favour of a needs-led approach through the process of Statementing of Special Educational Need. However, increases in the demands for documenting and processing the assessments of, and plans made for, children and young people, and the inevitable tensions between what might ideally be provided as a result of the Statements and what the local education authorities could afford, produced a rising agenda of work for educational psychologists. Not surprisingly, the wider roles that educational psychologists had played in conjunction with other disciplines reduced after 1980 in child guidance clinics.

Paradoxically, these changes to the roles of social workers and educational psychologists contributed to the rise in importance of nurses and clinical psychologists within child and adolescent mental healthcare. Until this point, the investment in nursing in CAMH had been largely restricted to day and in-patient units. In the last 20 years, there has been a very rapid growth of the number of nurses appointed to out-patient services, such that the Audit Commission showed in 1999 that nurses formed the single largest professional group in Specialist CAMHS.

When the Conservative Party returned to government in 1979, it responded to the universal healthcare challenges that it inherited by, first, endeavouring to get more order and productivity for the same finance by introducing general management into the NHS. Yet, our observations suggest to us that, before general management had had sufficient time to make sustained impacts, politicians were once again frustrated by the slow speed of getting to grip with increasing demand. The result was that, in the second half of the 1980s, the government began to look outside the UK for solutions and particularly to the USA. Thus was born the policies that led to the 'internal market' for which the legal, functional, and structural changes were achieved in the NHS and Community Care Act 1990. It is almost certainly unfair to summarize the next seven years in just a paragraph, but we see much of the remainder of the Conservative Party's governmental watch (until 1997) as characterized by it introducing structural change in the NHS consequent on its market concepts that were intended to drive down costs and increase productivity, efficiency, and effectiveness through regulated competition between providers of services. In effect, planning and strategic approaches to handling the big policy challenges to service delivery were replaced by regulating dynamic local tensions between demand, supply and cost.

As regards CAMHS, the new 'purchaser–provider split' for both health and social care did have some unfortunate effects. Different approaches to models of purchasing and commissioning contained within the 1990 Act led to a number of local authorities re-designating social workers as case managers, who commissioned programmes of care, rather than as practitioners. Consequently, it appeared to many within the NHS that increasing demands for therapeutic activity passed to it and to the voluntary sector.

Developments in England and Wales from 1990 to 1997

In retrospect, arguably, the 'internal market' built on and took further the changes to NHS and local authority functions and structures brought in from 1974. Thus, after 1990, the internal market separated responsibility for the healthcare of populations from managing healthcare provider agencies. Direct lines of responsibility and accountability for service provision between government and services were replaced by a system of regulation of the 'market'. The new health authorities became responsible for public health, and commissioning and purchasing healthcare from providers, but were also the conduit, through their 'contracts' with the new NHS Trusts, by which governmental regulation was brought to bear on the services delivered. This gave the contracts and health authorities a dual role in which there was great temptation for them to intervene recurrently in provider management. Interestingly, similar concerns are voiced about the current government micro-managing the NHS through its imposed performance management frameworks, and consequent adjustments in governmental approach are reflected in rationalisation of standards set by the government in England and Wales that is provided for in the Health and Social Care (Community Health and Standards) Act 2003. The way in which the system was constructed in the last decade of the twentieth century also took the responsible authorities away from a focus on longer term strategy.

Another, parallel, component of that government's approach was that of attempting to intervene centrally with demand by identifying health and social care priorities for the commissioning agencies. A product of this was the Department of Health's Health of the Nation (HoN) programme in England, which was developed by the government in the 1990s, in which it endeavoured to direct attention to priority groups of people who had, or were at greater risk of, certain diseases and disorders, by prescribing a public health approach to improved prevention and early intervention, but also to better provision of services for people with established ill health. The government's year-on-year priorities for its commissioners were delivered through annual statements of Priorities and Planning Guidance (PPG) for the NHS in England. Consequent on its publication of policy on CAMHS in 1995 (Department of Health), the specialty featured in the PPG in the middle years of the 1990s. Looking back in this way, we can see how the UK government adopted markets as its dominant mode of health and social care governance in the period but also retained key hierarchical approaches through which orthodoxy was expressed.

So far, we have portrayed dedicated child and adolescent mental healthcare in the UK as emerging over a period of 80 years driven largely by practitioners and local administrators rather than by policy. Our historical summary shows that, by the time that the Conservative Party returned to power in 1979, what we now know as CAMHS were going through a lean period in which there were very substantial pressures of resource, ideology, and competing priorities. And, all the while, it was evident that there was an absence of coherent policy. At the time when the 'internal market' was introduced, many practitioners feared that small services, as CAMHS usually were locally, would fair badly. In the event, it is probably appropriate to say that CAMHS were rescued by separate policy driven down the hierarchical command line from the competitive market frameworks for the NHS and local authority services that were introduced as a result of the NHS and Community Care Act 1990.

The speed of development of the potential capability of CAMHS contrasts with the picture of unplanned services that were failing to discharge their potential, growing demand and the setbacks that became increasingly apparent to policymakers, healthcare strategists, and practitioners in the UK in the 1980s. It was this that brought child and adolescent mental healthcare onto the political agenda in the early 1990s through the interest of a particular Secretary of State for Health in the UK government. Contrary to the predictions of many at the time, CAMH has had sustained political attention since then.

That Secretary of State, commissioned the NHS Health Advisory Service (the HAS was then an independent non-departmental public body that was responsible for reporting to the Secretary of State for Health on the state of mental health and eldercare services) to carry out a review of CAMHS with a view to making recommendations that would contribute to the formation of government policy for England and Wales and provide advice for the responsible authorities at local level. The outcomes were: influence on the Department of Health's Health of the Nation Handbook (1995), which produced the first coherent UK governance policy on CAMHS; a public report to ministers, Together we Stand (NHS Health Advisory Service 1995); and a 2-year ministerially-inspired and financed follow-up programme of advice to local commissioning and providing agencies on implementation of the policy and the HAS recommendations.

We summarize 3 years of the HAS' work in just three paragraphs. The findings of the subsequent review by the Audit Commission carried out against the framework set by the HAS report are summarized in Chapter 27. Briefly put, the HAS found in England and Wales:

absence of strategy;

ineffective commissioning;

poor collaboration between the NHS and local authorities;

patchy service provision that was unrelated to needs;

problems in the availability and accessibility of services;

limited standardization and replication of capability, of role and of interventions across different services in different parts of the country;

poor levels of general managers and low managerial knowledge of CAMHS;

widely varying expenditure per head of population between different authorities that was unrelated to assessed levels of need.

In addition that report indicated that:

the distribution of services owed more to historical patterns and local advocacy of service development than it did to assessed need;

access to services depended more on geography than on need;

good practice was being disseminated slowly but incompletely and not systematically;

the capacity of first-line, direct-access services, was very thin;

a general opinion that CAMHS (as provided by the social services departments, the special education services, paediatric services, and specialist child and adolescent mental health services) were valued but under enormous pressure; and

the commissioning arrangements were not suited to the more specialised of NHS services and CAMHS in particular.

A key component of the HAS' recommendations was conceptual. The HAS recommended that, to avoid the difficulties of language and the problems for general health, social care and education services staff at all levels in understanding CAMH and CAMHS, the government, services and practitioners should adopt a new four tier strategic framework to cross all sectors of care. That four-tier strategic framework, which is now in common use throughout CAMHS in the UK, arose from a number of different sources and pressures, and it did have the sustained advantage of enabling staff from a wide variety of agencies to engage with the topic of service commission and delivery. We return to the importance of strategic frameworks in the next three chapters.

In the second half of the 1990s, increased attention was given to CAMHS as a result of both of the Health of the Nation and PPG initiatives (e.g. the 1995 HoN Handbook Department of Health), though there is some evidence (Audit Commission 1999) that, without substantial new monies, the short-term impacts on CAMHS were limited. After 1997, these initiatives have been reinforced by the Labour government. Thus, in the late 1990s, a number of parliamentary, professional, charitable and voluntary bodies in the UK published guidance on CAMH and CAMHS in response to the challenge set by the government in England and Wales and the HAS (e.g. British Medical Association 1999; Chesson and Chisholm 1996; Craig *et al.* 1996; Green and Jacobs 1998; House of Commons 1997, 1998; Kurtz *et al.* 1995; Kurtz 1996; Leon and Smith 2001; Little and Mount 1999; Mental Health Foundation 1999, 2001; NHS Health Advisory Service 1996; Wardle 1991a,b). Also, stemming from enquiries set in hand in the latter half of the 1990s, the Office for National Statistics has reported, and continues to report on epidemiological funding from a cohort of young people that it researched in 1999 and subsequently (Meltzer *et al.* 2000, 2003a,b).

General policy developments from 1997 onwards

Current general policy

In 1997, the Labour Party formed a new government and inherited similar sets of tensions as did its predecessors. Early on, the new administration set about its manifesto commitment to explore devolution of governance to the nations that comprise the UK and, thereby, marked in high profile another underlying issue that has had powerful impacts on healthcare policy—the shift of executive responsibility for administering the country to more local levels, and a greater degree of involvement of sections of the population in it. Thus, while there have been four national health services and very many local authorities in the UK for some time, the policy distance between the four major jurisdictions in the UK has grown as a result. Now, these jurisdictions are moving progressively towards different structural solutions to similar problems.

Perhaps what surprised a substantial number of people was the way in which the incoming Labour administration in England's Department of Health at first held on to and then, if anything, further developed the notions of a mixed economy solution to healthcare delivery as one facet of a response to failure of public sector services to meet public expectation. Yet, at the same time, it is also apparent that, with overt policies to progressively devolve responsibility for local matters to local people, and the consequent changes in the structure of the health services in England and Wales, there also came challenges to how orthodoxy in healthcare and common approaches to policy could be sustained. In not dissimilar ways to its Conservative predecessor, the Labour administration has brought forward healthcare policy that has produced structures that devolve responsibilities, while also enacting other policies in which orthodoxy of response is defined centrally even to detailed levels.

Thus, while the Labour administration has enthusiastically embraced networking as its dominant mode of governance, we can also identify quasi-contractual and strong hierarchical modes in its repertoire. Interestingly, post-devolution, variations between the four jurisdictions that comprise the UK in the balance of their use of hierarchical, quasi-contractual, and networked modes of governance are becoming more evident. In particular, 'since before its election in 1997, the "New" Labour government has emphasised a collaborative discourse' in which 'partnership' is a widely used and recurring theme that appears central to the Labour approach to governance of the health and social welfare service (Powell and Glendinning 2002, p. 1). Chapters 1 and 15 of the book edited by Glendinning *et al.* (2002) examine the nature of partnerships in UK services as they have developed. They cite a report by the Audit Commission, which evidences the problems in defining partnerships, and cite the Audit Commission's definition and its summation of the qualities of effective partnership (1998). They have much in common with the summary findings of Williams and Salmon at the service and operational policy levels (2002). Rummery (2002) draws the conclusion that the hallmarks of mature partnerships include interdependence between organizations in partnership, in which their power and the benefits from collaborating are reasonably evenly balanced, with trust as the main mode of relating. However, she observes, from the evidence of the book, that the practical use of partnership does not map easily onto the characteristics of networks, with resulting ambiguity. On this basis, she is evidently sceptical about the nature of many recent partnerships and whether or not the government has really achieved a networked approach to governance. Despite these challenges, as we write, partnership remains a high-profile feature of the policies that are infusing the governance of CAMHS and the governments' expectations of their service and practice policies.

During the Conservative era, general management of the supply side was led through the internal market (in which there was central regulation of market-led local application of resources by providers and GP fundholders) and the Health of the Nation approach to orthodoxy in prioritizing demand (that was intended to align commitment across areas to centrally identified high priorities). More recently, the Labour governments have replaced these approaches with commissioning at local levels by primary care trusts (Local Health Boards in Wales), which are guided in their approach by centrally generated notions of healthcare priority, demand management, and performance management that are contained in National Service Frameworks (in both England and Wales) guidance from the National Institute for Clinical Excellence (NICE), and the Strategic and Financial Framework (SAFF) processes (Department of Health 1998 and, for example, NICE 2000). All of these structures are impacting on policies for CAMHS and their implementation.

The quality agenda: recent developments in the public sector service governance landscape

We have taken England and Wales as case studies against which to examine the development of over-arching policy frameworks for public sector-funded healthcare generally. In this account we have raised three key dynamic policy agendas. Recently, the governments in England and Wales have re-examined these very issues in what are referred as the Wanless reports (Wanless *et al.* 2002, 2004; Welsh Assembly Government 2003a). Each is shaping the landscape against which CAMHS are developing. The first refers to the scope and nature of what is considered by society, policymakers, and professionals to fall legitimately within healthcare how responsibilities are apportioned between the state and individuals and with non-discriminatory access to services. The second relates to the quantity of healthcare provision in which policymakers, healthcare strategists, service designers, service commissioners, and all who deliver services are endeavouring to balance demand, supply, and need, and ensure equity of access. Next we turn in more detail to the third agenda that is important to all stakeholders and to which we have already referred. It relates to assuring the quality of healthcare services. It is fascinating to note that, although the terminology may differ in different parts of the developing world, similar processes appear to be in play, and readers may consider that we are raising matters of wider generalization in what we have already said, as well as in the paragraphs that follow.

Earlier we referred to Salter's seminal paper (2001). While Salter looked at the increasing role of regulation in the governance of healthcare agencies and the dilemmas that exist for the professions, what he says could be applied to all public-sector agencies and professions. He has called for a re-examination of the relationship between the state and the public, between the state and the professions, and between the professions and the public. He drew particular attention to his perception of the need to put increasing energy into examining the relationship between the public and the professions.

The rise in the attention paid to the activities, performance, and probity of responsible bodies and authorities (such as health authorities, local authorities and NHS Trusts) has resulted in the concept of corporate governance. More recently, a parallel approach to assuring and raising the quality of clinical care in the NHS was developed in the UK in the closing years of the last century. Clinical Governance, the term now applied to this concept, has been defined by the Department of Health in England (Department of Health 1998; NHS Executive 1999) as 'a framework through which NHS organizations are accountable for continuously improving the quality of their services and safeguarding high standards of care by creating an environment in which excellence in clinical care will flourish'. Subsequently, this approach has been accepted throughout the UK.

According to the originators of the concept of clinical governance (Scally and Donaldson 1998), there are six core components of clinical governance. They are:

methods for improving quality;

approaches to risk avoidance;

affective mechanisms for dealing with poor performance;

improving organizational coherence;

attention to developing organizational culture; and

providing an infra-structure to enable access to evidence, training and information.

Thus, clinical governance covers a huge range of matters that bear on the quality of services and it includes the notions of performance management and evidence-based practice.

As a part of its quality assurance and improvement agenda, the Labour Government that was elected in 1997 created an agency to agree what might be legitimately provided within the state-funded health provision in England and Wales, and to set standards for healthcare delivery (the National Institute for Clinical Excellence or NICE), and another agency to monitor clinical governance in the NHS (the Commission for Health Improvement or CHI). CHI became the Commission for Health Audit and Inspection (CHAI) in 2004 and, more recently, the Healthcare Commission, and it has gained wider powers and responsibilities. Effectively, these organizations are responsible for defining and enforcing certain aspects of state orthodoxy in healthcare. Other components of the approach include improved appraisal and revalidation mechanisms, and continuing development for the professions. A number of the chapters in this book pick up and develop the themes identified here as they are being applied to CAMH.

More recently, there has been renewed interest in the organizational cultures of the environments represented by public sector-financed services, and the roles of values in healthcare policy, strategy, and delivery. These matters are developed in a number of the chapters in Part 1 of this book. Democratization of knowledge, increasing professional capability, and the greater involvement of patients and service users brings greater choice and, as Fulford and Williams (2003) show, with greater choice comes greater diversity of values and the need to look actively at working with values in clinical decision-making. Thus, has been generated the concept of values-based practice.

Child and adolescent mental health policy in the twenty-first century

England and Wales

The quality agenda issues apply in both Wales and England. We deal here with two key items; each is the subject of focus at policy and strategic levels. Neither is exclusively about CAMHS but each is likely to have a significant effect on future patterns of care.

The first major landscape issue that must be considered by all who develop policy for, and endeavour to develop, CAMHS concerns the workforce. It is apparent through the UK, as in many other countries, that the supply of professionals is insufficient to meet the volume of demand. Thus, in achieving both closure of the capacity–capability gap and in endeavouring to satisfy the drive to greater consistency of quality, there are enormous challenges to be overcome in recruiting, retaining, and ensuring the up-to-date training of all staff.

The second item concerns the safety of children in society at large, and particularly when in the care of the state. A series of allegations has been made in the last decade of services failing to protect children, either by not recognizing risk and intervening in time or by their failing to provide sufficiently safe environments (for example, Kendrick and Taylor 2000).

Thus, in Wales, we have the report of the judicial inquiry into allegations of the abuse of children while in the care of local authorities in North Wales (Waterhouse *et al.* 2000) and the subsequent Carlile review of services funded by NHS Wales. More recently, the Laming inquiry into the death of Victoria Climbié has already provoked considerable shifts in government policy. Each of these reports is likely to have significant impacts on policy for CAMHS and in a way in which they will develop.

The origins of the Carlile Review of safeguards for children and young people treated and cared for by the NHS in Wales (National Assembly for Wales 2002) lay in a substantial number of complaints made over a 20-year period about the quality of care of children and young people by a CAMHS in-patient unit in North Wales. The scope of the review included CAMHS but also went much wider to include the totality of public-funded healthcare. Consequently, the report provides a large number of recommendations. Just about all of them have been accepted by Welsh Assembly Government and they are already leading to policy developments. Key matters for CAMHS include:

the need to provide independent advocacy throughout services for children and young people;

the need to avoid isolation of all CAMHS facilities and, particularly, of their staff;

the importance of continuing professional development for all staff including managers;

the importance, in particular, of ensuring that up-to-date leadership and management is available to all CAMHS;

the priority of making appraisal, supervision, and mentoring available to all staff;

the importance of being aware of the potential impacts on staff of working with young people who have been abused and/or traumatized; and

the vital necessity to ensure that CAMHS are appropriately staffed and well-resourced.

Similar broad conclusions could be drawn from the Laming report, which 'exposed shameful failings in our ability to protect the most vulnerable children' (Department for Education and Skills 2003). In response, in mid-2003, the UK government launched a Green Paper called *Every child matters* (Department for Education and Skills 2003). *Every child matters* says that the government has consulted children, young people, and their families, and that that five items that matter most to them are:

being healthy;

staying safe;

making a positive contribution;

economic well-being; and

enjoying and achieving.

Despite the problems revealed by successive inquiries, the government has concluded that 'it has built the foundations for improving these outcomes'. It plans to build on them by:

creating sure start children's centres;

promoting extended schools;

increasing the focus on activities for children out of school through a new Young People's Fund;

increasing investment in CAMHS;

improving speech and language therapy;

tackling homelessness; and

further reforms to the Youth Justice Service.

To achieve these aims, the government proposes four main areas of action:

Supporting parents and carers;

Early intervention and effective protection;

Accountability and local, regional, and national integration; and

Workforce reform.

In particular, it plans to create posts in England for Directors of Children's Services and a Children's Commissioner for England.

All aspects of the Green Paper are planned to apply in England and the proposals for non-devolved responsibilities (e.g. Home Office services) will also apply in Wales. Otherwise, it is for the Welsh Assembly Government and the Scottish Executive to decide how to proceed in Wales and Scotland. As we write, it is too early to assess the responses to this Green Paper. However, at an informal level, many professionals have responded positively to the headline proposals, though they regard some of the detailed proposals as more controversial.

England

Since the election of the Labour Party to power in 1997, there has been a series of initiatives taken by central government for England in respect of CAMHS. The first of them was to make money available to develop better CAMHS.

Soon after its election, the Government in England confirmed the importance of CAMHS. Each year, the Department of Health produces, usually in the autumn, national priorities guidance. It was this that led in 1998 to the Department of Health providing new monies and requiring Health Authorities and Social Services Departments to deliver CAMHS objectives set out in the National Priorities Guidance for Health and Social Services and to confirmation of the ONS surveys in Britain. The government's assessment framework is also relevant to CAMHS (Department of Health *et al.* 2000a). In 1999, the Department of Health identified a 3-year plan for developing CAMHS (Department of Health 1999b). It restated its commands on heath and local authorities, and made available monies from the NHS Modernisation Fund and Mental Health Grant to support local developments. Our impression is that, despite some new money entering services and there being developments from the base-line of provision described by the Audit Commission in 1999 (compare chapters 27 and 28), there was also widespread concern in professional circles that it has been difficult to determine the actual sums of new money that entered the service and that they had arrived at their intended destinations.

In 2001, the Department of Health published the following guidance:

All health authorities and local councils must have an agreed joint CAMHS Development Strategy which sets out how local and national priorities are to be met, including 24 hour cover and outreach services increasing early intervention and prevention programs for children.
In particular they should provide:
advice, consultation, and care within primary care and local authority settings;
comprehensive assessment and a plan for treatment without a prolonged wait;
a range of treatments based on best evidence of effectiveness;
in-patient care in specialist settings appropriate to age and need;
local arrangements for 24 hour cover and emergency advice.

Subsequently, the Department of Health determined to bring forward a National Service Framework for children's services (NSF) and it split the contents into, initially, six modules.

One of those relates to mental health and psychological well-being of children and young people. The External Working Group (EWG) has produced its final report to government and the Department of Health is likely to produce a confirmed NSF for England in mid 2004. Emerging findings from the EWGs that were set up for each of the modules have been published (Department of Health 2003b). They are intended to give assistance to planners and practitioners by providing a picture of the way forward, and annexed is a brief paper on comprehensive CAMHS that should be a useful contribution to the library of those people who are responsible for developing services further.

It is evident to us that the health authorities and local councils in England have made variable progress with the targets set by National Priorities Guidance since their publication. While the original targets have evolved and been developed, they appear to have been overtaken by the more recent Public Service Agreement between the Department of Health and the Government, which was included in the Chancellor of the Exchequer's spending review of November 2002. The specific target for CAMHS included in that wide-ranging agreement is to 'improve life outcomes of adults and children with mental health problems through year on year improvements in access to crisis and CAMHS services, and reduce the mortality from suicide and undetermined injury by at least 20% by 2010'. This is coupled with expectations of:

increases in mental health promotion and early intervention services; and

increased support for CAMHS to meet the mental health needs of young offenders.

Specifically, the Department of Health's subsequent priorities and planning framework for mental health (Department of Health 2002) and its *Child and adolescent mental health service grant guidance* 2003/04 (Department of Health 2003a) require the children's NSF to set the standards and milestones for improvement in CAMHS and the core grant to be 'used to improve CAMHS according to the joint priorities in the local CAMHS Development Strategy and the Local Delivery Plan to achieve Priorities and Planning Framework targets'. The national capacity assumptions include the requirements that:

all CAMHS are to provide comprehensive services including mental health promotion and early intervention by 2006; and

there should be increases in CAMHS of 'at least 10% each year across the service according to agreed local priorities (demonstrated by increased staffing, patient contacts and/or investment)'.

In order to assist the health service and local authorities to meet these targets, the Treasury, through the Department of Health, has made substantial sums of new money available over a period of years, and the year-on-year allocations through, first, local authorities and, from 2004, the health service are available on the Department of Health website. Also, as we have noted, the Department of Health has issued the emerging findings of the EWG for the NSF's mental health and psychological well-being module (Department of Health 2003b).

In parallel, the Department of Health has promoted, among a number of other initiatives, actions to gain rather greater baseline detail on the financing, composition, and work of Specialist CAMHS through its CAMHS mapping exercise, which is being undertaken for it by the University of Durham. The results of the initial mapping exercise are available on the University of Durham website and are summarized in Chapter 28. We understand that it is the intention of the Department of Health to repeat this mapping exercise year-by-year to provide an evolving picture of the targeting of the new finance and the consequential development of services. In this setting, the publication of the NSF is likely to provide substantial advice to the health service locally and to local authorities on how they might allocate their new resource in order to deliver on the targets.

Wales

Earlier, we indicated that the renewed engagement of the Department of Health in the 1990s, following the previous policy vacuum for CAMHS, resulted in the work of the HAS across England and Wales and incorporation of many of its recommendations into Department of Health policy on CAMHS for England (Department of Health 1995). By comparison, the policy position in Wales (which has had a National Health Service that has been financed and managed separately from that in England for substantial number of years) has been less clear until recently.

CAMHS were included in the wide-ranging policy review published by the Secretary of State for Wales in 1987. However, Wales did not respond as rapidly to the work of the HAS as did England, and the detailed policy relating to CAMHS was insubstantial until the beginning of the present century.

In fact, work to create a detailed policy for CAMH was initiated by the Welsh Office under the incoming Labour Government for the UK prior to devolution and the election of a separate Government for Wales, which then had devolved responsibility for health and local authority services pertaining to CAMHS (among most other health and social care topics), delegated to it. The incoming devolved government, now known as Welsh Assembly Government, took over the commitment of the Welsh Office to develop much more detailed CAMH policy through, initially, an external advisory group.

In 2000, a report to government was published by the National Assembly for Wales as a consultation document and, thereafter, that document was developed into Wales' current comprehensive policy framework for CAMH and CAMHS in its document *Everybody's Business* (National Assembly for Wales 2001).

In the course of its work, the advisory group commissioned a content analysis of the substantial number of documents that had been published by many learned bodies in the 1990s (see p. 20 in this chapter) to give advice about developing CAMHS in the UK to build on the recommendations in Together We Stand (NHS Health Advisory Service 1995). Six common themes that can be regarded as core to developing modern value-based and needs-led CAMHS in the UK emerged. They are:

multi-agency ownership, in which all the agencies involved own a broad approach to the definition of CAMH and to resolving their problems and disorders;

the CAMHS concept, in which all agencies work together to deliver integrated and comprehensive services;

basing services on the assessed needs of the child and adolescent population in each locality, rather than the historical pattern of supply being based on individual advocacy;

audit and mapping of current services to determine local priorities for development;

adopting an evidence-based approach to practice and, thereby, targeting services according to more explicit criteria; and

adopting a strategic approach to designing and delivering CAMHS based on a common strategic framework used as a tool for future understanding and developments.

With regard to the CAMHS concept, *Everybody's business* said:

> ... we take the term CAMHS to mean all of the services provided by all sectors that impinge on the mental well-being, mental health, mental health problems and mental disorders of children and young people before their majority. This is what we term here 'the CAMHS Concept'. The adoption in Wales of such an approach would bring into the arena of CAMHS a number of services, on the basis of their ability to influence young people's mental health, that, previously have not considered themselves to be included.

Thus, we adopt in this book, the term CAMHS to imply the CAMHS Concept and the term 'Specialist CAMHS' to refer to those services that have often been referred to as child and adolescent mental health services in the past.

Policy for Wales has at its core the over-riding aims for services of providing:

> relief from current problems with the intentions of improving, as soon as possible, the mental health of children, adolescents and their families;

> longer term interventions to improve the mental health of young people as they grow up and when they become adults and thereby, to positively influence the mental health of future generations; and

> partnership with families, substitute families, and all those who care for young people.

The plan for Wales has 15 objectives and it identified 8 principles on which services should be based. They are that services should be;

> child-centred

> respectful and protecting of children and adolescents;

> lawful;

> equitable and responsive;

> comprehensive and appropriate;

> integrated;

> competent and accountable;

> effective, efficient and targeted.

The strategic vision for developing services that are consistent with those principles is that they should be built on three key components of;

> a multi-agency approach;

> the four-tier strategic framework; and

> partnerships between children, young people, their families, and professionals.

The policy for Wales required an implementation group to be set up by the government to provide more detailed plans and advice. That group has constructed detailed commissioning guidance, which has been issued as policy to Local Health Boards by Welsh Assembly Government (2003b). However, it remains to be seen how rapidly progress will be made. The intention of Welsh Assembly Government is to publish its own Children's NSF for consultation in 2003 and, within it, to set targets to drive implementation of *Everybody's business*. We think that, as in England, the limiting factors are likely to be the rate at which monies are made available to finance service developments and the volume of staff that can be trained to work in services to fill existing as well as any new vacancies.

The appointment of a Children's Commissioner for Wales, the first of its kind in the UK, was established by the Care Standards Act 2000. The Children's Commissioner for Wales Act 2001 broadened the scope of the post and the present, first, appointee took up the job later that year. In his report for 2002–3, the Children's Commissioner for Wales makes particular reference to CAMHS as his top-priority issue. While applauding Wales' policy for developing CAMHS, he criticizes particular failings of the service and expressed grave concerns about lack of progress with its implementation. In effect, he draws attention to the slow developments under dispersed local network and SAFF processes, and argues for greater initiatives from the centre driven by hierarchical command actions and by providing hypothecated new funds.

Formulating and implementing policy

We are forced, by writing this chapter at a particular time, to leave the policy story in both England and Wales incomplete. Events that are in the future as we write will determine how effective in developing CAMHS and closing the capability–capacity gap are the present governance policies of these two countries. But, perhaps obviously, we conclude from our analysis that modern public sector services require much greater integration between the public, policy-makers, and practitioners if the whole enterprise is not to become stalemated. Each is a stakeholder in the domain of the others. Thus, before we conclude, we think it appropriate to look, albeit briefly, at modern approaches to policy formulation and implementation with the intention of exploring common ground.

Policy formulation—evidence- and values-based policy?

Klein (2003) suggests that there are several different types of policy. First he identifies policies that involve structural change (e.g. the organization of the NHS), which he differentiates from policies formed as reactions to new shocks, such as the appearance of new disease or disorder (e.g. AIDS). Black (2001) distinguishes between practice policies (application of resources by practitioners), service policies (that determine the pattern of services), and governance policies (organizational and financial structures). We see these distinctions as useful.

Klein identifies a series of stages or steps in the process of policy formulation that are expressed in modified form by the following list.

To delineate and quantify, if possible more precisely, the nature of the problem.

To identify the policy options. This stage consists of two main parts:

considering the policy instruments or options available and their likely effectiveness; and

testing the implementability and political acceptability of the policy options.

Mapping out the implementation process for the chosen option by exploring what financial, managerial and organizational resources are required.

Earlier, we referred to the new concepts of evidence-based and values-based service design and policy. In much of practice, professionals are taking on the challenge of rather more rigorous evidence-based practice, but should, and can, policy formulation and implementation be similarly based? The obvious answer is 'yes' and 'the emergence of evidence-based medicine in the early 1990s led to some clinicians challenging managers and policy makers to be equally evidence-based in their policy making. This demand was shared by some health policy analysis…' (Black 2001). Black goes on to assert that 'the need to be seen to be making evidence-based decisions has permeated all areas of British public policy'. He continues, 'In essence, protagonists assume that the relation between research evidence and policy is linear; a problem is defined and research provides policy options'. It assumes research evidence can and should influence health policy. Klein's list almost assumes this too.

Black reviews several studies conducted on the relationship between research and policy-making in recent years. He suggests that the linear, rationalist model holds up quite well, with limitations, for practice policy, but he concludes that the relationship between research evidence and service policies is generally weak and he cites six main reasons. He goes on to opine that the direct influence of research on governance policies has been negligible. In this regard, he cites the re-organizations of the NHS in 1974 and subsequent to 1989 in which managed care was introduced. Consequently, Black believes that 'research has only a limited role because governance policies are driven by ideology, value judgements, financial stringency, economic theory, political experience and intellectual fashion'.

Klein, after examining similar issues as does Black, concludes that 'provided that we do not simplistically apply the evidence-based model, there remains a modest case for evidence-based policy'. In his opinion, the different types of policy and the different stages of the policy formation and implementation processes demand different types of evidence. He expresses the view that it is at the stage of delineating and quantifying the problems that scientific evidence may be most applicable (see, for example, Wallace *et al.* 1997 and Meltzer *et al.* 2000, 2003) though he warns that evidence, even scientific evidence, rarely speaks with a single clear voice about complex public issues. But, Klein emphasizes that 'scientific evidence may have very little to say about the implementability or political acceptability of a policy'. In this respect, organizational evidence, which is, in the case of health policy, 'the experience of those actually working in the NHS' (Klein 2003) may well be more significant (see, for example, NHS Health Advisory Service 1995).

Black suggests that 'evidence-based policy is not simply an extension of evidence-based medicine; it is qualitatively different. Research is considered less as problem solving than as a process of argument or debate to create concern and set the agenda'. Klein quotes a Cabinet Office paper on policy-making (Strategic Policy-making Team 1999), which says that:

> There is a tendency to think of evidence as something that is only generated by major pieces of research. In any policy area there is a great deal of critical evidence held in the minds of both frontline staff in departments, agencies and local authorities and those to whom the policy is directed. Very often they will have a clearer idea than the policymakers about why a situation is as it is and why previous initiatives have failed. Gathering that evidence through interviews or surveys can provide a very valuable input to the policy making process and can often be done much more quickly than more conventional research.

Arguably, the issue is not so much whether or not we should develop evidence-based policy but what sorts of information we are prepared to admit as constituting 'evidence' at each of the stages. A similar dialogue is underway with respect to evidence-based practice (Graham 2000; Hart 1997; Szatmari 1999; Williams 1999, 2000, 2002). Black asserts that researchers 'need to understand that there are many sorts of evidence, that sensible decisions may not reflect scientific rationality, and that context is all important, particularly with policies relating to services and governance'. He calls for 'those who fund and commission research... to review their conception of how research influences policy' and he says that 'policy makers need to be more involved in the conceptualisation and conduct of research... a closer relation between the groups needs to be sustained during the research and beyond if the work is to have any impact'.

The Cabinet Office paper and Klein's views support the notion of policymaking and practice being interactive. This loop can only be fully effective if policymakers are prepared to learn from, and be influenced by, practice, and if practitioners can see the value, in parallel with formal research, of extracting the wisdom and learning that may be derived from day-to-day practice.

Interestingly, and perhaps paradoxically in a world that appears, at first take, to be infatuated with scientific evidence, Bracken and Thomas (2001) argue that 'faith in the ability of science and technology to resolve human and social problem is diminishing'. They say:

> Psychiatry must move beyond its single 'modernist' framework to engage with recent government proposals and the growing power of service users. Post psychiatry emphasises social and cultural contexts, places ethics before technology, and works to minimise medical control of cohesive interventions.

Black asserts that 'one of the most useful roles for research is to make people review their beliefs and legitimise unorthodox views'. Klein points to the importance of ministerial values in selecting between the policy options (i.e. political acceptability). It is our view that, in the modern democratized world, these ministerial values should be overt and linked to the values involved in practice in a manner that runs parallel with evidence-based policy and evidence-based practice.

In respect of practice, Fulford and Williams (2003) have identified the importance and power of bringing together evidence-based practice with values-based practice in handling the diversity of values of the people who would use health services and the staff who provide health services, particularly when responding to the choices that flow from increasing scientific evidence. Similarly, Klein argues, for 'a more nuanced approach to strategy'. He suggests the importance of 'recognising the complexity of the policy process and the diversity of the kinds of relevant evidence'.

Our opinion is that, in parallel with developing broader but nonetheless rigorous approaches to evidence-based practice and evidence-based policy, we should also endeavour to develop virtuous loops between values-based policy and values-based practice. In our model, we advocate not only that policy should be more overtly connected to practice and, thereby the needs and experiences of the real service users and practitioners, but also that the combination of values-based practice and evidence-based practice should be reflected in their counterparts in policy-making. Figures 1.8, 1.9 and 1.10 have been created by adding the various processes to Fig. 1.2. Figures 1.8 and 1.9 show how we see evidence-based policy and evidence-based service design, and values-based policy and values-based service design, fitting into our overall approach, which more closely links policy with practice through strategy and service design. In similar terms, we think that performance management should include policymakers and service designers and their work within the feedback loop (Fig. 1.10).

Implementing policy

Now that both England and Wales are developing coherent governance policies for CAMH and CAMHS, there is an increasing need to concentrate on the crucial matters of developing service policies and clinical practice policies when formulating the in-depth local plans that will be expected to flow from the over-arching NSFs.

The role of policymakers does not stop with formulation but must, we believe, follow through into implementation. In the UK, implementation of policy and applying performance management and clinical governance in monitoring higher level and operational implementation are now becoming important matters for CAMHS.

Clifford, Professor of Social Work at the Norwegian University of Technology and Science in Trondheim, has identified four key issues with regard to implementing policy on parent training. We believe that these have wider applicability for policies for CAMHS. Graham's lessons for

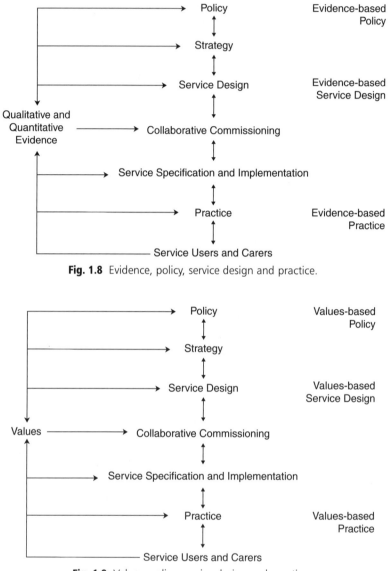

Fig. 1.8 Evidence, policy, service design and practice.

Fig. 1.9 Values, policy, service design and practice.

promoting success in implementing policy show the importance of:

Identifying the detailed practice programmes required to implement the policy and the training that staff will need to deliver the desired service programmes.

Lowering the threshold of resistance of the public and practitioners to implementing the governance and service policies. Graham sees the importance of policymakers and practitioners working together with users of services as a team to reduce the natural resistance to change that occurs in human systems.

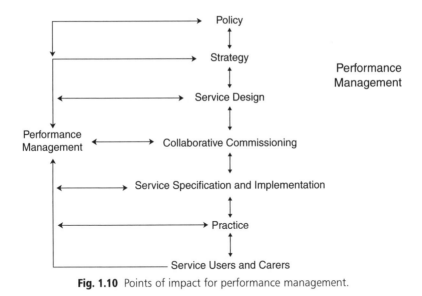

Fig. 1.10 Points of impact for performance management.

Ensuring programme fidelity so that drift away from the governance and service policies or their gradual decay or dilution in practice do not result in initiatives running aground; in this regard. Graham identifies the needs for:

clarity of the implementation plan;

maintaining steadfastness of purpose;

taking a step-by-step approach; and

sustaining long-termism.

Sustaining competence in the practices that are required to deliver identified policies, despite the possibility that plans to maintain high standards may open tensions between the timescales of politicians and practitioners.

Again, this suggests that we need much greater interaction between policymakers, managers, and practitioners if formulation of policy is to result in achievement of agreed aims.

Concluding comments

A recent review by Amnesty International on CAMHS in Ireland (Crowley 2003) draws attention to our opening assertion that policy challenges in delivering effective CAMH stretch well outside England and Wales and the United Kingdom.

For example, the report quotes the Chief Medical Officer in the Department of Health and Children in the Irish Government as saying in 2002:

> Approaches to the promotion and development of mental health for children, and the identification and treatment of psychological and psychiatric disorders have been patchy, unco-ordinated and under resourced.

The report from Amnesty International draws attention to similar challenges in providing adequate in-patient and community mental health services for young people in Ireland, as there are in the United Kingdom. It quotes the World Health Organization's summary of the position in 2003:

> In developed countries there are problems with mal-distribution, a declining enrolment in child psychiatry training programmes and a recent reduction in those working in community settings. In the developing world there is an almost universal lack of enough trained individuals to staff even basic child and adolescent mental health treatment facilities and certainly not enough to implement a full continuing of care as conventionally defined.

Yet the WHO reminds us that we cannot afford to fail to take on the challenge when it concluded that 'the lack of attention to the mental health of children and adolescents may lead to mental disorders with life long consequences, undermines compliance with health regimens and reduces the capacity of societies to be safe and productive'.

In 1998, the UN High Commissioner for Human Rights went further by saying that there are (see Crowley 2003):

> ...huge costs of failing children. Governments are fully aware from research findings that what happens to children in the early years, within the family and within other forms of care, significantly determines their positive or negative growth and development. This, in turn, determines their cost or contribution to society spread over the rest of their lives. As a consequence, the economic motive joins the moral and the social in providing conjoint reasons for all governments to record children as a high priority and careful attention. These may seem obvious points which derive from common sense. But they need to be convincing particularly with regard to governments if we are to promote child-centred societies.

Thus, there seems to be substantial evidence voiced by influential bodies that the issues that we have sketched out here in respect of two related jurisdictions in the developed world are probably reflected, albeit with different historical patterns and details, across a much wider range of the world's population. Evidently, there are serious challenges to be faced. However, it is clear that the will has to come from policy, be sustained through strategic vision and leadership and supported by investment of sufficient resource, but, vitally, be accompanied by adequate recruitment, retention and training of professional staff.

In the chapters that follow in this book, we look at a variety of aspects of the situation, and at the developing circumstances in the UK and elsewhere in endeavouring to summarize the knowledge-base that may help all stakeholders to move forward. What is the key is the importance to success of clarity of political purpose when formulating policy and certainty of political will in achieving implementation of change.

References

Allen, R.E. (ed.) (1990) *Concise Oxford dictionary of current English* (8th edn). Oxford: Clarendon Press.

Audit Commission (1996) *Misspent youth—young people and crime*. London: Audit Commission.

Audit Commission (1998) *A fruitful partnership: effective partnership working*. London: Audit Commission.

Audit Commission (1999) *Children in mind—a report on child and adolescent mental health services*. London: Audit Commission.

Black, D. (1993) A brief history of child and adolescent psychiatry. In *Seminars in child and adolescent psychiatry* (ed. Black D and Cottrell D). London: Gaskell.

Black, N. (2001) Evidence based policy: proceed with care. *British Medical Journal*, **323**, 275–8.

Bowlby, J. (1969, 1973, 1980) *Attachment and loss* (3 volumes). London: Hogarth Press.

Bracken, P. and Thomas, P. (2001) Post psychiatry: a new direction for mental health. *British Medical Journal,* **322,** 724–7.

British Medical Association (1999) *Growing up in Britain.* London: BMJ Books.

Bullock, R. and Little, M. (1999) The interface between social and health services for children and adolescent persons. *Current Opinion in Psychiatry* **12,** 421–4

Children's Commissioner for Wales (2003) *Report and accounts 2002–03.* Swansea: Children's Commissioner for Wales. http,//www.childcomwales.org.uk

Chesson, R. and Chisholm, D. (ed.) (1996) *Child psychiatric units at the crossroads.* London: Jessica Kingsley.

Craig, T.K.J., Hodson, S., Woodward, S., and Richardson, S. (1996) *Off to a bad start, a longitudinal study of homeless young people in London.* London: The Mental Health Foundation.

Crowley, F. (2003) *Mental illness, the neglected quarter—promoting the rights of the one in four Irish people affected by mental illness.* Dublin: Amnesty International (Irish Section).

Court, S.D.M. (1976) *Fit for the future, the report of the committee on child welfare services.* London: Department of Health and Social Security, HMSO.

Department for Education and Skills (2003) *Every child matters.* London: The Stationery Office.

Department of Health (1995) *Child and adolescent mental health services. The Health of the Nation Handbook.* London: Department of Health.

Department of Health, Social Services Inspectorate of the Department of Health and the Department for Education (1995) *A handbook of mental health—a text in the Health of the Nation series.* London: Department of Health.

Department of Health (1998) *A first class service—quality in the new NHS.* London: Department of Health.

Department of Health (1999a) *Consultation document on a framework for the assessment of children in need and their families.* London: Department of Health.

Department of Health (1999b) *HSC (1999)/126 , LAC (99) 22 NHS Modernisation Fund and Mental Health Grant for Child and Adolescent Mental Health Services 1999/2002.* London: Department of Health.

Department of Health (2002) *Improvement, expansion and reform. The next 3 years—priorities and planning framework 2003–2006.* London: Department of Health.

Department of Health (2003a) *HSC 2003/003, LAC (2003) 2 Child and Adolescent Mental Health Service (CAMHS) Grant Guidance 2003/04.* London: Department of Health.

Department of Health (2003b) *Getting the right start, National Service framework for children—emerging findings.* London: Department of Health. www.doh.gov.uk/nsf/children/gettingtherightstart

Department of Health, Department for Education and Employment, Home Office (2000) *Framework for the assessment of children in need and their families.* London: The Stationery Office.

Fulford, K.W.M. and Williams, R. (2003) Values-based child and adolescent mental health services? *Current Opinion in Psychiatry,* **16,** 369–76.

Glendinning, C., Powell, M., and Rummery, K. (ed.) (2002) *Partnerships, New Labour and The Governance of Welfare,* Bristol: The Policy Press.

Graham, P. (1976) Management in child psychiatry, recent trends. *British Journal of Psychiatry,* **129,** 97–108.

Graham, P. (2000) Treatment interventions and findings from research, bridging the chasm in child psychiatry. *British Journal of Psychiatry,* **176,** 414–9.

Green, J. and Jacobs, B. (ed.) (1998) *In-patient child psychiatry.* London: Routledge.

Ham, C. and Alberti, K.G.M.M. (2002) The medical profession, the public, and the government. *British Medical Journal,* **324,** 838–42.

Hart, J.T. (1997) Society for social medicine Cochrane lecture 1997, what evidence do we need for evidence-based medicine? *Journal of Epidemiology and Community Medicine,* **51,** 623–9.

House of Commons (1997) *Fourth report of the House of Commons Health Committee, child and adolescent mental health services.* London: HMSO.

House of Commons (1998) *Second report of the House of Commons Health Committee, children looked after by local authorities,* Vol. 1. London: HMSO.

Kanner, L. (1943). Autistic disturbance of affective contact. *Nervous Child,* **2,** 217–250.

Kendrick, A., Taylor, J. (2000) Hidden on the ward, the abuse of children in hospitals. *Journal of Advanced Nursing,* **31** (3), 565–73.

Klein, R. (2003) Evidence and policy, interpreting the Delphic Oracle. *Journal of the Royal Society of Medicine,* **96,** 429–31.

Kolvin, I. (1973) Evaluation of psychiatric services for children in England and Wales. In *Roots of evaluation* (ed. J.K. Wing and J. Hafner). Oxford: Oxford University Press.

Kurtz, Z. (1996) *Treating children well—a guide to using the evidence base in commissioning and managing services for the mental health of children and young people.* London: The Mental Health Foundation.

Kurtz, Z., Thornes, R., and Wolkind, S. (1995) *Mental health for children and young people in England. Assessment of needs and unmet needs.* London: Report to the Department of Health.

Leon, L. and Smith, K. (2001) Turned upside down, services for young people in crisis. *Young Minds Magazine,* **51,** 22–4.

Lister-Sharp, D., Chapman, S., Stewart-Brown, S., and Sowden, A. (1999) Health promoting schools and health promotion in schools, two systematic reviews. *Health Technology Assessment,* **3** (22), 1–207.

Little, M. and Bullock, R. (2004) Administrative frameworks for very difficult children and adolescents. Chapter 24 pp. 336–44. In *Adolescent forensic psychiatry* (ed S. Bailey and M. Dolan). London: Arnold Publishing.

Little, M. and Mount, K. (1999) *Prevention and early intervention with children in need.* Aldershot: Ashgate Publishing.

Meltzer, H., Gatward, R., Goodman, R., and Ford, T. (2000) *Mental health of children and adolescents in Great Britain (for the Office for National Statistics).* London: The Stationery Office.

Meltzer, H., Gatward, R., Corbin, T., Goodman, R., and Ford, T. (2003a) *Persistence, onset risk factors and outcomes of childhood mental disorders (for the Office for National Statistics).* London: The Stationery Office.

Meltzer, H., Gatward, R., Goodman, R., and Ford, T. (2003b) *The mental health of young people looked after by local authorities in England (for the Office for National Statistics).* London: The Stationery Office.

Mental Health Foundation (1999) *Bright futures.* London: Mental Health Foundation.

Mental Health Foundation (2001) *Turned upside down.* London: Mental Health Foundation.

Ministry of Health (1964) *In-patient accommodation for mentally ill and seriously maladjusted children and adolescents, HM(64)4.* London: HMSO.

National Assembly for Wales (2000) *Welsh index of multiple deprivation.* Cardiff: National Assembly for Wales.

National Assembly for Wales Statistical Directorate (2000) *Mapping social exclusion in Wales* (1999 edn). Cardiff: National Assembly for Wales.

National Assembly for Wales. Everybody's business—child and adolescent mental health services strategy document. Cardiff: National Assembly for Wales; (2001).

National Assembly for Wales (2002) *Too serious a thing—the Carlile review.* Cardiff, National Assembly for Wales.

NHS Executive (1999) *Clinical governance—quality in the new NHS.* London: Department of Health.

NHS Health Advisory Service (1986) *Bridges over troubled waters.* London: HMSO.

NHS Health Advisory Service (1996) *The substance of young needs—commissioning and providing services for children and adolescents who use and misuse substances.* London: HMSO.

National Institute for Clinical Excellence (2000) Guidance on the use of methylphenidate for attention deficit/hyperactivity disorder (ADHD) in childhood. *Technology appraisal guidance No 13.* London: National Institute for Clinical Excellence.

NHS Health Advisory Service (1995) *Together We Stand.* London: HMSO.

O'Neill, O. (2002) *BBC Reith Lectures 2002*—a question of trust, lecture 1—spreading suspicion; lecture 2—trust and terror; lecture 3—called to account; lecture 4—trust and transparency; lecture 5—licence to deceive? www.bbc.co.uk/radio4; 2002—20 April.

O'Neill, O. (2002) A question of trust: 2002 BBC Reith Lectures. Cambridge: Cambridge University Press.

Pendleton, D. and King, J. (2002) Values and leadership. *British Medical Journal,* 325, 1352–5.

Powell, M. and Glendinning, C. (2002) Introduction. In *Partnerships, New Labour and the Governance of Welfare.* (ed. Glendinning, C., Powell, M., and Rummery, K.). Bristol: The Policy Press.

Robertson, J. (1952) *A two year old goes to hospital* (film). Ipswich: Concord Films Council.

Robins, L. (1966) *Deviant children grown up.* Baltimore: Williams and Wilkins.

Roth, A. and Fonagy, P. (ed.) (2003) *What Works for Whom?* London: Guilford Press.

Rummery, K. (2002) Towards a theory of welfare partnerships. In *Partnerships, New Labour and the Governance of Welfare* (ed. C. Glendinning, M. Powell, K. Rummery). Bristol: The Policy Press.

Rutter, M., Tizard, J., and Whitmore, K. (1970) *Education, health and behaviour.* London: Longman.

Rutter, M. and Smith, D.J. (1995) *Psychosocial disorders in young people.* Chichester: Wiley.

Salter, B. (2001) Who rules? The new politics of medical regulation. *Soc Sci Med,* 52, 871–83.

Scally, G. and Donaldson, L. (1998) Clinical governance and the drive for quality improvement in the new NHS in England. *British Medical Journal,* 317, 61–5.

Steinberg, D. (ed) (1986) *The adolescent unit, work and teamwork in adolescent psychiatry.* Chichester: John Wiley.

Strategic Policy Making Team (1999) *Professional policy making for the 21st century.* London: Cabinet Office.

Szatmari, P. (1999) Evidence-based child psychiatry and the two solitudes [Evidence-based Mental Health notebook]. *Evidence-based Mental Health,* 1, 6–7.

Wallace, S.A., Crown, J.M., Berger, M., and Cox, A.D. (1997) Child and adolescent mental health. In *Health care needs assessment* (2nd series). (ed. A. Stevens, and J. Raftery) Oxford: Radcliffe Medical Press.

Wanless, D., Charlesworth, A., Walker, I., *et al.* (2002) *Securing our future health: taking a long-term view.* HM Treasury 2002. http://www.hm-treasury.gov.uk/wanless

Wanless, D., Jones, N., Anderson, R., *et al.* (2004) *Securing good health for the whole population.* HM Treasury and Department of Health. http://www.hmtreasury.gov.uk/media/867ED/Wanless04summary.pdf [25 May 2004].

Wardle, C. (1991a) Historical influences on services for children and adolescents before 1900. In *150 years of British psychiatry, 1841–1991.* (ed. G.E. Berrios, and H. Freeman). London: Gaskell.

Wardle, C. (1991b) Twentieth-century influences on the development in Britain of services for child and adolescent psychiatry. *British Journal of Psychiatry,* 159, 53–68.

Waterhouse, R., Clough, M., and le Fleming, M. (2000) *Lost in care—report of the tribunal of inquiry into the abuse of children in care in the former county council areas of Gwynedd and Clwyd since 1974.* London: The Stationery Office.

Welsh Assembly Government (2003a) *The review of health and social care in Wales.* Welsh Assembly Government 2003. http://www.wales.gov.uk/subieconomics/hsc-reviewe.htm

Welsh Assembly Government (2003b) *WHC (2003) 63 NHS Planning and commissioning guidance.* Cardiff: Welsh Assembly Government.

Williams, R. (1997) Setting the scene—the interaction between research and the strategic leadership of child and adolescent mental health services. *Current Opinion in Psychiatry,* **10**, 265–7.

Williams, R. (1999) Managing mental health care, risk and evidence-based practice. *Current Opinion in Psychiatry,* **12**, 385–91.

Williams, R. (2000) A cunning plan—the role of the evidence-base in translating policy into effective child and adolescent mental health services. *Current Opinion in Psychiatry,* **13**, 361–8.

Williams, R. (2002) Complexity, uncertainty and decision-making in an evidence-based world. *Current Opinion in Psychiatry,* **15**, 343–7.

Williams, R. and Salmon, G. (2002) Collaboration in commissioning and delivering child and adolescent mental health services. *Current Opinion in Psychiatry,* **15**, 349–53.

Williams, R. and Skeldon, I. (1992) Mental health services for adolescents. In *Youth policy in the 1990s.* (ed. J. Coleman and C. Warren). London: Routledge.

Winnicott, D. (1965) *The family and individual development.* London: Tavistock.

Chapter 2

The nature of strategy and its application in statutory and non-statutory services

Morton Warner and Richard Williams

Introduction

Strategy and strategic thinking have been around for a very long time. The writer of Proverbs 10 recognized 'where there is no vision, the people perish'. Perhaps Noah was one of the first people recorded to have seen that strategy implementation is at least as important as strategic initiation. This early example provides another lesson as well—that it is at the least desirable, if not imperative, to develop strategy in response to need. An ark proved more useful than a camel train as the means of transport! Form must follow function.

In this chapter, we will elucidate the nature of strategy, challenge often recounted conceptions of strategy as 'academic' or dry and impersonal, by showing how important are interpersonal skills to its formulation and implementation, and relate this to developing better child and adolescent mental health services (CAMHS). We begin with the most challenging question.

What is strategy?

At its simplest, the word 'strategy' means a plan. In other words, it is orientated to the future but also informed by current challenges. Plans are usual aspirational, yet they should also be realistic. The nature of what is desired must be related to what is possible, if seeking to rise beyond it. Strategy must be grounded in realizing that people will deliver the plans, but only if they share the values, are well led, and able to express their creativity and ambitions. Now, let us deepen this analysis.

The features of strategy

'Strategy' has its origins in ancient Greece (*strategos*) where it referred to organizing or disposing an army before the fighting began to give tactical advantage. Strategy relates to whole organizations. Also, good strategists must have intelligence about current circumstances and be able to identify the goals of their thinking and the direction of travel of the organization that is the subject of strategic change. Typical definitions embrace the notion that strategy is 'a longer term plan for how a desired goal is to be achieved'. The importance of linking purpose with means was identified by Mark Twain 'If you don't know where you are going, you won't know how to get there'.

The military origins and whole organizational scale of strategy link it to harnessing large numbers of people in pursuit of achieving an identified common goal. Far from being simply cerebral or arcane, strategy must be people-orientated. It allows for flexibility in implementation and recognizes the innate innovative capacity of real people when there are turns of events that may not be predictable once execution of the plan begins. Under these circumstances, it is now axiomatic of successful military campaigning and the doctrine of Mission Command that the senior commander's intentions are communicated to, supported, and maintained by the most junior soldiers, so that the goals are not lost if contact is lost with leaders. Communication, motivation, and alignment to common goals are key components of strategy. These are essential functions of leadership.

The leadership and motivational components of strategy have been identified by Billy Graham who said, 'You can't take people from where they aren't to where they don't want to go'. To avoid this, delegation of decision-making and necessary resources to those best equipped to make the decisions, at the lowest reasonable level sustains the involvement of the workforce, and values and develops their creativity.

The words of Maucher (Introduction to Jonassen 1999) provide a good summary of the leadership component of strategic thinking and acting:

> Any organization… looks to a leader for reassurance, for support, for guidance—but also for a challenge to make it go beyond what it believes it can do, to aim for excellence…. Corporate leaders succeed by freeing the creative drive that exists in the best leader elements of the organization, by letting these people stretch their wings and… try… new approaches. Yet, at the same time, leaders need to have their eye on the whole, on the strategic direction they have determined and on the goals they have set.

But, to drill down further, some years ago, one of the authors of a national report wrote the following. 'It is the function of leaders to ensure that staff want to go on the journey and do so with enthusiasm and commitment. It is the role of managers to ensure that staff are fully-equipped for the journey and that the full range of relevant factors has been taken into account when planning the route.' (NHS Health Advisory Service 1995). Strategy also involves management.

So far, we have identified strategy as a form of planning that is based on clear vision of the future (what might be and what could occur), and exercised through leadership and management. In the public sector, strategy also requires a lead from policies, preferably where there is clarity about what is required and which enables the intent and direction to be defined. Its functions (thinking and actions) can be divided into:

strategic vision—statesmanlike forethought, or the ability to perceive vividly in the imagination an idea for the future;

strategic planning—clear identification of the aims and definition of the functions required to achieve them;

strategic leadership—or ability to form, hold, develop, and galvanize a team (as the range of activities is so great that no one person can 'do' this kind of leadership without delegation); and

strategic management—predicting and prioritizing demands, finding and organizing resources (including, importantly, staff and training) from across the organization to be ready on a timely basis.

On the basis of this overview, we take an approach to strategy that identifies what we think are its three main components. They are:

the strategic processes of strategy formulation, implementation, and monitoring; and

the four strategic functions as defined in the previous paragraph;

the service user, carer, and workforce development and support activities that are required to develop and deliver strategy.

In the remainder of this chapter, we concentrate on the strategic processes by considering issues that are key to strategic thinking. The next chapter deals with the strategic functions and the workforce issues in more detail. First, we explore further strategy within the context of the public sector.

The public sector context

Until the decade of the 1990s, the National Health Service and its political masters, alongside the health professions and the unions, had all been rather content with re-organizing the supply side components. 'Structural conflict is ok! It allows for mutual recrimination followed by collective admiration' (Warner 1997). But now there is evidence of some real change in strategic thinking—the concept of *re-design*. It:

> begins with an articulation of strategic destinations that it is desired to achieve, and often include targets for long-term health and social gain, and for more immediate service delivery;

> views need (derived from medical, educational, and social epidemiological studies and studies of the impact and burden resulting from deviations from good health) and wants (consumer or patient-based views of their needs) for services in concert; and

> moves the supply-side towards consideration of programmes and the workforce necessary to run them first, with the facilities, or buildings question being subsidiary or supporting rather than leading matters.

The notion of investment in, or for, health improvement has become widespread (World Bank 1993; WHO 1998a; Warner 2000); and the most recent English NHS planning is based on it (e.g. Department of Health National Service Frameworks 1999—onwards). Our awareness of the requirement to use scarce resources effectively and efficiently challenges services to be planned that use the best available, but always incomplete, evidence. A mature approach to strategy should promote future health gain using evidence-based service (re-)design.

This provokes consideration of the kinds of evidence to be admitted into the strategic process. The concept of evidence-based practice began from a scientific standpoint. But Szatmari (1999) has drawn attention to the 'two solitudes of evidence' that divide service users and carers from practitioners. Very recently, the worlds of adult education and medical philosophy have begun to re-examine the nature of professionalism, and this has led to changes in professional education paradigms and identification of value-based approaches to designing practice responses to patients (see Fulford and Williams 2003).

Presently, the world is buzzing with developments of these kinds that seek to re-examine the triangle of relationships between the professions, the public, and the state, as if in answer to the challenge set by Salter (2001). All of these matters have implications for strategy.

Our analysis shows that strategists have an important role in helping staff who deliver services, service users, and carers to make choices. Their judgements should be supported by policy and both humanitarian and scientific evidence. Choice implies a baseline of thinking, values, and ethics; and so initiation of strategy pivots on the values expressed by senior leaders and their enaction and, particularly, on the values of the people who deliver services.

Mental health is a particularly complex public sector field. Its organization is complex and the impact upon sufferers of ill-health and their carers is major. Williams (2002) has considered in some detail complexity in respect of CAMHS (see also Chapters 3, 27, 28 and 32).

Strategic processes

Strategy formulation

There are a number of steps to be considered in order to identify the main thrust or intent of a strategy, and then to determine the directions that will be followed to ensure its achievement.

Establishing the value-base

The particular circumstances and needs of children have been recognized in many statements of rights, and of principles of good practice. The philosophy and values that they collectively represent are embodied in the Human Rights Act 1998 and a range of documents on children's rights produced at international, national, and sub-national levels (UN Convention on the Rights of the Child 1989; WHO HEALTH 21 1998b; Children Act 1989; National Assembly for Wales 2001; Chapter 1). Four groups of rights can be identified:

General Rights, where services should focus on the needs and wishes of children, and include:

non-discrimination of any kind;

the importance of families in supporting their offspring;

the right to be heard; and

protection from harm caused by other people or by their physical environment.

Right to Health, which implies three guiding principles:

life, with premature death reduced as far as possible;

health, at the highest possible level of attainment; and

development of the fullest potential.

Right to Health and Social Care, where the quality of service provision is assessed in terms of:

effectiveness of interventions;

equity, or equal treatment for equal need;

access to services;

relevance to the needs of whole communities, and for children and their families;

social acceptability to children and their parents; and

efficiency, or value for money.

Rights of 'Children in Need' looked after by local authorities directly or through the voluntary sector, who require an appropriate range and level of services for them and their families.

The Human Rights Act 1998 formulates in statute in the UK a number of general, absolute and relative rights. These are further explored in *Safeguards for young minds* (Williams *et al.,* 2004).

Together, these statements can be defined as representing the normative statement of equity—what is considered to be fair and just, and towards which any strategic developments should aim. The degree to which 'practice' does not secure achievement of these rights can be referred to as the 'equity deficit'. Methods for assessing this high-level item will be one of the subjects of the final section on monitoring and evaluation. Suffice it to say that the value-base from which strategy formulation begins, forms the bedrock for further developments. Paradoxically, it is often the least studied and understood component of the whole process.

The Welsh strategy for developing CAMHS (National Assembly for Wales 2001) takes these strands to identify eight principles. They are that services should be:

child-centred;

respectful and protecting of children and adolescents;

equitable and responsive;

comprehensive and appropriate;

integrated;

competent and accountable;

effective, efficient, and targeted; and

lawful.

Readers will see that each is underpinned by values and each is capable of contributing to both implementation of the plan and its evaluation through informing the development of standards, action points, and a performance management programme.

In recognition of the key importance to strategy of values, the term 'moral architecture' was coined a decade ago to refer to the values that are evident in whole organizations. The concept provokes a key question, when evaluating achievements, about the consistency between the values identified within a strategy and those of the organizations that deliver services. 'To be moral, the vision, values, priorities, structures, activities, use of funds, leadership and management processes and, critically, use of staff and their experience within an organization should be consistent with its espoused roles and values' (Williams 2000). We suggest that, where there is consistency of values between strategy and operational service delivery, true alignment of staff to the organization and its tasks is more likely to be achieved. Certainly, where there are schisms, the tensions are likely to be reflected in disharmony and unilateral actions.

Scoping and context: identifying the strategic intent

In spite of the landmark initiatives nearly 50 years ago in the field of social policy (Beveridge 1942), which identified the multiple interactive causes of social deprivation, government agendas in the UK have only recently faced squarely the fact that 'health' is determined by many factors beyond the health service. These are shown in Fig. 2.1 in a way that is challenging conceptually—both in terms of the range of determinants, and their relative positioning. Of importance in the initial scoping exercise is the detailed consideration of the evidence-base relating to the causal or associated relationship between each of the factors, singly or in combination, and the strategic health area under scrutiny.

This is particularly important in the field of mental health in which there is a range of areas—genetic, psychological, social, and environmental—that can influence, usually interactively, the vulnerability or resilience of individuals and groups of people to particular conditions. All have to be addressed when considering individual needs and service responses.

There is some clear evidence that must be taken into account as the scoping proceeds:

the interactive nature of people's mental health, physical health, developmental problems, and their family, educational, and social circumstances;

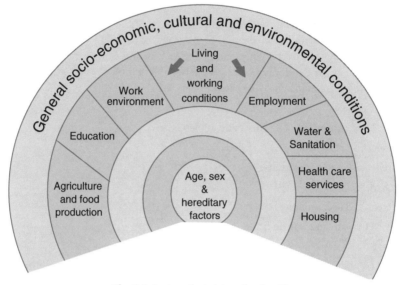

Fig. 2.1 Factors that determine health.

the fact that the culture and setting in which each person is cared for and treated can have a significant effect on the outcome; and

poor mental health impacts on people in different ways and the result can be profound in terms of long-term impact and disability for the individual and the burden experienced by others.

The socio-economic factors involved in mental dysfunction give enormous cause for concern and also present major challenges. Table 2.1 summarizes the evidence that requires consideration as the strategic journey gets underway. We illustrate this with regard to the mental health of children and adolescents by referring to the risk and resilience factors shared by mental disorder and substance misuse (and by a wide range of other problems) and by referring to common findings of co-morbidity.

While cause and effect cannot always be disentangled, some people are undoubtedly caught in a vicious spiral affected by one, and most often, more of the circumstances described.

The interactive circular model of causality that we have developed to link risk factors with psychological and physical developmental problems, psychiatric disorder and substance misuse is shown in Fig. 2.2. It reflects:

the interactive nature of a common pool of risk factors affecting mental health, physical ill health, social exclusion (including offending), substance use and misuse, psychosocial problems, and educational problems;

high levels of 'co-morbidity' in the child and adolescent population (Williams *et al.*, 2004); and

what we know of the interaction between psychiatric symptoms, significant psychosocial impairment, educational disadvantage, language, and other psychological and physical

Table 2.1 Socio-economic factors which are linked to mental health problems

Socio-economic factor	Schizophrenia	Manic depression	Depression	Anxiety	Personality disorders	Eating disorders	Suicidal behaviour
Gender			•	•		•	•
Ethnic background	•						
Age						•	•
Marital status			•	•			•
Social class	•		•	•		•	•
Urban/rural	•		•	•	•		•
Alcohol	•	•	•	•	•		•
Drugs	•		•	•	•		•
Homelessness	•	•					
Employment status	•		•	•			•

Source: adapted from Welsh Health Planning Forum/Welsh Office (1993). *Protocol for investment in health gain: mental health*. Cardiff, NHS Directorate.

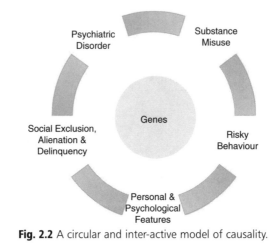

Fig. 2.2 A circular and inter-active model of causality.

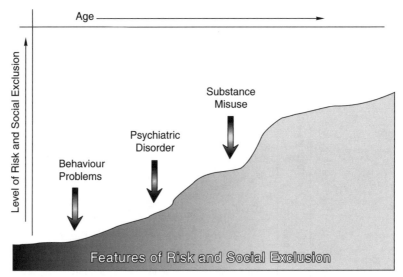

Fig. 2.3 The dynamic interaction of risk factors, substance misuse and mental disorder.

development disorders and problems, and cognitive delays (e.g. Gjaerum and Bjornerem 2003).

Similarly, Fig. 2.3 provides a graphical presentation of the association and dynamic interaction between risk factors in respect of substance misuse and mental disorder. It depicts evidence-based longitudinal links between escalating 'social exclusion' (as both cause and outcome effect) and mental disorder and substance use (Williams *et al.* 2004). In all probability, the link between substance misuse and mental disorder operates in both directions. Recent studies investigating longitudinal predictors of drug use claim that the concurrent existence of social exclusion and psychiatric disorder provides a pathway to substance misuse (Kuperman *et al.* 2001; Mullen and Barry 2001; Pedersen *et al.* 2001; Bushell *et al.* 2002). Ferdinand *et al.* (2001)

claim that risk factors can develop in a chain to form a pathway, which may first involve peer relationships, then delinquent behaviour, and finally drug use. Certainly, as readers will see in later chapters, the evidence for high levels of co-morbidity of mental disorder with many other conditions is overwhelming.

The shared pattern of risk and resilience factors predicts, correctly, that there are likely to be high levels of co-morbidity between substance misuse, psychiatric disorders, and many other health problems, including lower use of services; and education and social problems share overlapping risk and resilience factors. The triad of deprivation and poverty, psychiatric disorder and substance misuse holds together. Social exclusion and psychiatric disorders can also be the cause of non-recognition of substance misuse and co-morbidity, and non-attendance at services.

Co-morbidity is a professional conception that describes situations in which single syndromes do not adequately describe the common experiences and needs of the population at risk, making more than one diagnosis or a formulation important. However, patients/clients service users do not see or experience their problems as disjointed in this way.

The significance of co-morbidity to service design, as well as to professional practice, is that it emphasizes the importance of viewing people's needs from a broad perspective and providing articulated services that are able to respond to the real and inter-connected needs of the public. Indicative findings from several recent studies show that, where only substance misuse is treated, co-morbid behavioural conditions re-emerge in conjunction with higher levels of substance use after treatment than in non-co-morbid youth (Brown *et al.* 2001; Grella *et al.* 2001).

From all of this emerges the possibility of making a clear statement of strategic intent that can be used by any organization working in the mental health field. Cross-sectoral working is clearly obligatory and consideration of how to achieve it is important in strategic, operational, and practice thinking. The essential elements would include: 'working together'; 'a drive for better mental health on a level to compare with the best elsewhere'; 'pursuit of excellence and quality'; and 'within a reasonable time frame'.

Identifying the strategic directions

It is at this stage that the investment theme returns. It can be expressed through three questions:

What health and social gain is required?

How can services be more effective by being really people-centred (i.e. sensitive to the views of service users, their carers *and* the staff)?

What is the best way to use resources (the workforce and their associated equipment, buildings and other technologies)?

Health and social gain

At their highest level, health and social gain are measures used to indicate improvement in the quality of people's lives. This is the major reason for the existence of health and social services, although they also have a small role in preventing unnecessary premature death.

But to be more specific, and focusing on CAMHS, two overwhelming social purposes exist. The first was introduced under the 'rights' heading earlier and relates to the value we should place on children in a civilized society. The second addresses the consequences of *not* acting to prevent or deal with childhood mental health problems and disorders. Research on long-term

Disorder	Possible Onset In	Possible Consequences For Adolescence	Possible Consequences For Adulthood
Sexual abuse	Childhood →	• depression • suicidal behaviour • neurotic disorders →	• depression • suicidal behaviour • anxiety states • neurotic disorders
Emotional disorders	Childhood →	• school refusal • depression →	• depression • anxiety states
Conduct disorders	Childhood →	• delinquency →	• antisocial personality disorder • increased risk of offending
Eating disorders Manic depressive disorders (Bipolar affective disorders)	Childhood Adolescence →	• associated with increased mortality • associated with increased mortality →	• eating disorders • manic depressive disorders (bipolar affective disorders)
Psychotic disorders, e.g. schizophrenia	Adolescence →	→	• psychotic disorders, e.g. schizophrenia

Fig. 2.4 Linkages between mental disorder in childhood and mental disorder in adolescence and adulthood.

linkages of problems in childhood through into adult life provides strong evidence of serious implications of untreated disorder for an unhealthy adulthood. For example, the work of Knapp and his associates (see Chapter 9) has shown the long-term consequences and huge costs for a very wide range of public sector services of not being able to or not planning to intervene in childhood. Complementary evidence from studies of the effectiveness of currently available services stresses the importance of intervening in these linkages before children reach adolescence (Barton *et al.* 2002; Fonagy *et al.* 2002). Other examples are provided by Fig. 2.4.

Clearly any strategy that is being developed must address these major disorders, providing a rationale for their inclusion, incidence, prevalence, knock-on effects, etc.; and ultimately, in more operational terms, must identify effective interventions that are preventative/health promoting, diagnostic, treatment-based, and concerned with rehabilitation and monitoring (Welsh Health Planning Forum 1993).

Towards a more people-centred service

The highest possible level of return on investment will only be achieved when a service is seen as people-friendly. The NHS Health Advisory Service (1997) published a report on involving users and carers in mental healthcare. It produced a typology to summarize the various points in planning and delivery processes within which users and carers should participate. In recent times, much greater emphasis has been given to involving both sufferers and carers in the various aspects of planning and providing care. Strategically these should include their participation in:

> *Planning*, which involves sharing information and power, and an equal partnership between professionals, sufferers and carers in the processes ranging from individual care plans to local developments.

> *Quality Service Delivery*, which consists of providing the right type of service (from formal to informal), by the right provider (statutory or non-statutory), at the right time and place.

> *Facility Provision*, which is appropriate for good health promotion, preventive activities, diagnosis, treatment, and rehabilitation services.

> *Educating and Training Responsive Staff*, who are committed to a holistic approach to meeting the social, physical, and emotional needs of clients, patients, and carers.

> *Giving Lawful Consent*, based on providing the proper amount and depth of information that is tailored to fit the circumstances derived from an adequate risk assessment of both patients and carers, and presented in a language that is easily understood.

The natural consequence of following this particular strategic direction is that it enhances the needs-led approach to service development and provision, and results in a potentially productive partnership between sufferers, carers, and professionals—both clinical and managerial. An interesting practical consequence of this, which requires active management in strategic practice, is the apparent tension that can arise when planning services between needs-led strategists and practitioners and the diagnosis-led approaches of some other practitioners.

Effective resource use

CAMHS were reviewed by the NHS Health Advisory Service (Williams and Richardson 1995) and a detailed analysis made of the strengths and weaknesses of resource use. The concerns are reproduced in Tables 2.2 and 2.3.

Table 2.2 Concerns about provision expressed by primary health care professionals

....

- Problems in the availability and accessibility of CAMHS to provide advice, consultation and accept referrals from the primary care setting.
- Provision of basic information on CAMHS to primary care settings is poor, and feedback was limited.
- If training and support is not available, the demands of children, young people and their families with mental health problems on primary care staff generate problems about role adequacy, role legitimacy and role support.

Source: Williams, R. and Richardson, G. for NHS Health Advisory Service (1995). *Child and adolescent mental health services—together we stand: the commissioning, role and management of child and adolescent mental health services*. London, HMSO.

Table 2.3 Concerns about the provision of very specialized services

....

- Difficulties in relationships with local CAMHS:
  - difficulties of liaison with referrers;
  - difficulties of discharge planning;
  - disinclination to share specialist skills with secondary services.
- The vulnerability of very specialized services in the internal market:
  - lack of contracts for services creates difficulties of financial and service planning;
  - financial insecurity hampers development of new services and restricts their capacity to disseminate specialist skills.
- Inappropriate use of very specialized services in providing a source of less specialized interventions in districts with under-developed secondary level services.
- Inappropriate use of local specialist services to provide more specialized care, for example:
  - non-use of very specialized services, on grounds of their cost or insufficient capacity, lead to disruption of local CAMHS through disproportionate time and effort being diverted to difficult or extremely challenging cases.
- Poor systems of quality control and performance monitoring:
  - the absence of commissioning mechanisms often results in very specialized services not being subject to questions on monitoring of their activity effectiveness, and efficiency.

Source: Willaims, R. and Richardson, G. for NHS Health Advisory Service (1995). *Child and adolescent mental health services—together we stand: the commissioning, role and management of child and adolescent mental health services*. London, HMSO.

A strategic framework

In *Together We Stand* (1995), Williams and Richardson, its editors, proposed on behalf of a group of authors the now well-established four-tier strategic framework, which is described in more detail in Chapter 4. In general terms, and as a contribution to thinking about the strategic direction concerned with effective resource use, there are six priority areas that require consideration. They are all implicitly contained within the tiering arrangement:

> *balance of appropriate responses*, blending prevention and promotion, diagnosis, treatment, and care, and rehabilitation and monitoring;

balance of appropriate providers from within and outside the NHS, social services, and education departments;

motivation of staff, who represent 75% of service costs, to enable them to maximize their potential;

management of client contact at each stage, and to integrate services appropriately to reduce gaps and overlaps (to help create seamlessness in each family's journey through assessment, and intervention);

quality of service, with staff skills matched to client and carer need, alongside auditing mechanisms;

information management to assist integrated assessment, ongoing analysis of case management, and recording of outcome in terms of health and social functioning.

Strategy implementation

This chapter has set out the main tenets upon which strategy is constructed—value-based policy, a clear statement of intent, and a multi-faceted set of strategic directions. Additionally, we see a strategic framework as a device that aids recognition of the implications arising from complexity of need. It should promote dialogue between strategic and operational partners across organizational boundaries, and result in the re-design of better co-ordinated and more effective child-centred services. But all this is for nothing if implementation processes are not put into place.

It follows from what we have said so far that we believe that all organizations—private or public, statutory or non-statutory—need a strategy. And it is vital to get that strategy right: it determines both the map and the pathways to be followed for the longer term; and involves an irrevocable commitment of large-scale resources.

In this section, we look at the contribution that strategic thinking and behaviour should make when developing a service model.

Policy and strategy

Our position is that while the intent of public sector services must be driven at top levels of government, it should be informed constantly by the realities of service delivery. Strategy represents the point at which the two interact (see Chapter 1). It should fuel evidence-based service design and result in a practical service model that is shared by commissioners and practitioners alike.

Developing a model for any public sector service requires clear statements of the strategic intent and direction for the service relating to an identified client group. These considerations, taken together with explicitly identifying the value-set, should evoke the aims, objectives, and principles that underpin the design and delivery of the service. Strategy implementation is more assured if there is a high level of 'policy connect', a sort of double helix of policy and practice.

When combined with evidence about need, supply, demand, and service effectiveness, and the opinions of service users, carers, and practitioners, these strategic statements allow planners to prioritize service developments. In other words, a service model should draw on:

evidence-based policy;

values-based practice;

evidence-based practice; and

practice-based evidence;

in which are married critical aspects of vision and planning with research evidence and the clinical realities to help us to develop services that are appropriate, acceptable, realistic, effective, developing of staff, carers, and users and capable of further evolution (Fulford and Williams 2003).

Formulating a response strategy—priority setting

'You can't do everything' and 'It hurts!' These are the two guiding statements that envelope the process of strategy implementation. Up to this point, little in the way of boundary-setting, beyond the conceptual, has been required. Now comes the reality of having to connect strategic and operational thinking.

Figure 2.5 sets out in diagrammatic form the key questions that must be answered by planners, managers, clinicians, and social service educationalists and other professionals—whether from the statutory or non-statutory sectors—as they attempt to operationalize the high-level thinking behind the strategic intent and its associated directional pathways. See also the advice from the Welsh Health Planning Forum (1993).

The steps involve:

1. Developing a *current profile* of the present position, in terms of strengths and weaknesses, that is closely linked to the strategic directions identified.

2. *Assessment* of what would happen if nothing is done, and an examination of trends and projections to highlight opportunities and threats.

3. Focusing on *local issues* at the community level.

4. Identifying which *key issues* can be impacted on by agency action.

5. Identifying the *aims* it is intended to address in respect of the key issues.

6. Developing *specific objectives* for each aim.

7. Identifying all the *response choices* or actions available.

8. selecting and *evaluating* preferred response options.

This may appear to be a cumbersome process but it is worth the investment of time. Done properly, it involves all the stakeholders in a broad-ranging review of the current situation and reappraisal of thinking, and encourages their later ownership. Second, examining the whole field of activity in a systematic way avoids simplistic reductionism that often fails to face difficult issues with wide-ranging implications. Last, the final steps (6–8) demand examination of the evidence on both the effectiveness of interventions proposed and the most efficient of methods to be deployed in their delivery.

Need, supply, demand, and effectiveness

Need, supply and demand form a dynamic triangle of inter-locking forces. This book shows the high level of current morbidity but that only a fraction of children and young people in need receive a service. In other words, need greatly outstrips supply—the capacity of services to respond. A wide array of interventions could be delivered but presently there are substantial imbalances between the resources available, particularly well-trained staff, and demands for services. Gross imbalance in this triangle of forces provides a situation in which increases in service provision will provoke further demand.

A successful service model must recognize these and other system dynamics. It must balance perceptions of need, as seen by professionals, with the opinions and expectations of potential clients (here described as wants), but be realistically informed by present service capacities and

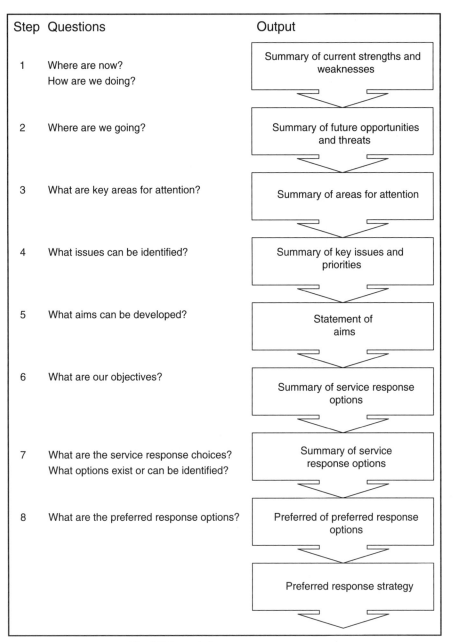

Fig. 2.5 Formulating a response strategy.

capabilities and the realities of clinical practice (Buston 2002). The client group anticipated for the service should be explicitly acknowledged by both strategy and model, which if mature and appropriate, should enable priority setting according to explicit criteria. The priorities chosen should be tempered by evidence of effectiveness of interventions from research which must include clients with complex problems who are likely to need the very services that are the subject of this chapter.

Using targeting

Targeting first came into prominence with the development of the 'management by objectives' approach (Drucker 1954). Here the emphasis was on how to structure and rationalize policy issues by focusing on strategy, productivity, marketing, innovation, and sales.

Health and social gain targeting borrow heavily on this but have a different orientation, particularly in tax-funded health and social care systems where the 'dividend' is stated more in terms of a reduction of unnecessary death or untoward incidents and improvements in quality of life, than monetary profit. However, the criteria by which targets are selected for inclusion in an organization's strategy probably vary very little. They must be:

inspirational and challenging—taking people beyond the status quo;

credible—in the sense of people believing they are worth attaining;

selective—seeking to achieve the most important things;

measurable—using soft and hard data approaches that are linked to processes and outcomes;

ethical—observing what a decent society believes ought to be done (Warner 1996).

Of importance is not to emphasize 'outcomes' alone; inclusion of 'process' brings a greater sense of both reality and possibility for all engaged in progressing target achievement. Interestingly, this advice, derived from experience, resonates with approaches to professional education and behaviour that flow from value-based practice and re-examination of professionalism in the modern context (see Chapters 5 and 6). An example is provided in Fig. 2.6.

In the past, as a contribution to achievement of a strategic intent, the NHS in Wales had one overall goal for mental health investment which was 'to improve the quality of life for people with mental health problems'. Under the heading 'People must be given an effective response at the right time' were set health gain targets, as outcomes to be achieved in the longer term and service (or process) targets to act as proxies. In respect of future policy relating to young people, targets of the types cited above are being hardened as we write into a set of Standards and Key Actions for the National Service Framework for children that is to come.

Several points arise from this example: first, the necessity of establishing baseline information to allow for later interim reviews of progress; second, the need to set a date for achievement; third, the introduction of the 'Monday morning' agenda to give a sense of immediacy that the job must be started now; and, fourth, recognition of the need for different perspectives, from 'prevention' to 'rehabilitation' to be included.

Those stakeholders responsible for monitoring at high level, tend to want a few indicator items and seek to minimize the number of targets. Managers are happy with a few more, but not too many! But perhaps it should be the practitioners who should ultimately be catered for; and experience has shown them to be personally motivated by targets specific to their own area of interest, providing that monitoring is not too heavy-handed (National Audit Office 1996).

Health Gain Target (Outcome)	Service Target (Process)
• Reduce illness due to emotional and conduct disorders in children and adolescents by early identification and intervention by 20% by 2002. (Baseline and methodology to be determined by 1995)	• By 1995, Health and Social Services should consider the development of approaches to care which allow the identification and treatment of both children and adults with psychological disorders and should include the consideration of: - 24-hour access to mental health services - crisis intervention teams - developing care registers - guidelines to facilitate early referrals to specialist care - multidisciplinary teams

Fig. 2.6 An example of outcome and process targets for CAMHS.

Inter-agency collaboration

After many years of rumination, the issue of collaboration has become the subject of formal legislation in the recent Health and Social Care Act (HMSO 2000). Now it is possible for money and resources to be used flexibly to meet need.

Scientific evidence supports the conclusion that the health needs of children and adolescents exacerbate their social needs and vice versa (Bullock and Little 1999; National Assembly for Wales 2002). Similar statements can be made with confidence about relationships between education problems, health and ill health, and social welfare factors (Meltzer and Gatward 2000; and see Chapter 10). Child and adolescence mental health is a zone of complexity and productive of substantial uncertainty (Sweeney and Griffiths 2002; Williams 2002). Thus, collaboration between agencies, disciplines, and teams has become a Holy Grail in policy, strategy and practice. It is difficult to conceive of a coherent plan for service for children that does not specify coherence between interlocking services provided by a range of agencies. However, achievement of this degree of collaboration remains illusory.

The traditional vertical approach to care provision, both by and within agencies, owes much to professional tribalism, and provides very poor integrated care. The common ground of considering how to achieve health and social gain targets, as part of the overall process of strategy formulation and implementation, can do much to move care patterns into a more horizontal arrangement.

Here, individual providers are asked not to provide a quantifiable level of service *per se*, but rather to indicate how, working with other agencies, they can help to achieve the long-term outcome targets. In this arrangement, the knowledge and skills of practitioners are drawn upon and combined with an increasingly available evidence base. Stakeholders are included from across the statutory and non-statutory sectors.

Experience shows that lack of collaboration leads to lack of shared vision, definitions, roles and tasks, and agencies making inappropriate assumptions about the roles of the others (Williams and Salmon 2002). This leads to case, cost, and responsibility shifting. Goodwill at the service delivery level, while vital, has been proven to be insufficient to change this all-too-well recognized

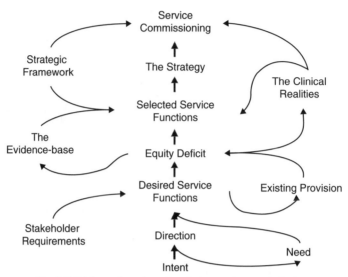

Fig. 2.7 Evidence-based service design and commissioning.

pattern in the public sector. This suggests that effective CAMHS also require collaboration to be driven through a strategy in which the corporate plan is shared by all relevant agencies. In turn, this requires a *Strategic Framework* as a reference point for dialogue and negotiation and to ensure continuing clarity and coherence of approach. (e.g. National Assembly for Wales 2000; Williams and Richardson 1995.)

Summary

Figure 2.7, hewn from experience in attempting to describe good commissioning and service design practice, provides a schematic summary of the contributions of strategic thinking and priority setting within a needs-led, evidence-based approach. It describes practical application of each of the steps identified in Fig. 2.5 and links formulation and implementation of strategy.

Monitoring and evaluating strategic developments

At the outset of this chapter strategic development was described as an important activity for all organizations because 'it determines both the map and the pathways to be followed for the longer term'. This should not be taken to mean, however, that once set, with implementation put in process, a period of calm can ensue. Quite the contrary is the case! In reality, the processes described in Fig. 2.7 are not linear but circular as we shall see in the next chapter.

Monitoring

Most often, even as the steps are being followed to formulate a response strategy, it becomes obvious that many of the questions raised can only be answered in an incomplete way, because of the quality or composition of the data currently available. Monitoring at best can only be partial, and is often seriously deficient for many programme areas. It could be said that the NHS and many social care and other agencies are awash with data but have failed to turn that data into information.

Why is this? The answer, perhaps, lies in the whole process of performance management which has tended to originate top down. On reaching the point at which practitioners become involved, the relevancy of the data required is often viewed as having insufficient bearing on patient or client care as to require only scant attention in its collection. The result? Meaningless or inaccurate data. The remedy? Build data and information systems up from the practice level and aggregate, as necessary and appropriate, for managers, policymakers and politicians.

Stakeholder evaluation

Across the statutory and non-statutory agencies, the variety of stakeholders can be enormous. At its broadest, the range may extend from: the individual volunteer working with a self-help group or community service organization; practitioners in daily contact with clients and their immediate problems; managers responsible for juggling the scarce resources at their disposal; chief executives and policymakers responsible for determining priorities for investment within a given cash envelope; and politicians who want an eye on everything because they are under pressure from the daily scrutiny of the media and because they receive representations from their constituents. No wonder that evaluation is a tricky business, especially given the long-term nature of strategy and the short term issues of political survival.

But the answers also lie in this conundrum. Evaluations in their various forms—from a personal view of the ability to derive gratification from volunteering, to an objective assessment of whether or not there are population improvements in child and adolescent mental health—will take place using different types of data, which are collected in many ways, over very varying times, and reflecting differing perspectives.

Evaluation pathways

Figure 2.8 identifies these components in a three-dimensional way, identifying the extremes for each item (e.g. soft and hard data).

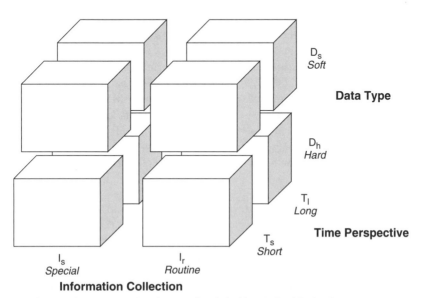

Fig. 2.8 The perceptual pathways of stakeholders in health development.

Table 2.4 Short-term perspectives of stakeholders in health development

Pathway	Perspective of data type and information collection	Study examples
(i) $I_sT_sD_s$	Crisis-oriented approach completed on a retrospective basis and within very limited time frames with a great sense of immediacy; of use principally to politicians, public and managers.	The Register introduced by the Department of Health in the 1990s
(ii) $I_rT_sD_s$	Case studies and summary of critical incidents, subjective client and professional programme assessments, studies of crises; and of use to all stakeholders.	The review of Part 8 Reviews (of adverse events in managing children and young people who are subject to the child protection procedures) conducted by Falkov A.
(iii) $I_rT_sD_h$	Utilisation data, worker activity levels, quality of care, special problem identification; of use to managers, central government managers, professional workers and to politicians.	Audits of referrals to Specialist CAMHS from GPs conducted by a variety of services in the last decade
		The CAMHS Mapping Exercise conducted for the Department of Health by the University of Durham from 2002 onwards
(iv) $I_sT_sD_h$	Best for identification of special target groups and short-term effectiveness measures; of use As for (iii) plus epidemiologists.	The review of funding of mental health services conducted by the Research Unit of the Royal College of Psychiatrists in 2003–4.

It is the interplay of the components that is of importance; and the evaluation pathways that can be constructed using them—eight in all—if data type and information collection are rotated around time, short- and long-term.

Tables 2.4 and 2.5 indicate both the pathways and the perspectives to which they best respond, together with descriptors of the type of data that might be collected for evaluative purposes. Some examples of work carried out by CAMHS is contained in the third column. Readers will, doubtless, be able to think of other examples.

The practical implications of these tables are that they enable strategists and practitioners alike to determine what emphases to give to any evaluative work that is carried out; and to be sensitive to the perspectives held by any particular stakeholder group.

High-level evaluation

High-level evaluation is the final stage in the evaluation process. The requirement is to make an assessment of whether the strategic intent to reduce, for example, inequities, is being achieved. This is done by comparing the actual state of practice with the policy principles that are generally accepted and that are represented in the value-base. In the case of CAMHS, this could be formed from the All Wales CAMHS strategy.

One writer's approach to equity (Dworkin 2000) can be paraphrased using the formula shown in Fig. 2.9.

Table 2.5 Long-term perspectives of stakeholders in health development

Pathway	Perspective of data type and information collection	Study examples
(v) $I_rT_lD_s$	This groups with (ii) and is the response to the demand by researchers that events be recorded at the time they happen.	Reviews of individual's Statements of Special Educational Need (including mental health and other healthcare needs) conducted by the education support services of the local education departments
(vi) $I_sT_lD_s$	Mainly consisting of a piecing together of programmes in a case study, historical way. This demands that soft data be stored systematically at the time of occurrence. Of use to researchers and government policymakers in better understanding of freak data situations.	Collection and review of information about clinical incidents by NHS Trusts
(vii) $I_sT_lD_h$	Data collected on retrospective or prospective basis on special target groups, or special problem areas. Can be used to develop needs/demands statements; of value to managers, researchers and consumer groups.	Data collected to audit/research the prevalence of co-morbid substance misuse and mental disorders in adolescents who attend clinics provided by Specialist CAMHS
(viii) $I_rT_lD_h$	Consistently collected data with previous definitions explicit; allows for a utiliser audit and a statement of health and social status indicator changes; of principle value to researchers, particularly epidemiologists, and public policy analysts.	The Children of the 90s cohort-based survey conducted by the University of Bristol

Source: Warner, M.M., New, P.K.M., and Pallan, P. (1976) *Towards a health centre evaluation model: a reality testing process approach*. University of British Columbia and Health and Welfare Canada.

$$\text{Inequality} \approx \text{Equal welfare level} - \text{Deviation from equal welfare level} = \text{Equity deficit}$$

(The value base-agreed policy & principles)   *(Practice)*   [evaluation]

Fig. 2.9 The equity formula.

A test of whether a strategy, policy or programme provides an improvement to the situation comes from a judgement that the equity deficit has been reduced; and this is based on minimizing the deviation from the equal welfare level.

Conclusions

And so we return to Noah. The problems facing him were enormous enough even at first sight—how to find two compatible animals and birds of each species and, then, to load them into the Ark. But, this was only the beginning: think of the range of food required; of the quantities of straw; of the need not to house cats and mice next to each other; and so on. It is evident that he formulated, implemented, and monitored his plan, and that it had clear aims and verifiable goals. What a visionary manager and leader! And the application of evidence? He had little to go on but his values and a will to perpetuate life.

References

Barton, H., Davey, I., Street, E., and Williams, R. (2002) *Mental health in childhood, children and young people who have mental health problems and mental disorders and mental health services for young people.* Health and Social Services Committee of the National Assembly for Wales. http://www.wales.gov.uk/assemblydata/3CBED339000BCF0700003BC400000000.rtf

Beveridge, W. (1942) *Social Insurance and Allied Services.* London: HMSO, cmnd 6404.

Brown, S.A., Amico, A.J.D., McCarthy, D.M., and Tapert, S.F. (2001) Four-Year Outcomes from Adolescent Alcohol and Drug Treatment. *Journal of Studies on Alcohol,* **62,** 381–8.

Bullock, R. and Little, M. (1999) The interface between social and health services for children and adolescent persons. *Current Opinion in Psychiatry,* **12,** 421–4.

Bushell, H.D., Crome, I. and Williams, R.J.W. (2002) How can risk be related to interventions for young people who misuse substances? *Current Opinion in Psychiatry,* **15,** 355–60.

Buston, K. (2002) Adolescents with mental health problems: what do they say about health services? *Journal of Adolescence,* **25,** 231–42.

Department of Health (1999) *A national service framework for mental health: modern standards and service models.* London: Department of Health.

Drucker, P.F. (1954) *The practice of management.* New York: Evanston, Harper and Row.

Dworkin, R. (2000) *Sovereign virtue: the theory and practice of equality.* Cambridge: Harvard University Press.

Falkov, A. (1996) *Department of Health Study of Working Together Part 8 Reports: Fatal child abuse and parental psychiatric disorder.* London: Department of Health Social Care Group, ACPC Series, Report 1.

Ferdinand, R.F., Blum, M. and Verhulst, F.C. (2001) Psychopathology in adolescence predicts substance use in young adulthood. *Addiction,* **96,** 861–70.

Fonagy, P., Target, M., Cottrell, D., Phillips, J., and Kurtz, Z. (2002) *What works for whom.* New York: The Guilford Press.

Fulford, K.W.M. and Williams, R. (2003) Values-based child and adolescent mental health services. *Current Opinion in Psychiatry,* **16,** 369–76.

Gjaerum, B. and Bjornerem, H. (2003) Psychosocial impairment is significant in young referred children with and without psychiatric diagnoses and cognitive delays. *European Child and Adolescent Psychiatry,* **12,** 239–48.

Grella, C.E., Hser, Y.-I., Joshi, V., and Rounds-Bryant, J. (2001) Drug Treatment Outcomes for Adolescents with Comorbid Mental and Substance Use Disorders. *The Journal of Nervous and Mental Disease,* **189,** 384–92.

Health and Social Care Act (2001) London: HMSO.

Jonassen, J.R. (1999) *Leadership—sharing the passion.* Alresford, Hants: Management Books Ltd.

Kuperman, S., Schlosser, S.S., Kramer, J.R., Bucholz, K., Hesselbrock, V., Reich, T., and Reich, W. (2001) Risk domains associated with an adolescent alcohol dependence diagnosis. *Addiction,* **96,** 629–36.

Maucher, H. (1999) *Introduction to Jonassen JR. Leadership—sharing the passion.* Alresford, Hants: Management Books Ltd.

Meltzer, H. and Gatward, R. for Office for National Statistics (2000) *Mental health of children and adolescents in Great Britain.* London: The Stationery Office.

Mullen, L. and Barry, J. (2001) An analysis of 15–19 year-old first attenders at the Dublin Needle Exchange 1990–97. *Addiction,* **96,** 251–8.

National Assembly for Wales (2000) *Children and young people. A framework for partnership—consultation document.* Cardiff: National Assembly for Wales.

National Assembly for Wales (2001) *Everybody's business—child and adolescent mental health services strategy document.* Cardiff: National Assembly for Wales.

National Assembly for Wales (2002) *Too serious a thing—the Carlile review.* Cardiff: National Assembly for Wales.

National Audit Office (1996) *Improving health in Wales: report by the Controller and Auditor General.* London: HMSO.

NHS Health Advisory Service (1995) *With care in mind secure—a report for the Special Hospitals Service Authority on the Services provided at Ashworth Hospital.* (ed. R. Williams, *et al.*) London: The Special Hospitals Service Authority.

NHS Health Advisory Service (1997) *Voices in partnership—involving users and carers in commissioning and delivering mental health services* (ed. R. Williams, G. Emerson, and Z. Muth). London: The Stationery Office

Pedersen, W., Mastekaasa, A., and Wichtrom, L. (2001) Conduct problems and early cannabis initiation: a longitudinal study of gender differences. *Addiction,* **96,** 415–31.

Salter, B. (2001) Who rules? The new politics of medical regulation. *Social Science and Medicine,* **52,** 871–83.

Sweeney, K. and Griffiths, F. (2002) *Complexity and healthcare: an introduction.* Oxford: Radcliffe Medical Press.

Szatmari, P. (1999) Evidence-based child psychiatry and the two solitudes. *Evidence-based Mental Health,* (Feb.) **1,** 6–7.

The Children Act 1989. London: HMSO.

The Human Rights Act 1998. London: HMSO.

United Nations (1989) *UN convention on the rights of the child.* New York: United Nations.

Warner, M.M. (1996) *Target setting for HFA in Wales.* Brussels, European Public Health Centre, North Rhine Westphalia.

Warner, M.M. (1997) Re-designing health services: reducing the zone of delusion. *The Nuffield Series No 1.* London: The Nuffield Trust.

Warner, M.M. (2000) Health gain investment for the 21st century: developments in Health for All in Wales. In *Exploring health policy development in Europe.* (ed. A. Ritsatakis and P. Harrington), European Centre for Health Policy, WHO Publications, WHO Regional Office for Europe.

Welsh Health Planning Forum/Welsh Office (1989) *Local strategies for health: a new approach to strategic planning.* Cardiff: NHS Directorate.

Welsh Health Planning Forum/Welsh Office (1993) *Protocol for investment in health gain: mental health.* Cardiff: NHS Directorate.

Williams, R. (2000) *A cunning plan—integrating evidence, judgement and passion in mental health strategy.* The Inaugural Lecture of Professor Richard Williams, Professor of Mental Health Strategy, given at the University of Glamorgan on 13 November 2000.

Williams, R. (2002) Complexity, uncertainty and decision-making in an evidence-based world. *Current Opinion in Psychiatry*, **15**:343–7.

Williams, R. and Richardson, G. (1995) *Child and adolescent mental health services—together we stand: the commissioning, role and management of child and adolescent mental health services.* London: HMSO.

Williams, R. and Salmon, G. (2002) Collaboration in commissioning and delivering child and adolescent mental health services. *Current Opinion in Psychiatry*, **15**, 349–53.

Williams, R., Gilvarry, E., and Christian, J. Models of service delivery. In *Young people and substance misuse.* London: Gaskell, in press.

Williams, R. (ed.) (2004) *Safeguards for young minds* (2nd edn). London: Gaskell.

World Bank (1993) *World development report: investing in health.* New York: Oxford University Press.

World Health Organization (1998a) *Investment for Health.* Copenhagen: WHO Europe.

World Health Organization (1998b) *HEALTH21: health for all in the 21st century.* Copenhagen: WHO Europe.

Chapter 3

Achieving service development by implementing strategy

Chris Heginbotham and Richard Williams

Introduction

In the previous chapter, this book identified the three core strategic processes of formulation, implementation, and monitoring. In this chapter, we consider how the processes presented graphically in Fig. 3.1 are conducted in practice.

Unapologetically, we take a no-nonsense approach to strategy. As in the last chapter, we aim to bring core matters of strategic behaviour in the public sector together with awareness of the position of child and adolescent mental health services (CAMHS) that has already been sketched in the opening two chapters.

This chapter establishes some key principles and certain good practice rules and considers briefly the four aspects of strategic vision, leadership, planning, and implementation. The discussion then:

turns to the key elements of a transformational approach to management of services run for human beings by human beings within this strategic framework;

describes briefly the components of a commissioning framework for CAMHS, linking this with a description of a process that can, and should, be used to structure health and social care responses to child and adolescent distress; and

ends by exploring the way the various elements described can be put together for the benefit of patients and practitioners alike through re-engineering organizations and empowering staff.

An approach to achieving change through strategy

Complicating the planning, development, and management of child and adolescent mental health care is very easy to do. The trick is to simplify, to be truly strategic—to look at the big picture and not to get dragged down into worthy detail, that detracts from taking necessary action to improve services. Over-complication can sometimes be a way of diverting attention from relatively straightforward problems that require tough decisions or hard choices. Valerie Iles, in her terrific book *Really managing healthcare* (Iles 1997) makes a valuable and critical distinction between the 'simple/hard' and the 'complex/easy'. Too many health service managers, she says, go for the seemingly complex problems that often have a relatively easy solution, and do not tackle the really difficult stuff, which may be easy to define but for which there is no easy answer.

Strategy is about common sense. Too much of the literature takes an arcane approach to the idea of strategic thinking and leaves many practitioners unsure of their own expertise.

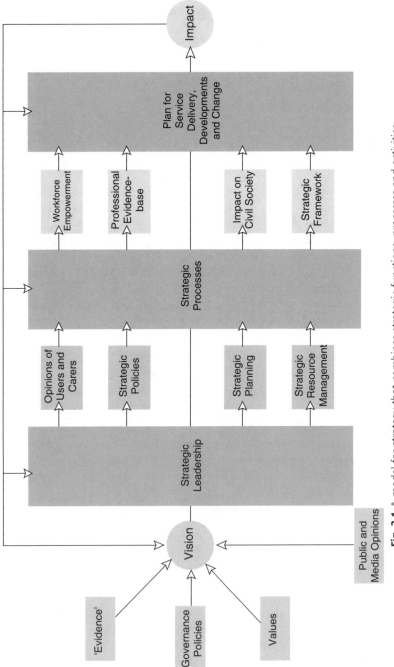

Fig. 3.1 A model for strategy that combines strategic functions, processes and activities.

In short, practitioners feel disempowered, unable to take the simple/hard decisions that they know need to be taken. By and large, what matters is to be clear about the main themes and to develop management arrangements that enable effective consideration of those themes. For many years, CAMHS have been characterized by well-meaning rhetorical support and far too little investment. It is now broadly accepted that many problems in adult mental health, including criminal and anti-social behaviour, have their beginnings in childhood, and that child and adolescent mental healthcare should be studied as logically prior to adult psychiatry, rather than as an after-thought considered only by those people who go into this branch of healthcare.

CAMHS have been given necessary attention during the last ten years; for example, through the work of the NHS Health Advisory Service, the campaigning activities of Young Minds, and, latterly, the attention of the Audit Commission, Welsh Assembly Government, Department of Health, and Department for Education and Skills. Even then, CAMHS are probably the most talked about and least well-established mental health services. There are many reasons for this: children with severe mental disorders are mercifully relatively rare; they do not usually draw great attention to themselves unlike, say, some adult mentally ill offenders; services are provided by a wide range of agencies, albeit in an inchoate and disorganized fashion; and there are simply too many other priorities for cash-strapped health and local authorities to cope with.

This lack of sustained concern for CAMHS should not distract us from either the very good work, which has been and continues to be done by many practitioners, or from the real opportunities that exist in many places for development and change. Sound well-considered advice and guidance is available, even if the resources do not match the needs of patients or the aspirations of staff. The reports of the NHS Health Advisory Service of the 1990s and the more recent Audit Commission and Welsh Assembly reports all testify to creative thinking and practical support for the development of CAMHS. But, one thing that has bedevilled attempts to improve CAMHS is the *perceived* complexity of the subject, coupled with some remarkable attempts, by health authorities especially, to *make* the subject complicated.

Tackling the simple/hard requires virtues, which many of us profess but which seem to desert us (or we claim have deserted our colleagues!) at important moments: clarity, honesty, courage, and abdication of sectional interests. Strategic thinking requires all these attributes allied with common sense, rather than a desire to make the subject too intricate. emphasizing this is important because, in respect of CAMHS, it is very easy to become overwhelmed by the sheer amount of detail and the extent of the potential 'problem' posed by young people.

We will see when we look at the epidemiology of child and adolescent mental disorders (see Part 2) that a case can be made (but should be examined carefully) for many thousands of children in the UK (as in other countries) to be considered either to be at risk or to have actual or incipient mental disorder. Often, the figures can be paralysing. Where do we draw the lines or set thresholds? Can we really provide for that group and not the other? For example, if we invest in Tier 4 services, will we be at fault in not providing for Tier 2? Can we make a change, if the other agency down the road can't or won't?

To overcome these problems, we have to live in the real world. The real world is messy, uncertain, and unclear; people can be more or less kind or horrid; can, by turns, be selfish or altruistic; and there are never enough resources to go round. By defining problems carefully and recognizing that there are no perfect solutions, we can give ourselves permission to take the best decision for today. There is rarely a correct decision; sometimes there is a right decision for today, but more often, it is the least worst.

What seems to have stymied CAMHS development in some parts of the UK, is the inability of senior managers to take necessarily pragmatic joint-agency decisions based on reasonable assumptions: a form of 'principled pragmatism' based in clearly articulated values but which recognizes the interplay of different professions, agencies, individuals and service users in a diverse multi-cultural and multi-ethnic society.

A strategic framework

Strategic vision

In an article in the *BMJ*, Pendleton and King (2002) define values as 'deeply held views that act as guiding principles for individuals and organizations. Trust flows from their being stated and followed. If they are stated and not followed then trust is broken. And broken trust is hard to mend'. We agree that trust is an essential factor in managing any complex organization, especially at times of change. Empowerment of staff requires managers to trust staff to get on with the job sensibly; staff must be able to trust managers to have their best interests at heart.

Six common themes can be identified that are regarded as essential or core in the development of modern value-led, evidence-based CAMHS in the UK (National Assembly for Wales 2001). Together, these themes form a vision for CAMHS:

Multi-agency Ownership of the CAMHS Concept. This means achieving shared, multi-agency ownership of a broad approach to the definition of children's mental health and, consequently, of approaches to resolving those problems.

Basing services on the *CAMHS Concept* in which all relevant sectors of care play their key and acknowledged roles to achieve the goal of delivering integrated and comprehensive services.

Basing service planning on the *Assessed Needs* of the child population in each locality in order to break away from provision built on historical patterns of supply or anecdotal levels of demand.

Conducting Audit and Mapping of Current Services in order to determine local priorities for development.

Adopting an *Evidence-based Approach* to practice and thereby *Targeting* services according to more explicit criteria.

Using a *Strategic Approach* to designing and delivering CAMHS based on a common *Strategic Framework* that is used as a tool for future understanding and development.

To these themes might be added a values-based approach to commissioning and practice, drawing on the ten principles of values-based practice (VBP) described by Fulford and Williams (2003) and developed further in Chapter 5. To be effective, this requires a shared vision and an agreed programme of action jointly owned by families and carers, the government, responsible authorities, and service providers. Each needs to be committed to a partnership in which the agencies work together to design and deliver shared local strategies and services. No sector can be absolved from the duty to play its full part in CAMHS and to co-operate across professional boundaries to better meet the needs of children and adolescents, and family adults, siblings, carers, and staff who work with children.

The concept of CAMHS thus needs to be inclusive; that is, the term CAMHS (the 'CAMHS concept') should mean all of the services provided by all sectors that impinge on the mental well-being, mental health, mental health problems, and mental disorders of children and young people before their majority (National Assembly for Wales 2001). Commonly, the term CAMHS has taken a narrower focus to imply those specialist services provided, mainly but by no means exclusively, by the NHS. These services are of key importance and they need to be developed in order to:

match contemporary demands better; and

support plans to develop those other services that should be drawn into CAMHS and developed to become part of an integrated and effective frontline of provision.

However, for our purposes here, we espouse the wider 'CAMHS concept' definition and think holistically about the needs of children and young people.

Strategic leadership

Although we do not wish to suggest that developing CAMHS is a form of warfare, there are some helpful analogies that illustrate our task. The military origins and whole organization scale of strategy are related to harnessing large numbers of people in pursuit of achieving an identified common goal. Far from being simply cerebral or arcane, strategy must be people-orientated. It must support flexibility in implementation and recognize the real abilities of real people, as the turn of events may not be accurately predictable once execution of the plan begins. For example, it has long been axiomatic of successful military campaigning that the senior commander's intentions are communicated to, supported by, and maintained by the most junior soldiers, so that the goals are not lost despite unpredicted turns of events or lapses in contact with leaders. It is also a truism that strategy barely survives the first hour of action. This is equally true of any complex implementation programme within public services and demands that managers and staff remain alert to emergent changes, while continuing to press towards the shared goal. Thus, communication, motivation, and alignment to common goals are also key components of strategy. These are leadership functions.

The leadership and motivational components of strategy give the lie to its perception as a pile of dust-covered documents. Similarly, delegation of decision-making and necessary resources, another strategic leadership principle, to those best equipped to make the decisions and down to the lowest reasonable level, sustains the involvement of the workforce by valuing and developing their creativity.

It should be obvious, but is worth making explicit, that, for leadership to be effective, there must be coherence between the stated aims of the leader and the managerial expectations placed on staff. To illustrate this point, we need to anticipate the critical elements of the commissioning framework described later in the chapter. Key components of the commissioning process are:

setting clear *objectives* for the service;

describing *need* and demand—the epidemiological framework;

having clarity about the *models* of care;

establishing *priorities* through robust process;

knowing the expected *outcomes*—what *success* will look like, and the performance indicators required to drive change.

Similarly, these are the components of a strategic planning and management process that must be articulated at the beginning of the process, re-emphasized throughout, and provides the necessary framework for action. We will return to this in the section on commissioning.

Strategic planning

Formulation, implementation, and monitoring of strategy require a plan to develop the organization and especially the workforce. Without it, plans remain plans and the written record (often erroneously described as '*the* strategy') will gather dust! At this point, we return to the link between strategic processes and what might be termed 'planning for performance'. Effective implementation of a strategy will almost certainly require a good deal of effort in organizational and workforce development. If the strategic processes have been established along the lines we describe, then there is available a strong link to the process of implementation.

Strategy relates to whole organizations. Also, good strategists must have good intelligence about current circumstances and be able to identify the goals of their thinking and the direction of travel of the organization in search of those defined goals. Through well-designed strategic planning processes, it is possible to link the high-level components of planning, as described in Chapter 1, with the practical 'hands on' planning of day-to-day functions. These tasks have enormous practical importance. They are not concerned simply with 'blueprint' planning— some sort of bureaucratic paper chase—but must be transformational, enabling real and lasting change to be achieved. Thus, synergy can be achieved between the early strategic processes and the practical managerial changes needed to create the future service.

Strategic management of implementation and delivery

Strategic processes can be integrated to give a transformational change management programme for service development. Table 3.1 modifies the literature (Beatty and Ulrich 1991) to make the language more appropriate to that used in this book. Here we take the ideas in the preceding chapter on another step in order to identify the stages of a transformational strategic implementation plan that unashamedly aims for what we call here 'sustained patient advantage'. Whether we use terms such as patient or service user (or client) what matters is to have a patient (or service user or client) focussed service that is informed by patient values.

In other words, strategic management brings the strategic vision and planning processes together into a coherent implementation plan. As Table 3.1 suggests, it is essential, if staff and service-users are to understand what is happening, for all three dimensions to be brought together into a consistent approach. This may sound rather obvious, but so often the strategic intentions do not match what is actually implemented. There are many reasons for this of which poor communication, lack of understanding, and deliberate obfuscation are the most common. This is why we stress, time and again, the need to remain strategic while dealing with some thorny day-to-day problems. Losing sight of the big picture will mean a lot of wasted

Table 3.1 Stages in transformational management (modified from Beauty and Ulrich 1991)

Restructuring organizational components to use resources effectively
Organizational development and processes to enable planned services to be provided
Continuous quality improvement and clinical governance
Workforce support, lifelong learning, and empowerment
Strategic cultural change, aiming for sustained patient advantage

effort and attention to the wrong detail, with the inevitable consequences of loss of staff morale and commitment, and a poorer service for the patients and service users.

Most organizations providing CAMHS have been in existence for many years, have been through many re-organizations, and are well established. They can be characterized as 'mature' organizations, certainly in the sense that there are strongly embedded individuals, attitudes, and cultures. The overall culture is an amalgam of separate clinical and managerial cultures that have grown up over time and to which staff will have firm attachment, even if they are not able to articulate the culture or know where it has come from. But changing, or attempting to change, the culture suddenly brings out defensive, almost immunological reactions. Staff coalesce around cultural icons, become agitated and angry (inflammation), and may react in highly protective ways to traditional work patterns and processes, and in so doing attempt to destroy the alien cultural transplant (rejection).

Tackling these issues requires explicit values, clarity of purpose (aims and objectives), sound evidence, carefully formulated models of care, established priorities, and proposals to achieve the stated outcomes—the critical success factors of the strategy. All are key points that we describe later. Additionally, it requires a transformational process, which draws from the strategic processes relating to resources, planning, policy and the workforce and creates a programme of change that is intended to achieve 'sustained patient advantage' (SPA).

SPA is akin to competitive advantage in industry, but here we are much less concerned with competition between providers (although this process will also give a distinct competitive edge if that is needed) than with providing the best possible care focused on the needs of each individual patient or service user. SPA draws on maximizing the use of assets to the patients' or clients' benefits, empowering the workforce, and focusing on clinical governance and continuous quality improvement. In short, it is about *'accountable care'*.

Commissioning as 'strategy in action'

Principled pragmatism

We have seen that strategic planning requires clarity, honesty, courage, and a certain selflessness. Equally importantly, it demands understanding and acceptance of some real tensions. These tensions (sometimes referred to as 'paradoxes') are perennial, they will not go away, and need to be tackled. Many fall into Valerie Iles' description of the 'simple hard'. Here are three:

Professional staff are essential to any service but the focus of any human service delivery must be on service users;

Improving services requires changes in behaviour but it is no good designing a service around ideal behaviours which, realistically, we know will not be achieved;

Resources need to be balanced across a service (e.g. across the tiers of the four tier model) but with the emphasis always towards the front line of distress.

It is a truism that the staff of a service are its main resource and the service could not be delivered without them. It is also the case that if people (in this case, children and adolescents) did not have needs, there would be no need of professionals. Just as children should be considered logically prior to adults, so the needs of users are logically prior to the needs of the organization or its staff, not withstanding the importance of those staff.

At the same time, we must live in the real world of individual personality and aspiration, hope and failure. We can say readily that so-and-so should do something, or do it differently, but if we know he or she can not or will not, then we will not design a service that will work.

Too often human services succumb to this triumph of hope over experience. This is not a counsel of despair; but it is a tension to be borne in mind in seeking to enshrine our principles pragmatically in an imperfect world. And imperfection is no reason for inaction.

A helpful way of tackling these differences of view is to consider the values of those involved in the service. Often in the past, this has been a rather sterile process of stating a set of 'motherhood and apple pie' values that are unexceptional and to which everyone can sign-up, irrespective of whether they believe they will make any difference. Instead, the process proposed here, and described in much greater detail in Chapter 5, is to follow a process of values-identification based on ten key principles, and then to use the diversity of values explicitly as a resource to actively negotiate differences. Making values open, transparent, and explicit enables everyone to understand and challenge the position taken by each other person—patient, carer, clinician, manager—and assists in dealing with the frequently hidden reasons for individuals' lack of commitment to the objectives articulated in the strategy. Values-based practice (VBP) complements evidence-based practice (EBP).

This may seems idealistic, but usually it is values and not evidence that really drive service delivery. Often, the evidence is patchy and, even where there is 'gold standard' evidence from good double-blind randomized control trials, the way in which the evidence is viewed, translated, and assimilated is critical. Evidence ignored for personal reasons; and, at other times, rather sketchy evidence, may be elevated to an unrealistically high status on the basis of individual value judgements (Hall 2002). But we are not naïve; no process is perfect. Nonetheless, making values explicit in order to negotiate a way forward that can be accepted and acted upon by all involved is a valuable process that can obviate difficulties. If left unattended, those difficulties can undermine even the best strategy, with detrimental effects on patients and staff alike.

Continuous improvement

Most health, education and social services staff will be familiar with the 'audit cycle', the 'plan-do-study-act' (PDSA) process. Less familiar perhaps is that the same cycle is apparent in nearly all activity associated with developing and shaping health and social care, from commissioning to performance evaluation. One way of describing the 'life cycle' of health services focuses on four stages:

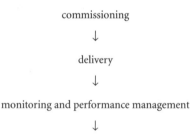

commissioning

↓

delivery

↓

monitoring and performance management

↓

proposing changes for improvement

... and back round the cycle!

Commissioning healthcare is necessarily an iterative and involving process. It cannot be achieved effectively through top–down imposition of ideas or propositions. Involving the providers and users of services is an essential pre-requisite, not simply to ensure 'ownership' but, more fundamentally, to ensure that they meet the real needs and aspirations of service users.

Thus, commissioning requires the following five stages:

1. An agreement of the *objectives* for the service, based on information about need and demand.

2. Consideration of epidemiological information relating to patient *need* and data on the historical use of current services on which to quantify the volume services and diversity required.

3. Developing *models* of service delivery incorporating effective ways of meeting perceived need and demand.

4. Agreement on the *priorities* for investment or development.

5. Clarification of the *outcomes* expected—the critical success factors—the targets and measures against which the performance of services is assessed.

Iteration between these stages is inevitable, if scarce resources are to be used to best effect. It is within this process that decisions on the relative importance of the identified needs are made and the investment in the four tiers of the service agreed. A critical problem that always surfaces at this stage might be summarized by the cliché 'the best is the enemy of the good'. In other words, there is no point in declining to make changes to improve a part of a service just because all of it cannot be improved. The next paragraphs consider each of these stages in order. Figures 3.2 and 3.3 summarise the processes as applied to CAMHS.

Objectives

Defining the aims and objectives of a service is vitally important. Our experience is that, often, the aims and objectives are assumed to be agreed when there are, in practice, significant differences of opinion. This is probably more so for CAMHS than other services because of

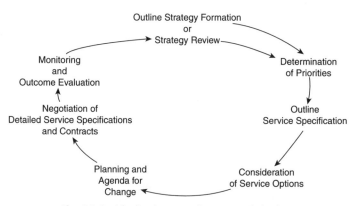

Fig. 3.2 An idealized approach to commissioning.

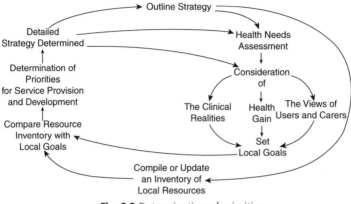

Fig. 3.3 Determination of priorities.

the interplay of disciplines, and the extensive and differential needs of the primary service users and their families. Lack of agreement about what a service is seeking to achieve will later hamper effective action to the disadvantage of the children for whom the service has been established.

Also, the wider boundaries of any service should be established early as a task. For example, is this a health service or an illness service? How is health defined? Is the service one that will integrate medicine, nursing, psychology, social services, education, and so on? Or will it be one of discrete entities? How will the service become genuinely child-centred?

Epidemiology, need, and demand

The literature on the epidemiology relating to children's mental health and ill health is huge. This provokes key questions such as 'are we concerned with the severe psychiatric illnesses or the wider but pervasive mental health problems that affect young people?'. And, 'are we concerned with therapeutic interventions for illness, or are we also concerned with promoting mental health?'. Problematically, the literature suggests that there is a very substantial morbidity across all age groups, social classes, ethnic groups, and diagnostic categories, to the extent that defining the proper boundaries of the service becomes very difficult. It is essential to cut through this to the critical elements. In this regard, it is crucial to define the thresholds of morbidity to be adopted for planning and service delivery purposes.

Epidemiological information is one input to identifying likely need, but must be translated into a service specification through a rigorous examination of realistic interventions. Implicit in this is the importance of making priority-setting decisions and this may be proved difficult.

Models

Many professional staff are sceptical about, and wary of, simple service organization 'models', believing that the needs of service users are too complex and multi-faceted to be shoe-horned into a single model of care. But models of care are intimately connected to need and the ability of staff to meet need. Sometimes for managers, it seems that this reaction is defensive and resistant to clarity, perhaps because it challenges professional mystique. Any approach that defines unambiguously the nature, purpose, and extent of a service, provides few hiding places for those who want to continue their traditional practice undisturbed by accountability to users, organization, or the taxpayer. This is not meant as a criticism of the genuine desire of some professional staff to develop niche skills for treating rare disorders; but it is a criticism of those who wish to continue undertaking such treatments once an organization has, through robust consultative processes, come to a decision that those particular treatments will be limited in their scope for sound reasons.

Present estimates of psychiatric, psychological, and social morbidity in children vastly exceed the resources available for their assessment and for intervention. This stresses the importance of achieving a holistic child-centred approach without unnecessarily medicalizing social and familial distress, some of which is profound and long-term or transient and self-limiting. But this requires another question to be answered, preferably at the beginning of the process: to what extent is the service holistic, multi-professional, multi-model, and multi-agency? Is the service genuinely child-centred? Where are the boundaries between home, healthcare, school, social services, and so on.

The ability of staff to meet defined needs is itself a complex matter. Some staff will have the necessary skills and can be deployed readily; others may need training; or individuals with specific expertise may need to be recruited. Yet, as we have already above, others may wish to continue with treatments or services, which are agreed now not to be a priority.

For many, managing this kind of scenario may be very difficult because it can bring managers into direct conflict with clinical staff and lead to arguments about clinical freedom and understanding. The best solution is to institute a properly constituted process in which *all* clinical staff are involved. 'Ownership' is an overused word, but the concept is critical. Staff must be encouraged to join in a process that is seen as robust, open, transparent and honest. But when a decision has been made through that process, a key principle must be that, everyone goes along with the result even if it does not accord with their personal view.

Priorities

The discussion on models is nested with that on priorities. The model adopted for any service will be influenced by the nature of the users' needs and opinions and the type of interventions to be provided. The model(s) adopted will influence the balance of resources to be invested in differing treatment modalities or arrangements. Deciding priorities can be time consuming and administratively difficult if all service users and their families, staff and others with a genuine and relevant interest are to be included. Nonetheless, involving all those 'stakeholders' is essential if the service is to meet the broad needs and demands of users and staff alike. Our experience is that time spent on what may appear as elaborate actually repays itself with interest later.

There is no 'correct' or perfect way to go about consultation, and experience, once again, shows that process is everything! Transparency, honesty, and mutual respect, even where there are fundamental disagreements, eventually pays off. This is where 'principled pragmatism' once again becomes necessary, as no perfect priority setting system exists. Things go wrong when individuals are excluded for whatever reason.

Priorities are determined on a basis of considering opinions from a number of sources. These include user and carer views, governmental planning and priorities guidance, local pictures of need from epidemiological studies, exploration of gaps in local services. A great deal has been said and written over the last 15 years or so and many diverse schemes devised for priority setting.

While it is right to use as good an evidence-base as possible, it is also essential to recognize local political and practical realities, and not to be too precious about less than perfect outcomes. If we wait until we have all the information, we won't do anything for 20 years and, by that time, our information will be out-of-date and the continuing impact of past need could be effecting future generations already. Doing nothing is worse than doing something, as long as there is a reasonable measure of agreement about the best course of action.

Of course, that does not mean anyone can, or should, be able to affect the outcome disproportionately, nor should a process be made foolishly complicated just because one or two individuals cannot agree. No organization should be held to ransom by a strong-willed person. There has to be a 'result', which can be implemented and tested and, if necessary, amended in due course. An earlier point bears repetition in a slightly different form: resources have been made available for CAMHS by government, on behalf of society, because young people have mental health problems and disorders. This gives all service staff a duty to use those resources in the most effective and efficient ways to provide the best possible care for young people and their families. We think that, to do otherwise would be unethical.

Outcomes and success factors

Integral to any strategic approach to service development and to management of change is the requirement to be clear about the outcomes that are expected—or what constitutes success. Usually, if the preparatory work has been done properly, the outcomes (the critical success factors) will marry up closely with the key objectives established for the service. For example, if a key objective is to ensure that all children between ages of 5 and 11 in the area, who display signs of developing psychotic disorder, are seen within five working days, then the success factor is the achievement of that goal.

However, not all success factors can be tied in a fully transparent way directly to the objectives of the service. Success can take a number of forms, such as improved morale of the staff, enhanced satisfaction of service users, more relevant service provision or improved patient functioning. Some factors may not be stated explicitly at the outset. Good objective setting is often a process of deciding the priorities that define success and then tailoring the objectives to the service's or team's view of how to achieve the priorities.

Establishing critical success factors enables a team to check outcomes against the original objectives, and also assists in defining the performance indicators against which the service should be judged. Performance indicators should be related directly to the objectives but may incorporate some latitude in their achievement. T o take the earlier example, achieving 100% of the target of seeing all children within five working days in year 1 may be difficult, if not impossible. So, performance targets may be set to reflect this: say, 80% in year 1, 90%, in year 2 and 100%, in year 3.

By now, we have come full circle in the cycle of service commissioning: Objectives (success factors) → Epidemiology and need → Models of care → Priorities → Success factors (performance management).

Strategic change: re-engineering organizations

If our strategy is right and our approach to commissioning effective, the next stage is for providers to make the necessary adjustments to their service provision. Of course it is not that simple. Commissioning is not an isolated process but requires careful debate with providers about what is possible, achievable, and affordable. So the strategy should have encompassed early in its formulation the providers' views on what can be achieved. However, it is essential for the providers to keep their side of the bargain when the strategy is implemented.

A plan to re-engineer the organization to achieve SPA has five main stages (set out in Table 3.1 above):

restructuring organizational components to use resources as effectively and efficiently as possible;

organizational development and process re-design;

workforce empowerment through training and education, staff development, and delegation to the 'lowest' level in the organization closest to patients;

continuous quality improvement and establishment of a clinical governance programme; and

overall cultural change to achieve sustained patient advantage.

Re-structuring organizational components

This first stage in re-engineering the organization requires a focus on the current deployment of resources, using whatever relevant analytic tools are available: performance indicators, benchmark data, good practice from elsewhere, innovative ideas drawn from the literature, and systems models. Outcomes of this part of the process could include gross structural change, such as 'delayering' and organizational re-design with the aim of associating those service components together that naturally form a better fit for the new strategic vision. This stage focuses on resource usage and links directly with effective priority setting processes that we describe later. Some tough decisions have to be taken, to be communicated to the staff and service users, and to be acted upon, especially when a current service or component of a service is to be abandoned altogether.

'Re-engineering' is a word that does not appeal to many clinicians. It smacks too much of manufacturing industry, of machines not people, of inanimate objects rather than patients. A term sometimes used to soften the impact is 'process re-design'. But we have to be careful to define our terms. Process re-design is part of re-engineering, but not the whole story. Re-organizing the enterprise may mean changing the structure fundamentally. To be effective, this should build on, or lead to, process changes, but may be warranted for other reasons, notably to force a change in the inter-relationship between departments or sections within the organization. A necessary approach to lasting workforce empowerment is maximum delegation of responsibility as close to the patient as possible.

Co-ordinating the best response to patients means linking departments or sections dynamically, removing unnecessary bureaucracy or boundaries, and giving frontline staff as much freedom as possible to create a service tailored to the needs of individual patients. Being innovative means being 'integrative' and vice versa (Kanter 1989)! By definition, this means sharing resources, and to work well, staff need feedback on whether the way they are using the resources is effective. Good measures are patient satisfaction (surveys and questionnaires), productivity indicators, and reduced response times (such as waiting times for clinics) (Ashkenas *et al.* 1995, p. 137). No one measure is sufficient and, in practice, may be misleading. The aim should be a 'balanced scorecard' (perhaps using 'spidergrams' for illustration) containing a judicious mix of input, process, output, and outcome measures, which staff themselves are involved in choosing, that assist in managing use of resources and which provide an overall picture of the organization.

Organizational development and process re-design

An organizational development (OD) programme can assist in developing the new structures and processes needed to deliver revised service models, and centres on process mapping, care process re-design, and the job profiles required in the 'new world'. Central to all of this is communication—a skill that is difficult to over-emphasize. Communication with staff and other interested groups is critical to the strategy and it's implementation. Agreeing priorities or negotiating values—whichever activity of the organization is picked—requires regular and deliberate attention to communication. That communication must be in all ways, between managers and staff, and vice versa, between clinicians and clinicians, between patients and their families with clinicians and managers, and between the service and the wider community.

OD is in itself a process of empowerment, of discovery, and of involvement. The best OD draws problems and solutions from the organization and assists in reformulating and reflecting ideas back to the organization. This is not the classic management consultant who 'borrows your watch to tell you the time'. Good OD: facilitates communication, openness, and interpretation; brings insights, suggestions, and models; assists integration through innovation and identifying emergent solutions; and reflects ideas drawn form the organization's own history, culture and objectives. Above all, an organizational development programme draws on the strengths and knowledge of staff to create a better environment in which to pursue the organization's remit.

Workforce empowerment

The most critical element of the whole programme is ensuring 'ownership' for the plans. All the staff should have an opportunity to contribute to the plan and to know not only what is being done to them personally but also to understand their essential role in delivering the plan. Empowerment is another of those often used but little understood words. Put simply, it means giving responsibility to the staff who are close to patients and trusting them to do their best to deliver appropriate care. This is not an abdication of management responsibility. True empowerment means support, help, training, education, and monitoring of delegated responsibility. It is onerous on managers, especially at first, but it pays off handsomely in the medium- and long-terms. Programmes, such as *Improving working lives* (Department of Health 1999b), provide a framework for this approach by emphasizing lifelong learning, support, involvement, and training.

Empowerment demands a flattening (or at least simplification) of hierarchy, decentralization, lateral as well as vertical communication, and creation of work groups or sections with delegated authority. These groups should be autonomous but integrated, independent but interdependent, and focused on their part of the business, yet linked horizontally with other similar groups. Successful integrative organizations are those 'that have a willingness to see problems as wholes and challenge accepted practices' and those that encourage a sense of pride in the organizations achievements (Kanter 1984, 1989, described in Pugh and Hickson 1996, pp. 121–2).

Continuous quality improvement

Clinical care is complex and demands a clinical governance framework that encourages both a continuous QA cycle—our ubiquitous plan-do-study-act (PDSA) cycle—and attention to the environment in which the activity takes place. The culture is highly important. An empowered workforce, with good risk-management procedures, effective clinical audit and feedback mechanisms, good training, and a commitment to the aims and objectives of the organization, will provide the 'accountable care' that is essence of clinical governance. Through patient and public involvement in service design, complaints monitoring, attention to outcome measures, and good communication, service programmes can achieve their objectives and lead to the workforce feeling fulfilled.

Strategic cultural change

The end result is a strategic shift in both the mindset of the organization and a new culture with patients at the centre. Achieving *sustained patient advantage* is the crucial and over-riding goal. But it needs continued hard work if it is to be embedded in a new culture and sustain improved practices. But, sometime in the future, the culture may have to change again. As Mintzberg *et al.* (1998, p. 36) put it:

> Explicit strategies are blinders designed to focus direction and thus block out peripheral vision. They can thus impede strategic change when it becomes necessary…. The more clearly articulated the strategy, the more deeply imbedded it becomes… breeding a resistance to later change.

The only solution is to remain alive to the emergence of a new strategic vision. From time-to-time, it is essential to use deliberately a different strategic model as a disrupter or catalyst for change. If the cycle of change advocated here is followed, then staff will have attended regularly to their changing circumstances and the changing needs of their patients. They should be picked up by the organization through clinical governance management processes.

In essence, the model proposed here is that of a 'learning organization' in which staff are seen as the pre-eminent resource. Above all, the workforce plan within the strategy must be practical incorporating active and real responses to the vital matters of recruitment, retention, training, and development in a planned way appropriate to the skills required of the service. Similarly, it must recognize that the world of work is changing. Many of the concerns of practitioners are about psychological survival and development in a world that has become more demanding, challenging, and exacting and much less forgiving.

In parallel with rising expectations of patients, politicians, professionals, and managers alike (National Assembly for Wales 2002), the real complexity of the problems facing clients and patients and, by transmission, the tasks before the staff, are becoming better recognized. Complexity science identifies that 'there is an insoluble paradox between the need for consistent and evidence-based standards of care and the unique predicament, context, priorities and choices of the individual patient' (Plsek and Greenhalgh 2001). Similarly, Szatmari has identified the two solitudes divided by the meaning of the term evidence (1999) in which what families want from services may not be delivered by applying the evidence as it is understood by practitioners.

Resolving the challenges requires greater investigation of what constitutes clinical judgement, clinical decision-making, and intuition through techniques such as critical reflection and reconstruction of narratives in practice and patients' lives, and for knowledge and clinical experience to be brought together in more transparent yet sensitive ways. Plsek and Greenhalgh talk of a 'zone of complexity' that lies between areas in which decision-making is predictable and circumstances in which there is 'so much disagreement and uncertainty that the system is thrown into chaos'. At the very least, the changing environment in healthcare involves more and not less uncertainty and practitioners must be assisted to function well in it if our plans are to be put into effect.

Hall reviewed the implications for healthcare professionals' education of intuition and uncertainty in decision-making (2002). She talks of the rules used by clinicians when making decisions, particularly in conditions of uncertainty, and uses Beresford's categorization of technical, personal, and conceptual sources of uncertainty. Fulford and Williams (2003) argue that, paradoxically, personal and conceptual of sources of uncertainty are likely to grow rather than decline as a consequence of increasing information, better evidence and consequent greater choice for patients and clients. Put another way, they call for good decision-making to be based on values-based practice set alongside traditional evidence-based practice. Similar considerations can be applied to supporting decision-making at all managerial levels. These matters are explored from different but overlapping perspectives in Chapters 5 and 6.

Conclusion

In this chapter, we have sought to provide a very practical approach to implementing strategy by focusing primarily, but not exclusively, on workforce issues and commissioning CAMHS. The over-arching message is of the need for simplicity, clarity, and consistency. Simplicity, because CAMHS are complex enough and complicating it further won't help; clarity, because staff and service users need to know what is being provided when and what is expected of them; and consistency, because everyone needs to be able to work to an agreed brief without constant change and disruption.

Thus, we have taken a people-based approach. Its importance is heightened by the recent shifts and, particularly since 1997, in the triad of relations between the public, the state, and the professions (Salter 2001). These changes, together with democratization of knowledge and social process, have resulted in the world now feeling much less certain to the staff of the public sector, than it did even ten years ago. Thus, one of the key tasks for senior managers is to sustain and develop the workforce in this cultural setting (Williams 2002). In this situation, work of the kind we have reviewed in this chapter should contribute to implementation of strategy by bringing together the complex worlds within healthcare of: science and practice; the professions and the public; and governments, managers and the professions.

We hope that our emphasis on sustained patient advantage will resonate with commissioners, staff, and service-users alike, and provide an exciting and motivating message for improving the quality of mental health care to children and adolescents. The challenge is to achieve sustained patient advantage as the goal of the service.

References

Ashkenas, R., Ulrich, D., Jick, T., and Herr, S. (1995) *The boundaryless organization: breaking the chains of organizational structure.* San Francisco: Jossey-Bass.

Bagshaw, M. and Bagshaw, C. (1999) Leadership in the twenty-first century. *Industrial and Commercial Training,* **3** (6), 236–9.

Beatty, R.W. and Ulrich, D.O. (1991) Reenergizing the mature organization. *Organizational Dynamics,* Summer 1991, 16–30.

Beresford, H.B. (1991) Uncertainty and the shaping of medical decisions. *Hastings Cent Rep,* **21**, 6–11.

Bullock, R. and Little, M. (1999) The interface between social and health services for children and adolescent persons. *Current Opinion in Psychiatry,* **12**, 421–4.

Dawson, S. (1996) *Analysing organizations.* Basingstoke: Macmillan Business.

Department of Health (1999a) *A national service framework for mental health: modern standards and service models*. London, Department of Health.

Department of Health, England (1999b) *Improving working lives* (incl DH Circular HSC1999/218). London: Department of Health.

Fulford, K.W.M. and Williams, R. (2003) Values-based child and adolescent mental health services? *Current Opinion in Psychiatry*, **16**, 369–76.

Goleman, D. (2000) Leadership that gets results. *Harvard Business Review*, March–April, 78–90.

Hall, K.H. (2002) Reviewing intuitive decision-making and uncertainty, the implications for medical education. *Med Educ*, **36**, 216–24.

Handy, C. (1999) Picture framing. In *Thoughts for the day* (ed. C. Handy), pp. 73–6. London: Arrow.

Iles, V. (1997) *Really Managing Health Care*. Buckingham: Open University Press.

Jonassen, J.R. (1999) *Leadership—sharing the passion*. Alresford, Hants: Management Books Ltd.

Kanter, R.M. (1984) *The change masters, corporate entrepreneurs at work*. New York: Allen and Unwin.

Kanter, R.M. (1989) *When giants learn to dance*. New York: Simon and Schuster.

Knapp, M.K., Scott, S., and Davies, J. (1999) The cost of antisocial behaviour in younger children, preliminary findings from a pilot sample of economic and family impact. *Clin Child Psychol Psychiatry*.

Kotter, J.P. (1998) What leaders really do? In *Harvard Business Review on Leadership*, pp. 37–60. Boston, MA: Harvard Business School Press.

Maucher, H. (1999) Introduction. In *Leadership—sharing the passion* (ed. J. R. Jonassen). Alresford, Hants: Management Books Ltd.

Meltzer, H. and Gatward, R. for Office for National Statistics (2000) *Mental health of children and adolescents in Great Britain*. London: The Stationery Office.

Mintzberg, H., Ahlstrand, B., and Lampel, J. (1998) *Strategy safari, a guided tour through the wilds of strategic management*. Hemel Hempstead: Prentice Hall Europe.

National Assembly for Wales (2000) *Children and young people. a framework for partnership—consultation document*. Cardiff: National Assembly for Wales.

National Assembly for Wales (2001) *Everybody's business—child and adolescent mental health services strategy document*. Cardiff: National Assembly for Wales.

National Assembly for Wales (2002) *Too serious a thing—the Carlile review*. Cardiff: National Assembly for Wales.

Pendleton, D. and King, J. (2002) Values and leadership. *BMJ*, **325**, 1352–5.

Plsek, P.E. and Greenhalgh, T. (2001) The challenge of complexity in healthcare. *BMJ*, **323**, 625–8.

Pugh, D.S. and Hickson, D.J. (1996) *Writers on Organizations*. London: Penguin.

Rawlinson, S. and Williams, R. (2000) The primary-secondary care interface in CAMHS—burden as a defining feature. *Current Opinion in Psychiatry*, **13**, 389–95.

Rutter, M. and Smith, D.J. (1995) *Psychosocial disorders in young people*. Chichester: Wiley.

Salter, B. (2001) Who rules? The new politics of medical regulation. *Soc Sci Med*, **52**, 871–83.

Sweeney, K. and Griffiths, F. (2002) *Complexity and healthcare, an introduction*. Oxford: Radcliffe Medical Press.

Szatmari, P. (1999) Evidence-based child psychiatry and the two solitudes [EBMH notebook]. *Evidence-based Mental Health*, **1**, 6–7.

The Human Rights Act (1998) London: HMSO.

Williams, R. (2002) Complexity, uncertainty and decision-making in an evidence-based world. *Current Opinion in Psychiatry*, **15**, 343–7.

Williams, R., White, R., and Harbour, A. (2003) *Safeguards for young minds* (3rd edn). London: Gaskell.

Williams, R. and Gale, F. (2003) Current approaches to working with children and adolescents. In *The handbook of community mental health nursing* (ed. B. Hannigan and M. Coffey). London: Routledge.

Williams, R. and Richardson, G. (1995) *Child and adolescent mental health services—together we stand. The commissioning, role and management of child and adolescent mental health services.* London: HMSO.

Williams, R. and Salmon, G. (2002) Collaboration in commissioning and delivering child and adolescent mental health services. *Current Opinion in Psychiatry,* **15**, 349–53.

Chapter 4

A strategic framework for child and adolescent mental health services

Greg Richardson

Introduction

The necessity for a strategy for Child and Adolescent Mental Health Services (CAMHS) has been detailed in the previous chapters, as have the complexities in developing a strategy within health services that is compatible across different statutory agencies. However, the well-being of children, and the adults they develop into, demands that these complexities are addressed and a clear strategy developed through formulation, implementation, monitoring, and review, much like any sound audit process.

In England the national vision for CAMHS improvements is set out in *Improvement, expansion and reform: the next three years priorities and planning framework 2003–2006* (Department of Health 2002). This document, along with The Child and Adolescent Mental Health Service (CAMHS) *Grant Guidance 2004–05* (Department of Health 2004) and the *Emerging Findings on CAMHS* from the National Service Framework for Children (Department of Health 2003a) point the way to how CAMHS should develop in line with local strategic plans. Such strategic development plans must incorporate the views and aspirations of partner agencies, indeed the release of funds as outlined in the *Child and Adolescent Mental Health Services* (CAMHS) *Grant Guidance 2003–4* (Department of Health 2003b) is dependent on interagency agreement on the development plan.

The strategic framework for CAMHS (NHS Health Advisory Service 1995) was developed to clarify the functioning of a small and untypical specialty operating in the health service environment, but needing to relate to other agencies working with children. The fact that no one agencies' CAMHS can be considered in isolation leads to 'the CAMHS concept', referred to in the previous chapter, of an inter-agency understanding of children's mental health needs, even if that agency does not consider mental health its primary agenda. A child-centred strategy must now incorporate the objectives of all those agencies in which preventive and Specialist CAMHS play a crucial part.

The idea of a tiered service is not new. The sufferers who do not seek help filter out the majority of mental health problems in adults. Of those who seek help from their general practitioners, the majority are dealt with by them operating a second filter, so that only a trickle are passed on to adult mental health services and even fewer to adult psychiatrists. The recognition and operation of such filters are essential to the operation and survival of the health service in general and an understanding of the tiered system in particular. The purpose of a strategic framework for CAMHS is to clarify roles, responsibilities, and structures, not to re-organize CAMHS. The strategic framework appears to be standing the test of time and is recognized as the most helpful way to understand CAMHS (House of Commons Health Committee 1997; Audit Commission 1999). *The new NHS* (Department of Health 1998) set a pathway for the development of health services, which was far more in tune with the interagency practice promulgated in *Together we stand* incorporating as it did:

the integration of primary care and community services;

the requirement for joint planning for health across agencies;

the exploration of pooled health and social service budgets;

the exploration of new organizational arrangements, e.g. primary care trusts and social care trusts;

the integration of care planning and communication across agencies;

an emphasis on co-terminosity between health and social service organizations;

local authority membership of primary care organizations;

the statutory duty on trusts to collaborate.

However, within CAMHS the development of the strategic framework has not produced a comprehensive, integrated service for young people and their families across the nation. The wide variations in service described in 1994 (Kurtz *et al.* 1994) remain (Audit Commission 1999). This variation in service appears to derive from the small but complex nature of CAMHS, which may lead to an absence of knowledge of the suggested frameworks for the organization of CAMHS, or call on disproportionate resources from commissioning organizations to develop a comprehensive inter-agency CAMHS strategy. There may be a belief that strategies can be bought off the peg from specialist consultants such as the NHS Health Advisory Service or Young Minds, rather than developed locally with users, carers, and providers who have vested interests in ensuring a good service and form a vital part of strategy development, implementations, and monitoring, which outside consultants cannot. The lack of local development of the strategy then militating against ownership by local practitioners. There are also misconceptions about the function and purpose of the tiers in the strategic framework, particularly that the tiers relate to skill level, the professionally pompous considering they only work at Tier 3 (presumably because they do not have the skills to work individually with young people or their families). Idiosyncratic practice that has thrived in CAMHS often avoids looking at effective methods of service delivery because of powerful therapists' personal interests. There has also been a certain view that a 'non-scientific' speciality has no real knowledge-base and can therefore be designed by users and carers, without professional input.

The commitment to strategy development and overcoming these obstacles will depend on local interest and determined commissioning upon which the mental health of young people is largely dependent. Only a systematic, inter-agency approach to young people's mental health will avoid the squandering of precious resource, so that preventive work is built in to the strategy along with the requirements for therapeutic interventions.

The strategic framework

The universal application of the strategic framework may go some way to addressing these issues and so it may be worth recapping the basics. The framework is built of filters and tiers. The first filter separates children and their families from the first tier of professionals with whom they come into contact during the routine course of their lives.

Tier 1 is CAMHS provided by these professionals, who do most mental health work with young people and their families, although often they do not recognize, or wish to take responsibility for, this role. Nevertheless teachers, health visitors, school nurses, social workers, and general practitioners have a considerable influence on children's psychological development and it is important that this role is recognized and supported by designated mental health professionals. These Tier 1 professionals operate Filter 2 by deciding when it is necessary to involve professionals from Tier 2, often in their own agency, so a teacher may refer to an educational psychologist and health professionals will tend to refer to a CAMHS. The finding that only 1% of CAMHS time is devoted to Tier 1 (Audit Commission 1999) clarifies that the majority of children and young people with mental health problems never see a mental health professional and that Tier 1 professionals working with children and families are largely unsupported in their attempts to address their mental health needs. The majority of children with identified mental health problems are never referred to Specialist CAMHS, as this is not considered necessary by a potential referrer or because they and their families have no wish to be involved with mental health services. This is fortunate in one respect, for CAMHS have not the resources to manage 15–30% of the child population. These children's only hope for improved functioning is by the day-to-day work of the Tier 1 professionals with whom they come into contact. The move to support those Tier 1 professionals in this work is currently the major challenge for CAMHS to ensure equity in meeting the needs of the populations served.

Tier 2 comprises mental health professionals working individually with children or young people or providing consultation. Such professionals need to work within a multidisciplinary CAMHS to ensure comprehensive service provision and to avoid idiosyncratic practice. This is the traditional work of mental health professionals when the skills, learned in their training, are used. However all individual children who comprise the 15–30% with mental health problems and their families are never going to see individual therapists of whatever profession, therefore methods of prioritizing young people and families for such provision have to be found using the evidence base (Goodman 1998). One of the most useful innovations in Tier 2 working in recent years has been the development of the primary mental health worker. Working in a locality of no more than 40 000 total population, they take all referrals, communicating with referrers to elaborate concerns, working with the other agencies in the locality and ensuring CAMHS interventions, through brief work with themselves, or referral to Tiers 2 or 3 is only used when absolutely necessary. Such work requires skilled and experienced professionals who command the respect of Tier 1 professionals in the locality and who network well. Already they are showing the impact they can make in increasing access to mental health expertise and avoiding referral to Specialist CAMHS (Clark and Robinson 1998). When Tier 2 intervention is insufficient or the Tier 2 worker feels further expertise to manage a situation is required, they may operate the third filter into Tier 3.

Tier 3 consists of members of Specialist CAMHS, who are also probably doing Tier 2 work, working together to meet the needs of specific groups such as those with eating disorders, attentional problems, or autistic spectrum disorders.

The fourth filter is the one through which young people with very specialist needs pass into Tier 4, such as those who require in-patient care or specialist liaison work because of the nature of their medical condition. The roles and functions of the tiers are now described in government documentation (Welsh Assembly Government 2003).

Limitations of the strategic approach

There is a perception that the CAMHS strategic model is health-based and does not easily integrate with other agencies. This is not the case, for the framework was designed to integrate with, and possibly provide a model for, other agencies. The child with mental health problems is usually the same child who has emotional and behavioural disturbance, in educational parlance, and is a child in need, in social service parlance. The situations these children find themselves in and their resultant behaviours are caused by, and present in, all areas of their functioning. The strategic framework recognizes that children's developmental needs cannot be subdivided into different educational, social, and health boxes and it is essential that all agencies work to support each other in providing a care pathway that meets all the child's developmental requirements.

There are some effective treatments for child and adolescent mental disorders (Fonagy *et al.* 2002), so restricting the practice of child and adolescent mental health services to certain specific areas where there is evidence of effective intervention has been proposed (Goodman 1998). Goodman gives graphic examples where the desire to meet mental health need has resulted in the considerable squandering of resource, although the interventions he quotes were based on therapy rather than systemic understanding and support directed at those working with young people, as the strategic framework would espouse. However certain interventions of proven effectiveness, such as multi-systemic therapy require for their success multidisciplinary and multi-agency input. Graham (2000) has detailed the difficulties in bringing the concept of evidence-based medicine to bear on interventions in young people, whose functioning is determined by and affects individual, family, and societal factors.

Advantages of the strategic framework

A strategy ensures that the functioning of CAMHS is easier to understand, which helps those who use the service, those who work with it, and those who manage it. The recognition that all agencies have similarly tiered structures aids understanding of them and working with them. The strategy clarifies that children with more complex problems, and hence more resource at higher tiers, are filtered, so that expensive resource is not used on more routine problems. Links between tiers are clarified, which enables care pathways to be defined, especially from Tiers 2 and 3 to Tier 4. This is intended to overcome the isolation of Tier 4 facilities, which is often reinforced by their specialist nature and their distance from community CAMHS. The strategic framework makes it clear that the young person's pathway of care should pass seamlessly through the tiers using procedures such as the Care Programme Approach (Department of Health 1990). The role adequacy, clarity, and legitimacy of each professional is more clearly defined by their place in the strategic framework, the specialist skills of each professional are optimally used, each taking personal responsibility and ownership for their own caseload, all professionals having the flexibility to operate at more than one tier. The deficits in a CAMHS are more clearly understood if it is viewed through the strategic framework, the current poor support to Tier 1 being a case in point. This enables the areas where the service needs to develop or change to be clarified.

Purpose of the strategic framework

The strategic framework must support the objectives of CAMHS by ensuring that professionals who work with children and families, from statutory and non-statutory agencies, work together in a co-ordinated manner for the greater benefit of those receiving services. There have been considerable initiatives in services for children and CAMHS must be networked into these, so that the mental health needs of the children served are recognized and met. There must be CAMHS links with Sure Start, Children's Fund, Connexions, Youth Offending Teams,

Paediatric Services, Services for Children Looked After, Services for Foster Carers, Services for Children leaving Care, Behaviour Support Services, Family Courts, Services for Drug misusers, and the Area Child Protection Committee. Such networks must be built on the principles of accessibility, multidisciplinary approaches, comprehensive CAMHS provision, accountability, and flexibility. Agencies may then provide support, supervision, and training for each other in the management and organization of their work. This should ensure that all those who work directly with children have access to information about services, as well as advice, support, and training for that role. This may be achieved by the appointment of primary mental health workers, Tier 1 specialization, consultation by CAMHS professionals, the provision of written guidelines on the management of common problems, or a consultation phone line. Information-sharing is an integral part of the strategy, so that all agencies working with young people and their families understand each other's functioning and use each other effectively. The operational policies of Specialist CAMHS will have been agreed with partner agencies and have incorporated the views of users and carers. Information on the operational policies should then be widely available to ensure that young people and families are fully aware of the support and services available to them through methods such as the development of an internet web-site, the publicizing of information help-lines or one-stop information phone-lines.

The strategy should ensure that the mental health needs of young people are assessed in a co-ordinated manner across agencies incorporating their social and educational needs. Case management then allows a key worker to co-ordinate care from all involved agencies so protecting the young person and their family from inter-agency barriers.

The strategy should define a management structure that can deliver it. Such a structure must recognize the diversity of activity in CAMHS and its difference from other health provision. More sophisticated commissioning should enable clearer specification of specialist services, recognize the value of work other than face-to-face contacts, be specific about priorities, evaluate and monitor work, and give greater stability to CAMHS. Health Act Flexibilities can now considerably assist the joint commissioning of services.

The strategy must ensure integrated systems across agencies are in place to guarantee regular user and carer feedback about the co-ordination of services from the family's perspective rather than through the procedures of each of the agencies. Young people and their families must be routinely and systematically involved by agencies in expressing their views on current services and how they would like services to develop. Audit questionaires are well-recognized but more innovative approaches such as the use of participatory appraisal are proving useful (Keir *et al.* 2003).

The CAMHS strategy should incorporate the promotion of the development of positive mental health, both as a product of the way they are organized (their process), as well as through the specific direct initiatives targeted at this goal (their content). Referral to Specialist CAMHS and consequent stigmatization may be avoided by integrating services into the work of Tier 1 professionals already involved with the young people or through joint initiatives with voluntary organizations or health promotion services. Parents may be empowered by developing parent advice services.

The strategy must pay attention to the training needs of those involved at every level in working with children and young people and ensure they are assessed and duly met by auditing training needs through annual review and the consideration of multi-agency training.

The strategy must also be aware of specialist need and account for it by providing a method by which services, such as those for young people in transition to adult mental health services, those with learning disability, those with specific sensory handicaps and those in and leaving care are commissioned.

Challenges in implementing the strategic framework

Anxiety, which children and young people frequently generate, tends to lead to linear thinking and the desire to refer the problem on to somebody else. Offering a more useful, supportive systemic intervention to the child and family requires inter-agency collaboration. This depends on the sophistication of the professionals involved in recognizing that there are no magic answers and that effective management of the problem comes from sharing perspectives and interventions. Workers in all agencies working with children must have the ability to develop a strategic plan for the young people and families with whom they come in contact. This work involves joint assessments, joint planning, agreement on treatment interventions to reduce disability and handicap, joint risk assessment and management, and joint evaluation. Robust joint protocols should ensure children sent away from the area are as few as possible because the local agencies have sufficient flexibility to provide innovative solutions to very difficult child care and education problems. Inter-agency collaboration should extend to senior management levels to ensure top of the office ownership of joint working, which not only provides better care but also is likely to be more economical as work is not repeated by the different agencies.

Referral rates to CAMHS are increasing all the time and families are continuing not to attend for appointments. This pressure upon CAMHS can lead to defensive, arcane practices, the most obvious being the waiting-list. The strategic framework clarifies that work in Tier 1 is the most efficient way to address this problem but this depends on clarifying to Tier 1 professionals that they will gain support from CAMHS to lighten their load, not make them feel burdened with an extra task. Tier 1 professionals' development must also ensure that they do not perceive primary mental health workers purely as referral conduits. They are gatekeepers to prevent children being damaged by well meaning professionals.

The challenge of information-sharing is not simply one of incompatible information systems across agencies. Medical confidentiality is highly regarded (General Medical Council 2000), but the methods used in child protection (Department of Health *et al.* 1999) may need to be used more widely. To do this they will have to develop a common language, so that they describe the same problems in the same terms, and understand the advantages and limitations of each other's interventions. The often conflicting views of users and carers will have to be incorporated into the ways the sharing of information are balanced against the welfare of the child through that inter-agency shared information.

It is generally accepted that CAMHS should be provided as close as possible to the young person and their family. That is they should be based on a locality. Weighed against this are issues of critical mass for a service to have sufficient professionals to provide good Tier 1 support, the full range of Tier 2 expertise and a comprehensive range of Tier 3 teams. Primary mental health workers provide an ideal locality resource based on a number of general practices or the catchment areas of certain adjacent secondary schools and their feeder primary schools. The primary mental health workers then provide the locality service while being supported by a wider area CAMHS. What determines a locality should be agreed between agencies, users and carers as part of their strategy development.

Congruent supervision and management is required across agencies and professions, so that staff are not expected to have differing priorities and practices when working in a CAMHS.

Similarly all agencies must be committed to supporting the multidisciplinary nature of CAMHS and avoid withdrawing resources to shore up deficiencies in other parts of their agency.

Tier 4 CAMHS were hit hard by the government reforms of the early nineties, commissioning was not taken seriously in view of the small numbers involved and health trusts could not risk making considerable investment-financial outlay providing beds for uncertain purchasers. Many beds closed, with the result that a good bed is hard to find (Anon 1997) and the independent sector has found a lucrative niche. There is currently no national strategy for in-patient psychiatric beds. Individual in-patient services operate as they think best but without common agreement on referral criteria, age ranges, or operational policies. The result is chaotic (National In-patient Child and Adolescent Psychiatry Study 2001). There is much work to be done in the standardization and clarification of Tier 4 CAMHS, ensuring their work and criteria for admission are clearly understood, so that young people experience Tier 4 provision as one part of a smooth care pathway across all the tiers and agencies. Fortunately standards are being produced for such facilities that can be incorporated into the strategy (Quality Network for In-patient CAMHS 2001).

Conclusion

A strategic framework is the essential tool to developing a CAMHS. No service can be considered to be realistically addressing the mental health needs of children and young people without such a strategy with all its components. Department of Health (1998b) and the proposed incorporation of CAMHS within the Children's National Service Framework recognize the need for inter-agency working, so there is now ministerial ownership for such collaboration. This should mean that jointly commissioned CAMHS strategies will flourish and blinkered agency managers founder, so that families and communities have the full range of skilled professionals available to them that they require.

References

Anon (1997) Emergency admissions: an open letter. *Young Minds Magazine*, **31**, 6–8.

Audit Commission (1999) *Children in mind*. London: Audit Commission Publications.

Clark, S. and Robinson, P. (1998) United we stand? working together in child and adolescent mental health services. Presentation to seminar on *Commissioning and delivering for child and adolescent mental health services'*. Health Services Management Centre, University of Birmingham.

Department of Health (1990) Joint health and social services circular: *The care programme approach for people with a mental illness referred to specialist psychiatric services*. HC(90)23/LASSL(90)11 DoH 1990.

Department of Health (1998) *The new NHS: modern, dependable*. London: The Stationery Office.

Department of Health (1998) *Our healthier nation: a contract for health*. London: The Stationery Office.

Department of Health (2002) *Improvement, expansion and reform: the next three years priorities and planning framework 2003–2006*. London: The Stationery Office.

Department of Health (2003a) Getting the right start: The national service framework for children-emerging findings. London: The Stationery Office.

Department of Health (2003b) Child and Adolescent Mental Health Service (CAMHS) Grant Guidance 2003–4. London: Department of Health.

Department of Health (2004) Child and Adolescent Mental Health Service (CAMHS) Grant Guidance 2004–5. HSC 2004/002: LAC (2004)2. London: Department of Health.

Department of Health, Home Office and Department of Education and Employment (1999) *Working together to safeguard children.* London: The Stationery Office.

Fonagy, P., Target, M., Cottrell, D., Phillips, J., and Kurtz, Z. (2002) *What works for whom? A critical review of treatments for children and adolescents.* London: Guilford Press.

General Medical Council (2000) *Confidentiality: protecting and providing information.* GMC Publications.

Goodman, R. (1998) *Child an adolescent mental health services: reasoned advice to commisioners and providers.* London: Institute of Psychiatry.

Graham, P. (2000) Treatment interventions and findings from research: bridging the chasm in child psychiatry. *British Journal of Psychiatry,* **176**, 414–9.

House of Commons Health Committee (1997) *Child and adolescent mental health services.* London: The Stationery Office.

Keir, C., Harris, J., and Webb, B. (2003) User participation. In *Child and adolescent mental health services: an operational handbook* (ed. G. Richardson and I. Partridge). pp. 55–60. London: Gaskell.

Kurtz, Z., Thornes, R., and Wolkind, S. (1994) *Services for the mental health of children and young people in England: a national review.* Maudsley Hospital and South Thames (West) Regional Health Authority.

NHS Health Advisory Service (1995) *Together we Stand: the commissioning, role and management of child and adolescent mental health services.* London: HMSO.

National In-patient Child and Adolescent Psychiatry Study (2001) *Key Findings Conference.* London: Royal College of Psychiatrists Research Unit.

Quality Network for In-patient CAMHS (2001) *Service standards.* London: Royal College of Psychiatrists' Research Unit.

Welsh Assembly Government (2003) *The four tier strategic concept for planning, commissioning and delivering child and adolescent mental health services (CAMHS).* NHS Planning and Commissioning Guidance, Annex A. 19–20.

Chapter 5

VBM²: a collaborative values-based model of healthcare decision-making combining medical and management perspectives

KWM (Bill) Fulford and John Benington

Introduction

In a book uniquely combining medical and management perspectives on child and adolescent psychiatry, a chapter on 'ethics' would not be out of place. This chapter is not about ethics. It is about the broader concept of values. More precisely, it is about what one of us has called elsewhere values-based practice (Fulford 2004).

Many of the problems between practitioners and managers in healthcare, we will suggest, arise from (largely unacknowledged) differences of values. Values-based practice offers practitioners and managers a set of theoretical principles and practical skills (summarized in Fig. 5.1) that allow them to build on the differences of values between them as a positive resource for healthcare decision-making. Values-based *medicine*, then, to anticipate the conclusion of our chapter, combined with values-based *management*, amounts to the VBM² model of collaborative decision-making of our title.

VBM²: values-based medicine and management

Child and adolescent mental health services (CAMHS) present many challenging ethical problems. These have been well-documented elsewhere (Graham 1999, ch.14; and several of the case studies in Dickenson and Fulford 2000). Management and leadership studies, too, raise many ethical issues. Bring the disciplines together, though, and an extra edge of difficulty is given to these problems by the different, and sometimes conflicting, value perspectives of their respective practitioners.

High-profile difficulties of this cross-disciplinary kind arise in such areas as resource allocation, for example (Dickenson and Fulford 2000, case 8.1). Lower profile but far more pervasive difficulties arise from the complexity of the task of integrating, across teams and agencies, responses to the problems faced by young people and their families (Salmon and Williams 2001; Williams and Salmon 2002). When child abuse is suspected, for example, the differing priorities of the child, his or her parents, social workers, psychiatrists, and the police, are often all too evident.

One response to such conflicting values is to search for ethical rules prescribing, in advance, by reference to 'right' values, the outcomes of healthcare decision-making. As an outcomes-oriented

The Theory

1st Principle of VBP
All decisions stand on two feet, on values as well as on facts, including decisions about diagnosis (the two feet principle).

2nd Principle of VBP
We tend to notice values only when they are diverse or conflicting and hence are likely to be problematic (the squeaky wheel principle).

3rd Principle of VBP
Scientific progress, in opening up choices, is increasingly bringing the full diversity of human values into play in all areas of healthcare (the science driven principle).

4th Principle of VBP
VBM's first call for information is the perspective of the patient or patient group concerned in a given decision (the patient-perspective principle).

5th Principle of VBP
In VBM, conflicts of values are resolved primarily, not by reference to a rule prescribing a right outcome, but by processes designed to support a balance of legitimately different perspectives (the multi-perspective principle).

The Practice

6th Principle of VBP
Careful attention to language use in a given context is one of a range of powerful methods for raising awareness of values (the values-blindness principle).

7th Principle of VBP
A rich resource of both empirical and philosophical methods is available for improving our knowledge of other people's values (the values-myopia principle).

8th Principle of VBP
Ethical reasoning is employed in VBM primarily to explore differences of values, not, as in quasi-legal bioethics, to determine what is right (the space of values principle).

9th Principle of VBP
In VBM, communication skills have a substantive rather than (as in quasi-legal ethics) a merely executive role in clinical decision-making (the how its done principle).

10th Principle of VBP
VBM, although involving a partnership with ethicists and lawyers (equivalent to the partnership with scientists and statisticians in EBM), puts decision-making back where it belongs, with users and providers at the clinical coal-face (the who decides principle).

Fig. 5.1 Ten principles of Values-Based Practice.

approach, this response to conflicting values is the basis of the growing body of codes and guidelines by which decision-making in healthcare is increasingly regulated (Fulford 2001a). VBP offers a different response. VBP starts from the premise that in many situations there may be no uniquely 'right' answer. This does not mean throwing in the decision-making towel, however. It means starting from respect for diversity of values, and then, where values conflict, relying primarily on 'good process' rather than 'good outcomes' for effective decision-making.

Child and adolescent mental health services, with their tradition of systemic working, offer many examples of good process. Management theory, correspondingly, which as we will suggest below is more hospitable to diversity of values than medical theory, offers a resource of skills and experience for effective decision-making where values conflict. Bring them together, therefore, as this book does, within the framework provided by VBP, and you have a powerful resource for healthcare decision-making.

In this chapter, then, we will start by outlining the theory of values-based practice. The key shift of focus in VBP from outcomes to process will then lead into a section on the skills-base of VBP as developed within values-based medicine. Finally, in the third section, the potential of values-based management as a resource of practical strategies for working with diverse (and hence sometimes conflicting) values, will be illustrated with the concept of adaptive work as developed by the American psychiatrist and management theorist, Ronald Heifetz (1994).

Values-based practice: the theory

When it comes to diversity, the very word 'values' is an instance of itself! It means different things to different people at different times and in different places. So, just what are values? Where do they come into clinical decision-making? And how does VBP differ from quasi-legal ethics as a response to the growing values-complexity of decision-making in healthcare?

What are values?

Values are broader than ethics. In modern healthcare, values are evident in the growing ethical complexity of practice. But values are also evident in the spread of charters and kite marks, of standards and performance indicators, and of procedural monitoring through audit, clinical governance, and clinical practice guidelines. The National Service Framework for Mental Health (NSF) (Department of Health 1999), the key policy document for service development in England and Wales, is defined by a set of key values (called 'standards').

Besides these explicit values, there are also implicit values. Less easy to identify, implicit values are no less influential in shaping practice. They range from the values of different professional groups, determining, in part, their respective models of disorder (Colombo *et al.* 2003; Fulford 2001b), through the values defining specific categories of disorder, for instance in the DSM's Criterion B for schizophrenia (Fulford 1994; 2002a and 2002b), to the epistemic values by which our core research programmes are guided (Sadler 1996).

Values, both explicit and implicit, come in many varieties, aesthetic and prudential, for example, as well as moral and ethical; and, importantly for healthcare, they take different logical forms— 'needs' are different from 'wants', for example, as any parent of a 2-year-old knows. VBP covers all these varieties and variations. VBP is concerned with values in healthcare, in the generic sense of the term, as covering any judgement of good and bad. The defining feature of such value judgements, as a former White's Professor of moral philosophy in Oxford, R M Hare, showed, is that they are 'prescriptive' or 'action guiding' (Hare 1952).

Values and decision-making

It is in virtue of their property of being action-guiding that values come into healthcare decision-making. We are familiar with the idea of decisions being evidence-based: and EBP, or evidence-based practice, understood broadly as encompassing both objective information and the experiential knowledge of individual practitioners (Sacket *et al.* 2000), is a response to the growing complexity of the facts bearing on decision-making in healthcare. But facts alone cannot determine action. Values provide the weightings by which facts form the basis of actions: and VBP is a response to the growing complexity of the *values* bearing on decision-making in healthcare.

Thus, even in as (relatively) simple a case as deciding what medication to prescribe, we balance benefits (effects) against disbenefits (side-effects); the balance, moreover, for a given drug, will vary from case to case according to the values (of all the kinds noted above) of a given patient; and our decision in a given case will be further constrained by decisions further back along the line about cost-effectiveness, decisions which are taken in part at a local and in part at a national level.

Decisions, then, *all* decisions, are values- as well as fact-based. In healthcare, this is not always clearly recognized, it being widely assumed that at least some decisions are 'purely' scientific and, hence, value-free. Decisions about diagnosis, in particular, are generally assumed to be based on value-free science. But a moment's reflection shows that this is simply not so (Fulford and Williams 2003). Thus, in child and adolescent psychiatry:

+ The differential diagnosis of many psychiatric disorders turns (in part) on value judgements: the diagnoses ADHD and autistic spectrum disorder, for example, turn on the assessments by a variety of adult observers of such value-laden concepts as 'aberrant' behaviour and 'functioning'.

+ Many of the individual criteria for diagnoses in child and adolescent mental health practice are overtly evaluative in form (e.g. conduct disorder).

In such cases, then, decisions about diagnosis, although of course based in part on facts, are also based in part on value judgements. Similar observations apply to the major adult psychiatric disorders, including the functional psychoses (Fulford 2002a; Jackson and Fulford 1997), and, in principle, though not always to the same degree in practice, to disorders in general.[1] And if diagnosis, ostensibly the most 'scientific' area of healthcare decision-making, is values-as well

---

[1] Thus the difference between decisions about diagnosis, in, say, cardiology and psychiatry, is not that cardiological diagnoses are 'purely' scientific while psychiatric diagnoses are value-laden, but that cardiological diagnosis, in general, involves shared values while psychiatric diagnosis, in general, involves values that are often *not* shared. What counts as good or bad functioning in hearts, for example, is more or less the same for everyone, hence the values involved in diagnoses of heart disorders are unlikely to be conflicting, hence they can be ignored in practice, and hence the operative values, although implicit, do not become explicit in our diagnostic manuals. But what counts as good or bad functioning in minds—in such areas as emotion, desire, volition, belief, sexuality, etc.—is very far from being more or less the same for everyone; hence the values involved in diagnoses of psychiatric disorders are very *likely* to be conflicting, hence they cannot be ignored in practice, and hence they tend to emerge, explicitly, although still not always recognized for what they are, in our diagnostic manuals (see generally Fulford 1989, chapters 3–6 and 8).

as fact-based, it seems likely that all areas of healthcare decision-making are, to some degree, values- as well as fact-based.

But if EBP is a response to complexity on the fact side of healthcare decision-making, how does VBP differ from the more familiar 'ethics' as a response to complexity on the value side?

VBP and bioethics as responses to complexity

As a theoretical discipline, bioethics encompasses a rich variety of scholarly traditions, philosophical, historical, and empirical (Fulford *et al.* 2002a, introductory chapter). In its connections with practice, though, bioethics has taken an increasingly quasi-legal form. As noted above, this has the consequence that bioethics is outcomes-focused. The rules and regulatory frameworks of modern bioethics seek to constrain decision-making by defining 'good outcomes'. Key values are identified—such as autonomy and confidentiality—and then codified in rule books (codes and guidelines), covering as wide a set of clinical situations as possible, and supported by regulatory bodies with executive powers to determine 'difficult' cases.

VBP, then, differs from quasi-legal ethics in that it starts from the premis of value diversity, switching attention from 'good outcomes' to 'good process'. VBP's response to complexity on the values side of decision-making is thus not to write more rules and regulations in an attempt to further constrain outcomes, it is rather to strengthen the skills, the clinical practice skills (summarized in Principles 6–9, Fig. 5.1), on which good process depends.

VBP, it is important to add, is not exclusive of quasi-legal ethics. To the contrary, VBP incorporates quasi-legal ethics for situations in which, for a given group, values are largely shared. In such situations, where everyone is signed up to a given value, it is helpful to have rules and regulations guiding the application of that value in particular cases. So understood, then, as expressing (largely) shared values, the rules and regulations of quasi-legal ethics, provide a framework for practice. By the same token, though, rules and regulations become inappropriate in situations in which values are *not* shared. In situations of value diversity, rules and regulations, expressing as they do *particular* values, will necessarily conflict with the *different* values of many of those to whom they are intended to apply.

As a response to complexity, quasi-legal ethics is thus not so much the wrong tool as the right tool in the wrong place. We do need a framework of shared values for practice, but we need a different approach to decision-making in the much wider range of circumstances in which legitimately different values are in play. In such circumstances, VBP suggests, it is good process not good outcomes on which we should rely, and good process means good clinical practice skills.

In CAMHS, the skills in question can be thought of as falling into two broad areas, respectively, individual child- and family-centred skills (Principle 4 in Fig. 5.1), and team-centred skills (Principle 5) (Fulford and Williams 2003).

Child- and family-centred skills

VBP's 'first call' is the perspectives of particular young people and their families concerned in a particular decision. Contemporary mental health practice—from politicians through managers to practitioners—is of course strongly child-centred (National Assembly for Wales 2001, 2002). In England and Wales, the principle of child-centredness is made explicit by the paramouncy principle in the Children Act 1989. In VBP, child-centredness, understood as paying particular attention to the values of individual children, follows directly from the premise of values diversity (Fulford and Williams 2003). If values are inherently diverse, decision-making must start from the *particular* values of those involved in a *particular* decision.

Multidisciplinary skills

The flip-side to child-centredness, though, in VBP, the flip-side to the premis of values diversity, is that disagreements about values are inevitable. In VBP, however, rather as in a political democracy, disagreements, as the key-stone of balanced decision-making, are to be welcomed. If disagreements are to work in a positive way, of course, they need to be supported by good process, and this is where the multidisciplinary team comes in. As a resource of intervention skills (social, psychological, medical, etc.), there is little disagreement that CAMHS should be founded firmly in multidisciplinary teamwork. Nonetheless, there are, all-too-often, uneasy tensions within teams that limit their effectiveness. Many factors lie behind these failures of collaboration (Williams and Salmon 2002). But an important factor is unrecognized or avoided differences of values (Colombo *et al.* 2003).

Values-based medicine: the skills base

The skills supporting good process in VBP, both child/adolescent-centred and multidisciplinary, fall under four broad headings: awareness, knowledge, ethical reasoning, and communication skills.

Skills area 1: awareness

Many of the problems with values in healthcare arise not so much from open conflicts of values, as from what may be called 'values blindness', i.e. a failure to recognize values (and differences of values) for what they are (Fulford 2004).

The first step, then, in working more effectively with values diversity, is to raise awareness. Each of the skills outlined in this section may contribute to this in different ways. A distinct and important skill, though, is greater attention to language. Although rooted theoretically in the rather abstract discipline of linguistic analytic philosophy (Fulford 1990), the effectiveness of attention to language as a practical training method for raising awareness of values in healthcare decision-making has been demonstrated in a joint programme between the Sainsbury Centre for Mental Health (SCMH) and the centre for Philosophy, Ethics and Mental Health (PEMH) at Warwick University.

SCMH and PEMH have piloted a values-awareness training session with groups of practitioners working in assertive outreach, community mental health, and acute in-patient settings. The response from such front-line practitioners to these training sessions has been very positive. Trainees have felt empowered, more confident in putting forward their views with other team members, and more attentive to the different and sometimes unexpected values of their clients and patients (Fulford *et al.* 2002b).

Skills area 2: knowledge

It is one thing to be more aware of values, it is another to understand the *particular* values bearing on a given case. Knowledge of the values likely to be involved in a particular situation may be derived from many sources, including:

First-hand narratives. There is now an extensive literature by patients, carers, and others, describing their experience of healthcare. Some of these are polemical in tone. But many are highly illuminating (see Fulford *et al.* 2002a for a wide selection). Luke Jackson's account of his experience of growing up as a child with Asperger's syndrome (Jackson 2002) is an exemplary example of the power of young people's own narratives in this respect.

Empirical research. Work in the social sciences—from surveys (Rogers *et al.* 1993) through ethnographic and anthropological investigations (Alderson 1990), to more traditional clinical studies (Morrow and Richards 2002)—offers a growing resource of information about the values different stakeholders bring to specific situations. Sometimes called 'empirical ethics', this connects with the wider development of combined philosophical and empirical methodologies in healthcare research (Fulford 2001b).

Analytic methods. Values are not always worn 'on the sleeve', of course. Besides psychoanalysis (Raphael-Leff 2002), there is a variety of text-based methods for revealing hidden meanings—hermeneutics (Widdershoven and Widdershoven-Heerding 2003), discursive psychology (Sabat 2001), and various schools of phenomenology (Fulford *et al.* 2003).

Quasi-legal ethics is at best ambivalent about the role of 'facts' in ethical decision-making' (Gillon 1996). VBP, by contrast, insists rather that we should draw as widely as possibly on the full range of sources of empirical information about values increasingly available. Relatively little empirical work has been done on the values—the actual needs, wishes, and preferences—of children and young people. In this area, perhaps even more so than with adults, the unspoken assumption is that someone else, a parent, a social worker, a doctor, 'knows best'. And in this area, of course, someone other than the child may well 'know best'. But decisions about what is 'best' should be based on fact not fancy. And there is evidence, in this as in other areas, that the 'facts about values' of young people are very far from being self-evident (Dickenson and Jones 1995).

Skills area 3: reasoning skills

Ethics offers a wide variety of reasoning skills, i.e. ways of reasoning about ethically problematic situations. These include: utilitarianism (a form of consequentialism), deontology (or rights-based ethics), relationship ethics, and communitarianism.

Each of these has applications in healthcare. For example, utilitarianism (balancing interests to achieve the maximum utility) is the basis of the QALY and other health economic models (Crisp 1994); deontology is important in defining duties, obligations, and responsibilities (Montgomery 1995); relationship ethics, although less familiar, has potentially fruitful applications in family therapy (Adshead 2000); and communitarianism, similarly, may be an essential tool for analysing ethical issues in the wider system of community-based services (Parker 1999).

At the level of practical decision-making, two approaches have proved particularly helpful: principles reasoning and casuistry (Fulford and Bloch 2000).

Principles reasoning. This is is a top-down form of reasoning in which general principles are applied to particular cases. The best known of such principles for healthcare use were defined originally by the American philosopher Tom Beauchamp and the theologian James Childress (Beauchamp and Childress 1994): Beauchamp and Childress' four principles are, autonomy (respecting patient choice), beneficence (acting as in the patient's interests), non-maleficence (avoiding harm), and justice (equal treatment of equal problem).

Casuistry. This is bottom-up reasoning, i.e. it starts from the concrete details of particular cases rather than from general principles. The basic idea with casuistry is to compare the case in question with other relevant cases in which the ethical 'solution' may be clearer.

This is done either by varying relevant details of the case in question, or by comparing it with different cases altogether.

In quasi-legal ethics, principles and casuistry, to the extent that they may produce different 'answers', are sometimes thought to be in competition. In VBP, they are complementary. Both, that is to say, offer ways of exploring what might be thought of as the 'space of values'. Both help us to understanding the values bearing on a given situation through the often very different perspectives of those involved. This active rather than passive use of ethical reasoning is particularly important in CAMHS. As the child psychiatrist, David Jones, and the philosopher, Donna Dickenson, have argued in relation to the assessment of 'best interests' under the Children Act (Dickenson and Jones 1995), actively involving children in making choices is one of the key ways in which they gain the competence to make choices for themselves.

Skills area 4: communication skills

Communication skills, although not traditionally part of 'ethics', are central to the processes that support VBP. This is indeed one of the key respects in which VBP is process rather than outcomes oriented. In quasi-legal ethics, the role of communication skills is executive—they help to make the rules 'stick'! In VBP, by contrast, communication skills have a substantive role. In VBP, a good decision is defined not only by *what* is done, but by *how* it is done.

Communication skills, in their own right and connected with ethical decision-making (Hope *et al.* 1996), have of course an important role in all areas of medicine. As a contributory skill for VBP, however, the medical model of communication has been focused particularly at the level of individual interactions. Management theory, by contrast, offers a rich resource of systemic approaches to working in a positive way with differences of values. It is to an example of such approaches that we turn in the final section of this chapter.

Values-based management: the skills of adaptive work

Management theory is more hospitable to diversity of values than medical theory. Medicine, although an essentially practical discipline, has a strongly scientific self-image when it comes to its theoretical basis. In science, we resolve conflicting views by getting more facts aimed at achieving consensus. One perspective is 'proven' to be right at the expense of competing perspectives. Quasi-legal ethics has adopted this approach too (Fulford 2002a). Its increasingly detailed codes are aimed at achieving consensus on what is 'right' at the expense of competing perspectives. This is why, as we argued above, quasi-legal ethics is the right tool but in the wrong place if it is used in situations of value diversity.

Management theory, on the other hand, has no 'scientific' self-image to protect. Hence, instead of assuming that agreement on values is to be expected, it has tackled head-on the need for effective decision-making where legitimately different values are in play. There are many in management, it should be said straightaway, who think that an organization can only be effective if it has 'shared values'. Certainly, to be effective an organization must have *some* shared values—the organizational equivalent of the shared values expressed by quasi-legal ethics and used, appropriately, to provide a framework for practice (see above). But management theory has been ahead of medical theory in tackling the problem of effective decision-making when values are *not* shared. Enter, by way of example, the concept of leadership as 'adaptive work' developed by Ronald A. Heifetz in his book, *Leadership without easy answers* (1994).

Values-based management—the theory

Formerly a psychiatrist, Heifetz now directs the Leadership Education Project at the John F. Kennedy School of Government at Harvard University. Adaptive work, as Heifetz describes in the opening chapter of his book, puts values, and conflicts of values, at the heart of leadership. 'Adaptive work', he writes (p. 22), 'consists of the learning required to address conflicts in the values people hold, or to diminish the gap between the values people stand for and the reality they face'.

Heifetz' concept of leadership as adaptive work shares two key elements with values-based practice: an emphasis on the importance of evidence (or facts) alongside values; and the recognition that differences of values, used in the right way, are a resource for, rather than an impediment to, effective action. 'Different values', Heifetz says, 'shed light on the different opportunities and facets of a situation. The implication is important, *the inclusion of competing value perspectives may be essential to adaptive success*' (p. 23, emphasis in original).

Heifetz identifies these two key elements at the level of organizations and management. Values-based practice identifies them at the level of clinical work. There is considerable potential, then, for two-way learning between clinical medicine and management in the area of value diversity. Heifetz, indeed, argues that his theory, as a theory of leadership, is applicable to doctor–patient relationships as much as to managers and business or political leaders. But how does 'adaptive work' work out in practice?

Values-based management—the practice

As a resource for healthcare decision-making, the importance of Heifetz' book is as much in the detailed case studies he provides as in the principles these illustrate. We can get a flavour of the strongly practical nature of his work, though, by taking one section of the applied part of his theory and showing how it illuminates some of the difficulties arising in child and adolescent mental health practice.

Thus, in his chapter on the use of authority, Heifetz outlines five strategic principles (p. 128). Heifetz illustrates these with a detailed study of President Lyndon Johnson's strategy, following Kennedy's assassination in 1965, to secure voting rights for black Americans. The relevance of Heifetz's principles, though, to child and adolescent practice is evident from the way in which they map directly on to many of the scenarios familiar in CAMHS. Thus:

Principle 1: identify the adaptive challenge

'Diagnose the situation in light of the values at stake and unbundle the issues that come with it' (p. 128).

The first principle of adaptive work maps directly on to the first principle of VBP (Fig. 5.1), namely that *all* decisions, *including* decisions about diagnosis, are values- as well evidence-based. We illustrated this above with the 'medical' diagnoses of ADHD and autistic spectrum disorder. Applied more widely, to the way in which a problem is assessed within a family setting for example, it is clear that understanding the operative values is a (perhaps *the*) key to effective intervention. Family therapists will identify with Heifetz when he writes that diagnosing the diverse and often contested values at stake within a situation of challenge requires an 'un-bundling' of their previous packaging, and a recognition of the tensions, pain, contradictions and conflicts locked or blocked within the 'bundle'.

Principle 2: regulating distress

'Keep the level of distress within a tolerable range for doing adaptive work.' Heifetz uses the pressure cooker analogy—'Keep the heat up without blowing up the vessel' (p. 139).

The effects of too much distress are all too evident in CAMHS! Heifetz notes among these effects, authoritarian rule (in a word, 'Doctor knows best'!), suppression of differences (domineering management styles), and fragmentation (factional in-fighting in multidisciplinary teams).

Principle 3: disciplined attention to the issues

Heifetz means by this, focusing on the tractable issues, thus counteracting 'work avoidance mechanisms like denial, scapegoating, externalising the enemy, pretending the problem is technical, or attacking individuals rather than issues' (p. 128).

Again, these mechanisms of avoidance are all too familiar in CAMHS. They include:

denial, e.g. in family work;

scape-goating: again, familiar in family dynamics, also within multidisciplinary teams;

externalizing the enemy: dissociative symptoms provide a dramatic example of this process;

pretending the problem is technical: substituting a dose of Ritalin for secure family relationships;

attacking individuals not issues: blaming 'the social worker' where the problem is lack of resources.

Principle 4: give the work back to the people with the problem (but at a rate they can stand)

Heifetz argues that people tend to push problems back to authorities when the work is really theirs to do. His concept of 'adaptive work' thus means helping people to help themselves.

This is an especially important principle in healthcare. Traditionally, 'the patient' has been a (passive) patient rather than (active) agent. In terms of therapy, though, many of the developments of the last 30 years have sought to move the emphasis away from passive therapies (notably drugs) to active learning strategies (such as cognitive-behavioural therapy). Family therapy, for example, depends critically on the therapist resisting demands from her client or client family to come up with 'answers' for them so that they are able to do the work of finding answers for themselves.

At the level of service organization, this principle is central to the difference between VBP and quasi-legal ethics as responses to conflicting values (see Fig. 5.1, Principle 10). Quasi-legal ethics looks to experts (ethicists, lawyers, ethics committees, regulatory bodies, etc.) for answers. VBP, while recognizing the value of expert input, puts decision-making back with 'users and providers at the clinical coal face' (Fulford *et al.* 2002a).

Principle 5: protecting voices of leadership without authority

'Give cover to those who raise hard questions and generate distress.' These 'leaders in the community' (p. 144) lack the authority of position; but this is their strength, for they 'have latitude to provoke rethinking that [leaders with authority] do not have' (p. 128).

What Heifetz has in mind here is rather more than 'my sharpest critic is my clearest guide'. In VBP terms, it is close to Principle 4, the principle of user-centrality. But it gives a particular cogency to this principle as applied to healthcare decision-making. It suggests that active dissenters, the leaders of dissent, may have a perspective that those 'in authority' lack. It is the unauthorized voice, then, to which we should 'give cover' so that, as a uniquely creative contribution to decision-making, it can be properly heard. And there are no more unauthorized voices than those of children!

There are many more examples that could be drawn from Heifetz' book. But we hope that these are enough to show the very direct way in which Heifetz' recommendations for working effectively in situations of value diversity, although derived from management rather than medical theory, map on to decision-making in child and adolescent mental health practice. It is of course no coincidence that Heifetz is a psychiatrist by training as well as a management theorist. As we noted, many of his examples are drawn from medicine. His dual background thus makes him a natural bridge between management and medicine. His concept of 'adaptive work' shows that there is useful traffic to flow across the bridge when it comes to the practical strategies required for effective action in situations of conflicting values.

Conclusions—from VBM-M to VBM²

In this chapter we have explored some of the issues arising from the diverse and hence often conflicting values operative in child and adolescent mental health from the perspective of values-based practice.

Values-based practice, as we noted in the first section above, is complementary to the more familiar 'bioethics'. Bioethics, in the predominately quasi-legal form which it takes in practice, seeks to define good outcomes. This is appropriate where values are shared and can thus provide a framework for practice. But *differences* of values, as we have seen, are the norm in mental health. Hence values-based practice starts from the premis of legitimate diversity of values and focuses on the skills that support good process rather than seeking to prescribe good outcomes. We outlined, in the second section of the chapter, four key skills areas essential to the 'good process' of VBP in medicine: awareness, knowledge, reasoning skills, and communication skills. Finally, in the third section of the chapter, we illustrated the potentially rich resources from management theory for building the skills-base of VBP, through Heifetz' concept of 'adaptive work'.

Traditionally, there has been something of a stand-off between practitioners and managers! Managers perceive practitioners as unrealistic and resistant to change. Practitioners perceive managers as penny-pinching and prone to fanciful reframing of their craft in jargon terms— brilliantly lampooned by the philosopher Michael Loughlin in his (1996) book, *Rationing, barbarity and the economist's perspective.*

From the perspective of values-based practice this traditional stand-off can be understood as being, essentially, a conflict between legitimately different value perspectives. It is legitimate that practitioners should be concerned primarily with the needs of their particular clients and patients. It is legitimate, equally, that managers should be concerned with the wider economics of supply and efficient distribution of resources. There is no quick 'ethical fix', then, no right or wrong principle prescribed in advance by a code of practice or ethical guideline, by which a given decision, at clinical, managerial or indeed policy level, should be governed. In values-based practice, by contrast, as Heifetz' concept of adaptive work so powerfully illustrates, the different values in play in healthcare between clinicians and managers cease to be a problem to be 'solved' and become a resource. The 'values problematic' environment of bioethics thus becomes, in VBP, an environment which is 'values rich'.

How we handle this values-rich environment, as we have shown in this chapter, is informed within values-based practice, equally by values-based medicine and by values-based management. Differences of values, then, between medicine and management, instead of reducing our effectiveness, as in the traditional stand-off between practitioners and managers, thus act to increase our effectiveness in the values-based practice model outlined here. In place of the reductive mathematics of the traditional stand-off, the bottom line of values-based practice is that our effectiveness, in all areas of healthcare decision-making, increases as the square of the differences between us.

Acknowledgements

Figure 5.1 was first published in Fulford, K.W.M. (2004) Ten principles of values-based medicine. In *The philosophy of psychiatry: a companion* (ed. J. Radden). New York: Oxford University Press, and we are grateful to Oxford University Press for permission to reproduce it here.

References

Adshead, G. (2000) Practitioner commentary. In *In two minds: a casebook of psychiatric ethics* (ed. D. Dickenson, and K.W.M. Fulford), pp. 233–6. Oxford: Oxford University Press.

Alderson, P. (1990) *Choosing for children: parents' consent to surgery.* Oxford: Oxford University Press.

Beauchamp, T.L. and Childress, J.F. (1994) *Principles of biomedical ethics* (4th edn). Oxford: Oxford University Press.

Colombo, A., Bendelow, G., Fulford, K.W.M., and Williams, S. (2003) Evaluating the influence of implicit models of mental disorder on processes of shared decision making within community-based multidisciplinary teams. *Social Science & Medicine,* **56,** 1557–70.

Crisp, R. (1994) Quality of life and health care. In *Medicine and moral reasoning* (ed. K.W.M. Fulford, G. Gillett, and J. Soskice), ch. 13. Cambridge: Cambridge University Press.

Department of Health (1999) *National service framework for mental health—modern standards and service models.* London: Department of Health.

Dickenson, D. and Fulford, K.W.M. (2000) *In two minds: a casebook of psychiatric ethics.* Oxford: Oxford University Press.

Dickenson, D. and Jones, D., (1995) True wishes: the philosophy and developmental psychology of children's informed consent. *Philosophy, Psychiatry, & Psychology,* **2/4,** 287–304.

Fulford, K.W.M. (1989) *Moral Theory and Medical Practice.* Cambridge: Cambridge University Press.

Fulford, K.W.M. (1990) Philosophy and medicine: the Oxford connection. *British Journal of Psychiatry,* **157,** 111–5.

Fulford, K.W.M. (1994) Closet logics: hidden conceptual elements in the DSM and ICD classifications of mental disorders. In *Philosophical perspectives on psychiatric diagnostic classification* (ed. J.Z. Sadler, O.P. Wiggins, and M.A. Schwartz), pp. 211–32. Baltimore: Johns Hopkins University Press.

Fulford, K.W.M. (2001a) The paradoxes of confidentiality. A philosophical introduction. In *Confidentiality and medical practice* (ed. C. Cordess), pp. 7–23. London: Jessica Kingsley.

Fulford, K.W.M. (2001b) Philosophy into practice: the case for ordinary language philosophy. In *Health, science and ordinary language* (ed. L. Nordenfelt), ch. 2, pp. 171–208. Amsterdam: Rodopi.

Fulford, K.W.M., (2002a) Values in psychiatric diagnosis: executive summary of a report to the chair of the ICD-12/DSM-VI coordination task force (dateline 2010). *Psychopathology,* **35,** 132–8.

Fulford, K.W.M. (2002b) Report to the chair of the dsm-vi task force from the editors of *ppp* on 'contentious and noncontentious evaluative language in psychiatric diagnosis' (dateline 2010). In *Descriptions & prescriptions: values, mental disorders, and the DSMs* (ed. J. Z. Sadler), ch. 21. Baltimore: The Johns Hopkins University Press.

Fulford, K.W.M. (2004) Ten principles of values-based medicine. In *Companion to the philosophy of psychiatry* (ed. J. Radden). New York: Oxford University Press.

Fulford, K.W.M. and Bloch, S. (2000) Psychiatric ethics: codes, concepts, and clinical practice skills. In *New Oxford textbook of psychiatry* (ed. M. Gelder, J. J. Lopez-Ibor, and N. Andreasen), pp. 27–32. Oxford: Oxford University Press.

Fulford, K.W.M. and Williams, R. (2003) Values-based child and adolescent mental health services? *Current Opinion in Psychiatry*, **16**, 369–76.

Fulford, K.W.M., Dickenson, D., and Murray, T.H. (2002) Introduction: many voices: human values in healthcare ethics. in *Healthcare ethics and human values: an introductory text with readings and case studies* (ed. K.W.M. Fulford, D. Dickenson, and T.H. Murray), pp. 1–19. Malden, USA, and Oxford, UK: Blackwell.

Fulford, K.W.M., Morris, K.J., Sadler, J.Z., and Stanghellini, G. (ed.) (2003) Past improbable, future possible: the renaissance in philosophy and psychiatry. In *Nature and narrative: an introduction to the new philosophy of psychiatry* (ed. K.W.M. Fulford, K.J. Morris, J.Z. Sadler, and G. Stanghellini), ch. 1, pp. 1–41. Oxford: Oxford University Press.

Fulford, K.W.M., Williamson, T., and Woodbridge, K. (2002) Values-added practice (a values-awareness workshop). *Mental Health Today*, October, 25–7.

Gillon, R. (1996) Editorial to JME issue which included Robertson, D. (1996) Ethical Theory, ethnography and differences between doctors and nurses in approaches to patient care. *Journal of Medical Ethics*, **22**, 292–9.

Graham, P. (1999) Ethics and child psychiatry. In *Psychiatric ethics* (3rd edn) (ed. S. Bloch, P. Chodoff, and S.A. Green), ch. 14, pp. 301–16. Oxford: Oxford University Press.

Hare, R.M. (1952) *The language of morals*. Oxford: Oxford University Press.

Heifetz, R. (1994) *Leadership without easy answers*. USA: Harvard University Press.

Hope, T., Fulford, K.W.M., and Yates, A. (1996). *The Oxford practice skills course: ethics, law and communication skills in health care education*. Oxford: Oxford University Press.

Jackson, L. (2002) *Freaks, geeks and asperger syndrome*. London: Jessica Kinglsey.

Jackson, M. and Fulford, K.W.M. (1997) Spiritual experience and psychopathology. *Philosophy, Psychiatry, and Psychology*, **4/1**, 41–66.

Loughlin, M. (1996) Rationing, barbarity and the economist's perspective. *Health Care Analysis*, **4**, 146–56.

Montgomery, J. (1995) Patients first: the role of rights. In *Essential practice in patient-centred care* (ed. Fulford, K.W.M., Ersser, S., and Hope, T.), ch. 9. Oxford: Blackwell Science.

Morrow, V. and Richards, M. (2002) The ethics of social research with children: an overview. In *Healthcare ethics and human values* (ed. K. W. M. Fulford, D. Dickenson, and T. H. Murray), pp. 270–4. Oxford: Blackwell Science.

National Assembly for Wales (2001) *Everybody's business—child and adolescent mental health services strategy document*. Cardiff, UK: National Assembly for Wales.

National Assembly for Wales (2002) *Too serious a thing—the Carlile review*. Cardiff, UK: National Assembly for Wales.

Parker, M. (ed.) (1999) *Ethics and Community in the Health Care Professions*. London and New York: Routledge.

Raphael-Leff, J. (2002) The 'kinder egg': some intrapsychic, interpersonal, and ethical implications of infertility treatment and gamete donation. In *Healthcare ethics and human values* (ed. K.W.M. Fulford, D. Dickenson, and T.H. Murray), pp. 201–5. Oxford: Blackwell Science.

Rogers, A., Pilgrim, D., and Lacey, R., (1993) *Experiencing psychiatry: users' views of services*, London: Macmillan.

Sabat, S.R. (2001) *The experience of Alzheimer's disease: life through a tangled veil*. Oxford: Blackwell Publishers.

Sackett, D.L., Straus, S.E., Scott Richardson, W., Rosenberg, W., and Haynes, R.B. (2000) *Evidence-based medicine: how to practice and teach EBM* (2nd edn). London: Churchill Livingstone.

Sadler, J.Z. (1996) Epistemic Value Commitments in the Debate over Categorical vs. Dimensional Personality Diagnosis. *Philosophy, Psychiatry, & Psychology*, **3/3**, 203–22.

Salmon, G. and Williams, R. (2001) A strategic model for co-operation, partnership and teamwork—the inter-agency challenge of the mental health of our children. In *The Welsh Institute for Health and Social Care—the first five years.*, pp.18–22. Pontypridd: University of Glamorgan.

Widdershoven, G. and Widdershoven-Heerding, I. (2003) Understanding dementia: a hermeneutic perspective. In *Nature and narrative: international perspectives in philosophy and psychiatry* (ed. K.W.M. Fulford, K. Morris, J.Z. Sadler, and G. Stanghellini), pp.103–11. Oxford: Oxford University Press.

Williams, R. and Salmon, G. (2002) Collaboration in commissioning and delivering child and adolescent mental health services. *Current Opinion in Psychiatry*, **15**, 349–53.

Chapter 6

Where is the wisdom? Professional education and the realization of healthcare

Colin Coles

Summary

In this chapter I examine the recent literature on professional development, and consider the implications both for the education of the healthcare professions and for the realisation of healthcare services. I describe how professionals are asked to engage in complex and unpredictable tasks on society's behalf, and in doing so must exercise their discretion in situations of uncertainty, that is they must make judgements—decide what is 'best' in the particular situation rather than what is 'right' in some absolute sense. Inevitably some of these judgements will lead to 'error', which is endemic to professional practice.

This challenges some current ideologies in healthcare regarding the primacy of evidence-based practice and the application of protocols.

Underpinning professional judgement is a form of knowledge—called practical wisdom—which is not formally taught and learnt but is acquired largely through experience and informal conversations with respected peers. Wisdom develops through 'the critical reconstruction of practice'. Central to this is 'deliberation', which is distinguished from mere reflection on practice.

The fundamental implication for education is that professionals need to engage in the appreciation of their practice—not just to understand what underpins their own practice but also to consider critically the contestable issues endemic to practising as a professional. For the delivery of healthcare services, the implications are even more wide-ranging, not least as the concept of 'delivery' devalues professional practice. Professionals practice within 'communities'. There is the need for them to have a sense of 'collegiality', and to engage in 'criticality'.

All of this is fundamentally counter to the prevailing view that healthcare services and healthcare education are technical matters that require technical approaches to solve technical problems. The chapter concludes by arguing that there is the need for a fundamental re-think on the part of policy makers, since the current climate is not in society's best interests.

Introduction

Current approaches to healthcare education rest on the need for accountability and performance review. Central to my argument in this chapter is an alternative view that holds this thinking up to critical scrutiny in the light of today's understanding about what it means to be professional, the kind of knowledge that underpins professional practice, and the manner in which this knowledge is acquired, shared and developed.

The nature of professional practice

Society asks certain of its members to be professionals—to undertake particular tasks and perform roles that others cannot or will not do. The caring professions are not in any way 'better' than other occupational groups. Rather they are different, 'special' in particular ways. As one writer (Friedson 1994) puts it:

> Professionalism… is not just any kind of work…. [It] is esoteric, complex and discretionary in character: it requires theoretical knowledge, skill, and judgement that ordinary people do not possess, may not wholly comprehend and cannot readily evaluate…. The work they do is believed to be especially important for the well-being of individuals or society at large, having a value so special that money cannot serve as its sole measure…. It is the capacity to perform that special kind of work which distinguishes those who are professional from most other workers.

Wilfred Carr (1995) notes that professional people are marked out by the acquisition of—and an adherence to—the traditions of their chosen profession:

> To 'practise'… is always to act within a tradition, and it is only by submitting to its authority that practitioners can begin to acquire the practical knowledge and standards of excellence by means of which their own practical competence can be judged.

Golby and Parrott (1999) put this another way: 'professions represent the social embodiment of key aspects of human welfare'. Lave and Wenger (1991) also emphasize the social nature of any professional practice, and point out that through both formal and informal educational processes practitioners become members of what they call 'communities of practice', which they see occurring through a process of 'absorbing and being absorbed' into those communities. Carr also notes that any profession is influenced by social, historical, and ideological constraints. Both professional practice and the education of practitioners are inevitably politically located.

Donald Schön (1983, 1987) coined the term 'the swampy lowlands' to characterize the uncertainties of the work of professional people. He noted that many of the problems that professionals face are complex and often indeterminate—sometimes having no clear solution. Others (e.g. Plsek and Greenhalgh 2001) call this 'complexity science', and contend that 'in complex systems unpredictability and paradox are ever present, and some things will remain unknowable'.

Writers (e.g. Eraut 1994; Fish and Coles 1998; Tyreman 2000) widely point out that professional practice involves practitioners not so much in finding the 'right' answer (which probably does not often exist in some absolute sense) but rather in deciding what is 'best' in the situation in which they find themselves. As Carr (1995) puts it:

> [Professional action] is not 'right' action in the sense that it has been proved to be correct. It is 'right' action because it is *reasoned* action that can be defended discursively in argument and justified as morally appropriate to the particular circumstances in which it was taken.

A judicial enquiry into the homicide committed by a schizophrenic patient being supervised in the community reported (Bart *et al.* 1998):

> Each decision made in the care and treatment of a mentally disordered patient involves risk…. There are no simple answers. The complexity and the difficulty of the balancing exercise which clinicians have to make daily as the guardians of the patient's health and the public safety, should not be underestimated…. Clinicians are often placed in an

Table 6.1 Technical/rational and professional artistry view of practice

Technical/rational	Professional artistry
Practice is concerned with certainty	Uncertainty is endemic to practice
Complexity must be reduced	Complexity is inevitable
Factual knowledge is required	Some things will remain unknowable
Protocols are needed to drive practice	Judgement is central to practice
Quality is measurable	Quality lies within each professional
Services are to be delivered	Care can only be realised
Performance management is essential	Professional self-regulation is needed
Regulatory mechanisms are required	Development achieves high quality
Staff training is needed	Professional education is required

invidious position forced to choose between options which are not ideal.... Even the most eminent can be tested to the utmost of his skill and occasionally fail.

One writer (Mintzberg 1983) offers this definition of professionalism: 'the exercise of discretion, on behalf of another, in a situation of uncertainty'. This recognizes that professional practice quite fundamentally involves the practitioner in making *judgements*. Without 'judgement' professional practice is merely 'technical' work.

Schön suggested that this view—that professional practice is 'judgement-based'—is not universally, nor indeed widely, held in today's world. He argued that a much more prevalent view was that professional practice is seen as what he called a 'technical/rational' matter. To view it as involving 'the exercise of discretion in situations of uncertainty' is to hold what he called a 'professional artistry' view. This distinction is shown in Table 6.1.

Here statements about healthcare (including education and clinical service) are paired to show the different language used to articulate particular ideas. More significantly, the language of technical/rationality is used largely by commentators in the popular press and media, and often in 'official' documents and reports. On the other hand, the language of 'professional artistry' is more often used by practitioners, who find the technical/rational language not only uncomfortable but unable to represent their practice as they experience and understand it. As we will see later, Schön's analysis is very significant not just for healthcare education but also for the realisation of healthcare services.

Support for Schön's view comes from another, perhaps even more compelling, source. The ancient Greeks, and particularly Aristotle (see Carr 1995), distinguished between two forms of human action—*poesis* and *praxis*. *Poesis* referred to those actions where the outcomes (the 'ends') were known before the action began, and where the ways of achieving that outcome (the 'means') were minutely prescribed. This can be seen in the construction of objects and artefacts. *Praxis* on the other hand was reserved, by the Greeks, for those actions where the people involved had to make decisions about both the 'ends' and the 'means' of those actions. For Aristotle, the work of caring professionals clearly came into this second category, and required a particular form of knowledge.

The knowledge that underpins professional judgement

Many contemporary writers (e.g. Eraut 1994; Fish and Coles 1998) have noted that there are different kinds of 'knowledge'. Epstein (1999), writing about medical practice, comments:

> Clinical judgement is based on both explicit and tacit knowledge. Medical decision making… is often presented only as the conscious application to the patient's problem of explicitly defined rules and objectively verifiable data…. Seasoned practitioners also apply to their practice a large body of knowledge, skills, values and experiences that are not explicitly stated by or known to them…. While explicit elements of practice are taught formally, tacit elements are usually learned during observation and practice. Often, excellent clinicians are less able to articulate what they do than others who observe them.

Carr sees this form of knowledge to be a way of thinking:

> Since the ends of a practice always remain indeterminate and cannot be fixed in advance, it always requires a form of reasoning in which choice, deliberation and practical judgement play a crucial role·

Others (e.g. Atkinson and Claxton 2000) have used the term 'intuitive knowing' to characterize the knowledge that underpins professional judgement.

This immediately transforms the debate into something much more substantial: judgement involves a form of reasoning. Again the ancient Greeks were aware of this. For Aristotle *techne* (or technical knowledge) only enabled *poesis* (making things) to occur but *phronesis*—which today we would translate as 'practical wisdom'—was required for professional action or *praxis*.

Carr asserts that practical wisdom is 'the supreme intellectual virtue and an indispensable feature of practice'. He adds that someone who lacks *phronesis* 'may be technically accountable, but can never be morally answerable'. This sentiment has not been lost in the literary arts either when T. S. Eliot asks (in *The four quartets*):

> Where is the wisdom we have lost in knowledge?
> Where is the knowledge we have lost in information?

To which we might add: 'And where is the information we have lost in data?!'

How is practical wisdom acquired?

At the heart of this discussion about professional practice and the knowledge that underpins it there is an implicit message about how professionals learn to do what they do, and more importantly to be what they are.

First, and quite fundamentally, professionals acquire practical wisdom through the process of becoming members of a profession, and only they know what they know, which is of course the basis of professionals' claims for autonomy and self-regulation.

But this raises a huge set of questions for professionals to answer, as shown by the considerable public disquiet concerning recent clinical mishaps and misdemeanours, which in the UK have led central government to ask: 'Why wasn't the problem identified earlier? Why wasn't something done about it? Why were people unwilling to raise it with the powers that be? How could such a situation have been allowed to prevail?' (Department of Health 1999). These are natural concerns. Society can so easily see professionalism becoming a 'self fulfilling prophecy'.

Carr's response to these concerns directly challenges the professions:

> … the authoritative nature of a tradition does not make it immune to criticism. The practical knowledge made available through tradition is not mechanically or passively reproduced: it is

constantly being reinterpreted and revised through dialogue and discussion about how to pursue the practical goods which constitute the tradition. It is precisely because it embodies this process of critical reconstruction that a tradition evolves and changes rather than remains static or fixed. When the ethical aims of a practice are officially deemed to be either uncontentious or impervious to rational discussion, the notions of practical knowledge and tradition will tend to be used in a wholly negative way.

Here Carr is arguing that the understandable right of professionals to regulate their own practice rests on there being a constant re-interpretation and revision of practice through continued dialogue and discussion, with professionals developing their professionalism through 'the critical reconstruction of practice'. What is the evidence to suggest that this occurs?

Research in North America over the past decade by Davis and his colleagues (1999) supports this view. Doctors have been shown to change their practice (and perhaps even more importantly to improve healthcare) largely through conversations with respected peers rather than through formal educational programmes or even sustained (particularly unfocused) reading. Similarly a study (Coles and Mountford 1999) in the UK of clinical units that were highly acclaimed by medical trainees as places to receive good training (and which the trainees saw as providing high quality healthcare) showed these units to be characterized by:

a sense of community—feeling that you belonged there;

a sense of collegiality—feeling that you were a colleague;

a sense of criticality—feeling that anything that happened there could be openly and honestly discussed.

The judicial review cited earlier noted (Bart *et al.* 1998):

> … the importance of clinicians not being so overburdened that they do not have time for mature reflection or to foster appropriately strong links with their teams.

The thread running through these accounts is that professional practice changes when practitioners engage in 'the continuous dialectical reconstruction of knowledge and action'— a process that some writers (Fish and Coles 1998) note involves 'deliberation'.

> Deliberation… is more than the critical *consideration* of one's practice for three reasons. First, it is concerned with practice 'as a whole' rather than one's own practice—with the critical reconsideration of the *traditions* of one's practice…. Second, reconstruction fundamentally involves 'building again', and not…merely the mechanical or passive reproduction of practice…. Third, critical reconstruction involves a perspective beyond current practice (and even its traditions), and takes the professional into the wider consideration of [his or her] actions. Here not just other people's views on one's practice but the accumulated views of the profession itself… are taken into account in reconstructing what one does and says.

Thus, practical wisdom develops when practitioners critically reconstruct their practice, when they 'deliberate', and this occurs often quite naturally through the everyday 'professional conversations' they have with their peers. However, as we will see, this does not always occur, is not always encouraged, and while necessary may not entirely be sufficient.

Professional education and the development of practical wisdom

If what I have been saying so far has wide support in the literature, what are the implications for professional education? In particular, what will this mean for teaching and learning, and for the methods of assessment that validate practice?

Teaching and learning

I have chosen to deal with teaching and learning together rather than as separate entities, and I have done this for a purpose: they are two sides of the same coin.

The most fundamental point to make is that 'practice' is (or rather should be) central to programmes of education in the health professions. By 'practice' I mean not just what practitioners *do* (and choose not to do) but also what they *are*. And as such it includes the knowledge and thought that underpins their actions as well as the actions themselves.

This fundamentally challenges some conventional assumptions about healthcare education. It suggests that education is likely to occur at any time (indeed is occurring all the time), and that 'protecting' time for education might not be the wisest course of action. It certainly implies that 'formal' educational programmes may miss the very essence of professional practice simply because they are most often located in situations of certainty rather than uncertainty. By its very nature, formal education is most often *planned*. Yet professional practice—in the sense that professionalism begins when certainty ends—can never be fully pre-planned.

In addition, to locate professional education in professional practice means we need to make different assumptions regarding the nature of knowledge. Earlier I showed how 'implicit', as well as 'explicit', knowledge underpins professional practice, and that there is a very real role for 'intuition'. As we will see shortly when considering 'assessment', this has huge implications for how we can tell if someone's practice is acceptable. We need to abandon the cosy distinction often made between objective knowledge and subjective impressions.

Related to this, we must also question traditional views as to the place of 'theory' in the practice of healthcare. Often people assume that theory should precede practice, and many educational programmes are built on that assumption, of which the so-called 'pre-clinical' part of many undergraduate courses is a clear example, where there is a large 'front loading' of curricula with theory teaching.

Another highly questionable assumption is that theory can be applied to practice, in the sense that once you have acquired some theory you can then utilize this to inform your practice. In situations of uncertainty we do not actually know what to do—simply because they are uncertain. A widely accepted view of learning is that in these situations we 'construct' the necessary theory for our actions. Only after the event do we articulate what we feel we 'knew' that enabled us to act the way we did.

A third assumption about theory is that it is in some way 'derived from' practice. We might 'put into words' what we believe we 'knew' when making a professional judgement, but that 'theory' can never inform other subsequent actions, precisely because they too will involve uncertainty.

Rather theory and practice are 'mutually constitutive and dialectically related domains'(Carr 1995). In other words, they both exist but only in relation to each other. More particularly in professional education programmes and initiatives, theory and practice need to be taught and learnt together.

This is where the concept of deliberation is so important. Earlier I argued that this involves the critical *reconstruction* (not simply the critical *consideration*) of practice. Teaching people 'critical thinking' will not be enough. Critical reconstruction involves practitioners in several related actions and resources:

absorbing and being absorbed into communities of practice;

becoming immersed into the traditions of practice;

traditions must not be merely replicated but critically reconstructed anew by each professional;

conversations between professionals are crucial;

professionals learn *from* talk but they also learn *to* talk;

access to the related writings of others, which form the recorded history of professional practice, is crucial too.

Teaching and learning in professional education and development, then, require an appreciation of one's practice. The role of the teacher is simply crucial here, and it has been suggested (Atkinson 2000) that professional development requires high levels of support and structure but as little 'direction' as possible, which is a difficult balance to achieve. The implications for teacher development (and in particular the development of teachers in the practice setting) are huge.

What is quite certain, though, is that traditional views of teaching and learning, especially when these assume that the teacher must be active and the learner passive, are quite inappropriate. More appropriate is a 'relationship' between more experienced and less experienced practitioners who engage in 'professional conversations' about their professional work together. In common parlance, this relationship is often referred to as 'an apprenticeship', though the term suggests something more to do with learning a set of replicable skills or crafts or perhaps entry into some guild or other. Learning about professional practice is much more than that. While professional practice does, of course, involve practical skills and procedural knowledge, its very essence rests on the possession (and continuing development) of practical wisdom to be able to deal with complex (and unpredictable) professional responsibilities.

Assessing professional competence

In many ways, the above discussion on teaching and learning can only be made complete if we now consider the vexed issue of assessment. Again, this will inevitably challenge some firmly held assumptions. The first is that assessment should be taken away from the practice setting (with all its messiness) and located where the 'variables' can be tightly (and neatly) 'controlled'. The very language here is of course 'technical/rational', and the notion of 'objectivity' is not far away.

However, my earlier discussion clearly suggests that if we are to say whether professionals' practice is appropriate, then we must focus on the judgements made *in the course of their practice* rather than how they deal with the inevitably 'sanitized' situations presented to them in conventional assessments that occur largely outside their practice.

A further assumption we need to challenge is that knowledge and skills (and even attitudes) are somehow separate (and can be assessed in isolation) from one another. Again, this is a technical/rational view, and is located within reductionist thinking. Rather, knowledge skills and attitudes are all involved in professional practice, and are inseparable from each other in the course of that practice. The knowledge that we have carries with it certain attitudes in its use, and so do any skills we possess. Wisdom is the fusion of all three—and is greater than the sum of the separate parts.

In addition, we must recognize that a practitioner's professional actions cannot be understood let alone appreciated without taking into account the thinking that lies behind them. Again, wisdom does not distinguish between what we do and what enables us to do it. It requires us to examine not just a practitioner's actions (including the actions they choose not to take) but crucially the practitioner's own account of the reasons for those actions.

Articulating one's practice in this way means deliberating on it—engaging in its critical construction (and not simply its critical consideration). This shifts the responsibility for assessment away from the examiner asking questions (to which the candidate responds) towards the candidate asking critical questions of his or her own practice (to which he or she, and maybe the examiner, then responds). The examiner then becomes a party to this critical reconstruction, and the judgement that the examiner makes about the candidate (which is just as much a professional judgement though in this case an educational one), will need to be based on the candidate's capacity to engage in that critical reconstruction. In short, there are few right answers in professional education (just as there are no right answers in professional practice) mostly best ones.

This suggests that we must recognize that examiners engage in acts of judgement when they assess another's practice. At that moment, the examiner's 'professional practice' is their examination of the candidate, and as such involves them in the exercise of discretion in situations of uncertainty for which they require 'practical wisdom'.

All along I have argued that this 'practical wisdom' (in this case, to assess someone's practice appropriately) comes about (or rather ought to come about) through 'deliberative reasoning'. How might this happen? (For a fuller discussion of this see Coles 2000.)

It seems only reasonable that, in the context of educational assessment, as in that of clinical practice, writing down accounts of one's practice (whether as an examiner or a candidate) should be part of the deliberation needed not just to develop one's practice but quite fundamentally in order to assess someone's professional capability.

This means, then, that we need to question quite seriously the notion of 'objectivity', and look to improve our subjectivity. At all costs, we must avoid the more accurate measurement of what is least important in favour of the less accurate appreciation of what is more important.

To illustrate this rather different approach to assessment, let me refer to a very typical (and practical) situation. A junior doctor is going about his or her clinical work. A more senior doctor is 'on call', that is, he or she can be called at any time by the junior doctor if something to do with the clinical work proves problematic. In our example here, the junior doctor, who we can assume is correctly following protocols for dealing with the majority of the patients in his or her care, recognizes that a situation has arisen with a particular patient that is not routine, cannot be dealt with in line with the protocols, and that he or she cannot cope alone, so calls the senior doctor.

This is entirely understandable. The consultant has more 'experience'—has seen (and had to deal with) more cases of this nature, and (in the terms I have used already) has acquired the capacity 'to exercise his or her discretion in situations of uncertainty'.

Now, in such a situation, the consultant inevitably comes to a view as to the quality of the more junior doctor's thinking and actions. It is also worth noting that no *measurements* of the junior doctor's performance have been undertaken. Neither, probably, was either the junior or the senior doctor conscious that an assessment was taking place—yet, inevitably, it most certainly was.

How, then, can such a situation be rendered useful as an assessment? Here are some thoughts:

> Both the senior and junior doctor should recognize that 'assessment is going on all the time', and that this is 'normal'.

> They should see that assessment has a dual role: while it needs to be regulatory, it should also be developmental; it is possible to learn in and through the critical reconstruction of one's practice.

They should recognize that assessment is not separate from but part of the educational process, and that both educational processes and clinical processes are each specific forms of professional practice.

They should understand more clearly the nature of professional practice—that it involves exercising discretion for someone's good in situations of uncertainty—that there are few 'right' answers in such situations, largely best ways forward.

They should understand that the purpose of medical education (at all stages) is for less experienced doctors to become more experienced—that is for them to develop their practical wisdom—and for them to appreciate that situations of uncertainty are not only 'normal'—they are to be expected—but they can be enormously valuable learning experiences.

The junior doctor should be encouraged to develop ways to make explicit his or her thinking processes regarding how he or she attempted to deal with the situation, the call for assistance, and what happened subsequently.

The senior doctor should, by all of his or her actions, facilitate the junior doctor in this.

Both should find ways of learning from the situation—the junior doctor to learn how to proceed next time, the senior doctor to appreciate his or her educational role in such situations (educational in two ways; regulatory and developmental).

Both should find ways to record their experiences (of the situation, of their interaction one with the other, and the learning that has occurred).

The implications for healthcare services

So far in this chapter I have set out the view from current literature that locates professional practice in what some have called 'the zone of complexity'. Professionals are placed (by society) in a position where they must exercise their discretion in the interests of another person less fortunate than themselves. To do this, they must develop the capacity for professional judgement, and this rests on what has been called 'practical wisdom', which develops in and through professionals deliberating (critically reconstructing) their practice. I have argued that this has huge implications for both teaching and learning, and for assessing whether or not someone is capable of independent professional practice.

Support for my argument comes from the 2002 Reith lecturer, Onora O'Neill, who, speaking to the theme *A question of trust*, says:

> Perhaps claims about a crisis of trust are mainly evidence of an unrealistic hankering for a world in which safety and compliance are total, and breaches of trust are eliminated. Perhaps the culture of accountability that we are relentlessly building for ourselves actually damages trust rather than supporting it. Plants don't flourish when we pull them up too often to check how their roots are growing: political institutional and professional life too may not go well if we constantly uproot them to demonstrate that everything is transparent and trustworthy.

Overall, this discussion has involved us in questioning and seriously challenging some long-held assumptions, and I have argued that these assumptions are themselves based on whether or not the person making those assumptions sees professional practice (whether clinical or educational) as a technical matter or something more akin to artistry (see Table 6.1).

There is much that I could say here but I will restrict myself to some issues that are both topical and central to the argument: the first is the notion of 'service delivery' and the second concerns the term 'clinical governance'. Once I have considered these I will draw out some implications.

'Service delivery'

My first consideration, which is crucial here, is to challenge the term 'service delivery', a term that has become something of a shibboleth in today's world. Ten or more years ago we wouldn't have heard the term in the context of healthcare. Now it is commonplace. But what does it mean, and more importantly what does it imply?

The word 'delivery' suggests two things: first, that something is transferred from one person to another through some agreed mechanism, and second, that the person making the delivery does not tamper in any way with what it is that is being delivered. Examples of delivery in these terms would be the postal service or a milk round (perhaps more commonly today a pizza!).

Now, this notion of 'delivery' suggests that, not just the ends of the action are agreed in advance (you will receive your letters, milk, or a pizza) but, the means for doing so are pre-determined also (as to the mechanism of delivery, the time, and timing, etc.).

Not just this, but the agent of delivery—the person making the delivery—is a minor player in all of this—almost anyone could do it with a little training. Certainly you would not associate any of these occupations as being professional (though this is not to say that the people might not conduct themselves in a highly organized and socially very acceptable manner, nor that the public would not expect them to do so). But they would not be expected to change the ends, nor even the means, of their actions in any way. Indeed, tampering with the goods could in certain circumstances be seen as a felony.

This analysis of the term 'delivery' shows just how far professionals have become devalued in recent years. My discussion above concerning the nature of professional practice (as crucially involving judgment) and the nature of professional knowledge (as being practical wisdom) puts a very different complexion on the term.

Earlier I showed that the Ancient Greeks saw *praxis* (which is the equivalent of professional practice) as requiring the individual to exercise judgement over both the means and the ends of his or her actions. Indeed, society requires this of the professional. Without this discretionary power, society's interests cannot be at all well served.

Carr (1995) puts it this way:

> ... the end of a practice is not to produce an object or artefact but to realise some morally worth-while 'good'.... Practice is not a neutral instrument by means of which this 'good' can be produced. The 'good'... cannot be 'made', it can only be 'done'.... Its ends are neither immutable nor fixed. Instead, they are constantly revised... and can only be made intelligible in terms of the inherited and largely unarticulated body of practical knowledge which constitutes the tradition within which the good intrinsic to a practice is enshrined. To practise is thus never a matter of individuals accepting and implementing some rational account of what the 'aims' of their practice should be. It is always a matter of being initiated into the knowledge, understandings and beliefs bequeathed by that tradition through which the practice has been conveyed to us in its present shape.

What Carr is clearly setting out here is the argument for professionals determining both the means and the ends of their practice—which in common everyday parlance is what we understand by the term 'professional self-regulation'. However, as I argued earlier, professionals cannot assume that self-regulation will be given to them automatically by society. The traditions of practice must not be passively and uncritically reproduced in an unthinking way from genera-tion to generation. Maybe this is where the healthcare professions have fallen short of the ideal in some instances. Rather, professional people have to accept the responsibility of critically reconstructing their practice through, as I described above, a process of deliberation.

The term 'delivery' is thus a technical/rational one. It not only limits the scope of professional people to use their judgement but it places strict control over what they can and cannot do. The rise of the protocol as a way of determining professional practice is a direct result of a shift in society more generally towards seeing professionals as instruments in carrying out technical tasks.

Much, of course, follows from this view of healthcare. When something goes wrong (as it inevitably will, given that healthcare will always involve situations of uncertainty), then practi-tioners can be held to account—why were the protocols not followed? But this misrepresents the nature of practice, and the centrality of judgement, and the wisdom that underpins it.

We need a better term than 'delivery' to describe healthcare—one which captures more truth-fully the realities of being professional—and I suggest we speak more of 'the fulfilment' or 'the realization' of practice than its 'delivery'.

'Clinical governance'

The notion of 'clinical governance' is also of recent origin, and like the term 'delivery' has become widely used. And similarly, it can attract very different interpretations. If you see pro-fessional practice in a technical/rational way, it can mean 'performance management' and 'league tables', but see it in terms of professional artistry, then clinical governance has more to do with learning and development.

Turning first to the technical/rational interpretation of clinical governance, the danger here lies in society seeing healthcare (and indeed education) as a commodity—a service to meet a general need (and hence its delivery), and the 'need' is a deficit (disease is a lack of health, igno-rance is a lack of knowledge) that can be 'made up' through application of that commodity.

This thinking very quickly gives rise to what is commonly termed 'the blame culture': if something goes wrong, someone is at fault, and must 'pay' for this in some way. But, as I showed earlier in the judicial review I cited, 'even the most eminent can be tested to the utmost of his ability and occasionally fail'. Where professional practice is seen as artistry, then professionals are expected to exercise judgements because they are working in situations of uncertainty.

What seems to have gone wrong is that society has developed an inaccurate view of professional practice. More seriously, the current technical/rational view has been fuelled by some sections of the media (notably the so-called popular press), and it has served some politicians to re-inforce this view. A more measured approach is now needed, and both the media and politicians must come to recognize that it is in society's best interests to develop a view of professional practice that accords with what Schön called an artistry approach, recognizing the complexities involved, and the inevitability of error in the caring professions, which are judgement-based.

Interestingly, and perhaps ironically, this alternative view of practice can be seen quite clearly in the Department of Health's own definition of clinical governance (1998):

> Clinical governance can be defined as a framework through which NHS organizations are accountable for continuously improving the quality of their services and safeguarding high standards of care by creating an environment in which excellence in clinical care will flourish.

Three points are worth highlighting here. First is the notion of 'continuous improvement'. This suggests a developmental approach. Second is the reference to 'safeguarding', which seems to link with my earlier discussion about the traditions of practice. Third is the statement concerning the creation of an environment in which excellence will flourish. This suggests a biological (certainly botanical) imagery of the conditions for healthy growth.

The Department of Health also links clinical governance with professional self-regulation and life-long learning—again concepts that I have been dealing with in my analysis earlier in this chapter. But through what mechanism is all of this to be realized (rather than 'delivered')?

Again, the Department of Health (1999) suggests a way forward. In their publication *Supporting doctors, protecting patients* it is suggested that the mechanism for development will be what they term 'appraisal', and it is quite clear what the intention of this is:

> Appraisal is a positive process to give someone feedback on their performance, to chart their continuing progress and to identify development needs. It is a forward looking process essential for the developmental and educational planning needs of an individual.... It is not the primary aim of appraisal to scrutinise doctors to see if they are performing badly but rather to help them consolidate and improve on good performance aiming towards excellence.

So far, so good! Perhaps it was a pity that in the delivery (and I use the term advisedly here!) of the scheme for consultant appraisal they confused this clear developmental message by suggesting that there might be a hidden regulatory one (for example, by saying that the scheme was mandatory and that failure to engage in it would be viewed as a disciplinary matter, and that it would be closely linked to re-validation—a regulatory mechanism).

Some implications

What then are the implications of these terms 'service delivery' and 'clinical governance'? In the light of my earlier discussions, perhaps a more appropriate question would be to consider what the implications are of taking either a technical/rational or an artistry view of the practice of health professionals.

If you view professional practice as a technical matter, then very quickly you are into the delivery of service through pre-determined means to achieve pre-set ends, and failure to achieve this is the 'fault' of the staff involved. Quality is external to the professionals involved, and is set by those who govern healthcare, and the achievement of quality is a matter of driving up standards through regulatory mechanisms—hence performance management and league tables. 'Naming and shaming' quite naturally follows on from this. In this blinkered view, development is unnecessary. Only some form of technical training is required.

However, if you view professional practice as the exercise of discretion in situations of uncertainty, which naturally involves the use of judgement and the utilization of practical wisdom, then quality resides in the practice of the professional—only he or she has the capacity for quality, and it is only in their practice that it can be seen, particularly in how they cope with complexity and uncertainty. Development is necessary and essential. Education is required. Anything less is not in society's (which means patients') best interests.

Conclusions

In this chapter I have examined the nature of professional practice and the knowledge that underpins it, and then at what the literature says about how this is acquired.

Inevitably, this has raised a number of issues to do with professional development, and I have considered the implications for healthcare education (teaching, learning and assessment) and healthcare services (delivery and clinical governance).

I have suggested that quite fundamentally, deliberation is required, and that this occurs through professionals holding conversations with one another in the development of their 'communities of practice', by critically reconstructing the traditions that give substance to, and a basis for, their professional practice.

Throughout this discussion I have challenged some firmly held assumptions, and pointed out that these rest on interpretations in the light of whether one takes a technical/rational or an artistry view of professional practice.

Very clearly, my analysis of the literature aligns my argument with the artistry view, and in conclusion may I offer these suggestions for the future?

Healthcare professionals must be supported in their endeavours.

Currently many feel undervalued—a view which has been created by certain sections of the media and sustained by some politicians.

Not just the language of technical/rationality but the assumptions and values that lie behind it need to be challenged.

A developmental rather than a regulatory approach is needed to ensure that high quality healthcare is realized through the actions of the professionals involved.

Professional conversations lie at the heart of healthcare development, and these need to occur within 'communities of practice'.

A very practical way of achieving this would be to 'ensure that professionals are not so over-burdened that they do not have time for mature reflection or to develop strong links with their teams'.

This means making resources available for these reflections and links to occur.

References

Atkinson, L. (2000) Trusting your own judgement (or allowing yourself to eat the pudding). In *The intuitive practitioner: on the value of not always knowing what one is doing* (ed. T. Atkinson, and G. Claxton), pp. 53–65. Buckingham: The Open University.

Atkinson, T. and Claxton, G. (2000) *The intuitive practitioner: on the value of not always knowing what one is doing.* Buckingham: The Open University.

Bart, A., Kelly, H., and Devaux, M. (1998) *The Report of Luke Warm Luke Mental Health Inquiry.* London: Lambeth, Southwark and Lewisham Health Authority.

Carr, W. (1995) *For education: towards critical educational inquiry.* Buckingham: The Open University.

Coles, C. (2000) Developing our intuitive knowing: an alternative approach to the assessment of doctors. In *Credentialing physician specialists: a world perspective* (ed. P.G. Bashook, S.H. Miller, J. Parboosingh, and S.G. Horowitz), pp. 93–108. Proceedings of the conference held in Chicago, June 8–10. conference held in Chicago, June 8–10, 2000. The Royal College of Physicians and Surgeons of Canada, and The American Board of Medical Specialties.

Coles, C. and Mountford, B. (1999) *Supporting education in a service environment: a report to the Wessex Deanery.* Winchester, Wessex Deanery for Postgraduate Medical and Dental Education.

Davis, D., O'Brien, M.A.T., Freemantle, N., Wolf, E.M., Marmanium, P., and Taylor-Valsey, A. (1999) Impact of formal continuing medical education: do conferences, workshops, rounds, and other institutional continuing educational activities change physician behaviour or healthcare outcomes? *Journal of the American Medical Association*, **282**, 857–74.

Department of Health (1998) *A first class service: quality in the new NHS.* London: Department of Health.

Department of Health (1999) *Supporting doctors, protecting patients. A consultation paper on preventing, recognizing and dealing with poor clinical performance of doctors in the NHS in England.* London: Department of Health.

Epstein, R.M. (1999) Mindful practice. *The Journal of the American Medical Association,* **282,** 833–9.

Eraut, M. (1994) *Developing professional knowledge and competence.* Brighton: The Falmer Press.

Fish, D. and Coles, C. (1998) Developing Professional Judgment. In *Healthcare: learning through the critical appreciation of practice.* Oxford: Butterworth Heinemann.

Friedson, E. (1994) *Professionalism reborn: theory, prophecy and policy.* London: Policy Press.

Golby, M. and Parrott, A. (1999) *Educational research and educational practice.* Exeter: Fairway Publications.

Lave, J. and Wenger, E. (1991) *Situated learning: legitimate peripheral participation.* Cambridge: Cambridge University Press.

Mintzberg, H. (1983) *Structures in fives.* New York: Prentice Hall.

O'Neill, O. (2002) *A Question of Trust: The BBC Reith Lectures 2002,* Cambridge: Cambridge University Press.

Plsek, P.E. and Greenhalgh, T. (2001) The challenge of complexity in healthcare. *British Medical Journal,* **323,** 625–8.

Schön, D. (1983) *The reflective practitioner.* London: Basic Books.

Schön, D. (1987) *Educating the reflective practitioner.* London: Basic Books.

Tyreman, S. (2000) Promoting critical thinking: phronesis and criticality. *Medicine, Healthcare and Philosophy,* **3,** 117–24.

Chapter 7

The mental health agenda from an educational perspective

Ted Cole, Harry Daniels, and John Visser

> It is our firm belief that if we want to change things, school has to be the place to do it.
> (MHF, 1999, p.31)

Potentially, teachers and their learning support colleagues have an extended daily opportunity to create school systems and cultures that foster children's emotional well-being and are responsive to mental health difficulties. We will argue that this opportunity is sometimes not grasped by educators, nor supported by colleagues in the health services. When it is, improved mental health is promoted for all children and young people, including those with specific difficulties in this area. In this chapter, we use the educational descriptor 'emotional and behavioural difficulties' (EBD) as the base from which to discuss the mental health agenda in educational settings.

The chapter opens with a short historical account of educational interventions with pupils with EBD. Discussion then moves to contemporary issues as highlighted by recent literature (including: NHS Health Advisory Service 1995; Audit Commission 1999; Mental Health Foundation 1999) and the work of our Emotional and Behavioural Difficulties Research Team[1]. The chapter ends with some suggestions for national, local, and institutional strategies for mental health promotion in schools.

Definitions/terminology

Despite some reservations about the terminology employed,[2] we adopt the following definition of mental health problems (Department of Health 2000, p.25):

> Mental health problems in children and young people are broadly defined as disorders of emotions, behaviour or social relationships sufficiently marked or prolonged to cause suffering or risk to optimal development in the child, or distress or disturbance in the family or community.

This definition overlaps substantially with descriptors attached to the term 'maladjustment', used in education circles, following the Second World War, to encompass many pupils with

---

[1] Since 1995, the School of Education EBD Research Team, University of Birmingham, has conducted a range of national and local projects funded by government agencies as well as by the Nuffield Foundation.

[2] Some terms commonly used in CAMHS (including 'mental health') were not routinely used in DFEE guidance in the 1990s. Nor in our experience, were they part of the normal discourse of teachers and support workers, whether in mainstream or special settings. The word 'difficulties' is generally employed instead of 'disorders'.

mental health problems. It also overlaps 'EBD', the term that came to replace 'maladjustment' in the 1980s. We worry about the imprecision of EBD and how this label is given to pupils, perhaps used on occasion as a smokescreen for school or staff shortcomings. However, EBD is in common use and children deemed EBD are defined by the Department for Education (1994a) as follows:

> Children with EBD are on a continuum. Their problems are clearer and greater than sporadic naughtiness or moodiness and yet not so great as to be classed as mental illness.

These pupils' problems range from 'social maladaptation to abnormal emotional stresses' (Department for Education, 1994a, p.7); 'are persistent and constitute learning difficulties' (p.7); involve emotional factors and/or externalised disruptive behaviours; and general difficulties in forming 'normal' relationships. Social, psychological, and sometimes biological factors, or commonly interactions between these three strands, are seen as causing pupils' EBD (Cooper *et al.* 1994; Department for Education 1994a). Department for Education (1994a) briefly described a minority of pupils deemed EBD, who need specialist psychiatric services. The DFE description of EBD covers many of the detailed Health of the Nation Outcome Scales thirteen areas of mental health (Audit Commission 1999). Thus to discuss effective responses to pupils with EBD, is to discuss the addressing of many, although not all, mental health problems (see next section) in educational settings.

The extent of EBD

Our research team's work (Daniels *et al.* 1998a, b; Cole *et al.* 1999, 2000; Cole and Visser 2000) suggests both that pupils can be unfairly labelled as EBD but also that some pupils with substantial EBD are not at present recognized in schools, particularly those whose difficulties are 'internalizing' rather than 'externalizing' (Achenbach 1991). Those overlooked include some who might merit Tier 3 or 4 interventions. Furthermore, if pupils' difficulties are noticed, these young people are not necessarily placed on the special educational needs register 'stages' required by the then current first 'Code of Practice on the Identification and Assessment of Special Educational Needs' (Department for Education 1994c). The NHS Health Advisory Service (1995) believed that the code provided school staff with 'an ideal method' for recognizing mental health problems' (p.9). Our data suggest that the reality falls short of this. In some local education authorities (LEAs), the time-consuming bureaucracy of taking a child through to Stage 3 or even to a 'statement' of special educational needs (Stage 5), is not merited given the meagre provision of additional resources that the LEA can make available (Daniels *et al.* 1998a, b).

Rates of assessing pupils as having EBD vary from school to school and from LEA to LEA. This variation is sometimes related to the services the LEA is able to offer (see Galloway *et al.* 1994) and sometimes to the particular meanings individual teachers or supporting professionals attach to an imprecise and at times perhaps *unhelpful* label (Thomas and Glenny 2000). What might qualify for a 'Stage 3' intervention in one area will elicit a statement of special educational needs in another (Daniels *et al.* 1998a).

These factors may explain the wide discrepancy between health service accounts of the numbers of children with mental health problems (between 10 and 30%, NHS Health Advisory Service 1995) and educational writers' estimates of the numbers of pupils presenting significant EBD. Cole *et al.* (1999) indicate that, nationally, under 5% of the school population receive additional educational service interventions because they are deemed to have EBD (although individual schools serving difficult areas may have a much higher proportion of pupils said to have EBD). Amongst this, 4–5% will be some of the 2% said by the NHS Health Advisory Service (1995) to have severe and disabling mental health problems. While most of the 5% are in the mainstream schools, an estimated 0.3–0.4% of the compulsory school-aged population (over 20 000 pupils) is placed in EBD special schools, off-site special units called Pupil Referral Units (PRUs), and other alternative settings. These pupils include many of those excluded from mainstream schools (Cole *et al.* 1999; Parsons 1999) and school phobics likely to be in receipt of Tier 2 help.

Nationally, in 1998, boys outnumbered girls by about twelve to one in the EBD special schools, while in the PRUs, by over three to one. CAMHS have sometimes recommended that pupils with mental health difficulties should be placed in EBD special schools and PRUs (Cole and Visser 2000).

Historical overview

By 1930 it was possible for LEAs to finance the placing of children with mental health problems, by then starting to be called 'maladjusted', at a few pioneer independent residential schools (Cole 1989).

The first LEA-run child guidance clinic (CGC) opened in Birmingham in 1932 and by 1954 there were 300 CGCs, 204 run by LEAs and the rest by health or voluntary authorities. These were usually staffed by 'the Holy Trinity' (Redl 1966) of psychiatrist, psychologist, and psychiatric social worker. Following the 1944 Education Act, children showing evidence of emotional instability or psychological disturbance could be formally categorized as 'maladjusted' with LEAs having a duty to make appropriate provision for them (Cole 1989).

After a 5-year enquiry, the Underwood Report (Ministry of Education 1955) noted difficulties in diagnosing maladjustment and widely differing reported incidence rates. Maladjustment was sometimes seen as a 'within child' medical problem but also as 'a term describing an individual's relation at a particular time to the people and circumstances which make up his environment' (p.22). The report found an incomplete range of provision with about 3000 pupils deemed maladjusted attending:

45 special hostels, while going to mainstream day schools;

153 boarding schools created for 'normal' pupils;

'off-site' 'tutorial classes' in London with part-time attendance at mainstream schools and teachers devoting a day a week to working with pupils' families;

32 specialist residential schools (some run on permissive therapeutic lines, guided by a psychodynamic approach; others rejecting this 'medical' approach);

3 day-schools for the maladjusted.

For some pupils, placement in small, non-competitive classes was believed to help in the solving of their emotional problems. The role of teachers working with the maladjusted was seen in starkly different terms to the Office for Standards in Education's (OfSTED's) expectations of teachers in 1990s schools for pupils with EBD: then the teacher's primary function was 'not to teach, but to help each child to release the emotional tensions' that prevented him from learning (para.208). Today OfSTED expect the primary stress to be on *teaching* these pupils.

The Underwood report urged the expansion of child guidance as 'the principal means of attacking the problems of maladjustment in children' (para.161). However, CGCs needed to move away from a clinic-based orientation. Guidance should 'have roots in the schools' (p.41); be closely connected to other health services and involve work with the child's family. Also recommended was the establishment of schools' psychological services that should be primarily non-medical and run by LEAs. The report recommended that CGCs or schools psychological services should help to retain more maladjusted children in mainstream schools, perhaps with these children spending some of their time in CGCs. Boarding schools were seen as alien to many families and to be avoided.

Doubts raised in the report about the value of psychiatry in helping many children persisted amongst Ministry of Education officials through to the transfer of the Schools Medical Services from the new Department of Education and Science to the Department of Health in 1974. Department of Education and Science (1974) questioned the value of time-consuming psycho-therapeutic methods that tended to ignore neurological and socio-cultural considerations (Department of Education and Science 1974) and noted a lack of evidence for the effectiveness of CGCs. It urged reform, asking for:

psychiatrists to use their time more effectively by helping to train teachers and social workers in methods of assisting the maladjusted;

CGC staff to work *in schools* with children;

more preventive work to be undertaken by teachers in primary schools;

CGCs to use the 'potential skills of other personnel, beginning with the teachers' (p.17) but also social workers and general practitioners.

These recommendations were largely repeated by the NHS Health Advisory Service (1995).

The 1970s witnessed a rapid expansion of day and residential facilities for maladjusted pupils. A national survey for the Schools Council (Wilson and Evans 1980), agreeing with aspects of the Warnock Report (Department of Education and Science 1978), stressed the importance, for children deemed maladjusted, of:

'normal education' as a therapeutic tool;

addressing their pronounced educational underachievement ;

building pupils' self-esteem through successful achievement;

working through closer personal relationships to ameliorate emotional and externalizing behaviour difficulties

schools working closely with parents.

Wilson and Evans (1980) noted the teacher worries about the wisdom of 'drug therapies' (reflected in continuing teacher doubts about the use of methylphenidate for the treatment of children said to have attention deficit/hyperactivity disorders: see Cole *et al.* 1998; Baldwin 2000). Department of Education and Science (1978) also stressed the need to develop the skills of teachers in mainstream schools in recognizing and supporting maladjusted children.

The 1970s also saw an explosion nationally in the numbers of new special units for children deemed disaffected or disruptive, many of whom had unrecognized mental health problems (Visser 1980; Her Majesty's Inspectorate 1978). By 1983 there were 226 units catering for 3800 pupils in the Inner London Education Authority alone (Cole 1989).

Special educational provision in 1980s and 1990s

Some pupils deemed EBD were placed in residential schools and an increasing number of day special schools, following assessments leading to statements of special educational needs (SENs) by educational psychologists to which health service staff should but too often do not significantly contribute. By 1983 there were 220 of these state- and charity-run schools in England.

While some LEA schools have since closed, others have opened, so that a similar number continued to exist in 1998 (Cole *et al.* 1999). An independent sector burgeoned but was in sharp decline by 1990. As the NHS Health Advisory Service (1995) suggested, the use of the latter indicated an *ad hoc* expediency 'the very reverse of an active needs-led, community based service' (p.2). In addition 'off-site' special units, often called 'tutorial centres' for disaffected pupils (including school phobics), continued in existence, some being transformed into pupil referral units in the 1990s. Over 300 PRUs existed in 1998 (Cole *et al.* 1999), as well as some 'tutorial centres', which might or might not be PRUs devoted specifically to 'emotionally vulnerable' children with distinct mental health difficulties in parts of the country (Cole *et al.* 1999; Cole and Visser 2000).

The 'traditional' attitude towards the role of teachers in special schools and units, in part fostered by the Underwood Report, came under sustained attack. Stressing emotional and social education at the expense of delivering a broad, balanced, and 'normal' school curriculum, in the guise of a compulsory National Curriculum, was not acceptable to Department of Education and Science (1989) or OfSTED (1995). The mid-1990s were perhaps the heyday of the 'schools effectiveness/school improvement' movement, whose 'silence on affective areas' was acknowledged as a weakness by Stoll and Fink (1994, p.166).

Cole *et al.*'s (1998) national survey of English EBD special schools found most accepting the National Curriculum and believing that, on balance, it had assisted in raising standards, if slightly, at the expense of staff finding 'quality' time and resources for addressing the emotional and social needs of their pupils. In line with Department of Education and Science (1978) and Wilson and Evans (1980), most senior staff in these schools favoured an eclectic, humanistic approach that stressed the importance of working through positive relationships, listening, and talking to children, as well as education as therapy (Cole *et al.* 1998). The use of behaviourist systems of points and rewards, to motivate and control pupils, was common but was mixed with cognitive approaches that sought to adjust skewed patterns of thinking, encouraging internal locus of control. While EBD special schools received some valued support from educational psychologists, their contact with CAMHS was often minimal (Department of Education and Science 1989; Cole *et al.* 1998). OfSTED (1999) noted that the input of psychiatrists into LEA EBD schools was almost non-existent.

Managing EBD in mainstream schools

Accounts of secondary schooling, before the impact of the quasi-market reforms of the Thatcher era, suggested many schools' lack of responsiveness to the mental health needs of many children. For example, Schostak's research (1983) indicated ill-devised and delivered curricula, overstressing the academic and contributing significantly to 'maladjusted schooling', which exacerbated disaffection, attacked pupil self-esteem, and neglected pupils' affective needs. Galloway (1990) extended Schostak's findings in relation to the lack of time teachers found for talking and listening to pupils about their social and emotional concerns. He found it necessary to write:

> Parents are entitled to expect that their child will be known reasonably well by at least one teacher and have ready access to this teacher. Yet the organisation of some comprehensive schools makes this impossible.

Many writers fear that the major Education Acts of the 1980s and 1990s, requiring published examination league tables, parental choice, and initially rigid National Curriculum, have created school cultures that are even less responsive to pupils' affective needs (Cooper 1993; Cooper *et al.* 1994; Parsons 1999; Munn *et al.* 2000). As a result of these reforms, many headteachers are thought to have accorded a low priority to creating inclusive environments in which pupils with EBD meet with tolerance and support (Booth *et al.* 1998; Parsons 1999; Mental Health Foundation 1999). With the introduction of local management of schools, LEAs found themselves with reduced powers, able only to stress to schools the need for a mental health agenda likely to be of benefit to pupils in need of Tier 1 services.

Despite the above, we are aware of both primary and secondary schools keeping social development and personal well-being to the fore. These schools have an understanding of EBD needs and try to address mental health difficulties (Daniels *et al.* 1998a, b; Cole *et al.* 1999, 2000; Cole and Visser 2000; Cole *et al.* in press). Our research findings on the approaches used in these schools are close to those of other research reported in the last decade (e.g. Cooper 1993; Cooper *et al.* 1994; Hallam and Castle 1999; Mental Health Foundation 1999; Munn *et al.* 2000).

Redl (1966), in describing therapeutic milieux for disturbed young people, stressed the importance of appropriate values; that is, attitudes and feelings of staff 'that really fill the place, that are lived' (p.86). Lindsay (1997) and Daniels *et al.* (1998a, b) re-emphasized this in relation to mainstream schools. Schools that minimize EBD, and thus promote mental health, have leaderships supported by a critical mass of teachers who are genuinely committed to the welfare of all their pupils, including those who resist the schools' systems. Children and young people with EBD still feel valued members of their school community. As Galloway (1990) and later the Mental Health Foundation (1999) advised, personal, social, and health education are not merely 'bolted-on': they permeate most areas of the taught and of the 'hidden' curriculum. In these schools, as Greenhalgh (1994) and Davie and Galloway (1996) advise, time is found to listen to and to talk to children regularly, providing the emotional support and understanding that is essential for pupils with EBD. Echoing the Audit Commission's (1999) findings, we found that the label EBD tended to be avoided (Daniels *et al.* 1998b) and staff tried to match school experience to the children's individual needs (see Cooper's 1993, call for 'Schools for Individuals'). If necessary, curriculum demands were adjusted to play to the pupil's strengths and to build on the satisfactory relationships he or she may have with particular members of staff. A collaborative approach between teacher and child to planning work was employed. Whether the adoption of these approaches was brought about by the literature is uncertain but these approaches were in accord with the advice offered by, for example, Department for Education (1994 a, b), Cooper *et al.* (1994) and Munn *et al.* (2000). Providing structure and limits to behaviour was important, but skilful staff managed to provide 'clinical elasticity' (Redl 1966; Cole *et al.* 1998) that allowed for particular pupil idiosyncrasies. These schools, unlike some described by Power (1996), managed to achieve a suitable balance between pursuit of the academic and attendance to the pastoral needs of pupils despite the demands of the quasi-market. In recognition of the close links between under-achievement, learning difficulties, and EBD, close communication and collaboration existed between pastoral staff responsible for 'discipline' and specialist staff, particularly the Special Educational Needs Co-ordinator (SENCo). Such schools worked hard to provide achievements that boosted the self-worth of pupils with EBD, sometimes in areas beyond the requirements of the National Curriculum (as advised by Mental Health Foundation 1999).

Our research suggests that schools that manage pupils with EBD effectively also show a respect for parents and are enterprising in their approaches for enlisting the support of parents. Some hosted parent clubs and creches on-site (as a means of offering parenting skills)

(Cole *et al.* 2000) or encouraged parents to participate in parenting classes offered locally by voluntary organisations (Daniels *et al.* 1998b).

Schools involved in our research projects held to the above principles and practices but not without considerable difficulties. Indeed, some schools are under intense and perhaps increasing stress, reducing teachers' capacity for taking time and trouble with individual students with mental health needs (e.g. Cole and Visser 2000). If teachers are to become effective Tier 1 contributors, as the NHS Health Advisory Service (1995) hoped, the call of the Mental Health Foundation (1999) for reductions in the pressures on the nation's schools, particularly in areas of high social deprivation, needs heeding.

But what of services from CAMH professionals to mainstream schools? The NHS Health Advisory Service (1995) noted the retreat of educational psychologists from working alongside health service staff in for example, the Child and Family Services. The Audit Commission (1999) found that CAMHS staff devote a meagre 1% of their time to developing Tier 1 professionals. Our research since 1995 would seem to reflect these findings. Alterations to management, funding mechanisms, and acute constraints on quantity of funding have widened the gulf between CAMHS professionals and educationalists in many parts of England. Generally, psychologists, headteachers, deputy headteachers, heads of year, and SENCos interviewed in the course of our research have depicted flawed services, similar to the criticisms of CAMHS made in NHS Health Advisory Service (1995) and to an extent in the Audit Commission (1999). In particular, long waiting-lists, difficulties in making referrals, and an alleged lack of perseverance by CAMHS with families in need who did not attend a first appointment, were cited. School staff also reported a perceived lack of respect by many medical professionals for teachers' concerns. The links between LEAs, schools, and CAMHS in LEA behaviour support plans (Cole *et al.* 1999) seemed similarly patchy. Our data suggest that where good trans-disciplinary working has occurred, it has tended to rest upon informal networks or time-limited additional government grants for particular projects.

A strategy for mental health promotion in schools

To move forward, developments in relation to mental health needs are required at four levels: national, local government, institutional, and at the level of the individual child.

National

The English government should continue its review of the legislative and guidance framework to raise the profile of mental health promotion in schools. More importance, and therefore time, should be attached to personal and social education as well as to pastoral support for vulnerable children. The recommendation of the Mental Health Foundation (1999) for a mental health co-ordinator for each school is worthy of investigation by central government. There are signs that emotional and social development and citizenship are gaining in importance in the eyes of politicians but as the Mental Health Foundation (1999) point out, only limited progress can be made without reform of present ways of publicizing schools' success and failures. We endorse recommendations that league tables (if they are to continue) and other measures of schools performance should use a range of indicators extending beyond academic success. The Mental Health Foundation (1999) suggests that these measures should allow for the extent to which schools promote children's social and emotional well-being, including pupils with EBD, and recognize pupil achievement in creative and sporting achievements. Recent press reports suggest that OfSTED now plans to move in this direction by publicly recognizing school achievement in difficult-to-quantify areas (Cassidy 2001).

To create a teaching profession more aware of, and skilled in, mental health, the initial training of teachers should provide fuller coverage of children's emotional and social development, as well as stressing competence in delivering specialist academic subjects. For established teachers, further professional development on recognizing and responding to mental health difficulties is needed (as argued in Mental Health Foundation 1999).

The government should press forward with strategies for more 'joined-up' working (e.g. Department for Education and Employment 1997, 1998) between local agencies. Central government could encourage further examples of local authority children's departments drawing together schools and social services into single directorates. Divisions between health services and local authorities should similarly start to be bridged, e.g. through government doing more to foster the creation of locality-based multi-agency CAMHS. Efforts are of course being made to do this with indications of progress in some areas since the NHS Health Advisory Service (1995) (Audit Commission 1999; Cole *et al.* 1998).

Local government level

Health Advisory Service (1995) called for closer working between CAMHS and local authorities, urging Directors of Education to see mental health as a major responsibility of schools. Although LEAs now have restricted powers, they can and should draw headteachers' attention to mental health issues and exercise influence, where possible, through their control of SENs, social inclusion, and other budgets. Given LEAs' limited mandate, Tier 1 and Tier 2 CAMHS should find other ways of establishing needs and of delivering services to single schools or perhaps clusters of schools. Creating clear referral and intervention pathways from senior school staff to local CAMHS would seem a priority. The creation of easily-accessed, locality-based multi-agency CAMHS, with primary health care-workers known, welcomed, and respected in the local schools, would be an important step forward. Local CAMHS might even share sites with schools. Given practice in other countries (Mental Health Foundation 1999), it might not be an impossible dream for co-ordinated educational, health, and social services to be delivered from 'full-service' school-sites, as Mental Health Foundation (1999) hoped. For the necessary holistic, multi-agency approach, social service resources and priorities would also need reviewing and changes made to enable social worker activity beyond 'fire-fighting' in response to child abuse procedures and beyond the needs of the tiny but important proportion of children who are 'looked after'.

Institutional level

Given current mandatory central government demands, it is difficult to create school communities that are significantly more responsive to pupils with EBD and more general mental health needs. However, as noted earlier, some schools are more successful than others in this area. These effective schools are communities with an underlying value base of collaboration and inclusion that stresses the pastoral as well as the academic. They have clear policies and practice in relation to behaviour management. Approaches are used that build self-esteem and the emotional resilience of particularly the less academic, for example, through anti-bullying policies, Circle Time, Circle of Friends, use of peer and non-teacher adult mentors, training in anger management and conflict resolution. Academic standards are valued but there is a flexibility and breadth of curricular approach, particularly for Key Stage 4 pupils, that plays to pupils' strengths and avoids re-inforcing pupil failure. There is on-going staff development in relation to recognizing and addressing pupils' affective, as well as their cognitive, needs. Proactive work happens with the families of pupils designated 'at risk'. These schools are open to support from other professionals, for example, having a welcoming attitude to advisory teachers, psychologists. Schools in which these features are weak should be helped to follow the example of schools where these features are embedded in their normal practice.

CAMHS staff could clearly bring a range of interventions that would supplement and develop the skills of staff in special schools and PRUs. Their expertise in family work and counselling could be of particular benefit.

Individual level

The proposals above should impact significantly on the many pupils who might be viewed as needing Tier 1 services, as well as those requiring more intensive help. In addition, Tiers 2, 3 and 4 services should be more readily accessible. It would be a sign of respect by the medical profession, and would remove a common grievance, if referral mechanisms could be reviewed to allow senior educationists (e.g. headteachers and SENCos) to make direct referrals of individual pupils to CAMHS. Routing through over-worked educational psychologists with their own long waiting-lists, or general practitioners who might lack interest or expertise in mental health issues (Health Advisory Service 1995; Daniels *et al.* 1998b), can be unsatisfactory. Waiting-lists for appointments, of course, need to be cut. Services should be offered locally when possible: schools generally appreciate CAMHS professionals offering services to individuals on school sites (where this complies with client wishes). In short, many of the recommendations made by the NHS Health Advisory Service (1995), Audit Commission (1999), and Mental Health Foundation (1999) should have benefits for mental health promotion in schools. The distinct lack of CAMHS support to individual pupils in special schools and units has been noted and clearly needs correcting.

Conclusion

Given evidence offered in the historical section above, this strategy has a somewhat old ring to it but is no less important for that. It is not surprising that progress has been slow given that education, health, and social services are beset by intractable financial, organizational, and perhaps philosophical dilemmas. Nevertheless, because attempts to create better co-ordinated approaches have foundered in the past does not mean that they will necessarily fail in the future. A new drive for promoting better mental health in schools as part of a co-ordinated community-based approach is overdue and seems timely given a new interest in citizenship, social inclusion, and Goleman's (1995) 'emotional intelligence'. All schools should be helped to see the importance of 'promoting the well-being of the whole-child alongside that of academic success' (Mental Health Foundation 1999, p.31) and assisted in turning recognition of this into effective practice.

References

Achenbach, T.M. (1991) *Manual for the teachers' report form & 1991 profile of the child behaviour checklist.* Vermont: University of Vermont.

Audit Commission (1999) *Children in mind: child and adolescent mental health services.* London: Audit Commission.

Baldwin, S. (2000) 'How should ADHD be treated: a discussion with Paul Cooper'. *The Psychologist,* **13** (12), 598–602.

Booth, T., Ainscow, M., and Dyson, A. (1998) England: inclusion and exclusion in a competitive system. In *From them to us* (ed. T. Booth and M. Ainscow), pp. 193–225. London: Routledge.

Cassidy, S. (2001) OFSTED chief moots 10-year inspections. *Times Educational Supplement*, p. 3, 16.2.01.

Cole, T. (1989) *Apart or a part? Integration and the growth of British special education*. Milton Keynes: Open University Press.

Cole, T. and Visser, J. (2000) *EBD policy, practice and provision in Shropshire LEA and Telford & Wrekin LEA*. Birmingham: University of Birmingham.

Cole, T., Visser, J., and Upton, G. (1998) *Effective schooling for pupils with emotional and behavioural difficulties*. London: David Fulton Publishers.

Cole, T., Daniels, H., and Visser, J. (1999) *Patterns of educational provision maintained by LEAs for pupils with behaviour problems*. Sponsored by Nuffield Foundation. Birmingham: University of Birmingham.

Cole, T., Visser, J., and Daniels, H. (2000) *An evaluation of 'in-school centres'*. Report for Dudley LEA. Birmingham: University of Birmingham.

Cole, T., Visser, J., and Daniels, H. (2001) Inclusive practice for pupils with emotional and behavioural difficulties in mainstream schools. In *International Perspectives on Inclusive Education: Emotional and Behavioural Difficulties* (ed. J. Visser *et al.*) London: Elsevier/JAI.

Cooper, P. (1993) *Effective schooling for disaffected pupils*. London: Routledge.

Cooper, P. (1996) Giving it a name: the value of descriptive categories in educational approaches to emotional and behavioural difficulties. *Support for Learning*, 1 (4), 146–59.

Cooper, P., Smith, C., and Upton, G. (1994) *Emotional and behavioural difficulties*. London: Routledge.

Daniels, A. and Williams, H. (2000) Reducing the Need for Exclusions and Statements for Behaviour. *Educational Psychology in Practice*, 15 (4), 221–7.

Daniels, H., Visser, J., Cole, T., and de Reybekill, N. (1998a) *Emotional and behavioural difficulties in mainstream schools*, Research Report RR90. London: Department for Education and Employment.

Daniels, H., Visser, J., Cole, T., de Reybekill, N., Harris, J., and Cumella, S. (1998b) *Educational support for children with mental health issues: including the emotionally vulnerable*. Report for City of Birmingham/Birmingham Health Authority. Birmingham: University of Birmingham.

Davie, R. and Galloway, D. (ed.) (1996) *Listening to children in education*. London: David Fulton Publishers.

Department For Education (1994a) *Emotional and behavioural difficulties*, Circular 9/94. London: Department for Education.

Department For Education (1994b) *Code of practice on the identification and assessment of special educational needs*. London: Department for Education.

Department for Education and Employment (1997) *Excellence for all children: meeting special educational needs* (Green Paper). London: Department for Education and Employment.

Department for Education and Employment (1998) *LEA behaviour support plans*, Circular 1/98. London: Department for Education and Employment.

Department of Education and Science (1974) *Report of the chief medical officer for 1971–2*. London: HMSO.

Department of Education and Science (1978) *Report of the committee of enquiry into the education of handicapped children and young people* (the Warnock Report) London: HMSO.

Department of Education and Science (1989) *Special schools for pupils with EBD*, Circular 23/89. London: Department of Education and Science.

Department of Health (2000) *Promoting health for looked-after children: a guide to healthcare planning, assessment and monitoring*. London: Department of Health.

Galloway, D. (1990) *Pupil welfare and counselling: an approach to personal and social education across the curriculum.* London: Longman.

Galloway, D., Armstrong, D., and Tomlinson, S. (1994) *The assessment of special educational needs.* London: Longman.

Goleman, D. (1995) *Emotional intelligence.* London: Bloomsbury.

Greenhalgh, P. (1994) *Emotional growth and learning.* London: Routledge.

Hallam, S. and Castle, F. (1999) *Evaluation of the behaviour and discipline pilot projects (1996–1999).* Research Report, RR163. London: Department for Education and Employment.

Hargreaves, D, Hester, S., and Mellor, F. (1975) *Deviance in classrooms.* London: Routledge & Kegan Paul.

HMI (1978) *Behavioural units: a survey of special units for pupils with behavioural problems.* London: Department of Education and Science.

Mental Health Foundation (1999) *Bright futures: promoting children and young people's mental health.* London: Mental Health Foundation.

Ministry of Education (1955) *Report of the committee on maladjusted children* (the Underwood Report). London: HMSO.

Munn, P., Lloyd, G. and Cullen, M. (2000) *Alternatives to School Exclusion.* London: Paul Chapman.

NHS Health Advisory Service (1995) *Together we stand–the commissioning, role and management of CAMHS.* London: HMSO.

OfSTED (1995) *Annual Report of Her Majesty's Chief Inspector of Schools.* London: OfSTED.

OfSTED (1999) *Principles into practice: effective education for pupils with EBD.* London: OfSTED.

Parsons, C. (1999) *Education, exclusion and citizenship.* London: Routledge.

Powers, S. (1996) *The pastoral and the academic.* London: Cassell.

Redl, F. (1966) *When we deal with children.* New York: Free Press.

Schostak, J. (1983) *Maladjusted schooling: deviance, social control and individuality in secondary schooling.* Lewes: Falmer Press.

Stoll, L. and Fink, D. (1994) School Effectiveness and School Improvement: Voices from the Field. *School Effectiveness and School Improvement,* **5** (2), 147–77.

Thomas, G. and Glenny, G. (2000) Emotional and behavioural difficulties: bogus needs in a false category. *Discourse: Studies in the Cultural Politics of Education,* **21** (2), 283–98.

Visser, J. (1980) *Issues involved in the provision in the secondary school of school-based units for children with behaviour problems.* Unpublished M Ed thesis University College Cardiff.

Visser, J., Daniels, H., and Cole, T. (ed.) *International perspectives on inclusive education: emotional and behavioural difficulties in mainstream schools.* London: Sage/JAI, in press.

Wilson, M. and Evans, M. (1980) *Education of disturbed pupils.* London: Methuen.

Chapter 8

Partnerships between health and local authorities

Michael Kerfoot

The issue of what constitutes a child or adolescent mental health problem is difficult to determine. Concepts of health and illness are influenced by, among other things, physical, psychological, and social processes, and are dynamic and subject to change. Mental health problems arise from diverse sets of circumstances and from widely varying contexts. Often a problem can be detected through changes in a child's emotional state (increasing anxiety or distress) or through changes in behaviour towards other people or property. Features of a problem that facilitate the assessment and understanding of what is happening include the intensity and seriousness of the problem, its frequency of occurrence, its duration over time, and its effects on the child and those close to the child. When mental health problems become severe, persistent, or associated with other problems, they may be referred to as a 'disorder'. A mental disorder is, therefore, a mental health problem that has become severe or persistent, and seriously disrupts normal functioning.

The social dimension to understanding mental health is important because it acknowledges the diverse contexts in which children and young people develop, and attempts to understand and address the issues that arise from these. It offers a unique contribution to the multidisciplinary diagnostic process by presenting the social model of functioning and dysfunction at individual, familial, and societal levels. It considers roles and relationships, and particularly the structures within which these develop and function, and the influence that environmental factors such as low employment opportunities, poor neighbourhoods, and inadequate or inappropriate public service provision have upon them. It considers the ways in which the social mix in neighbourhoods, in terms of social class, economic stability, and ethnic and cultural diversity, reflects the power relationships locally and how particular groups become prominent or powerful while others remain powerless. These wider societal influences are mediated through families and may have a profound influence upon the mental health of children and young people. Social services departments have traditionally been the first port of call for people experiencing 'social' problems, a term that encompasses a wide range and diversity of predicaments.

It is self-evident that social service agencies and educational establishments will encounter many examples of mental health problems in young people and steps may be in place to assist and support staff in helping those children. A difficulty arises around determining whether or not a problem has become a disorder and how, when, and where to seek specialist help. Social services staff have always had the potential to be high users of CAMHS for those children who are 'looked after' but, in practice, the likelihood is that a referral will only be made when the child has become unmanageable or when some other crisis has occurred. In view of this it is probably fair to say that the children usually referred to specialist services by social services and education, often have a serious and entrenched disorder. These agencies will generally have coped with their difficult children for as long as they can, containing the problem while simultaneously trying to think of management strategies and interventions. The decision to refer to specialist services rarely occurs at an opportune time and is frequently driven by a crisis of some kind. From the specialist service side the prospect is hardly an encouraging one: the child's disorder is likely to be acute or even chronic, a number of interventions will have been tried without success and there may well be quite unrealistic expectations about what specialist referral can achieve.

Policy background

Disturbances in child and adolescent mental health range in degree and complexity from very mild to extremely severe. A growing body of evidence indicates that the number of children and young people with mental health problems is rising and that about 20% of all children and young people, aged 0–18 years, suffer from a wide range of disorders to varying degrees. The Audit Commission Report *Children in mind* (1999) identified a number of groups of children as being at greater risk of developing mental health problems. They reported that:

40% were living with only one natural parent compared with around 21% of all families with dependent children in Great Britain in 1996;

34% were living in families where the main breadwinner was unemployed, a figure greatly in excess of the national average;

27% of children has some form of learning disability;

19% were living with a parent who had mental illness;

9% of children were 'looked after' by the local authority as compared with 0.5% in the general population.

We also know that the following groups of children are particularly vulnerable to the development of mental health problems when compared with other children (Department of Health 1995). These include:

children with emotional and behavioural difficulties;

young people who have recently left local authority 'care';

young offenders and children from a criminal background;

children with physical disability and/or sensory impairment;

children who have been abused;

children excluded from school;

children with a chronic physical illness;

children of parents with a substance abuse problem;

children who have experienced sudden loss or trauma;

children who are refugees.

When these findings are viewed in the context of factors more likely to occur in families from areas of social deprivation or disadvantage, one can see clearly the link between the government's social inclusion strategies and the drive to improve child and adolescent mental health.

Recognition of the need to modernize and make improvements to CAMHS is reflected in the large number of policy documents and directives issued in recent years, and culminating in special funding being made available over a 3-year period through Modernization Funds and the Mental Health Grant for Child and Adolescent Mental Health Services. This sets out the requirements on health and local authorities to submit jointly agreed strategies and to focus on improvements in specialist multidisciplinary services to ensure that there are sufficient trained CAMHS professionals with an appropriate range of skills organized in a manner that avoids professional isolation. The number of recent reviews and circulars specific to CAMHS or with a direct relevance perhaps says more than anything about previous service neglect and the urgency of action required to repair and improve the service. This emphasis, however, is only part of a total strategy to improve the health, welfare, and educational opportunities of children and young people across all agencies as envisioned in the quality protects initiative in social services departments and the development of behavioural support services and pupil referral units in education authorities.

In addition, the requirement for 'joined-up' thinking and multi-agency strategies is a key part of government policy on social exclusion, a policy that will address itself to the issue through an attack on problems such as low income, low skills, poor physical and mental health, family breakdown, bad housing and high crime rates. Regeneration schemes, health and education action zones, and programmes such as Sure Start are examples of this policy in action.

Bringing together health, social services, and education

Fragmentation of provision for children has meant that there have been many gaps in services and separate planning procedures within authorities has led to overlapping or duplication of services. The picture that emerged was one of three separate structures, each with its own policy directives and resources, working in the same context but independently of each other. For some children and families this must have created a chaotic and unfathomable mix of personnel and practices, and with few points of contact where parents or carers might clarify plans and procedures or register their own views about the situation.

A number of key documents, notably the NHS Health Advisory Service thematic review of child and adolescent mental health services *Together we stand* (NHS Health Advisory Service 1995) and the Health of the Nation Key Handbook on child and adolescent mental health (Department of Health 1995b), highlighted the need for health authorities and local authorities to work together to provide comprehensive mental health services for children and adolescents. Critical to the notion of 'working together' was the concept of joint commissioning of services between these two sectors. The impetus for moving towards joint commissioning arose, in part, from governmental interest in promoting the provision of comprehensive services for children and adolescents. As a lever towards ensuring that joint activity occurs, measures to encourage sectors to engage in joint planning were introduced as part of the performance management targets by the NHS Executive. These enable the executive to judge to what extent health authorities have been meeting with the local authority sector in joint planning forums. On the social services side, the Audit Commission and the Social Services Inspectorate have scrutinized annual childrens service plans produced by social services departments, for evidence of joint activity with health and education. Guidance for health and local authorities on moving towards joint working, and eventually joint commissioning, had been made available (Department of Health 1995a), and subsequently a development pack for joint commissioning was produced (Gorman 1996). However, getting authorities to move from the stage of aspirational statements based on published 'guidance', to 'real action', is a major endeavour and, as will become apparent, is one to be approached with some trepidation.

It is possible to bring different sectors of the health and local authority services spectrum together to engage in sustained joint activity regarding children and adolescents, and the Department of Health has urged health authorities to develop partnerships with local authorities for this purpose (Department of Health 1998). In 1997, the University of Manchester reported to the Department of Health on a development project that had been commissioned by the department regarding joint commissioning (Kerfoot and Huxley 1995). The original commission had been to write 'guidance' for health and local authorities but subsequent contact with authorities discouraged us from pursuing this and we presented an alternative proposal to the Department of Health. In this proposal we agreed to work with a number of identified authorities (health, social services, education and voluntary sector) around the country to help them towards joint working. To help us identify authorities whose thinking was already moving towards joint working we were permitted to interrogate the database established by Zarrina Kurtz and colleagues at South Thames Health Authority, and which formed the substance of their national review of child and adolescent mental health services (Kurtz *et al.* 1994). On the basis of this evidence, we made initial visits to seven authorities and these enabled us to connect with a variety of service commissioners and providers in a number of settings. Within each visit, therefore, meetings were arranged with social services, health authorities, provider trusts, and education authorities, these being the main stakeholders in the joint commissioning field. We then formulated a development plan for work with three of these authorities in the belief that undertaking development work, rather than formulating guidance, would generate insights about the key elements in joint commissioning, and provide valuable clues towards the promotion of joint working. The selected authorities were equally concerned not to be given further guidance since this would be occurring in a 'planning vacuum' and they welcomed the prospect of having external consultation, and monitoring of their work towards joint commissioning.

The three authorities selected included a county area, a Metropolitan Borough and a London Borough. Six whole day sessions were provided to each authority over a 9-months period. All interested parties were invited to the initial meetings in order to establish the constitution and membership of the working group, and its preliminary agenda. Each authority had issues and problems that were specific to its own geographical area and current service configuration, and the working group had, of necessity, to devote some of its time to addressing some of these issues in order to clear the way for developmental work. As is usually the case, each authority brings its own agenda into a joint working group and, if not dealt with, activity becomes diverted into important but peripheral issues, and the energy for developing the CAMHS joint working initiative becomes dissipated.

In order to structure and summarize the information and insights gained from the project we adopted an approach suggested by Grant (1995). Grant analyses the conditions required for organizations to be successful in achieving their primary goals. In the case of joint working we are concerned with the ways in which a multiple set of agencies can successfully deliver an integrated and comprehensive service for children and adolescents with mental health problems. The analysis used by Grant is useful in enabling agencies to move beyond the very early stages in which most of them have found themselves, in relation to joint working. He argues that there are four key aspects to the development and successful implementation of strategy. These are: having clear goals (often expressed in very simple terms); understanding of the external environment; appreciation of internal strengths and weaknesses; and effective implementation. To date there has been no evidence of CAMHS development having been seen in these terms, yet if this approach reflects the collective evidence of success in other fields, it ought to be applicable to CAMHS too. Grant's key points, as applied to CAMHS, are summarized in Table 8.1 and emphasize the importance of developing a strategy for taking forward CAMHS service development.

In addition to applying the key features of successful strategies, Grant distinguishes between corporate and business strategies. The former is concerned with the overall scope of the enterprise, and in CAMHS terms, means *all the stakeholder agencies coming together to have a corporate view of the prospective shape of the service*. The latter is concerned with how to actually implement the joint approach once established, and is sometimes referred to as the 'functional strategy'. In many instances agencies were unable to move to a co-ordinated functional approach because of the absence of a corporate agreement. Indeed one might locate authorities in terms of a continuum of strategic development, from those who on the one hand are still unable to agree the corporate approach, through those who have achieved this state and have developed service specifications, to those who are experimenting in different kinds of implementation (see Table 8.2). The first group 'worst' are operating the functional implementation of services on an entirely separate basis, coming together only to respond to crises in budgetary or inter-agency matters. The second group, 'developing', are beginning to align their services to improve delivery and achieve the corporate objectives, and may have established mechanisms for achieving this. The third group, 'best', not only have joint commissioning structures in place, but may also have joint budgetary arrangements, and jointly operated services with single referral points and unitary assessment procedures.

The corporate, business and functional strategies need to be in harmony in order to deliver an effective CAMH service. The corporate approach can be jointly agreed but this must not be

Table 8.1 Conditions required for organizational achievement of primary goals

- A clear statement of the goals set for CAMHS strategies.
- An analysis of the strengths and weaknesses of inter-agency and intra-agency work as it applies to CAMHS.
- A description of the ways in which agencies are responding to the external environment, in this case to central government and purchasing initiatives.
- A description of examples of the effective implementation of joint commissioning and joint service development at a local level.

Table 8.2 A joint commissioning spectrum

	Worst	Developing	Best
Corporate strategy	None	Interim	Agreed
Agency (business) strategy	Independent Isolated	Aligning	Co-ordinated Consistent
Functional strategy	Crisis-led	Partial co-operation (e.g. At Tier 4)	Joint projects Budget management

at odds with agency's (business) approach, and both must be consistent with the functional strategy which will inevitably include both joint operations and service alignments.

In Grant's model the strategy is located between the agencies and the external environment (as in Fig. 8.1). It reveals the need for inter-agency arrangements in order to develop the corporate strategy, and lists a number of the external factors to which the strategy has to respond. How they can do this will be considered later when examples from practice will be given. Strategy forms a link between agencies and their environment. The strategy development and the development of a service specification involves a number of decisions and choices about priorities for action. In Fig. 8.1 the strategy has to include decisions about which of the many environmental imperatives it is going to respond to, and in which order. Local circumstances will determine which of these demands is more pressing. It may be, for example, that inspectors have reported unfavourably on progress to joint commissioning or the development of children's service plans, and so this assumes the number one priority. Alternatively, it may be that out-of-borough placement budgets of the main agencies are under severe pressure and so the decision is taken to start with agreements about Tier 4 complex cases. There may be such demand pressures that functional strategies to deal with these have to be put into place first, even before a full strategy can be developed. Finally, the purchasing intentions of social services, health authorities and fund-holding GPs may need to be made explicit (and aligned) before the priorities within the functional strategy can be put into chronological sequence.

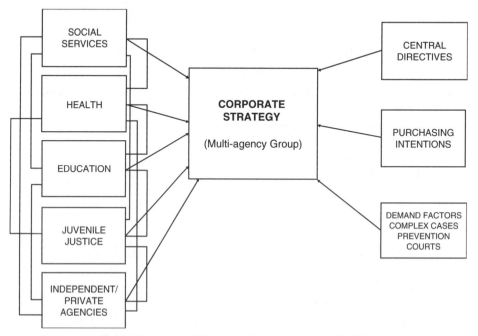

Fig. 8.1 Strategy and the external environment in CAMHS.

I want now to consider in more detail, and with some practical examples, each of the aspects of development outlined in Table 8.1.

Aspect 1: clear goals

In order to have a corporate approach in such a complex area as CAMHS it is necessary to define the scope of the strategy. To illustrate the complexity, one authority in our study had developed separate approaches for each of the following services but did not address any mental health needs in the process. The service plans related to: children in need; children with disabilities; early years; child protection; looked-after children; education of children in need; private fostering; young people 16–21; adoption; and youth justice. No real inter-agency approach was evident in the authority's documentation and it was clearly not yet ready to proceed with development work on joint commissioning of CAMHS. A number of agencies had intended to work with us in the developmental phase of the project but then withdrew once the scope and focus of the project was explained in detail. Interestingly, the planning material forwarded to us by these authorities contained hardly any material about the goals of the service or about the joint approach. Examples of goals formulated by authorities, and which are insufficiently clear include:

> 'There needs to be further consultation with GPs on the shape of the service they would like to see.'
> 'Need to explore the possibility of expanding the role of primary and community services especially for primary prevention and early secondary prevention and management.'
> 'Need to improve liaison services.'
> 'The service should be integrated with other services dealing with this client group. This will include primary care, child health, paediatrics, adult psychiatry, and substance misuse services.'
> 'The service should be accessible by users in terms of location, time of operation, ease of referral routes and equity.'
> 'The service should ensure that all agencies work together in the best interests of the child by sharing resources and skills with each other.'

As a set of 'aspirational' statements these are acceptable but as a set of goals for service development they are unclear, vague, tentative, over-inclusive, and over-ambitious. Agencies that are ready for joint development work have usually worked through issues concerning resource allocation, service demand, staff roles and responsibilities, prioritizing patient need, and preventive work, so that they have an informed view on these aspects of service, and are often ready to move to service specification (the functional strategy stage). At this stage goals become more clearly specified and the following are examples of this greater clarity of purpose:

> 'To maintain the child within the family setting wherever possible and when in-patient admission is required to keep this brief.'
> 'To produce agreed care plans, defining the needs to be met, and identify the practitioner with lead responsibility and a named key worker.'
> 'To strengthen the multidisciplinary team by appointing new staff.'
> 'To establish a central referral point with a clear referral protocol.'
> 'To provide a staff development profile for all professionals in CAMHS.'
> 'To establish the integration of the clinical psychology services.'

It can be argued that it may be necessary to go though the stages of more global agreement before greater specificity can be achieved, and that even these more clearly stated goals are still not sufficiently specific for implementation purposes. A critical element in achieving goal specificity is about defining the scope of the strategy. It is important to establish that the strategy covers Tiers 1–4, but that within each tier it will be important to identify the kinds of problem that are to be given priority.

Aspect 2: strengths and weaknesses of inter-agency work

Regular and intensive work with joint working groups revealed a number of problems and issues which, though not insurmountable, proved to be serious obstacles to progress in joint working and joint commissioning. These have been grouped under the headings of 'political/organizational', 'prioritization', 'financial', 'professional', and 'partnership'.

Political/organizational

Co-terminosity of boundaries greatly facilitates joint activity. The creation of unitary authorities has produced boundary problems for some authorities who were considering joint working.

Internal re-organization within health authorities has meant discontinuity in the personnel representing the health view on joint working groups.

Prioritization

Too great a focus on adults and community care, to the exclusion of children and adolescents. CAMHS is not regarded as a priority.

Some authorities withdraw from priority-setting and allow their agenda to become crisis-driven.

Priority setting needs to be a joint activity otherwise it generates disagreement and non-co-operation.

The volume of child protection work means that this often dominates the agenda for child and adolescent services.

The volume of demand for court assessments seems to take precedence over other priority areas.

Financial

No identified budget for CAMHS spending.

Lack of investment by commissioners in the CAMHS infrastructure.

Clear need for extra resources either as bridging monies to see providers through reorganization of services, or as more general development funding.

Professional

Changing services or shifting the balance of resources can result in a loss of control for some personnel.

The shortage of child psychiatrists has produced recruitment problems in some areas and an unavoidable skills gap.

There is no common language, terminology or usage between professionals.

The skills issues associated with the different tiers of service in CAMHS must be addressed.

There is a need to link with other professionals and to acknowledge and utilise their abilities and influence (e.g. the influence of schools around bullying policy is undervalued).

Partnership

A low resource base and increasing waiting lists leads to mutual blaming between purchasers and providers.

Purchasers need to utilize the knowledge providers have in order to inform service planning, purchasing intentions, and subsequent contracting.

Joint Children's Service Panels are a good model of joint working.

Progress is difficult and time is wasted on skirmishing where there are persistent or unaddressed inter-agency problems, and lack of trust.

'Top of the organization' ownership is essential if the initiative is to be driven successfully, and a real sense of partnership is to develop.

Uneven representation on joint working groups often represents uneven commitment by the partners, and the debate can be hampered if there is poor understanding of the legal and financial basis for joint working. It follows that all representatives must be of equivalent status and must have the power to commit resources.

The problems and issues summarized here are familiar to many authorities but, interestingly, do not always stifle progress in all areas. For example, important ground work has occurred quite often in a policy vacuum at field level, anticipating a time when an agreed policy would legitimise the activities that were already taking place.

Aspect 3: responding to the external environment

The external environment often impinges upon authorities in the form of initiatives or directives from central government and in order to respond to these effectively health authorities and local authorities need to establish a forum on child and adolescent mental health services. A CAMHS strategic group would address some of the issues listed under 'partnership' in the previous section, but the components of joint commissioning that such a group can address should include:

(1) joint needs assessment and service mapping;

(2) development of a joint strategy for CAMHS;

(3) joint service planning;

(4) care planning for individual cases;

(5) joint commissioning; and

(6) evaluation and monitoring of services.

The joint commissioning framework needs to address all four tiers of CAMHS, although in practice Tier 1, which has a strong preventive focus, and Tier 4, which caters for extremely complex cases, are often considered after Tiers 2 and 3.

Joint strategy development needs to be preceded by a needs assessment so that service requirements can be reliably and efficiently prioritized. For many years, mental health services for children have been developed incrementally with little attention to the needs of the local population but in recent years attempts have been made to develop more rational ways of planning. In particular, the information required to develop a needs-led child mental health service has been documented, as have the criteria to be considered in determining priorities (Harrington *et al.* 1999). A good needs assessment can take up considerable time and resources and will inevitably be ongoing while other activities are progressing. It is an essential element of the process of developing a strategy, although it may take some time for a strategic direction to become clear, particularly where there is an inability to agree shared priorities or where there are fears of being bound to a strategy that will inevitably run over a 5-year cycle. An alternative way of proceeding with strategy development is to begin with the types of outcomes that are desired and a means of measuring these. Once agreement has been reached on these measures, the rest of the development of the strategy works back to the means required to deliver the outcomes, and the resource and service organization that is needed, and a determination of the priority groups. Joint planning and joint commissioning are key tasks for the CAMHS strategic group and clearly the membership of this group will be critical in terms of representation and status of members. All 'stakeholders' should be represented from health authorities, health trusts, social services departments, local education authorities, and voluntary sector agencies, and all representatives should be, insofar as is possible, of equal status within their respective organizations. In particular, representatives should have the authority and power to commit resources if a purposeful dialogue is to ensue, and the business of the group is to move forward. Within the strategic group, the roles of 'leader' and 'driver' are of particular importance. The leadership role is one that can be assumed alongside other professional responsibilities, since it relates particularly to managing the business of the group during its meetings. The role of the 'driver', which should be seen as distinct from that of the 'leader', assumes its particular importance outside of the formal group meetings. The 'driver' is charged with responsibility for 'driving' the whole CAMHS joint initiative. This is the person who works to keep the group functioning jointly, and who tries to ensure that the decisions taken within the formal group meetings are translated into action and followed through between meetings. The role is essential precisely because motivation, initiative, and application are likely to fluctuate markedly without the presence of a driving force to back up the formal meetings. Clear evidence of the commitment to joint working can be seen in those stakeholders who have jointly recognized that the 'driver' needs to be a dedicated post, and have then agreed to jointly fund such a post. Critical to the success of a 'driver' post is the postholder's ability to develop a common language for transactions within the CAMHS group. Professional terminology can be used to confuse as well as convince, but a shared language means that all the stakeholders are clear about what the issues are, and what they are signing up to.

Aspect 4: examples of effective joint responses

Service saturation factors are an important component of strategic thinking and there are several external stressors to CAMHS that, if unchecked, are a potential source of saturation within a service. For example, service personnel need to take an early decision on how they will manage a high volume of referrals in a particular problem category such as 'conduct disorder' or, perhaps, how they will manage the demand from other sectors such as social services, for consultation, advice or opinion. Conduct-disordered adolescents, for example, often have complex needs coupled with a history of being 'batted' from service to service, simply because their problems are so established and entrenched at the time of referral, there is no straightforward solution to their difficulties. Examples from practice of positive responses to these demands might include:

(1) setting up a joint social services and education panel to respond to children and adolescents with complex needs and to facilitate appropriate placement based on health, education, and social care needs; or

(2) regular input from a psychiatrist or clinical psychologist regarding the management of young people with complex needs who are in social services residential provision.

With regard to child protection, few social services departments consider themselves to have the skills in-house to undertake effective therapeutic work with these children and their families. If it is to be effective, such work will be time-consuming and will place quite long-term demands on those who undertake it. The strict legislative framework within which child protection services operate means that all these cases have to be given priority over other work, and the treatment arm is the most poorly served part of child protection services. A positive response from practice to the scarcity and long waiting-lists for treatment in specialist child protection units might be for social services to undertake a skills inventory among its child care workers. A number of authorities are beginning to rediscover the value of good child care practice and family casework, as evidenced in the skills and talents of its own workforce, rather than assuming that automatic referral to a more specialised resource is always necessary. Finally, the demand for psychiatric assessments and reports for courts has increased dramatically in the last decade and can result in a serious drain on scarce time within CAMHS. Since many court cases referred for psychiatric assessment are in adjournment, there is some urgency to the task and this has to be accommodated alongside the ever-present waiting-list and within the already over-stretched resources. Creative responses from practice have included, for example, involving magistrates and court personnel in social services information days to brief them on the scope of existing assessments, and the special circumstances in which a psychiatric opinion should be sought. Court liaison committees are another useful forum in which excessively high demands for court reports can be addressed, and constructive solutions sought.

Increasingly, service providers are recognizing that the mental health needs of seriously disturbed children are being neglected and that fragmented services contribute to this neglect. A response to service fragmentation, and one that has attracted growing interest in the USA, is to have integrated child mental health services. A wide range of developments in case (care) management for emotionally and behaviourally disturbed children has taken place in the USA and a number of programmes have been established using intensive case management services to co-ordinate the community treatment of children and adolescents with emotional disturbance and a need for long-term care (Wagner 1987; Cheung 1991; Dollard 1991; Fertman 1991; LeCroy 1992).

Although the large health and social care institutions in the UK appear to be relatively homogenous and fragmentation has not occurred on the scale that is has in the USA, there is, however, fragmentation both within and between the major health and social care services. It is appropriate, therefore, to consider care management as a possible solution to the same problems of fragmentation and multiple purchasers found in the USA. This is especially true for children with severe emotional and behavioural disorders spanning the age range from infancy to young adulthood. When considered longitudinally in this way, the fragmentation of care for this age group becomes all too apparent. Within services, care management models are deployed on only the most difficult and costly cases and, therefore, caseload sizes are deliberately small and care management services are clinical, intensive, and expensive, although not as costly as expensive residential solutions. Services are based on individual assessment and care planning, and when compared to the cost of 'out of town' residential placements, care management is likely to be the preferred option. Effective care management systems require integrated planning mechanisms and integrated funding arrangements, and there are clear links here with joint commissioning initiatives. Mechanisms that clearly facilitate the development of joint activity and joint funding arrangements, perhaps through pooled budgets, would, therefore, be a key feature of care management programmes. Thus far there have been few studies evaluating the effectiveness of care management programmes when compared to other service models but the widespread adoption of the model in US services would indicate that cost savings have accrued as a result of its introduction and that case outcomes are as good, if not better, than under the previous 'placement' system. Research is, however, needed into the style, form, content, and outcome of care management programmes for children and adolescents, and its absence highlights the need for demonstration projects to be funded in those areas where a joint approach is reasonably established, and is working well.

In the past, there has been little evidence of co-ordinated or aligned thinking between health and local authorities regarding the mental health needs of children. Services for children with emotional or behavioural problems have been especially vulnerable to short-sighted and unilateral planning as a result of failure to reconcile differences between agencies, and between the professionals within the agencies providing the services. The drive from the Department of Health urging health authorities to develop partnerships with local authorities around the definition of 'need', and the development of a joint children's strategy to meet this, has been particularly welcome. With appropriate representation and purposeful management of the strategy group, the planning process could become an effective vehicle for change.

References

Audit Commission (1999) *Children in mind.* London: Audit Commission.

Cheung, K.M. (1991) Competency-based evaluation of case-management skills in child sexual abuse intervention. *Child Welfare,* **70**, 425–35.

Department of Health (1995a) *Practical guidance on joint commissioning for project leaders.* London: HMSO.

Department of Health (1995b) *A handbook on child and adolescent mental health.* London: HMSO.

Department of Health (1998) *Our healthier nation: a contract for health.* London: The Stationery Office.

Dollard, N. (1991) *Evaluation of New York State's children and youth intensive case management programme.* Albany: New York State Office of Mental Health.

Fertman, C.I. (1991) Aftercare for teenagers: matching services and needs. *Journal of Alcohol and Drug Education,* **36**, 1–11.

Gorman, P. (1996) *A development pack for joint commissioning.* Wetherby: Department of Health.

Grant, R. (1995) *Contemporary strategic analysis.* London: Blackwell.

Harrington, R., Kerfoot, M., and Verduyn, C. (1999) Developing needs led child and adolescent mental health services: issues and prospects. *European Child & Adolescent Psychiatry,* **8**, 1–10.

Kerfoot, M. and Huxley, P. (1995) *The Personal Social Services Contribution to the Joint Commissioning of Child and Adolescent Mental Health Services.* A Report to the Social Services Inspectorate. University of Manchester: Mental Health Social Work Research Unit.

Kurtz, Z., Thornes, R., and Wolkind, S. (1994) *Services for the mental health of children and young people in England: a national review.* London: South Thames RHA.

Le Croy, C.W. (1992) Enhancing the delivery of effective mental health services to children. *Social Work,* **37**, 225–31.

NHS Health Advisory Service (1995) *Together we stand: the commissioning, role and management of child and adolescent mental health services.* London: HMSO.

Wagner, W.G. (1987) Child sexual abuse: a multidisciplinary approach to case management. *Journal of Counselling and Development,* **65**, 435–9.

Chapter 9

What is best value? The health economic evidence

Sarah Byford and Martin Knapp

Introduction

Demands for economic insights

Growing awareness of the need to improve, not only the effectiveness but also the cost-effectiveness of health care, social care, and other services and interventions, has generated various demands for economic evidence (summarized in Box 9.1) in all sectors of society. One set of demands has been for descriptions of the resource consequences of different illnesses, problems, or behaviours. An associated demand is for measures of the overall cost impact of a particular health problem. In the child and adolescent mental health field, for example, recognition of the often quite considerable effects of some behaviour problems of childhood and adolescence has encouraged a number of such cost studies. However, whilst service utilization descriptions can be informative, this rather reductionist focus on costs can be misleading and is unable to provide evidence upon which to base 'best value' assessments.

Of more interest are economic evaluations of particular policy or practice interventions that explore costs and effects (outcomes) simultaneously. Such evaluations generate evidence of cost-effectiveness that can guide decision-makers on how they might make more efficient use of the resources under their control. In other words, they explore how to achieve better outcomes for young people and their families for a given level of resources or how to minimize expenditure whilst maintaining the same outcomes. In addition, there are demands for information on the equity implications of these different distributions of resources across the population.

Each of these demands for economic evidence is as pertinent in the child and adolescent mental health area as in any other. Given the complexity of supports and services used by some young people and their families, it is not surprising that there should be calls for basic descriptive studies that can begin to map the patterns of utilization and the associated costs. Nor is it surprising, given the widely acknowledged scarcity of resources, that budget-holders are continually on the lookout for more efficient treatments and service arrangements.

Economics: the science of choice

Economics is explicitly concerned with issues of resource scarcity, resource allocation, and the consequences of different distributions of resources for individuals, organizations, and society more generally. Every care system in the world operates under conditions of scarce resources (whether skilled staff, buildings, drugs, expertise, etc.) relative to the needs or demands for

Box 9.1 Demands for economic insights

What are the service and cost implications of mental health problems in childhood, both now and in the future?

What services are available for young people with mental health problems and their families and what do they cost?

What personal, family, or situational circumstances in childhood increase or reduce the need for services?

Is the money spent on child and adolescent mental health services related to treatment effectiveness?

Which services for children and adolescents with mental health problems are the most cost-effective?

What is the impact of mental health services on the use of services elsewhere, for example social and education services?

What are the distributional impacts of funding mental health services for young people? In other words, which young people benefit?

Will higher investment in child and adolescent mental health services today reap longer-term benefits?

them and has always done so. However, questions concerning the best use of scarce resources are more frequently voiced today, or certainly more explicitly stated, reflecting a more widespread recognition of scarcity and a greater willingness to target services where needs are believed or assessed to be greatest. Economics is the study of how these priority-setting choices can be made—how to improve what can be achieved from available resources in the face of scarcity.

Performance criteria

Four performance criteria dominate the theoretical underpinnings, conceptual structures, and empirical endeavours of economic evaluation. These are summarized in Box 9.2. Economy and effectiveness are important issues in evaluation, but fundamentally, economists are more interested in efficiency and equity, since the study of costs in isolation of the effects, or of the effects whilst ignoring the costs, is not enough to answer questions of resource allocation. Indeed, the definition of an economic evaluation demands that we look at both the cost and outcome sides of a health system, social care service, educational policy and so on.

Chapter structure

This chapter describes the purpose and methods of economic evaluation and the application of these techniques to the evaluation of child and adolescent mental health services (CAMHS). The next section introduces the main modes of economic evaluation and some more descriptive tools. The third section runs through three areas of application of these techniques: descriptions of service utilization and cost patterns, evaluations of

Box 9.2 Economy, effectiveness, efficiency, and equity

Economy relates to the saving of resources. The pursuit of economy requires detailed and accurate cost information but pays no heed to the impact of lower expenditure on individuals, their families, or the wider society.

Effectiveness, on the other hand, pays no particular regard to costs but relates to the enhancement of health or quality of life or other chosen objectives.

Efficiency combines both cost and effectiveness and involves reducing the cost of producing a stated level of outcome or effectiveness, or improving the level of effectiveness or the volume and quality of outcomes achieved under fixed budgets.

Equity refers to the fairness of an allocation and is particularly associated with the targeting of services on needs.

interventions, and long-term follow-up studies. The concluding section considers future directions for research and touches on some of the design challenges that should be addressed to improve the quality of economic evaluations in this field. Throughout the chapter we use empirical examples from the UK to illustrate the concepts and arguments presented, although the methods employed are readily transferable to other systems and contexts.

Economic evaluation

What is an economic evaluation?

An economic evaluation involves a systematic attempt to identify, measure, and compare all relevant costs and effects (outcomes) of alternative policies or interventions. It must, therefore, fulfil two basic requirements: the measurement of both costs and outcomes, and the comparison of two or more interventions.

By this definition, comparing the costs of one treatment with another, without any evidence of outcomes for children or families, does not constitute an economic evaluation. Such an exercise might be an interesting description of service utilization patterns and associated costs, and it might be conducted with considerable skill, but it does not provide enough information to assist service professionals, managers, or others facing the choice between two or more alternatives, for it tells them nothing about the outcome consequences of choosing one over the others. Similarly, calculating the costs and outcomes of a single service could be interesting but cannot be classed as an economic evaluation, unless those costs and outcomes are compared with equivalent data for another service, or even compared with the option of 'doing nothing'.

Economists have developed a number of evaluation tools, meeting both of the requirements listed. Those developed to evaluate healthcare interventions and policies provide an excellent starting point for work in the field of child and adolescent mental health. Among the better textbooks in the field are Drummond *et al.* (1997) and Gold *et al.* (1996). A useful introduction to economic evaluation can be found in a series of brief papers by Robinson (1993).

Methods of economic evaluation

All methods of economic evaluation measure costs in monetary units. They differ, however, in their approach to measuring the outcomes.

Cost-benefit analysis

The best known, but most rarely conducted method of economic evaluation in the mental health field, is cost-benefit analysis (CBA), which measures both costs and outcomes in the same monetary units. The CBA approach is unique among economic evaluation methods in that it addresses the extent to which a treatment or policy is socially worthwhile in the broadest sense. If benefits exceed costs, the evaluation would recommend providing the service or treatment, and vice versa. With two or more alternatives, the evaluation would recommend the one with the greatest net benefit (benefit minus cost) as the most efficient.

CBAs are intrinsically attractive, but due to the difficulties associated with valuing outcomes in monetary terms, conducting them in any area—including CAMHS—is problematic.

Methodologies are being developed by economists working in proximate fields, which aim to obtain direct valuations of health outcomes from users, relatives, or the general public. One example is that of 'willingness-to-pay' techniques, where an individual states the amount they would be prepared to pay (hypothetically) to achieve a given health state or health gain. Olsen and Smith (2001) offer a (cautionary) review of CBAs in health care more broadly, opining that the theoretical robustness of the approach is still running a little way ahead of the empirical achievements of many studies to date.

Cost-effectiveness analysis

Cost-effectiveness analysis (CEA) is a more commonly adopted approach to the economic evaluation of mental health services and is concerned with ensuring that the resources allocated to, say, the child and adolescent mental health sector are used to best effect. CEA is usually employed to help decision-makers choose between alternative interventions available to specific user groups. CEA involves the measurement of outcomes in a single 'natural' or 'disease-specific' measure such as level of depression or family functioning. Where one intervention is found to dominate the others (i.e. is more effective and less costly, more effective and equally costly, or equally effective and less costly), relative cost-effectiveness is straightforward. However, where one intervention is found to produce greater effectiveness for greater cost, an incremental cost-effectiveness analysis is required, involving the calculation of the ratio of additional costs to additional outcomes produced by one intervention in comparison to another. This cost-effectiveness ratio can then be compared to other interventions employing the same measure of effect, and preference should be given to those with the lower incremental cost-effectiveness ratios.

CEA is easily transferable to CAMHS and some examples are provided below, but CEA does have its weaknesses. First, it is impossible to make comparisons across a diverse spectrum of interventions competing for a share of a finite budget. CAMHS are extremely varied and the aims and outcomes of services provided will often differ and be multiple. Comparisons of cost-effectiveness using disease-specific units can only be made between interventions whose outcomes can be measured on the same scale. For example, a CEA would not help us choose between spending more on drug treatments for hyperactive children or interventions for self-harming adolescents, since outcomes measured are likely to differ. Second, it is difficult to capture all possible effects of an intervention on a single outcome scale. CAMHS will often influence many areas of an individual's life and the lives of other family members, but combining costs with multi-dimensional outcomes measured on a number of different scales makes interpretation difficult, particularly if improvements are seen on some scales but not others. For this reason, a CEA will often be based on the outcome measure considered to be of greatest importance to the purpose of the evaluation (the primary outcome), requiring some judgement to be made about the relative value of the alternative outcomes of interest.

Cost-consequences analysis

Where the omission of other outcomes could be misleading, studies may present a range of outcomes (or consequences) alongside the costs, using cost-consequences analysis (CCA). Rather than one single ratio, a number of ratios of outcome to costs are presented, allowing the decision-maker to weigh up the different outcomes in relation to the costs and to make a decision on the basis of value judgements about the relative importance of each outcome scale presented. Although CCA is clearly limited by an inability to rank interventions in terms of cost-effectiveness, the method does allow policies and practices to be evaluated in a way that comes quite close to the everyday reality of decision-making. The presentation of all costs and consequences can greatly enhance the understanding gained from a CEA and thus a supplementary CCA should be encouraged even when a primary outcome measure has been selected and a CEA carried out.

Cost-utility analysis

An alternative solution to the real world challenge of multiple outcomes is to condense them into one generic measure, which is the approach adopted in cost-utility analysis (CUA). As with CEA, a cost-effectiveness ratio can be calculated, but outcomes are now measured in terms of health-related quality of life. The value of the quality-of-life improvement is measured in units of 'utility', expressed by a combined index of the quality (morbidity) and quantity (mortality) of life-effects of an intervention. One example of a utility-based measure is the quality adjusted life-year (QALY). The calculation of QALYs involves the use of quality adjustment weights (utilities) for different health states. The utility weights are then multiplied by the time spent in each health state and summed to provide the number of quality adjusted life-years. The results are expressed in terms of the additional cost per QALY gained from undertaking a particular intervention, providing a common measure of output that allows comparisons to be made between any number of diverse interventions.

CUAs avoid the potential ambiguities of multi-dimensional outcomes and can be applied to a broad range of treatments or diagnoses and across different areas of healthcare. The transparency of the methods used to derive utility scores is a particular strength, but utility measures are obviously more general than a single outcome measure and thus may not be as sensitive to change. In addition, the measures that are currently widely in use are intended for application across the widest diagnostic range and are focused more on physical than psychological functioning and more on adults than children. Their validity and reliability for use in CAMHS as the sole indicator of impact is therefore questionable, and it is recommended that such measures are used alongside more sensitive and child-focused disease-specific measures (cf. Chisholm *et al.* 1997, for a discussion in the broader mental health context).

Cost studies

Cost-offset and cost-minimization analyses

Cost-offset and cost-minimisation analyses are the simplest of procedures and are concerned only with the comparison of costs. By the definition offered above, these are not economic evaluations *per se* unless health or quality-of-life outcomes have been well-established in previous research. A cost-minimization approach proceeds in the knowledge that previous research has shown outcomes to be equal in the treatment groups being examined (in which case it could probably be more usefully described as an 'interrupted cost-effectiveness analysis'). Its principal aim is to look for the lowest cost alternative, given equality of outcomes. A cost-offset analysis compares costs incurred with other costs saved, and is sometimes conducted as part of a fuller evaluation such as a cost-effectiveness study.

Cost-of-illness studies

Cost-of-illness (COI) studies are commonly used to assess the overall resource impact of a particular condition or disease, but they are not economic evaluations. The aim is to identify and measure all the costs of a particular disease, which may include such elements as health and social care service utilization, special educational support, parents' lost employment or productivity, and less tangible family impacts. The output, expressed in monetary terms, is an estimation of the total burden of a particular disease to society (Rice 1994). An example is provided by a recent study that estimated the economic consequences of autism in the UK (Järbrink and Knapp 2001).

COI studies can be helpful because they allow broad comparisons with other health problems and draw attention to what could be a major societal cost, and by implication they suggest the amount that could be saved if the condition was eradicated. Such information is often used to help guide research and funding priorities by highlighting areas where inefficiencies may exist and savings may be made (Ament and Evers 1993; Rice 1994). Aggregate cost measures, however, often over-simplify the complexity of the real world and such calculations can never be seen as evaluative exercises, since they say nothing about how to improve efficiency or reduce inequity. In particular, a high-cost illness is not necessarily amenable to treatment or may not have cost-effective treatments available, so that savings may not be achievable (Byford *et al.* 2000). Another difficulty is attribution. A child with both a depressive disorder and conduct disorder is likely to be a heavy service user (Knapp *et al.* 2002), but how are the associated costs to be attributed?

Cost measurement

A core requirement of all methods of economic evaluation is accurate cost information. Before costs can be calculated, all relevant services used by individuals over the period of a study must be identified. This is not always straightforward, particularly in mental health contexts, where many agencies may be involved in the care of one individual or family. Box 9.3 lists some of the costs that may be relevant to young people with mental health problems.

To some, it may seem more sensible (and less time-consuming) when conducting an evaluation, to focus on the use of CAMHS services only, but in fact this may be detrimental to the purpose of the exercise. For example, a new CAMHS intervention that is shown to be more effective than routine care may still be discouraged if the additional cost cannot be justified by the gain in patient outcomes. It is quite plausible, however, that these improvements in outcome may lead to cost savings elsewhere through reduced reliance on services outside CAMHS, such as social care and education services. Thus total costs of the new intervention may in fact be lower from a wider perspective than a narrow one.

Once a list of likely services has been drawn up, there are a number of methods available to record the use of these services by study participants, including questionnaires, diaries, or

Box 9.3 Costs that may be relevant to young people with mental health problems

Primary healthcare services (e.g. GP, practice nurse).

Secondary healthcare services (e.g. in-patient, out-patient, day-patient, or accident and emergency services).

Social services (e.g. local authority care and accommodation, social work).

Education services (e.g. educational psychologists, education welfare officers).

Voluntary sector services (e.g. ChildLine, Barnardos).

Private sector services (e.g. private inpatient treatment for anorexia).

Youth justice services (e.g. youth offending team, youth custody).

Patient and family costs (e.g. travel and child care).

Productivity costs (e.g. parent taking time off work to care for young person).

searches of case notes. Service-use questionnaires can be self-reported or completed by researchers at interview, and a number of these questionnaires have been designed for use within health economic evaluations. One example is the Client Service Receipt Inventory (CSRI), which includes sections on accommodation, employment, income, service receipt, informal support, and satisfaction with services (Beecham and Knapp 2001). Such questionnaires often need to be adapted to the particular study, as some services may only be used by specific patient groups, and indeed the CSRI has been adapted for use in evaluations based in CAMHS (e.g. Beecham *et al.* 2002).

The disadvantage of questionnaires is the need to rely on the memory of interviewees. Service-use diaries are one method of improving recall and involve asking participants to record their use of services prospectively over the period of a study. Diaries are likely to be more accurate than questionnaires, but will also place a greater burden on patients and therefore are not always completed (cf. Stone *et al.* 2002). An alternative method of enhancing accuracy is to collect information directly from case notes, although this can be a time-consuming process. In addition, the data will often be limited to the use of services provided by the agency to whom the case files belong. A multi-sector picture can thus only be built by exploring the case files of many different agencies. Again there will always be some worries about how accurately such file notes are completed by busy professionals.

The total cost of supporting an individual is calculated by multiplying service-use data by appropriate unit costs. In many instances, local service-providers may be able to supply unit cost information or the raw data needed to calculate the costs directly. However, this will not always be the case and direct calculation may be needed. Direct calculation requires detailed information on all inputs into a service (staff, equipment, buildings, and so on) with each element costed individually. Direct calculation is recommended for 'key' services—those that are central to the evaluation such as the experimental intervention itself or services that contribute to a significant proportion of total costs. For further information on direct calculation see, for example, Netten and Beecham (1993), Beecham (1995, 2000), and Brouwer *et al.* (2001). Where local data are unavailable, or for services that add little to total cost, it may be possible to use published national or regional unit cost. Examples include CIPFA (2001a, b) and Netten *et al.* (2001).

Outcome measurement

An economic evaluation measures both costs and outcomes. As described above, the various modes of evaluation can be distinguished by their approaches to outcome measurement. Cost-effectiveness and cost-consequences analyses employ outcome measures of the kind familiar to clinical, social work, and educational researchers. Cost-utility analyses measure health-related quality of life as a catch-all indicator of outcome, and cost-benefit analyses calculate the monetary values of the consequences of a treatment or service. We do not go into further detail here, but standard health economics textbooks offer excellent accounts of how these outcomes are measured in practice (e.g. Drummond *et al.* 1997; Gold *et al.* 1996).

Applications and illustrations

Intervention studies

A comprehensive review of the international literature a few years ago revealed no more than a handful of economic evaluations of interventions for mental health problems in childhood and adolescence, most of them methodologically weak (Knapp 1997). Since then a few UK studies have been published that give a rather better indication of the potential of economic evaluation in this area and the appropriate methods to use, although weaknesses are still in evidence. Encouragingly, there are also a number of economic evaluations of interventions currently underway.

Social work intervention for deliberate self-poisoning

Byford and colleagues (1999) carried out a cost-effectiveness analysis of a home-based social work intervention for children and adolescents who have deliberately poisoned themselves. The evaluation was part of a randomized, controlled trial carried out between 1994 and 1997. One hundred and sixty-two children aged 16 years and under, referred to child and adolescent mental health teams with a diagnosis of deliberate self-poisoning, were randomly allocated to either routine care ($n = 77$) or routine care plus the social work intervention ($n = 85$). The primary outcome measures, assessed at baseline, two and six months, were suicidal ideation, hopelessness, and family functioning. The economic analysis took a broad focus and included data on the use of all NHS, education, social and voluntary sector services over the period of the study, collected from the parents at the six-month follow-up interview. Unit costs were calculated for the financial year 1997/98.

No significant differences were found between the two groups in terms of the main outcome measures or costs, although parental satisfaction with treatment was significantly higher in the social work group at the two-month assessment ($p < 0.001$). In a sub-group of young people without major depression, suicidal ideation was significantly lower in the social work group than the control group at the six-month follow-up ($p = 0.01$), with no significant differences in cost, suggesting that the new intervention may be cost-effective for this particular group. The study is a good example of an economic evaluation in the CAMHS field, discussing the reasons for carrying out such an evaluation and providing detailed information on the methods used to calculate costs. In addition, the service utilization data are presented along with useful sources of cost data and the unit costs themselves.

Parental education groups for behavioural disorders

Another useful guide to carrying out an economic evaluation in the CAMHS field is provided by Harrington and colleagues (2000), who undertook an economic evaluation of community and hospital-based mental health services for children with behavioural disorders, as part of a randomized, controlled trial. The intervention, parental education groups, was the same in both groups but the location varied. The starting point for the evaluation was increasing concern that hospital-based services are inaccessible, stigmatizing, expensive, and poorly integrated with community services. The authors thus hypothesized that a community-based service would be more effective and less costly than a hospital-based service. One hundred and forty-one eligible parents entered the trial (72 in the hospital service and 69 in the community). The primary outcome was parental report of the child's behaviour, and assessments were carried out at baseline, three and twelve months.

Economic data included the children's use of NHS, social services, education, voluntary and private sector services over the period of the trial. Given the parental focus of this trial, the use of services by the primary carer (usually the mother) was also recorded, as well as family costs, such as travel and childcare. Information was collected at follow-up using a resource-use questionnaire designed for the purpose of the study. The evaluation found no significant differences in either costs or outcomes, suggesting that location of CAMHS may be less important than the type of services that they provide. Observed differences in cost were, in fact, large, with the hospital group costing 30% less than the community group. The authors acknowledge that the trial sample may not have been large enough to detect a statistically significant difference in cost because the study was powered to detect differences in outcome not cost.

Psychotherapy for sexually abused girls

A more recent study evaluated the cost-effectiveness of group psychotherapy compared to individual psychotherapy for sexually abused girls. Unlike the previous examples, this economic study was carried out retrospectively after the main randomized, controlled trial was completed, with service-use data collected from case records only (McCrone *et al.* 2004). The perspective of the economic analysis was thus narrower than for the studies described above, being limited to the cost of the psychotherapy interventions (including supervision). Outcomes, including psychopathology and functioning, were assessed one and two years after trial entry.

Both groups 'showed a substantial reduction in psychopathological symptoms and an improvement in functioning'. There were no significant differences between individual and group therapy except that girls who had individual therapy had 'a greater improvement in manifestations of post-traumatic stress disorder'(Trowell *et al.* 2002, p. 234). Individual psychotherapy was found to be significantly more expensive than group psychotherapy. It was therefore concluded that group psychotherapy is more cost-effective than individual psychotherapy from the narrow perspective employed in the study though the authors argue that the use and cost of other services is unlikely to differ between the two groups given equality of outcomes. This study was also limited by small sample sizes and retrospective design. Nevertheless, the study provides valuable information in an area where no economic data are available, information upon which future research can be built.

Descriptive studies

Descriptive studies of service utilization patterns and their associated costs have been more common in the UK than full economic evaluations in CAMHS. Although not evaluative, such

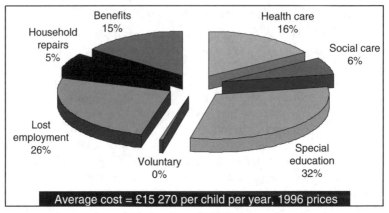

Fig. 9.1 The cost implications of childhood conduct disorder.

studies can provide contextual data to inform policy and practice discussions of effective, cost-effective, and well-targeted interventions. Together, a number of (generally small) studies are beginning to paint pictures of childhood service needs, utilization, and costs.

Examples of descriptive studies

For example, Knapp *et al.* (1998) estimated the broad cost implications for services, families, and the economy of childhood conduct disorder in a small pilot sample. Over a one-year period these costs averaged £15 282 per family (range £5411–£40 896) and fell quite broadly across different sectors (see Fig. 9.1). Although diagnosed as a health problem and treated by special-ist child mental health services, in fact only 16% of the total cost fell to the NHS. In the follow-ing section, it can be seen that the scale and breadth of the resource impact of many child and adolescent mental health problems are both considerable, and that both can continue well into adulthood. The challenges for integrated and long-term working are many.

Other recent examples include studies of: pre-school children with oppositional defiance disorder (Beecham and Topan 1997); children with cerebral palsy and other severe disabilities (Curran *et al.* 2001); young adults with hemiplegia (Beecham *et al.* 2001); children with intel-lectual (learning) disabilities (Beecham *et al.* 2002); and children with autistic spectrum disor-der (Järbrink and Knapp 2001; Järbrink *et al.* 2003).

Predicting cost studies

An alternative method of exploring the cost of a particular disorder or health problem is to analyse factors that influence cost (Knapp 1998). Such analysis can be used to determine which types of young people are likely to be costly to treat, providing useful information to support budgetary decisions, and can give an insight into the appropriateness of such expenditure by determining whether expenditure is being driven by need or other factors. Multivariate regression analysis is used to explore the relationship between cost and such variables as socio-demographic, family, and clinical characteristics of young people with a particular condition.

One example is provided by Byford *et al.* (2001) who used data from their evaluation of a social work intervention for young people who have deliberately poisoned themselves, described above (Byford *et al.* 1999). Baseline characteristics in the sample found to be significantly associated with relatively more expensive care packages included a definite intention to die, the existence of current problems, being in foster care, poorer parental well-being, and not having a diagnosis of conduct disorder. No significant relationships were found between cost and measures of illness severity, including suicidal ideation, hopelessness, and severity of depression. The authors conclude that, although costs are not influenced by clinical measures of severity, service provision does appear to respond to more 'practical' notions of severity, such as intent to die and the existence of current problems.

Long-term follow-up studies

There is a great deal of evidence linking mental health problems in childhood with enduring difficulties into adolescence and adulthood (Fombonne *et al.* 2001; Maughan and Rutter 1998). Attention has recently turned to the economic consequences of these adulthood sequelae, partly because—individually and in aggregate—they are often so devastating to the people concerned and to society at large, and partly because it is sometimes easier for strategic decision-makers and the general public to appreciate the sheer enormity of these problems when aggregated and couched in monetary terms.

Recently, two published UK studies have identified and charted some of the key adulthood implications of childhood or adolescent mental health problems. In each study, costs were calculated for service use over and above standard or basic provision (for example, special needs education was costed, but not mainstream education). Costs were measured as comprehensively as possible, although only counted at all if there was a sound information base. In other words, the estimates are conservative. All figures presented are at 1998 prices for 1998 service arrangements. The main costing dimensions are education, healthcare, social care services, social security benefits, criminal justice, and the court costs of domestic violence. Missing costs thus include patient and family costs, and the victim costs of crime, for example. Moreover, the studies do not quantify the wider psychological or social impacts of disorders or their sequelae.

Conduct disorder

The Inner London Longitudinal Study looked at 10-year-olds in state primary schools in one London borough in 1970 ($n = 2281$), and selected a sub-sample after screening (Maughan 1989). The sub-sample excluded children from ethnic minorities, who were separately studied. Teachers rated problems in children, and interviews were also conducted with parents for a selected group. Children were allocated to one of five groups: no problems at school and no clinical diagnosis ($n = 65$); emotional problems as rated by the teacher, but not clinically diagnosed (32); emotional disorder as clinically diagnosed following interview with parent (8); anti-social problems at school, as rated by the teacher (61); and conduct disorder as clinically rated following interview with parent (16).

By age 28, compared to those with anti-social problems and those with no problems, the group with conduct disorder were more likely to have experienced broken cohabitations, had a greater incidence of depression and anxiety disorder, more alcohol problems, a greater likelihood of anti-social personality disorder, greater levels of criminality, and higher utilization of a number of services. When consequences in adulthood could be costed, it was found that the conduct disorder group were considerably more expensive by age 28 than people who, as children, had been in the other categories (Scott *et al.* 2001a). Figure 9.2 summarizes the cost differences.

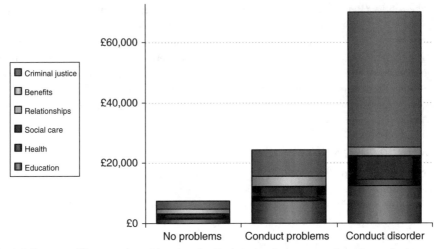

Fig. 9.2 The cost differences found in a longitudinal study of young people with conduct problems and disorders.

Depression and comorbid conduct disorder

A second follow-up study looked at 140 adults who, as children, had been treated at the Maudsley Hospital during 1970–83, of whom 91 had major depressive disorder in childhood, and 53 had depression *and* conduct problems. They were followed-up in 1997–99, and an economics component was built into the data collection. In adulthood, the group with depression *and* conduct disorder were found to have more alcohol dependence, more drug abuse, greater personality dysfunction, higher conviction rates for criminal offences, and poorer social and family adjustment. When the costs were calculated, the comorbid group also accrued much higher costs than the group who, in childhood, had depression only (Fombonne *et al.* 2001; Knapp *et al.* 2002). Total service costs per year were £631 for the depression (only) group compared to £1372 for the comorbid group ($p = 0.015$). The annual costs of crime since age 17 were £32 for the depressed (only) group, but £179 for those who also had conduct disorder ($p < 0.001$). In-patient services accounted for the lion's share of the service costs (57% for the depression group, 51% for the comorbid group).

Implications

Methodologically, it is clear from both these studies that mental health problems in childhood and adolescence have enduring economic implications well into adulthood, and research needs to be designed so as to identify and explore these consequences. It is particularly important to examine the links between childhood problems and their personal and societal impacts in adulthood. In terms of policy and practice, the strong threads of continuity running from childhood to adolescence, and on to adulthood, need to be broken. This is obviously far easier said than done, but there are encouraging signs that effective interventions can be used (Scott *et al.* 2001b), whose cost-effectiveness now needs to be examined.

A second implication is for policy and practice, and is the need to tackle the perverse incentives that arise in a context where, not only are multiple agencies affected by child and adolescent mental health problems, but affected over the course of many years. A successful but potentially expensive investment by the health service in childhood may not save the NHS vast sums of money over that person's lifetime (although the amounts are nevertheless worth pursuing), but the savings to other parts of the public sector, and to society more generally, could be substantial. More importantly, successful interventions should bring about potentially significant improvements to personal and societal quality of life.

Conclusions

One of the fundamental points to take from this chapter is that well-conducted economic evaluations can make significant contributions to our understanding in almost every aspect of policy and practice development in the child and adolescent mental health field. They can support decisions relating to the funding and provision of services and can help to improve the efficiency with which scarce CAMHS resources are allocated. Although a number of descriptive cost studies have been undertaken in this area, few full economic evaluations exist, although the number of studies in progress is increasing.

Ensuring *quality* in the evaluation process is imperative. Evaluators need to pay especial attention to cost measurement, outcome conceptualisation and measurement, and research design.

The measurement of service costs has generally been quite good in economic studies of child and adolescent mental health, covering a broad range of service providers and sectors. However, some cost areas have thus far been neglected, including informal family care, lost employment and productivity, and (where relevant) premature mortality. Continuing disputes in broader health economic contexts concerning the inclusion of such costs, however, mean that these same topics in child and adolescent mental health studies are going to be sources of future debate and differences of opinion.

Outcome measurement represents a tougher challenge because—as we noted earlier—different policy questions require different modes of evaluation, and in turn generate a need to develop the techniques that would allow the construction of reliable clinical or social outcome indicators, utility scores or monetary valuations of outcomes. These methodological ideals come on top of the broader need to continue to improve effectiveness measurement in (some) child mental health study areas, as discussed in other chapters.

A third area where child and adolescent mental health researchers may need to pay particular attention is in relation to the overall design of their studies. Economic evaluations are particularly suited to experimental designs, such as the randomized, controlled trial (RCT). However, RCTs—for all their many advantages—may not reproduce the service-use patterns of everyday practice or may be so narrow the sample of children for inclusion as to make generalization of findings difficult because 'high cost children' are excluded. To improve the usefulness of results, pragmatism in the design of trials should be encouraged. Sample size is another concern in the economic evaluation of mental health services, since the sample required to detect a significant difference in costs is often larger than that needed for outcomes, due to high variability in the data (Sturm *et al.* 1999). Studies that are powered on outcomes alone, however, will often be underpowered in relation to costs.

On all three counts—cost measurement, outcome measurement and research design—the quality of economic studies in the child and adolescent mental health area has been improving noticeably. However, the number of such studies remains too low; there are too many pressing policy and practice decisions whose cost and cost-effectiveness implications can only be guessed at rather than predicted from a sound evidence base.

References

Ament, A. and Evers, S. (1993) Cost of illness studies in healthcare: a comparison of two cases. *Health Policy*, **26**, 29–42.

Beecham, J.K. (1995) Collecting and estimating costs. In *The economic evaluation of mental healthcare* (ed. Knapp, M.R.J.), pp. 61–82. Aldershot: Ashgate Publishing Limited.

Beecham, J.K. (2000) *Unit costs: not exactly child's play*. London: Department of Health.

Beecham, J.K. and Knapp, M.R.J. (2001) Costing psychiatric interventions. In *Measuring mental health needs* (2nd edn) (ed. Thornicroft, G.), pp. 201–24. London: Gaskell.

Beecham, J.K. and Topan, C. (1997) Costs and treatment for pre-school children with oppositional defiance disorder, *Mental Health Research Review*, **4**, 26–9.

Beecham, J.K., O'Neil, T., and Goodman, R. (2001) Supporting young adults with hemiplegia: services and costs. *Health and Social Care in the Community*, **9**(1), 51–9.

Beecham, J.K., Chadwick, O., Fidan, D., and Bernard, S. (2002) Children with severe learning disabilities; needs services and costs. *Children & Society*, **16**, 168–81.

Brouwer, W., Rutten, F., and Koopmanschap, M. (2001) Costing in economic evaluations. In *Economic evaluation in healthcare: merging theory with practice* (ed. M. Drummond, and A. McGuire), pp. 68–93. New York: Oxford University Press.

Byford, S., Harrington, R., Torgerson, D., Kerfoot, M., Dyer, E., Harrington, V., *et al*. (1999) Cost-effectiveness analysis of a home-based social work intervention for children and adolescents who have deliberately poisoned themselves: the results of a randomised controlled trial. *British Journal Psychiatry*, **174**, 56–62.

Byford, S., Torgerson, D.J., and Raftery, J. (2000) Cost of illness studies. *British Medical Journal*, **320**, 1335.

Byford, S., Barber, J., and Harrington, R. (2001) Factors that influence the cost of deliberate self-poisoning in children and adolescents. *Journal of Mental Health Policy and Economics*, **4**, 113–21.

Chisholm, D., Healey, A., and Knapp, M.R.J. (1997) QALYs and mental healthcare. *Social Psychiatry and Psychiatric Epidemiology*, **32**, 68–75.

CIPFA (2001a) *Personal social services statistics: 1999–2000 actuals*. London: Chartered Institute of Public Finance and Accountancy.

CIPFA (2001b) *Health service financial database*. London: Chartered Institute of Public Finance and Accountancy.

Curran, A., Sharples, P., White, C., and Knapp, M.R.J. (2001) Time costs of caring for children with severe disabilities compared with caring for children without disabilities. *Developmental Medicine and Child Neurology*, **43**, 529–33.

Drummond, M., O'Brien, B., Stoddart, G., and Torrance, G. (1997) *Methods for the economic evaluation of healthcare programmes*. Oxford: Oxford University Press.

Fombonne, E., Wostear, G., Cooper, V., Harrington, R., and Rutter, M. (2001) The Maudsley long-term follow-up of child and adolescent depression, *British Journal of Psychiatry*, **179**, 210–17.

Gold, M.R., Siegel, J.E., Russell, L.B., and Weinstein, M.C. (ed.) (1996) *Cost-effectiveness in health and medicine*. New York: Oxford University Press.

Harrington, R., Peters, S., Green, J., Byford, S., Woods, J., and McGowan, R. (2000) Randomised comparison of the effectiveness and costs of community and hospital based mental health services for children with behavioural disorders. *British Medical Journal*, **321**, 1047–50.

Järbrink, K. and Knapp, M.R.J. (2001) The economic impact of autism in Britain. *Autism*, **5**, 7–22.

Järbrink, K., Fombonne, E., and Knapp, M.R.J. (2003) Measuring the parental, service and cost impacts of children with autistic spectrum disorder: a pilot study. *Journal of Autism and Developmental Disorders*, **33**(4), 395–402.

Knapp, M.R.J. (1997) Economic evaluations and interventions for children and adolescents with mental health problems. *Journal of Child Psychology and Psychiatry*, **38**, 3–25.

Knapp, M.R.J. (1998) Making music out of noise: the cost function approach to evaluation. *British Journal of Psychiatry*, **173** (Supplement 1), 37–45.

Knapp, M.R.J., Scott, S., and Davies, J. (1998) The cost of antisocial behaviour in younger children. *Clinical Child Psychology and Psychiatry*, **4**, 457–73.

Knapp, M.R.J., McCrone, P., Fombonne, E., Beecham, J.K., and Worstear, G. (2002) The Maudsley long-term follow-up of child and adolescent depression: impact of comorbid conduct disorder on service use and costs in adulthood. *British Journal of Psychiatry*, **180**, 19–23.

Maughan, B. (1989) Growing up in the inner city: findings from the inner London longitudinal study. *Paediatric and Perinatal Epidemiology*, **3**, 195–215.

Maughan, B. and Rutter, M. (1998) Continuities and discontinuities in antisocial behaviour from childhood to adult life. In *Advances in clinical child psychology* (ed. T.M. Ollendick and R.J. Prinz), pp. 1–47. New York: Plenum.

McCrone, P., Weeramanthri, T., Knapp, M.R.J., Rushton, A., Trowell, J., Miles, G., *et al.* (2004) Cost effectiveness of individual versus group psychotherapy for sexually abused girls. *Child and Adolescent Mental Health, in press.*

Netten, A. and Beecham, J. (1993) *Costing community care.* Aldershot: Ashgate Publishing Limited.

Netten, A., Harrison, G., and Rees, T. (2001) *Unit costs of health and social care.* University of Kent at Canterbury: Personal Social Services Research Unit.

Olsen, J.A. and Smith, R.D. (2001) Theory versus practice: a review of 'willingness to pay' in health and healthcare. *Health Economics*, **10**, 39–52.

Rice, D.P. (1994) Cost-of-illness studies: fact or fiction? *Lancet*, **344**, 1519–20.

Robinson, R. (1993) Economic evaluation and healthcare. *British Medical Journal*, **307**, 728–9; 793–5; 859–62; 924–6; 994–6.

Scott, S., Knapp, M.R.J., Henderson, J., and Maughan, B. (2001a) Financial cost of social exclusion: follow-up study of antisocial children into adulthood. *British Medical Journal*, **323**, 191–4.

Scott, S., Spender, Q., Doolan, M., Jacobs, B., and Aspland, H. (2001b) Multicentre controlled trial of parenting groups for childhood antisocial behaviour in clinical practice. *British Medical Journal*, **323**, 194–8.

Stone, A.A., Shiffman, S., Shwartz, J.E., Broderick, J.E., and Hufford, M.R. (2002) Patient non-compliance with paper diaries. *British Medical Journal*, **324**, 1193–4.

Sturm, R., Unützer, J., and Katon, W. (1999) Effectiveness research and implications for study design: sample size and statistical power. *General Hospital Psychiatry*, **21**, 274–83.

Trowell, J., Kolvin, I., Weeramanthri, T., Sadowski, H., Berelowitz, M., Glasser, D., *et al.* (2002) Psychotherapy for sexually abused girls: psychopathological outcome findings and patterns of change. *British Journal of Psychiatry*, **180**, 234–47.

Part 2

The challenges to be overcome

Chapter 10

The nature and scale of the problem—the prevalence of mental health problems and mental disorders in childhood and adolescence

Howard Meltzer

Introduction

This chapter is divided into three sections. In the first of them, the use of the terms, mental health problems and mental disorders, in relation to young people is discussed with respect to how they are operationalized in large-scale survey research. This is followed by a review of studies that have attempted to measure the prevalence of mental health problems and disorders among children with particular emphasis on the national study of childhood mental disorders in Great Britain. The chapter ends with a brief summary of the implications of national prevalence data for a comprehensive child and adolescent mental health service.

Concepts and their measurement

Estimates of the prevalence of psychiatric morbidity among young people depend on the choice of concepts, how they are operationalized, and the target population. This point needs emphasizing because it means that estimates from one study will not necessarily be comparable with those obtained from other studies using different concepts and methods or using samples which may not be representative of the total population of children and adolescents.

Definitions of mental health problems and mental disorder

The use of the terms, mental health problems and mental disorders, can cause concern because of what they imply about their aetiology and their consequences. In 1995, the NHS Health Advisory Service said:

> First such terms can be stigmatising, and mark the child as being different. However, unless children with mental health problems are recognised, and some attempt is made to understand and classify their problems, in the context of their social, educational and health needs, it is very difficult to organise helpful interventions for them. The second concern is that the term mental disorder may be taken to indicate that the problem is entirely within the child. In reality disorders may arise for a variety of reasons, often interacting. In certain circumstances, a mental or psychiatric disorder, which describes a constellation or syndrome of features, may indicate the reactions of a child or adolescent to external circumstances, which, if changed, could largely resolve the problem.

It is important to define terms relating to the mental health of children and adolescents because experience shows that lack of terminological clarity leads to confusion and uncertainty about the suffering involved, the treatability of problems and disorders and the need to allocate resources.

Mental disorders imply a clinically recognizable set of symptoms or behaviour associated, in most cases, with considerable distress and substantial interference with personal functions. Children with mental health problems also exhibit symptomatic behaviour but are not necessarily socially impaired, i.e., having a significant impact on their social relationships and classroom learning or placing a burden on their parents and teachers.

Prevalence

In psychiatric epidemiology, rates of disorders are often expressed in terms of a particular period: past month, past year, or lifetime. These need to be made explicit in order to aid comparative analysis. Prevalence should not be confused with incidence, which is normally defined as new cases arising within the past twelve months. Rates of childhood disorders based on the same data will also vary according to whether the research diagnostic criteria are based on the ICD10 or DSM1V classification systems.

Co-occurrence of disorders

Instruments used for clinical assessments of psychiatric disorders often allow for several possible diagnoses to be made. Although it would be possible to impose a hierarchy among different disorders, for statistical purposes it is more meaningful to present their prevalence without the imposition of a hierarchy. Co-occurrence of disorders can be examined by a more detailed analysis at a later stage.

Childhood and adolescence

What age range is appropriate for the assessment of childhood mental disorders? In survey research in the UK there is a general acceptance that children and adolescents are aged under 16. Given that many of the epidemiological instruments developed for measuring the prevalence of childhood mental disorders propose an age range from 4 to 17, and that teacher data can be a helpful adjunct to parents' reports, many research projects look at 5–15-year-olds or focus on a particular age group, for example, 10-year-olds.

Single versus multiple informants

While single-informant investigation characterized nearly all of the early epidemiological studies, more recent studies have broadened data collection to include information gathered from parents, teachers, and the subjects themselves. Hodges (1993) has pointed out that children and adolescents can respond to direct questions aimed at enquiring about their mental status and that there is no indication that asking these direct questions has any morbidity or mortality risks. A well-established fact is that information from many sources is a better predictor of disorder than just one source. Many experienced clinicians and researchers in child psychiatry believe that information gleaned from multiple informants facilitates the best estimate of diagnosis in the individual case (Young et al. 1987). At the population level, information from multiple informants enhance the specificity of prevalence estimates.

Angold (1989) states:

> In general, parents often seem to have a limited knowledge of children's internal mental states and to report less in the way of depressive and anxiety symptoms than their children would report. On the other hand adults seem to be better informants about externalised or conduct disorder items such as fighting and disobedience. Teachers are good informants about school behaviour and performance, whilst parents are informative about home life.

Hodges (1993) comments that agreement between child and parent has varied, depending on type of pathology, 'There appears to be more agreement for behavioural symptoms, moderate agreement for depressive symptoms, and poor agreement for anxiety'.

Presentation of prevalence data

One of the problems of collecting information from various sources is finding the best way to integrate the information, which may show a lack of agreement. One method has been to accept a diagnosis irrespective of its source (Bird *et al.* 1992). Others have promoted 'case vignette' assessments where clinical judgements are made on detailed case histories from several sources (Goodman *et al.* 1996).

The prevalence of childhood mental disorders in Great Britain

The findings described in this section focus on the prevalence of mental disorders among 5–15-year-olds and summarize the results of a national survey of the mental health of children and adolescents in Great Britain (Meltzer *et al.* 2000). The prevalence of mental disorders were based on ICD10 diagnostic criteria without the imposition of a hierarchy from data collected from parents, children aged 11–15, and teachers about symptoms occurring in the past six months.

As well as presenting prevalence rates, based on 10 438 interviews, associations between the presence of a mental disorder and biographic, socio-demographic, socio-economic, and social functioning characteristics of the child and the family are presented.

Prevalence of mental disorders

Overall, 10% of children aged 5–15 years had a mental disorder: 5% had clinically significant conduct disorders; 4% were assessed as having emotional disorders—anxiety and depression—and 1% were rated as hyperactive. As their name suggests, the less common disorders (autistic disorders, tics, and eating disorders) were attributed to 0.5% of the sampled population.

However, a report by the Audit Commission in 1999 gave the rate at about 20%. This is because they were looking at mental health problems as distinct from clinically recognised mental disorders with strict impairment criteria (Audit Commission 1999).

Among 5–10 year olds in Great Britain, 10% of boys and 6% of girls had a mental disorder. In the older age group, the 11–15-year-olds, the proportions of children with any mental disorder were 13% for boys and 10% for girls.

The prevalence rates of mental disorders were greater among children:

in lone-parent compared with two-parent families (16%, 8%);

in reconstituted families rather than those with no step-children (15%, 9%);

in families with five or more children compared with two-children (18%, 8%);

if the interviewed parent had no educational qualifications compared with a degree level or equivalent qualification (15%, 6%);

in families with neither parent working compared with both parents at work (20%, 8%);

in families with a gross weekly household income of less than £200 compared with £500 or more (16%, 6%);

in families of social class V compared with social class I (14%, 5%);

whose parents were social sector tenants compared with owner occupiers (17%, 6%); and

in a household with a striving rather than a thriving geodemographic (ACORN) classification (13%, 5%).

Children with a mental disorder compared with other children were more likely to be boys, living in a lower income household, in social sector housing, and with a lone parent. They were less likely to be living with married parents or in social class I or II households.

Physical health, education, and social functioning characteristics

Children with mental disorders were more likely than non-mentally disordered children to have a co-occurring physical illness (as reported by their mothers): bed-wetting (12% compared with 4%), speech or language problems (12% compared with 3%), co-ordination difficulties (8% compared with 2%), and soiling pants (4% compared with 1%).

Although one in five children had officially recognized special educational needs, those with a disorder were about three times more likely than other children to have special needs: 49% compared with 15%. More specifically, among children with officially recognized special educational needs, 28% of those with a disorder and 13% without a disorder had been issued with a statement of SEN by the local authority (Stage 5).

Given that the rate of specific learning difficulties (SpLD) was set at 5%, children with a mental disorder were three times more likely than those with no disorder to have SpLD: 12% compared with 4%.

Of all the topics included in the national survey, those relating to the social functioning of the family were most strongly related to the childhood mental disorders:

Of children assessed as having a mental disorder, 47% had a parent who scored 3 or more on the GHQ12 (the 12-item General Health Questionnaire), approximately twice the proportion of the sample of children with no disorder, 23%.

Children with a mental disorder were twice as likely to live in families with family discord compared with children with no disorder: 35% and 17%, respectively.

Children with mental disorders were far more likely to be frequently punished than children with no mental disorder: 18% compared with 8% were sent to their rooms; 17% compared with 5% were grounded, and 42% compared with 26% were shouted at.

Of children with a mental disorder, 50% had at one time seen the separation of their parents, compared with 29% of the sample with no disorder. The corresponding figures for problems with the police were 15% and 5% and for a parent or sibling dying—6% compared with 3%.

Two factors associated with the highest prevalence rates of mental disorders were: children (aged 13–15) who had split with a boyfriend or girlfriend (24%) and children whose parent had been in trouble with the police (22%).

The role of comprehensive child and adolescent mental health services

The national survey of children's and adolescents' mental health in Great Britain has shown that one in ten children have a mental disorder and that these children compared with others were more likely to have:

poorer physical health;

special educational needs;

special learning difficulties;

parents with mental health problems;

family discord;

been more frequently punished by their parents;

experienced several stressful life events.

Therefore a comprehensive CAHMS needs to address all these issues in terms of the magnitude and nature of the problem.

Further reading

This chapter describes the key findings from the ONS study. Since publication of the core findings, further analysis of the data and additional follow-up studies have led to further publications that are relevant to the subject matter of this chapter. Readers are referred to the list of publications that follows for more information.

Fombonne, E., Simmons, H., Ford, T., Meltzer, H., and Goodman, R. (2001) Prevalence of pervasive developmental disorders in the UK nationwide survey of mental health. *Journal of the American Academy of Child and Adolescent Psychiatry*, **40**, 820–7.

Ford, T., Goodman, R., and Meltzer, H. (2003) Service use over 18 months among a nationally representative sample of British children with psychiatric disorder. *Clinical Child Psychology and Psychiatry*, **8** (1), 37–51.

Gledhill, J., Ford, T., and Goodman, R. (2002) Does season of birth matter? The relationship between age within school year (season of birth) and educational difficulties amongst a representative population sample of children and adolescents aged 5–15 in Great Britain. *Research in Education*, **68**, 41–7.

Goodman, R., Ford, T., and Meltzer, H. (2002) Mental health problems of children in the community: 18 month follow up. *British Medical Journal*, **324**, 1496–7.

Heyman, I., Fombonne, E., Simmons, H., Ford, T., Meltzer, H., and Goodman, R. (2001) Prevalence of obsessive-compulsive disorder in the British nationwide survey of child mental health, *British Journal of Psychiatry*, **179**, 324–9.

References

Angold, A. (1989) Structured assessments of psychopathology in children and adolescents. In *The instruments of Psychiatric Research*. (ed. C. Thompson), pp. 271-304. New York: John Wiley & Sons Ltd.

Audit Commission (1999) Children in mind: child and adolescent mental health services. London: Audit Commission for Local Authorities and the National Health Service.

Bird, H.B., Gould, M.S., and Staghezza, B. (1992) Aggregating data from multiple informants in child psychiatry epidemiological research, *Journal of the American Academy of Child and Adolescent Psychiatry*, **31**, 78–85.

Goodman, R. and Scott, S. (1999) Comparing the Strengths and Difficulties. Questionnaire and the Child Behavior Checklist: Is small beautiful? *Journal of Abnormal Child Psychology*, **27**, 17–24.

Goodman, R., Yude, C., Richards, H., and Taylor, E. (1996) Rating child psychiatric caseness from detailed case histories. *Journal of Child Psychology and Psychiatry*, **37**, 369–79.

Hodges, K. (1993) Structured Interviews for assessing children. *Journal of Child Psychology and Psychiatry*, **34**, 49–68.

McMunn, A., Bost, L., Nazroo, J., and Primatesta, P. (1998) Pychological well being. In *Health survey for England: the health of young people '95-'97.* (ed. P. Prescott-Clarke and P. Primatesta), pp. 339-62. London: HMSO.

Meltzer, H., Gatward, R., Goodman, R., and Ford, T. (2000) *The mental health of children and adolescents in Great Britain.* London: The Stationery Office.

NHS Health Advisory Service (1995) *Child and adolescent mental health services: together we stand.* London: HMSO.

Rutter, M., Tizard, J., and Whitmore, K. (1970) *Education, health and behaviour.* London: Longmans.

Verhulst, F.C., Berden, G.F.M.G., and Sanders-Woudstra, J.A.R. (1985) Mental health in Dutch children: (II) the prevalence of psychiatric disorder and relationship between measures. *Acta Psychiatrica Scandanavia Supplement* **324**, 1–45.

Vikan, A. (1985) Psychiatric epidemiology in a sample of 1510 ten-year-old children. *Journal of Child Psychology and Psychiatry*, **26**, 55–75.

World Health Organization (1993) *The ICD-10 classification of mental and behavioural disorders: diagnostic criteria for research.* Geneva: World Health Organization.

Young, J.G., O'Brien, J.D., Gutterman, E.M., and Cohen, P. (1987) Research on the clinical interview. *Journal of the American Academy of Child and Adolescent Psychiatry*, **26** (5), 613–20.

Chapter 11

The impact of the new genetics on planning and delivering child and adolescent mental health services

Rajesh Gowda, Jane Scourfield, and Anita Thapar

Introduction

The Genome Project and genetic research has excited scientists, health providers, the media, and the general public. There are, however, many myths as to the extent genetic research will change medical practice and services in the near future. At present, there would appear to be little 'on the ground' effect by genetic research on general psychiatric services, and even less on child and adolescent mental health services (CAMHS). The role of an evidence-based approach in CAMHS has been highlighted (Williams 2000) but the application can be difficult (Ramchandini *et al.* 2001; Harrington 2001). Knowledge and evidence-based medicine and its application is fraught with hurdles.

In this chapter, we aim to outline realistically the future challenges that CAMHS may face. By reviewing the present effect of our genetic knowledge on services in medicine and outlining the key research findings, it is possible to estimate how genetic research may impact on services in the future. There are many logistical and ethical dilemmas that will need to be addressed as knowledge on genetics increases.

Methods

Application of new research and knowledge into a service requires some understanding of the methods that have been previously used and the innovative techniques that are presently being applied. There is now an air of change from 'if genes are important' to 'how genes work'.

Quantitative genetic designs namely: family, twin, adoption, and 'combination' studies, are used to examine the contribution of genetic and environmental influences to specific disorders. These methods have been described in detail elsewhere (Thapar and McGuffin 2000).

Family studies involve examining the prevalence of a psychiatric disorder among the relatives of probands (affected individuals) and comparing this with the rate of disorder in relatives of a control group. Family studies are relatively easy to carry out but separating the genetic and shared environment aetiological factors is not really possible. That is, disorders can run in families because of shared environmental risk factors (e.g. family adversity that impinge equally on all members of the family), as well as genes. However, they are important in providing information that can be used to assess the risk of an individual for a particular illness or disorder.

Twin studies allow assessment of both environmental factors and genetic factors, and enable us to distinguish the effects of shared environmental factors and genes. Inferences are based on the fact that monozygotic (MZ) twins have the same genetic material and dizygotic (DZ) twins share, on average, 50% of their genetic material. Thus, phenotype differences amongst MZ twins could be said to be due to non-shared environmental factors. Similarly, if DZ- and MZ-twin similarities are substantial (usually presented as concordance rates or correlation coefficients) and similar, it could be concluded that shared environmental factors are important. Conversely, if MZ concordance rates are very much higher than DZ concordance rates, genetic factors are more important. In making such conclusions, certain assumptions have been made. These are numerous and have been the subject of criticism. Each study design has its own pattern of methodological strengths and weaknesses, and thus greater confidence is usually placed in findings that are consistent across different study designs.

Adoption studies are particularly useful for assessing the contribution of environmental influences. One example of study design involves comparing the risk of a specific disorder in MZ twins who have been reared apart in two separate environments. Most adoption studies have focused on comparing the similarity of adoptive relatives compared with biologically related family members. For disorders that are genetically influenced, we would expect the biologically related relatives of affected individuals to be more commonly affected than the adoptive relatives. If shared environmental factors make a significant contribution, we would expect high rates of disorder among the adoptive relatives. Caution again is needed, in interpreting results, as there are drawbacks to the adoption methods, such as selective placement. Combination studies, although more complex, are useful. These involve using different sets of relatives, for example, twins and siblings and step families. By using siblings the special status of being twins can be lessened.

Molecular genetic designs are becoming increasingly advanced. There are several strategies that have been used. The merits and pitfalls are complex and disputed (Rutter *et al.* 1999). Here, we will only outline the main principles. Two main types of study design are used in molecular genetics: allelic association and linkage.

Allelic association studies use a case control design and involve comparing the frequency of a particular gene variant among affected individuals with the frequency amongst controls. The main drawback of association studies is the potential for confounding factors (unmeasured differences between cases and controls, and population stratification) that could cause false-positives. Family based association studies utilize genetic information from both parents and do not require an external control group. This removes the problem of stratification. Linkage studies rely on meiosis not affecting recombination of two markers that lie close together on a chromosome. Thus, if a DNA marker is located close to a specific disease-susceptibility gene on a chromosome, there will be a tendency for that marker variant to co-segregate with the disorder. The affected sib-pair method is the most suitable type of linkage method used in psychiatric genetics. This involves collecting samples where at least two siblings show the disorder of interest (e.g. autism) and examining whether the siblings more commonly share specific variants of a large number of genetic markers that span the whole genome than expected. Association and linkage studies can be very complex and have been discussed in more detail (e.g. Baron 2001).

Complex and innovative methods used by geneticists include new automated laboratory methods that allow for the rapid, relatively economical genotyping of a huge number of genetic markers that span the entire genome.

Genetics of childhood disorders

The following outline some of the key research findings in recent years.

Autism

Autism was initially attributed to environmental factors for many years and most specifically thought to arise from 'refrigerator parents'. Family studies have now shown that the risk to siblings of children with autism is about 3–5%, which represents a 100–150-fold increase in risk compared to the general population. Twin studies (Bailey *et al.* 1995), have provided evidence that autism is strongly influenced by genetic factors. Molecular genetic studies on autism are now underway but so far there have been no major consistent findings other than linkage with a marker on chromosome seven. It seems likely that susceptibility genes for disorders such as autism will individually be of small effect size but may interact to greatly increase the risk of disorder. It should be noted that even in a highly genetic disorder, such as autism, prevalence rates have increased; this is unlikely to be as a result of genes changing, thus highlighting the importance of the environment and methods of diagnosis.

Attention deficit hyperactivity disorder/hyperkinetic disorder

Much interest has also focused on the genetics of attention deficit hyperactivity disorder/ hyperkinetic disorder (ADHD). Again there is consistent evidence from family, twin, and adoption studies that ADHD is familial and appears to be influenced by genetic factors (Biederman *et al.* 1992). Molecular genetic study findings are emerging with most consistent findings of an association with a variant of the D4 dopamine receptor (DRD4) and the dopamine transporter gene (Cook *et al.* 1995; LaHoste *et al.* 1996). Several research groups have independently replicated the DRD4 findings and a meta-analysis of these findings has also shown a significant association. However the effect size is small with a reported odds ratio of 1.9 for case-control studies and 1.4 for family-based studies (Faraone *et al.* 2001). A meta-analysis of the DRD5 has also shown significant association with ADHD, with a reported odds ratio of 1.24 (Lowe *et al.* 2004).

Depression

Findings for depression and anxiety in childhood have been much more mixed. Depression occurring in childhood and adolescence has a tendency to run in families with a recent meta-analysis revealing a relative risk of approximately four, among first-degree relatives (Rice *et al.* 2002). As mentioned earlier, this may not be necessarily due to genetic influences but may be a result of shared environmental factors or over-recognition and awareness of depressive symptoms in these families (Chilcoat and Breslan 1997). Although twin studies of depressive symptoms suggest the importance of genetics and the environment, there have been no twin studies of depressive disorder in adolescence, and much work is needed. Adoption studies (Eley *et al.* 1998; van den Oord *et al.* 1994) have, however, detected no genetic effect. The contradicting results should not be seen as a flaw in genetic research but more of a challenge to scientists to hypothesise possible reasons for the discrepancies.

Schizophrenia

Schizophrenia, like depression, can present in early adulthood and adolescence, but rarely before puberty. Notably, the earlier age of onset, the higher the genetic influence (Kendler *et al.* 1987). The cumulative evidence of a genetic component in schizophrenia is strong. Most estimates put the figure over 75% (McGuffin *et al.* 1994). However, new findings are extremely encouraging with replicated findings that favour Neuregulin1 (NRG1) and Dysbindin (DTNB1) as susceptibility genes (Owen *et al.* 2004).

Conduct and oppositional disorder

Conduct and oppositional disorder has been associated within families and has been shown to be global (Rutter *et al.* 1998). The heterogeneity of the disorder has provided more clues to its aetiology but also may be responsible for some of the inconsistencies of recent published work. Interestingly, several studies found that antisocial behaviour was more heritable when hyper-activity or inattention were also associated with the antisocial behaviours. Moreover, there is also evidence that early onset conduct disorder symptoms that persist in adult life are more likely to have a genetic bias.

The aims and purposes of genetic research

Mental illnesses, like physical illnesses, are influenced by both genetic and environmental factors. Although we will have sequenced the human genome, we have limited knowledge on how genes work and produce differences in human beings. From before conception, the environment has an influence on how that genetic information becomes the phenotype. The assumption or belief that some disorders are primarily genetically or environmental in aetiology is being made obsolete. It could be said that new genetic research will, rather than diminishing the role of the environment, increase our understanding of its mechanism on the pathogenesis of psychiatric disorders (Ottman 1996). It has the potential to confirm the role of psychological and social factors in the role of pathogenesis but may also exclude hypotheses that have little or no evidence-base. The role of gene and environment interaction is increasingly recognized as important in explaining, for example, antisocial behaviour and depression (e.g. Silberg *et al.* 2001; Caspi *et al.* 2002). There is evidence that the impact of environmental adversity is greater when genetic risk factors are also present (Bohman 1996). Genes may also be important in the limiting of potential environmental risks (Plomin *et al.* 1990). Gene–environment correlation (e.g. Ge *et al.* 1996; O'Connor *et al.* 1998) highlights the complexity of how genes and environment act.

Our understanding of disorders is bound to increase, and with it new therapies should be developed and become utilized. One aspect that is overlooked is the potential for treatment to be more specific, depending on phenotype allied with genetic information.

Environmental modification to those at risk is one area that is often neglected in discussion when genetic knowledge is being utilized. It may be possible to limit the risk of a disorder, not with prophylactic medication, but for example with behavioural programmes. Together with the redefinition of phenotypes, it should be possible to direct psychological and social intervention more appropriately.

The genetic research that has influenced the health services and the possible ways it may influence interventions and services

New genetic knowledge has already markedly changed what is known about certain illnesses to an extent that could be called revolutionary. This applies to physical diseases and to a limited number of illnesses that affect the mind. Examples of illnesses include cystic fibrosis (Riordan *et al.* 1989), polycystic kidney (European Polycystic Kidney Disease Consortium 1994) and Huntington's disease (Huntington's Disease Collaborative Group 1993). These illnesses are, however, very different from psychiatric disorders, in that they are caused by a single gene. Identifying the 'gene' in a patient for these disorders can significantly affect the risk of develop-ing the disorder by up to 100%, i.e. they have a largely deterministic role in the pathogenesis of the illness. This is clearly not the case for complex disorders, including psychiatric disorders, that are influenced by a number of different genes and by environmental influences that are likely to interact as well as co-act. Moreover, it is the understanding of mechanisms by which genes influence disorder that will be pivotal to how the health services respond to evidence derived from genetic research.

Understanding pathogenesis

The pathogenesis mechanisms have become clearer in a number of physical illnesses, not from identifying a 'gene' but from elucidating how certain 'genes' operate (Roses 1995). The number of people with early-onset Alzheimer's disease is relatively small, but its association, for example, with Apo E4, has led researchers to understand some of the pathogenesis of late-onset Alzheimer's disease.

We urge caution coupled with excitement given that, although genes have been identified for an increasing number of single-gene disorders, there has been a delay in moving this forward into developing new methods of treatment. There are still no effective methods of intervention available for many of these disabling conditions.

The impact of new genetics on more complex disorders, where several aetiological factors have been identified, is less distinct. There have been a number of false dawns in the identification of susceptibility genes in psychiatric disorders, although replicated findings are now beginning to emerge for some disorders, e.g. ADHD. These 'genes' may alter the risk of development of the disorder depending on other genes and the environmental risks. They are thought to act by a complex interaction. Many psychiatric disorders are complex mixture of 'inherited tendency and pathogenic exposure'. Some question the relevance of genetics in such disorders as schizophrenia. The lack of any pathogenetic basis may appear, to some scientists, as if the researchers were 'stabbing in the dark', and yet this is also a compelling reason to pursue research focused on better understanding the aetiology of these disorders.

It is hoped that new genetics will not necessarily just help us determine the risk of a particular illness for a patient but also change services in other ways. New genetics should probably be regarded as a new technique to aid our understanding of illnesses such as ADHD and autism. It has the potential to help health professional understand causes of psychiatric disorders, change previous attitudes to some illnesses, and remove some of the unfounded attribution placed by professionals and the public onto patients and their families.

Classification

The classification systems (DSM-IV-TR, American Psychiatric Association (2000) and ICD-10, World Health Organization (1993)) used by mental health professional to diagnose mental illness are based on symptoms and functioning. Furthermore, the phenotype boundaries are not well-defined. Depressive disorders are classed by symptoms and level of functioning. The different forms of schizophrenia are based on groups of symptoms. By understanding the mechanisms of these illnesses it may be possible, in the near future, to reclassify many of these 'less worked out' illnesses by aetiology, much in the same way that the different dementias are classified by their main aetiological factor, for example, vascular dementia.

Pharmacogenetics

The pharmaceutical industry is investing in the field of pharmacogenetics for a number of reasons. Besides the obvious development of new drugs, there is a role for directing medication to individuals who are more likely to respond. There is potential for selective use of drugs, based on genetic screening, e.g. adverse side-effects. By clarifying any biochemical mechanisms by which certain phenotypes are exhibiting their symptoms, it may be possible to streamline certain patients to specific medical or psychological treatment (or both), i.e. assigning treatments according to genotype. The role of treatment may become less of a lottery. Interventions would be based on clear rationale. Even where a disorder is strongly influenced by a gene(s), the mediating mechanism may be an environmental factor.

Genetic counselling and genotyping

One area of present and future challenges is undoubtedly the field of genetic counselling and testing. Genetic testing is a hotbed of ethical, moral, social, and legal debate. It has the potential to stigmatize and destigmatize mental illness. On the one hand it could be seen as 'bad blood', and the other, it could remove some of the layman's beliefs about mental illness (God's judgment and immorality). It is also likely that much of genetic counselling about mental disorder will be to dispel some of the myths, such as the one-to-one relationship of gene and disorder. Knowledge of one's genetic makeup may also make one feel flawed. It is vital to ascertain the view of the patient and family to what questions they need clarifying.

Genetic counselling and testing is non-paternal and non-directive. Like any screening test, genetic testing, should be justified, on the grounds of importance, prevalence, therapeutic choices, and economics, amongst other considerations, such as sensitivity and specificity. At present, the biggest failing of genetic testing of mental illness, in even highly heritable common mental disorders, is the inability of the clinician to use the test to reliably predict the individual risk. The reality is that assessing the genetic status at best only increases the accuracy of predicting risk, slightly above what is known from empirical data from family studies. However, in some illnesses previously novel genetic tests will become part of the clinical diagnostic process, for example, following the British Government's announcement that genetic testing for breast cancer (BRCA1 and 2) will become available on the National Health Service. We could learn many lessons from other innovative service providers who have been impacted by new genetics.

Genetic tests open debate on various subjects such as eugenics. The effects on reproductive decision, either voluntarily or involuntary, requires consideration before we embark on genetic testing. One example of the complexities of genetic testing is highlighted by the low uptake (10–20%) of widely available genetic testing for Huntington's disease (HD). The reasons include insurance implications, treatment availability, inadvertently showing HD status of parents of those offspring tested, and psychological consequences of both negative and positive results (Meiser and Dunn 2000). Due to these considerations the counselling process for HD is rightly thorough (Crauford and Tyler 1992).

In the USA it is possible to have genetic predictive testing for early-onset Alzheimer's but take-up has been low. This is probably for a number of reasons including that noted by The Nuffield Council on Bioethics (1998) which 'recommends that genetic testing for susceptibility genes providing predictive or diagnostic input of certainty to, or lower than, that offered by Apo E tests for Alzheimer's disease should be discouraged unless and until the information can be put to effective preventive or therapeutic use'. The potential of discrimination in education, employment, insurance, housing amongst other areas, is immense.

In Britain, the Association of British Insurers (ABI) and the British Medical Association (BMA) joint guidelines (2002) key points include that no one will be asked to undergo genetic test but will be asked to reveal results on any known tests. Only those results of genetic tests that been approved by the Genetics and Insurance Committee (UK), in the course of a clinical diagnostic process, would be requested. The insurance industry appears to have taken a responsible line, but would, for example, some employers exclude those who had genes that implied susceptibility to stress? Exclusion from mainstream society is a theoretical but valid concern.

The logistics and economics of any future genetic counselling and testing are immense. At present, there are approximately one to two consultant geneticists per million population. How can genetic counselling and predictive/diagnostic testing be incorporated into present services? Can primary care services develop the expertise to provide such a service? Like any relatively new service, it needs to have evaluated, planned, developed, training devised, implemented, and managed.

Serious ethical and consent concerns arise out testing of minors. Genotyping for conditions such as psychosis may not define the exact risk of the illness but it may provide enough information to justify increased surveillance and screening for those at increased risk. However, predictive genetic testing could be potentially harmful; for example, stigmatizing the individual and their family, and causing negative psychological effects. We cannot assume an individual's motivation to change their behaviour (Evans *et al.* 2001), for example, if one is at risk of developing schizophrenia to abstain from using cannabis.

Should parents or appropriate children have the right to consent to testing (Cohen 1998)? Matters become further complicated by what constitutes treatment and 'in the best interests' as this has legal implications to consent. Should child testing be banned when some illness such as schizophrenia may first affect the individual as a teenager (especially those with higher genetic loading)? Early intervention in psychotic disorders is widely held to be effective in reducing disability incurred by a first episode psychosis (McGlashan 1996). What about the effect on relatives and siblings? It is possible to detect the carrier status of siblings of, for example, a girl having confirmed Fragile X syndrome. Should we breach confidentiality by informing those at obvious risk?

The challenges specifically for CAMHS will be multi-directional; the probable advances are difficult to prophesize. We can make reasonable suggestions in what areas CAMHS will have to readjust to meet the demands of the new knowledge and technology. The following imaginary cases illustrate hypothetical interventions (Table 11.1) based on general knowledge.

Table 11.1 An illustrative imaginary case

The case history	Possible points of intervention include the following:
Referral of 7-year-old girl for genetic for counselling	Preconception counselling
	Antenatal testing
	Genetic testing (when, whose consent?)
Father said to have been hyperactive as a child and later developed antisocial personality disorder	Advise abstinence from alcohol or illegal drugs
	Hypervigilance to detect symptoms
Mother stable, no mental illness	Behavioural programme or other treatment as prophylaxis for disorder(s)
Daughter has symptoms of ADHD only at home	Appropriate therapy based on new knowledge derived from research (both genetic and non-genetic)

Summary

Challenges are, at present, the misconceptions by both professionals and the public of the role of new genetics in the health service. It will be important for health professionals to keep abreast of the new findings, so as to provide accurate information for patients and their families, who may have a misguided understanding about genetics. The role of much genetic research is not the identification of 'genes for disorders' but in determining the role of genes in the pathogenesis of a disorder.

What will determine the challenges for CAMHS depends on present and future research findings, not only in the genetic field but, also in the environment and socio-economic fields, which have undoubtedly a major role in the development of pathology that we see in our clinics.

The genetic research revolution impacting on CAMHS is not imminent but is certainly creeping into services at various levels from primary care to Tier 4.

Acknowledgments

We would like to thank Mr Tom Fowler for comments on an earlier draft.

References

American Psychiatric Association (2000) *Diagnostic and statistical manual of mental disorders* (4th edn). Washington, DC: American Psychiatric Association.

Association of British Insurers and the British Medical Association (2000) *Medical Information and Insurance*, pp. 11. London: BMA.

Bailey, A., Le Couteur, A., Gottesman, I., Bolton, P., Simonoff, E.E., and Rutter, M. (1995) Autism as a strongly genetic disorder: Evidence from a British twin study. *Psychological Medicine,* **25**, 63–77.

Baron, M. (2001) The search for complex disease genes: fault by linkage or fault by association? *Molecular Psychiatry,* **6**, 143–9.

Biederman, J., Faraone, S.V., Keenan, K., Benjamin, J., Krifcher, B., and Moore, C. (1992) Further evidence for familial-genetic risk factors in ADHD: Pattterns of comorbidity in probands and relatives in psychiatrically and paediactrically referred samples. *Archives of General Psychiatry,* **49**, 728–38.

Bohman, M. (1996) Predispostion to criminalty: Swedish adoption studies in retrospect. In *Genetics of criminal and antisocial behaviour* (ed. G.R. Bock, and J.A. Goode), pp. 99–114. Chichester: Wiley.

Caspi, A., McClay, J., Moffitt, T.E., Mill, J., Martin, J., Craig, I.W., *et al.* (2002) Role of genotype in the cycle of violence in maltreated children. *Science,* **297**(5582), 851–4.

Chilcoat, H.D. and Breslau, N. (1997) Does psychiatric history bias mothers' reports? An application of a new analytic approach. *Journal of the American Academy of Child and Adolescent Psychiatry,* **36**, 971–9.

Cohen, C.B. (1998) Wrestling with the future: should we test children for adult-onset genetic conditions? *Kennedy Institute of Ethics Journal,* **8**, 111–30.

Cook, E.H., Stein, M.A., Krasowski, M.D. *et al.* (1995) Association of attention-deficit disorder and the dopamine transporter gene. *American Journal of Human Genetics,* **56**, 993–8.

Crauford, D. and Tyler, A. (1992) Predictive testing for Huntington's disease: protocol of the UK Huntington's Prediction Consortium. *Journal of Medical Genetics,* **29**, 915–8.

Eley, T.C., Deater-Deckard, K., Fombonne, E., Fulker, D.W., and Plomin, R. (1998) An adoption study of depressive symptoms in middle childhood. *Journal of Child Psychology and Psychiatry and allied disciplines,* **39**, 337–45.

European Polycystic Kidney Disease Consortium (1994) The polycystic kidney disease 1 gene encodes a 14 kb transcript and lies within a duplicated region on chromosome 16. *Cell,* **77**, 881–6.

Evans, J.P., Skrzynia, C., and Burke, W. (2001) The complexities of predictive genetic testing. *British Medical Journal*, **322**, 1052–6.

Faraone, S.V., Doyle, A.E., Mick, E., and Biederman, J. (2001) Meta-analysis of the association between the Dopamine D4 Gene 7-repeat allele and attention deficit hyperactivity disorder. *American Journal of Psychiatry*, **158**(7), 1052–7.

Ge, X., Conger, R.D., Cadonet, R.J., Neidersier, J.M., Yates, W., Troughton, E., and Stuart, M.E. (1996) The developmental interface between nature and nurture: a mutual influence model of child antisocial behaviour and parenting. *Developmental Psychology*, **32**, 574–89.

Harrington, R. (2001) Commentary: evidence-based child and mental health services. *Child Psychology and Psychiatry Review*, **6**(2), 65.

Huntington's Disease Collaborative Group (1993) A novel gene containing a trinucleotide repeat that is unexpanded and unstable on Huntington's chromosomes. *Cell*, **72**, 971–83.

The International Classification of Diseases-10 (1993) *Classification of mental and behavioural disorders*. World Health Organization, Geneva, Switzerland.

Kendler, K.S., Tsaung, M.Y., and Hays, P. (1997) Age at onset in schizophrenia: a family perspective. *Archives of General Psychiatry*, **44**, 881–90.

LaHoste, G.J., Swanson, J.M., Wigal, S.B., Glabe, C., Wigal, T., King, N. and Kennedy, J.L. (1996) Dopamine D4 receptor gene polymorphism is associated with attention deficit hyperactivity disorder. *Molecular Psychiatry*, **1**, 121–4.

Lowe, N., Kirley, A., Hawi, Z., Sham, P., Wickham, H., Kratochvil, C.J., *et al.* (2004) Joint analysis of the DRD5 marker concludes association with attention-deficit/hyperactivity disorder confined to the predominantly inattentive and combined subtypes. *Am J Hum Genet*, **74**(2), 348–56.

McGlashan, T.H. (1996) Early detection and intervention in schizophrenia: research. *Schizophrenia Bulletin*, **22**(2), 327–45.

McGuffin, P., Asherson, P., Owen, M., and Farmer, A. (1994) The strength of the genetic effect: is there room for an environmental influence on the aetiology of schizophrenia? *British Journal of Psychiatry*, **164**, 593–9.

Meiser, B. and Dunn, S. (2000) Psychological input of genetic testing for Huntington's disease: an update of the literature. *Journal of Neurology, Neurosurgery and Psychiatry*, **69**, 574–8.

Nuffield Council on Bioethics (1998) Clinical applications of genetic information about mental disorders: ethical and legal issues. *Mental disorders and genetics: the ethical context*, pp. 38–9. London: Nuffield Council on Bioethics.

O'Connor, T.G., Deater-Deckerd, K., Fulker, D., Rutter, Plomin, R. (1998) Genotype-environment correlation in late childhood and adolescence: antisocial behavioural problems and coercive parenting. *Developmental Psychology*, **34**(5), 970–81.

Ottman, R. (1996) Gene-environment interaction: definitions and study designs. *Preventive Medicine*, **25**, 764–70.

Owen, M.J., Williams, N.M., and O'Donovan, M.C. (2004) The molecular genetics of schizophrenia: new findings promise new insights. *Mol Psychiatry*, **9**(1), 14–27.

Plomin, R., Lichtenstein, P., Pedersen, N.L., McClearn, G.E., and Nesselroade, J.R. (1990) Genetic influence on life events during the last half of the life span. *Psychology and Ageing*, **5**, 25–30.

Ramchandini, P., Joughin, C., and Zwi, M. (2001) Evidence-based child and mental health services: oxymoron or brave new dawn? *Child Psychology and Psychiatry Review*, **6**(2), 59–64.

Rice, F., Harold, G., and Thapar, A. (2002) The aetiology of childhood depression: review of genetic influences. *Journal of Child Psychology and Psychiatry and Allied Disciplines, Annual Research Review*, **43**(1), 65–79.

Riordan, J.R., Rommens, J.M., Kerem, B.S., Alou, N., Rozmahel, R., Grezelczak, Z., *et al.* (1989) Identification of the cystic fibrosis gene: cloning and characterisation of complimentary DNA. *Science*, **245**, 1066–73.

Roses, A. (1995) Apolipoprotein E genotyping in the differential diagnosis, not prediction, of Alzheimer's disease. *Annals of Neurology*, **38**, 6–14.

Rutter, M., Giller, H., and Hagell, A. (1998) *Antisocial behaviour by young people.* Cambridge: Cambridge University Press.

Rutter, M., Silberg, J., O'Connor, T., and Simonoff, E. (1999) Genetics and Child Psychiatry: I Advances in Quantitative and Molecular Genetics. *Journal of Child Psychology and Psychiatry and allied disciplines*, **40**(1), 3–18.

Silberg, J., Rutter, M., Neale, M., and Eaves, L. (2001) Genetic moderation of environmental risk for depression and anxiety in adolescent girls. *British Journal of Psychiatry*, **179**, 116–21.

Thapar, A. and McGuffin, P. (2000) Quantitative Genetics. In *New Oxford textbook of psychiatry* (ed. M.G. Gelder, J.J. Lopez-Ibor, and N. Andreasen), pp. 233–42. Oxford: Oxford University Press.

van den Oord, E.J.C.G., Boosma, D.I., and Verhulst, F.C. (1994) A study of problem behaviours in 10- to 15-year biologically related and unrelated international adoptees. *Behaviour Genetics*, **24**, 193–205.

Williams, R. (2000) A cunning plan: The role of research evidence in translating policy into effective child and adolescent mental health services. *Current Opinion in Psychiatry*, **13**(4), 361–8.

World Health Organization (1993) The ICD-10 Classification of Mental and Behavioral Diseases. Geneva: World Health Organization.

Chapter 12

Mental health promotion, prevention, and early intervention in childhood and adolescence

Peter Hill

Introduction

Child mental health promotion or, restated with a slightly different emphasis, the prevention of child and adolescent mental health disorders, is something that health authorities are expected to include in commissioning. The Health Advisory Service includes it in its standards, for instance (Health Advisory Service 2000). It is conventionally recognized as a different activity from clinical assessment and treatment.

Various authorities have argued that it needs to be expanded, since existing resources for assessment and treatment are inadequate for their task, yet are also unlikely to expand sufficiently to treat all cases. There will never be enough resources for treatment, it is said. This can be linked to the fact that most children (here taken to be a term including school-age teenagers) with mental health disorders are not going to be referred to, or seen by, secondary care specialist clinical services. There are opportunities within primary care (Hill and Spender 1996; Spender and Hill 1996) but, in general, community- and school-based projects have been promoted, especially in North America.

The classical approach to reducing the level of disorders in a population is by means of primary, secondary, and tertiary interventions:

primary prevention stops conditions occurring;

secondary prevention applies the promptest and most effective treatment to curtail duration and limit severity;

tertiary prevention reduces disability and deterioration.

This scheme is well-recognized and has close links with epidemiology. Graham (1994) pointed out that primary prevention (the attempt to stop disorders happening) is effectively an attempt to reduce incidence. Secondary prevention, which aims to shorten the duration of established disorder, is equivalent to reducing prevalence; since the condition lasts less long, there is simply less of it about. Tertiary prevention, it might similarly be argued, is indistinguishable from good clinical practice in rehabilitation.

An alternative perspective views such an approach as overlapping with ordinary clinical assessment and treatment: early detection of prodromal clinical concerns, early treatment, and good quality longer term care (Hill 2000). Because of these criticisms it has been argued that *early intervention* is a better term to apply, at least to what has previously been known as primary and secondary prevention.

The distinction between levels becomes more blurred when one considers what is being prevented. Obviously the purpose of prevention in this context is to stop childhood psychiatric disorder happening or enduring. Yet disorder is not that easily distinguished from normality; the boundary between normality and pathology is not clear-cut. Pathology or caseness is usually defined according to the number of symptoms or a level of impairment. Yet epidemiology demonstrates that these two aspects do not necessarily correlate: a child can be substantially impaired, even when only a few symptoms are present. What is more, impairment is not a single threshold and can be measured on a scale, as in DSM-IV. Symptoms are distributed unimodally, not bimodally, and there is effectively a dimensional gradient of severity from normal to abnormal with no clear cut-off. This is in spite of a categorical approach to diagnostic classification. The reasons for this are not absolute but pragmatic: diagnoses are helpfully conceptualized as categories when it comes to quantifying population morbidity or clinical activity, for instance.

Primary prevention thus becomes, not so much a question of stopping something happening but, an activity that moves psychopathology from a level of severity that is on the point of becoming clinically significant to a point that is well below this on a scale of severity. It is to establish a process that progressively moves clinical symptomatology or impairment away from the threshold of a diagnostic entity. This is clearly comparable with treatment and supports the early-intervention concept. On a notional 10-point scale, which measures severity and identifies caseness as a score over 6, moving a score of severity from say 5 to 3 is likely to involve similar activities to moving a score from 7 to 5, which would be considered a successful treatment.

This approach is perhaps not always going to be correct: there may be some diagnoses or clinical entities in which the distinction from normality is clear-cut (schizophrenia, perhaps) but across the broad range of child mental health it seems usually applicable.

Health promotion

Prevention—stopping something happening—is often equated with health promotion, a more fashionable phrase. The difficulty is that mental health can be characterized in various ways.

A popular approach has been to describe optimal psychosocial development. In *Together we stand* (Williams and Richardson 1995), a definition drawn up by Hill's group was cited and has been widely adopted. In this, mental health in children and adolescents is indicated by:

a capacity to enter into, and sustain, mutually satisfying personal relationships;

continuing progression of development;

an ability to play and learn, so that attainments are appropriate for age and intellectual level;

a developing sense of right and wrong;

the degree of psychological distress and maladaptive behaviour being within normal limits for the child's age and behaviour.

This is broadly equivalent to promoting normal psychosocial development but could reasonably be criticized as being Utopian. It also encroaches upon moral and spiritual well-being without any qualification as to how these might be manifest in different cultures. Furthermore, although some child psychiatric disorder is reasonably conceptualized as equivalent to distorted psychosocial development (e.g. autistic spectrum disorders), this is not always so (e.g. post-traumatic stress disorder). Prevention of child and adolescent mental health disorder based solely on the promotion of psychosocial development will, therefore, be incomplete.

An alternative approach, arguably complementary, regards mental health in childhood and adolescence as a commodity. A mentally healthy child will have enough health to cope successfully with adversity. In other words he or she will have enough of a capacity for satisfying personal relationships, sufficient defences against overwhelming emotions, adequate self-esteem to withstand disappointment, and a repertoire of strategies with which to manage challenges without resorting to immature or self-defeating responses. Mental health is not just the absence of disorder but also of resilience. In such a view, a mentally healthy young person is one who, when faced with adversity, can survive it and possibly also be strengthened ('steeled') by it.

The main difficulty with such an approach is that not all components of resilience can be taught or promoted—high intelligence and benign temperament, for instance. Furthermore, not all child or adolescent psychiatric disorder arises from exposure to adversity. As with the former definition, it cannot provide a path to total prevention.

Both the above approaches indicate that child and adolescent mental health promotion is closely associated with socialization so that the quality of parenting and education become key issues. Not surprisingly, most attempts to promote child mental health have focused upon these areas.

However, there is a further consideration. It may sometimes be appropriate to identify a state of less-than-adequate mental health on the basis of an inherent predisposition to future disorder. Genetic vulnerability to the later development of schizophrenia, bipolar disorder, or Tourette's syndrome, are examples. Children with such genes might be considered less healthy because of such a risk factor, intrinsic to them. This sort of thinking becomes relevant if types of prevention/promotion are considered.

Very little work has been done on the prevention of child and adolescent psychiatric disorders as such but there is a reasonable volume of work on such topics as adolescent antisocial behaviour or substance misuse, which can stand as proxies for disorder. With this in mind, the terms promotion and prevention are used interchangeably in this chapter.

More modern approaches to classification

Two broad approaches may be taken to provide early intervention and reduce the incidence of a condition. If the whole child population in a particular area receives an intervention, this is termed a universal approach. But if the intervention is addressed to a sub-population, it is said to be *targeted*. This itself may be *selective* (when groups of children are defined because they have been exposed to a risk factor for psychiatric disorder, such as being offspring of parents known to have depression). Alternatively it may be *indicated*, when index children are the recipients, chosen by virtue of possessing a biological predisposition (as in genetic counselling) or early, prodromal, signs of disorder, as in mild antisocial behaviour.

Risk, vulnerability, and protective factors

Targeting can be on the basis of individual vulnerabilities, situational factors, or events. Central to this principle are the concepts of risk and vulnerability. These concepts are the fruit of the conceptual approach known as developmental psychopathology, which draws upon developmental psychology, clinical science, and epidemiology to describe influences on the onset and course of childhood psychiatric disorders.

Risk factors are present before the onset of a disorder and increase the likelihood of the disorder occurring in children exposed to them. Some are intrinsic to the individual; constitutional or experiential, and increase the vulnerability to disorder of some children as opposed to

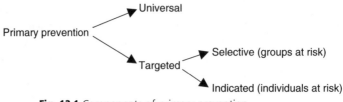

Fig. 12.1 Components of primary prevention.

others (see Fig. 12.1). Other risk and vulnerability factors are environmental: family factors, peer group influences, schooling, and neighbourhood. Although a number of intrinsic factors are fixed (e.g. male gender), many of the environmental factors are potentially modifiable.

Only some children exposed to a risk factor will develop a psychiatric disorder. Those that succumb will have vulnerability factors but, conversely, those that escape will have protective factors such as high self-esteem. These precede the appearance of the disorder and reduce the adverse impact of a risk factor.

In principle, the more is known about risk, vulnerability, and protective factors, the better informed a preventive approach will be. Yet there is a further technical consideration. In order to target a preventive intervention, a sub-population will need to be identified by screening. How effective a screening instrument, such as a questionnaire, is will depend upon sensitivity and specificity, in particular its positive predictive value. From the standpoint of clinicians, a high predictive value is relevant because it identifies how many of the sub-population will develop disorder. But from the public health point of view, the sensitivity is important because it will indicate how many of those children who develop disorder were picked up by the screen. There is a trade-off between the two attributes.

Choosing between universal and targeted approaches

The early population approaches to prevention in medicine tended to be based on an 'inoculation' model. A single intervention provides some protection against the future occurrence of a disorder. The universal immunization of young children has been a potent example. Yet most authorities in child mental health consider this an inappropriate example and, in an analogy to malnutrition prevention, favour a 'nutritional' model (e.g. Barnes 1998). This requires building protective strengths over a longer period. Parent management training has been a popular instance of this because it has demonstrable value in reducing antisocial behaviour in children in experimental studies. But such 'nutritional' interventions will be protracted and thus expensive, so that a targeted intervention might be preferred over a universal one. How does one make a choice between universal and targeted approaches?

Universal approaches do not stigmatize participants, have the advantage of including well-educated or influential families who will demand the programme be well-run, and avoid Rose's (1998) paradox. The latter refers to the fact that, although high-risk groups do, by definition, yield a high proportion of disorder within their own sub-population, this will usually be a minority in the population as a whole and more cases, numerically, will come from the low-risk remainder of the whole population. Put simply, more cases arise from low-risk populations than from high-risk groups because the latter are comparatively small.

Consider, for instance, the provision of parent management training aimed at reducing the incidence of conduct disorder. Given that this is more common in socially disadvantaged families, it might be thought sensible to target these. Yet they are in a minority in the population as a whole and more cases of conduct disorder will come from less socially disadvantaged families, since they are vastly more common. The ultimate impact of the programme will thus be small, even if it succeeds within the targeted sub-population.

On the other hand, whole-population approaches will, because of this, benefit mainly those at lowest risk; something that can increase inequality between high- and low-risk subgroups (often the richest and poorest) within a population (Offord and Bennett 2002). There may be poor compliance, if opting-in is required, because the perceived benefit for most of the whole population will be small.

A targeted approach, although cheaper, has the difficulty of stigmatization and technical problems with selecting and implementing screening. High-risk groups for a number of child and adolescent psychiatric disorders are likely to be less compliant with screening devices such as questionnaires.

Not all universal approaches require active opting-in. Major changes in social values, such as intolerance of abuse and neglect, can have an impact. If these are to be intentionally implemented as child mental health promotion, then clear thinking is required in order to ensure that the mechanism whereby they reduce mental disorder is understood.

Having said all this, it needs to be appreciated that the choice between universal and targeted interventions is rather academic, since it has not yet been shown scientifically that any intentional universal approach has in fact reduced the burden of child and adolescent psychiatric disorder. There are promising studies in targeted intervention but these are untested as major interventions beyond demonstration or experimental projects. Nevertheless some principles seem to be emerging and are now addressed.

Interventions should be active and persistent

The recipient of any preventive measure should be a participant. Although the provision of information is logically necessary, it is not likely to prove sufficient. It needs to be actively considered. For instance, Beardslee et al. (1997) attempted to prevent the later development of depression in adolescence among children with a depressed parent. Active participation in discussions about the impact of depression in a parent was more successful than hearing lectures.

In a number of studies, positive effects of promotion programmes wash out after a year or so. This was true, for instance, in a study of intensive home visiting (mainly by health visitors) in the UK (Nicol et al. 1993). That the period of intervention may need to be quite long is suggested by the Montreal Longitudinal Experimental Study (Tremblay et al. 1995), directed towards high-risk kindergarten boys. This provided both school-based social skills training together with home-based parent training for two years. A reduction in antisocial behaviour for the experimental group at the end of the programme was no longer evident at age 15. There are other examples, which lead most authorities to argue strongly for protracted involvement. As most studies have addressed antisocial behaviour there is the possibility that this may not apply to internalizing disorders, since a 5-year programme of home visiting in early childhood was effective in reducing internalized symptoms (not psychiatric disorder) in adolescence without intervention in the intervening years (Aronen and Kurkela 1996). Similarly, a 10-week programme for selected anxious 3–7-year-old Australian children produced a small reduction in anxiety disorders two years later compared with controls (Dadds et al. 1999).

Targeting young children

In a review of prevention of antisocial behaviour problems, Offord and Bennett (2002) demonstrate the relative effectiveness of parent training and social skills promotion in children under the age of 5, compared with programmes directed at older children. In the field of emotional disorders, one of the very few studies to actually show a reduction in psychiatric (anxiety) disorders specifically targeted pre-school children (Aronen and Kurkela 1996).

Most of the work on prevention of future antisocial behaviour has targeted pre-school children. The Perry/HighScope parent training project is perhaps the best known and showed an effect but, as is so often the case, the size of this was modest.

Children's psychiatric disorders are usually chronic and the question arises whether the factors maintaining them would be better targets than those known to initiate them. Peer-group factors might become more relevant with age compared with parenting factors for instance yet most studies have addressed parenting.

Interventions should include both the child and the child's environment

Most attempts at prevention of child psychiatric disorder have included schooling and parenting. When it has been possible to assess the relative contributions of environmental change (usually enrichment) and interventions direct to the child, environmental input has seemed to be more powerful.

Most schemes that have included both approaches to children and environmental input have focused on social skills training. It has been unusual to provide social skills training alone. One instance is the study by Selman *et al.* (1993), which promoted social adjustment through joint counselling of pairs of aggressive and withdrawn boys, provides only preliminary results with modest gains.

Recent studies have examined combinations of interventions directed at parents and children, since this 'multi-component' approach is now generally considered to be more powerful and preliminary results appear to support this (e.g. in the Fast Track project: Conduct Problems Research Group 1999; or the Tri-Ministry Helping Children Adjust Project, Boyle *et al.* 1999).

On the other hand, the take-up of parent management training in such programmes can be poor (see Boyle *et al.* 1999) and undermine the programme, whereas children can always be found in the school classroom. Home visiting (as in Fast Track) can assist parental involvement but is expensive. Alternatively, a prevention project intentionally involving the community or parents of children attending local schools (e.g. The School Development Program: Comer 1985) can motivate parents, presumably through peer support and minimal stigmatization. These issues are addressed below.

Home visiting and outreach are important

As a general rule, high-risk families are hardest to reach. Those families who are most likely to gain from interventions, such as parent management training, for example, are also those least likely to attend training sessions. With this in mind, home visiting or ways of making professional advice and assistance to parents are often considered. The programme for health visitors in South London (Davis and Spurr 1997) is an oft-cited evaluated example of an early intervention (though not strictly a prevention) project. There is quite widespread use of home visiting schemes in the UK, based on health visitors (Elkan *et al.* 2000) though the mental health component of this activity is variable and the ultimate impact on future psychiatric disorder either insignificant (Nicol *et al.* 1993) or untested by formal trial. Although resolution of behaviour problems can result from such work (Davis and Spurr 1997; Nicol *et al.* 1993), the longer term benefit is less certain. Nevertheless, because of encouraging results from schemes such as Olds' group (see e.g. Olds *et al.* 1999) or Aronen and Kurkel (1996), some centres have thought it worthwhile to promote health visitor training in child mental health (e.g. Earle and Hill 1998).

The school is an important potential arena for mental health promotion

There have been a number of studies that have attempted to capitalize upon the facts that all children attend schools and can thus be found there, and that many of the social processes that take place in schools can affect behavioural development and would, in theory, be susceptible to school-based interventions. The Good Behavior game (Kellam *et al.* 1994), the Montreal Longitudinal Experimental Study (Tremblay *et al.* 1995), and the PATH curriculum of the Fast Track programme (Conduct Problems Prevention Research Group 1999) are all examples of school-based projects that reduce antisocial behaviour, at least at school. There are other, less controlled studies but generally speaking, the gains are rather small.

There has been less work with emotional disorders, though the Queensland Early Intervention and Prevention of Anxiety Project (Dadds *et al.* 1999), a school-based programme intended to reduce anxiety disorder in mildly affected children through teaching cognitive coping strategies, did show an effect, maintained at follow-up, though somewhat modest in size. The expense of the project makes replication unlikely.

Prevention is not harmless

Harrington and Clark (1998), reviewing possibilities for the prevention of adolescent depression, drew together some of the possible adverse effects of prevention. Screening creates ethical problems and may be counterproductive by providing a 'certificate of health' for those only just below risk threshold. Programmes cost money, which could be spent on proven treatments, bearing in mind most cases currently go untreated. Educational programmes to prevent suicide may upset students or normalize suicidal behaviour. Some well-intentioned programmes, such as the Cambridge-Somerville study (McCord 1992), have eventually produced a worse outcome than routine care or no intervention. Interventions of proven effectiveness may be too expensive in terms of resource consumption to implement.

Conclusions

Child mental health promotion/prevention activity is in its infancy. The distinction between prevention and treatment is blurred. By and large, programmes have been expensive and gains, where demonstrable, modest. There is still no robust, replicated programme shown scientifically to prevent the development of disorder. Nevertheless, a number of initiatives show promise in furthering mental health, psychosocial development and social functioning (see Offord and Bennett 2002). Interventions need to be selective, early, intensive, multi-modal, persistent, participative, and involve outreach. UK initiatives have generally been targeted at pre-school children and this has been enhanced by Sure Start, though the absence of scientific outcome evaluation and the diversity of local initiatives means it will be hard to know what to make of it in child mental health terms. Nor is prevention harmless (Hill 2000), since it consumes resources that could be spent elsewhere and may actually be harmful. Although it seems appropriate to promote promotion, caution and careful evaluation remain watchwords.

The contribution of treatment services to the reduction in population morbidity is beginning to be evaluated but early signs are that it will come to a similar conclusion. Once effectiveness in limiting psychiatric morbidity in children is established, questions will follow as to whether adverse effects outweigh benefit, and whether the financial cost is warranted compared with an alternative policy of increased expenditure on treatment services.

References

Aronen, E.T. and Kurkela, S.A. (1996) Long-term effects of an early home-based intervention. *Journal of the American Academy of Child and Adolescent Psychiatry*, **35**, 1665–72.

Barnes, J. (1998) Mental health promotion: a developmental perspective. *Psychology, Health and Medicine*, **3**, 55–89.

Beardslee, W.R., Wright, E.J., Salt, P., Drezner, K., Gladstone, T.R.G., Versage, E.M., *et al.* (1997) Examination of children's responses to two preventive intervention strategies over time. *Journal of the American Academy of Child and Adolescent Psychiatry*, **36**, 196–204.

Boyle, M.H., Cunningham, C., Heale, J., and Hundert, J. (1999) Helpng children adjust: a Tri-Ministry study. I. Evaluation methodology. *Journal of Child Psychology and Psychiatry*, **40**, 1051–60.

Comer, J.P. (1985) The Yale-New Haven primary prevention project: a follow-up study. *Journal of the American Academy of Child and Adolescent Psychiatry*, **24**, 154–60.

Conduct Problems Research Group (1999) Initial impact of the Fast Track prevention trial for conduct problems: II. Classroom effects. *Journal of Consulting and Clinical Psychology*, **67**, 648–57.

Dadds, M.R., Holland, D.E., Laurens, K.R., Mullins, M., Barrett, P.M., and Spence, S. (1999) Early intervention and prevention of anxiety disorders in children: results at 2-year follow-up. *Journal of Consulting and Clinical Psychology*, **67**, 145–50.

Davis, H. and Spurr, P. (1997) Parent counselling: an evaluation of a community child mental health service. *Journal of Child Psychology and Psychiatry*, **38**, 365–76.

Earle, J. and Hill, P. (1998) *Research into practice: promoting the mental health of young children*. A Distance Learning Pack for Health Visitors. London: St George's Hospital Medical School.

Elkan, R., Kendrick, D., Hewitt, M., Robinson, J.J.A., Tolley, K., and Blair, M. (2000) The effectiveness of domiciliary health visiting: a systematic review of international studies and a selective review of the British literature. *Health Technology Assessment*, **4**, 13.

Graham, P. (1994) Prevention. In *Child and adolescent psychiatry: modern approaches* (3rd edn) (ed. M. Rutter, E. Taylor, and L. Hersov). pp. 815–28. Oxford: Blackwell Science.

Harrington, R.C. and Clark, A. (1998) Prevention and early intervention for depression in adolescence and early adult life. *European Archives of Psychiatry and Clinical Neuroscience*, **248**, 32–45.

Health Advisory Service (HAS) (2000) *Standards for child and adolescent mental health services*. Brighton: Pavilion Press.

Hill, P. (2000) Prevention of mental disorder in childhood and other public health issues. In *New Oxford textbook of psychiatry* (ed. M. Gelder, J. Lopez Ibor, N. Andreason). pp. 1705–11. Oxford: Oxford University Press.

Hill, P. and Spender, Q. (1996) Secondary prevention of childhood mental health problems. In *The prevention of mental illness in primary care* (ed. T. Kendrick, A. Tylee, and P. Freeling), ch. 9, pp. 149–66. Cambridge: Cambridge University Press.

Kellam, S.G., Rebok, G.W., Ialongo, N., and Mayer, L.S. (1994) The course and malleability of aggressive behavior from early first grade into middle school: results of a developmentally epidemiologically based preventive trial. *Journal of Child Psychology and Psychiatry,* **35**, 259–81.

McCord, J. (1992) The Cambridge-Somerville study: a pioneering longitudinal experimental study of delinquency prevention. In *Preventing antisocial behavior* (ed. J. McCord and R. Tremblay), pp. 196–206). New York: Guilford Press.

Nicol, A.R., Stretch, D., and Fundudis, T. (1993) *Preschool children in troubled families.* Chichester: John Wiley.

Offord, D.R. and Bennett, K.J. (2002) Prevention. In *Child and Adolescent Psychiatry* (4th edn) (ed. M. Rutter and E. Taylor). pp. 881–99. Oxford: Blackwell Scientific.

Olds, D.L., Henderson, C.R., Kitzman, H., Eckenrode, J., Cole, R.E., and Tatelbaum, R.C. (1999) Prenatal and home infancy home visitation by nurses: recent findings. *Future of Children,* **9**, 44–65.

Rose, G. (1998) Sick individuals, sick population. *International Journal of Epidemiology,* **14**, 32–8.

Selman, R.L., Schultz, L.H., Nakkula, M., Barr, D., Watts, C., and Richmond, J.R. (1993) Friendship and fighting: a developmental approach to the study of risk and prevention. *Development and Psychopathology,* **4**, 529–58.

Spender, Q. and Hill, P. (1996) Primary prevention of childhood mental health problems. In *The prevention of mental illness in primary care* (ed. T. Kendrick, A. Tylee, and P. Freeling), ch.2, pp. 21–40. Cambridge: Cambridge University Press.

Tremblay, R.E., Kurtz, L., Musse, L.C., Vitaro, F., and Pihl, R.O. (1995) A bimodal preventive intervention for disruptive kindergarten boys: its impact through mid-adolescence. *Journal of Consulting and Clinical Psychology,* **63**, 560–8.

Williams, R. and Richardson, G. (1995) *Together we stand.* NHS Health Advisory Service. London: HMSO.

Chapter 13

The impact of parental mental disorder on children

Peter Hill

A substantial challenge

In the last decade or so the increasing emphasis on mental health care in the community has meant that a number of adults with psychiatric disorder or substance misuse problems are treated while they continue to live with their families. At least a quarter of the adults who are so treated will be parents of children of school-age or below. In Nottingham, 25% of women seen by mental health services had a child under the age of 5 years (Oates 1997).

It is also the case that about one-fifth of admissions to psychiatric hospital are for women of child-bearing age (Dover *et al.* 1994). Conversely, one-third of the parents of children referred to child and adolescent mental health services have a psychiatric disorder, though this does not meant that their condition will necessarily be known to health services (Blanch *et al.* 1994). A similar figure arises from epidemiological surveys: children with a parent with a mental disorder are three times as likely to have a mental disorder themselves as those with mentally healthy parents, and the risk to the child rises with the severity of the parental disorder (Meltzer *et al.* 2000).

This association between parental psychiatric disorder (taken here to include alcohol and substance misuse) and childhood psychiatric disorder has been recognized for nearly forty years (Rutter 1966). The association also applies to child abuse: about one-fifth of children known to child protection agencies will have alcohol or drug misuse problems and about one-sixth will have a mental illness (Bell, Conroy and Gibbons 1995).

The most frequent conditions affecting adults who are parents of school-age or younger children are depression, alcohol and drug misuse, and personality disorder. Psychosis is less common and may actually impair ordinary parenting less than personality disorder, but it is more likely to be lethal to the child. Although most mentally ill parents do not harm their child, when this does occur and the child dies, there is a 50% chance that the parent will be suffering from a psychotic disorder (Falkov 1996).

A crude stereotype of the mentally ill parent most likely to be encountered is that of a woman with multiple social disadvantages. She is more likely than chance to be from an ethnic minority. About one in three of women so described will have a psychotic disorder and they will have been admitted compulsorily under the Mental Health Act at some stage (Falkov *et al.* 1998).

The reasons for the association between psychiatric disorder in the parent and mental health problems in the child

There is no inevitable link between parental and child psychiatric disorder in any individual case. Disorder in the parent is best conceived of as a risk factor for the child's mental health.

There are various types of causal link:

psychiatric disorder (here taken to include substance misuse) in a parent causes disorder in the child;

psychiatric disorder in the child causes disorder in the parent;

a common factor causes psychiatric disorder in both.

These may co-exist and multiply the effect of each other, systemically. There are several possible causal pathways, listed and discussed below.

Genetics

Various conditions are heritable and can exist in both parent and offspring: schizophrenia, and bipolar and unipolar affective disorders are clear examples, but in general this is unusual because they are rather more likely to appear at an age after childhood itself. Attention-deficit hyperactivity disorder (hyperkinetic disorder) is probably a commoner example but is not yet widely recognised in adults.

Neglect or sub-optimal care

The tasks of parenting are various and psychiatric disorder in a parent can compromise or impair any of these. Chronic intoxication or abnormal preoccupations, anxieties, or mood can adversely affect parenting tasks across the board. Parental provision for a child's development includes a range of activities: nutrition, protection, supervision, instruction, opportunity for emotional attachment formation, setting an appropriate example of social and moral behaviour, discipline and emotional support, and so forth. Should a parent's psychiatric disorder lead to poor quality of the child's physical, interpersonal, cognitive and emotional environment, then the child's physical and psychological development can be impaired or distorted. In turn this can predispose or directly cause psychiatric disorder in the child.

Alternatively, the parental responses to the child may be less sensitive or delayed because of parental psychiatric disorder. This can place the child at physical risk or, in young children, lead to a relative failure in the formation of secure attachments. Because secure attachment is associated with less anxiety and distress in the child, unresponsive parenting can be associated with a higher risk of childhood emotional disorder. In later childhood, inadequate parental supervision of a child places them at risk for accidents, abuse by strangers, or other inappropriate experiences. Truancy, delinquent activities, and drug or alcohol misuse within the peer group are less likely to be detected and increase the risk of conduct disorder in particular.

Physical abuse

The majority of parents who abuse their children are not psychiatrically disordered but there is an increased risk of abuse when a parent is so disturbed (see Falkov 1996). This may reflect less tolerance by a parent, less vigilance as to possible abuse by a partner, or a malignant parental belief that the child is inherently wicked. Physical abuse can, in turn lead to permanent physical injury through, for example, shaking in infancy. It is also a risk factor for either exceptionally aggressive or avoidant behaviour in the child.

A higher rate of adverse life events for the child

This particularly applies to separation of young children from a parent when she has to be admitted to hospital or when the child has to be taken into local authority care. Such separation experiences, when multiple, are a risk factor for the development of psychiatric disorder in the child through various mechanisms.

Adults with psychiatric disorders are themselves prone to a number of adverse life events, some of which will also affect their children. As a generalization, adverse life-events increase the risk of psychiatric disorder in a child, even though the impact of single, short-lived events is not great.

Distortions of care as a result of abnormal parental beliefs

Delusional beliefs, exaggerated concerns (as in obsessional disorders), or distorted ideas (as in anorexia nervosa) may not so much impair parenting as distort its practice. The child may be exposed to the parent's beliefs directly and come to believe them (as in *folie à deux*) or be the subject of them (as in philanthropic murder or Munchausen's syndrome by proxy).

Reversed dependency and young carers

The normal pattern of dependency means that immature and vulnerable children are cared for by adult parents. Yet sometimes it falls to the child to care for an adult parent who is psychiatrically disordered. The burden of physical care—shopping, obtaining prescriptions and so forth—can cause fatigue and loss of time at school. But it is emotional dependency that is especially pernicious—extreme worry on the child's part about the parent's welfare, fuelled by the parent turning to the child for reassurance or by the child's experience of suicidal behaviour or talk by the parent. Children often simply cannot carry such a burden of concern if their normal source of comfort and reassurance is unavailable because the tables are turned, though an emotionally warm, supportive relationship with another parent can offer some protection.

Conflictual family relationships

Adult mental health disorders, especially personality disorder, alcohol or drug misuse, and irritability associated with affective and anxiety disorders, are generally associated with an increased risk of discordant relationships with other family members.

It is well-established that discordant, conflictual relationships within the family are a potent risk factor for the common psychiatric disorders of childhood. Epidemiologically, discord at any level of relationships between family members is an aetiological factor for child psychiatric disorder but the association is strongest when it exists between parent and child. More precisely, high levels of hostile criticism and an irritable, nagging tone of voice addressed to children (as researched under 'expressed emotion') is closely associated with the development of antisocial behaviour disorders generally. Emotional rejection is an extreme form of this and is likely to be associated, under such circumstances, with emotional symptoms, desperate attempts to appease the parent alternating with anger, stealing from parents, and poor self-esteem. When such parental behaviour is associated with extreme threats, the resulting chronic fear has a corrosive effect on a young mind.

In parallel with this, open discord between parents with the child as bystander also has an adverse effect on child mental health. In extreme cases there will be violence between parental figures, which can disturb children by inducing post-traumatic stress disorder or anxiety. Flight by a parent from a violent partner will lead to an abrupt change of life circumstances for the children if she takes them with her. There is the possibility of loss of a parent by flight, desertion, imprisonment, or death.

Deviant example

Part of normal socialization is the experience of observing how a parent solves interpersonal or resource crises. Children model themselves on parental behaviour and standards. This might be tempered somewhat in adolescence but even then parental influence is more substantial than popularly supposed.

If the parent uses maladaptive coping strategies (overdosing or other self-harm, intoxication with legal or illegal substances, advertising helplessness, disproportionate aggression) then there is an increased chance of the child learning these too.

Loss or distortion of social contacts

Children may well want to conceal a parent's eccentric or abnormal behaviour from friends. They are less likely to invite them back to the family home and are at risk for increasing social isolation within the peer group. Having a parent with noticeable mental disorder can be a focus for teasing or even bullying at school. 'Cussing' a child's mother is a frequent cause of playground fights.

Loss of family stability

Admission of a parent to psychiatric hospital very commonly results in the children having to go and live somewhere else (Hawes and Cottrell 1999). They may stay with relatives or be received into local authority care. A given child may thus experience a number of caregivers over the years and in the very young this can prejudice the formation of secure emotional attachments.

Loss of family income

Chronic adult psychiatric disorder is likely to drain family resources, emotional and material. It is usually the case that there is less income; something that tends to prejudice optimal parenting.

Bereavement

Because there is a higher rate of mortality among adults with psychiatric disorders, children of affected adults who are parents will experience a higher rate of bereavement, particularly through parental suicide. This is again a risk factor for psychiatric disorder in childhood.

Circular processes within families

Although the main burden of this section is to stress how parental psychiatric disorder or its treatment can be a risk for childhood mental health, there are grounds for thinking the reverse is also true.

Disruptive behaviour disorders in childhood seem particularly prone to exhaust parents and produce parental tension or anxiety. A possible outcome is the situation in which such disorder in the child angers or exhausts the parent who then takes it out on the child, exacerbating his uncontained or angry behaviour, which further irritates the parent or drives them into despair in a circular, systemic process. There are ethical issues in all this since there may be a call for the child to be effectively sedated for the sake of the parent (or vice versa) and a balance of needs has to be considered.

Dangerousness

Many psychiatrically disordered adults who are parents of young children are particularly concerned that their altered state of mind may lead them to neglect or harm their children. They worry that their children may be removed by a social services department.

In fact the number of such instances is small. It exists but should not distort the overall picture. Most instances in which a child's welfare is compromised by adult psychiatric disorder are relatively mild. Severe cases in which a child is physically harmed or killed are rare. There is a spectrum of severity from which can be projected a triangle (see Fig. 13.1).

The impact on the child of treatment for the adult parent

Treating the adult should, in theory, improve their functioning, including their capacity to be a competent parent. However, there are components of treatment that may have an adverse effect on the child.

Admission to psychiatric hospital is one such instance, especially if done as an emergency. There is a clear risk to continuity of parenting if the patient is a lone parent. Services need to have admission protocols that include consideration of the children's needs beyond the immediately expedient. Almost certainly this will require some joint planning between health and social services.

The timing of follow-up or medication clinics does not usually take the needs of parents into account. However it is usually possible to ensure that parents attending these can be given appointments with times that do not conflict directly with child care responsibilities.

Some medication for adult psychiatric disorder will sedate or at least impair physical and emotional responsiveness to children. There may be alternatives that have less adverse effects on parental energy and sensitivity.

An extension of this is the possible adverse effects of medicines on pregnancy or, through lactation, on breast-fed babies. At one level this is about finding ways for mentally sick mothers, who need to be in hospital, to be able to continue to breast-feed their babies. At another it indicates a need for hospital pharmacies and prescribing doctors to have guidelines on safe medication in pregnancy and lactation.

Good practice

Logically, a number of recommendations follow from the above. These can be considered according to whether they would affect professional practice or service organization.

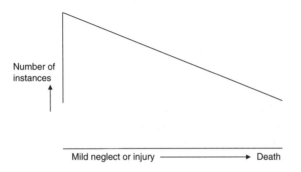

Fig. 13.1 A continuum of safety.

The professional practice of clinical mental health professionals who see predominantly adult patients

They should be aware that every adult they see may be a parent whose parenting capacity may be compromised by their condition, or that they fear it may be. To this end, they need to:

ascertain whether their patient has children and list their names, ages, and where-abouts ;

ask questions about the patient's capacity to parent;

enquire as to the mental health of the children.

They should be prepared to talk with their patient about parenting. All parents want to be good parents and some are painfully aware that they are not as good as they would like to be, per-haps because of their psychiatric condition or its treatment. It may be helpful to discuss aspects of parenting with the patient's partner.

There is no need for those clinicians who are predominantly concerned with adult patients to be experts on parenting or child mental health to do this and to explore key areas. A few aspects, rather than the total picture need addressing. A key issue here is ascertaining whether the patient, as a parent, has an appropriate capacity for concern for her children (see Fig. 13.2). With respect to the tasks of parenting, the further issues are whether she can:

ensure the general safety, health, and welfare of their child;

provide adequate child-rearing in areas such as discipline, education, and opportunities to socialize;

have a positive, loving relationship with their child.

As part of their practice, mental health professionals who predominantly treat adults should also be prepared to:

refer or act as an advocate for their patient as a parent and for the family as a whole, so that appropriate services from various agencies are deployed;

activate child protection procedures when these are required (only occasionally).

This does not mean that clinical professionals need to become inquisitorial. For practical pur-poses, a simple grid can be completed within the case-notes to organize appraisal and enable practice to be audited.

It may also be that the burden of parenting is affecting the adult patient's mental health or its treatment. Enquiry along the above lines will expose this.

An area for consideration is the extent to which the practical and emotional burden of care for the patient, who is a parent, falls upon her children. Practical questioning about who cares for younger children, who cooks and shops, who picks up prescriptions, and so forth, can illuminate this.

If there are grounds for concern but the situation is still obscure, further information can be obtained from a spouse/partner, general practitioner, health visitor, or, if allocated, social worker. Doubts about the children's mental health can be discussed with a child mental health professional. Concern about children's safety or welfare should lead to invoking child protec-tion procedures. Staff need training in this.

When parenting has been impaired by psychiatric disorder, it is important to recognize that a return to reasonable mental health does not necessarily mean that there will be an automatic return to adequate parenting.

	Due to disorder	Due to in-patient treatment	Due to out- or day-patient treatment
Children's safety, health and welfare			
Care-giving and general child-rearing tasks			
Positive, supportive, loving relationship			

Fig. 13.2 A simple grid, suitable for audit purposes.

The professional practice of clinical mental health professionals who predominantly see child and adolescent patients

It is reasonable to expect such staff to be capable of assessing parenting. They should be responsive to requests for assistance from colleagues who predominantly see adults, and be prepared to attend CPA meetings, if appropriate.

In their own right, they should be alert to evidence of mental health problems in the parents of the children they see and refer accordingly. They will ordinarily be accustomed to taking a systemic view of interactions between children's emotional or behavioural symptoms and parental mental state.

Mental health services

Clearly services should support, facilitate, and encourage the auditing of clinical practices described above. They also need to consider the following:

Provision of child-friendly physical environments adjacent to clinics or wards, where patients who are parents may bring or be visited by their children.

How ward staff can make sensitive decisions about visiting arrangements, so that children who visit are not frightened or put at risk by the behaviour of other patients. Aspects of this are addressed in the Mental Health Act (1983) Revised Code of Pactice (para. 26.3).

How children's interests can best be met by the timing of clinics, home visits, and visits by children to a parent who is an in-patient. Clashes with school or child-care arrangements can often be avoided, given forethought.

The provision of straightforward, understandable information for children about their parent's mental health problems or crises (admission to hospital, overdoses, etc.) arising from these.

Similarly, parents who are also patients need information about how local services and agencies can help them continue to be competent parents, satisfied in their role as such.

Prescribing policies for patients who are pregnant or breast-feeding.

Ensuring that each service has within it, or access to, a named person who can answer clinicians' questions about children's welfare, safety, and protection. It might be possible for this person to be a liaison nurse who can promote liaison between adult mental health, child and adolescent mental health, paediatrics, and primary care. That individual can also drive audit in the areas of safe and fear-free visiting by children, provision of information and sensitive management of clinical crises. She (it probably will usually be she) also can advise management about administrative and resource implications in the area.

Prevention

There are opportunities in this area to develop preventive policies for children's mental health problems, given that a number of the latter can be associated with adult parental mental health disorders. For instance, post-natal depression is an obvious topic, though screening for this will ordinarily be carried out in primary care. However, it should follow that specialist services provide a prompt secondary care response to referral of a depressed new mother.

Conclusion

This is an area in which collaboration between, at least, adult- and child-centred mental health services needs to happen. This will not necessarily occur without active promotion. It leads to active collaboration with other agencies—primary care, social services, and paediatrics are clear instances. Striving for practices that promote both the mental health and happiness of children, as well as supporting their parents, who would like to practice optimal parenting, need not be expensive.

At the time of writing (2001/2), a Royal College of Psychiatrists working party on patients as parents is completing a paper, which will probably be published as a council document . It will contain more detail and recommendations than this chapter can include.

References

Bell, C., Conroy, S., and Gibbons, J. (1995) *Operating the child protection system: a study of child protection practices in english local authorities.* London: HMSO.

Blanch, A.K., Nicholson, J., and Purcell, J. (1994) Parents with severe mental illness and their children: The need for human services integration. *The Journal of Mental Health Administration,* **21**, 388–96.

Dover, S., Leahy, A., and Foreman, D. (1994) Parental psychiatric disorder: Clinical prevalence and effects on default from treatment. *Child Care Health and Development,* **20**, 137–43.

Falkov, A. (1996) *Department of Health study of working together 'part 8' reports: fatal child abuse and parental psychiatric disorder.* London: Department of Health Social Care Group, ACPC Series, Report 1.

Falkov, A. Murphy, M., and Antweiler, U. (1998) In *Crossing bridges* (ed. A. Falkov), p. 11. London: Department of Health.

Hawes, V. and Cottrell, D. (1999) Disruption of children's lives by maternal psychiatric admission. *Psychiatric Bulletin,* **23**, 153–6.

Meltzer, H., Gatward, R., Goodman, R., and Ford, T. (2000*) The mental health of children and adolescents in Great Britain.* London: Office for National Statistics, The Stationery Office.

Oates, M. (1997) Patients as parents: the risk to children. *British Journal of Psychiatry,* **170** (suppl. 32), 22–7.

Rutter, M. (1966) *Children of Sick Parents.* Maudsley Monograph No. 16. Oxford: Oxford University Press.

Chapter 14

Client groups that challenge services
Suicide and deliberate self-harm

Michael Kerfoot

Definitions

In general, suicidal behaviour is made up of two separate phenomena but with a marked degree of overlap between them. In one group can be included those individuals who intentionally kill themselves (suicide), or who harm themselves with the clear intention of ending their lives, but who unexpectedly survive (attempted suicide). In the other group are those who intentionally harm themselves but in the reasonably secure belief that death will not result from their action (deliberate self-harm). However, just as some suicides survive their actions, so some acts of deliberate self-harm do have a quite unintended fatal outcome.

Epidemiology

In the UK suicide is now one of the leading causes of death among young people aged 15–24 years (Office of National Statistics 1999) and similar trends have been observed in the USA. Rates of deliberate self-harm (DSH) among British 15–19-year-olds are higher than in almost all European countries (Hawton et al. 1998), and may be increasing (Hawton et al. 1997). Referrals to hospital because of DSH remain at a high level in this age group (Hawton and Fagg 1992), and child and adolescent mental health services (CAMHS) spend a great deal of time in the assessment and aftercare of overdose cases, which, in some areas, account for up to 20% of all referrals (Kerfoot 1988). Moreover, although the risk of subsequent suicide following an episode of DSH appears to be low (Pfeffer et al. 1993), it is notable that around one-third of adolescents who kill themselves have a history of DSH (Martunnen et al. 1993).

Suicide in children under 12 years of age is rare (Shaffer 1974; Hawton and Goldacre 1982) and is a relatively unusual event in the under 15s. However, suicide rates since the 1970s have shown a particular increase for 15–19-year-old males. This increase is also reflected in rates for 'accidental' and 'undetermined' deaths (McClure 1994), and is associated with the increase in more lethal methods, such as hanging and poisoning by vehicle exhaust gas. In contrast, over the same period the rates for young women fell by nearly a half. The reasons for this are unclear but social factors, such as the increasing rate of divorce, may be important. Misuse of drugs and alcohol by young people has also increased, and both are related to suicide among the young (Martunnen et al. 1991). There is increasing evidence to suggest an important link between psychiatric disorders, such as depression, and suicide in young people (Brent et al. 1994b). Suicide among the young is often preceded by psychosocial difficulties of one kind or another. It is probably the culmination of chronic difficulties, which include depression, drug or alcohol use, psychosocial stress, and/or behavioural problems. The effects of suicide on family and friends have also been highlighted in research (Brent *et al*. 1994a) where friends of young suicide victims experienced significant psychiatric morbidity after the death, and grief reactions which persisted for some months.

On the basis of rates found in Oxford (Hawton and Fagg 1992), it has been estimated that around 20 000 young people will be referred to general hospitals each year in England and Wales, as a result of deliberate self-poisoning or self-injury. Rates are higher for older teenagers than for younger ones (under 16s) and rates for females have continued to increase, while those for males have tended to remain stable. There are few reports of DSH in children under the age of 12, although it does occur from time to time. DSH is far more common among girls than boys, the sex ratio being around 4:1, and by far the method of choice in DSH is self-poisoning, usually by an overdose of tablets. Frequently these are tablets that can be bought over the counter, such as analgesics (Hawton and Goldacre 1982), but in younger adolescents at least half of the overdoses that occur involve the use of prescribed medication (Kerfoot 1988). Other forms of self-harm, such as the cutting of wrists and arms, is more common in older adolescents, and does not usually result in serious risk to life.

Causation

Several factors have been linked to DSH in young people. For example, our previous research (Kerfoot 1988; Kerfoot *et al*. 1996) has found a strong and robust association between childhood DSH and (1) parental problems such as criminality and reliance on welfare benefits; and (2) a disrupted upbringing caused by, for example, periods in local authority 'care', or parental marital problems resulting in separation or divorce. There is also a strong association with on-going family relationship problems (which are the most common precipitant of an overdose) and with factors intrinsic to the child, such as behavioural problems, hopelessness, and depression.

Depression is important because around one-half of children and adolescents presenting with DSH score positively for major depressive disorder (Andrews and Lewinsohn 1992; Kerfoot *et al*. 1996) and children who have harmed themselves have many features in common with depressed children (Pfeffer 1992; De Wilde *et al*. 1993). Moreover, some follow-up studies find that the outcome of childhood DSH is similar to that of childhood depression (Lewinsohn *et al*. 1994), and that repetition of DSH is often linked to episodes of depression (Pfeffer *et al*. 1993). These findings suggest that in many cases DSH is best conceptualized as a symptom of major depressive disorder. However, our work shows that major depressive disorder often remits very rapidly following DSH (Kerfoot *et al*. 1996), raising the possibility that depression has a different significance when it occurs in the context of DSH. Childhood DSH is strongly linked with family dysfunction, behavioural problems, and psychosocial stressors, such as poverty (Kerfoot 1988; Kerfoot *et al*. 1996). Stressful relationships with parents, particularly mother–adolescent relationships, have been shown to be significantly related to depression and suicidal ideation (Adams *et al*. 1994), with families showing dysfunction in areas such as problem-solving and crisis avoidance. Substance misuse is becoming increasingly cited in research reports as a serious risk factor for completed suicide and deliberate self-harm in adolescents (Buckstein *et al*. 1993).

Assessment

Offers of treatment must always follow a rigorous psychosocial assessment of the individual, and the immediate family or caretakers. Assessment is crucial, both in calculating current or potential suicide risk but also in deciding the most appropriate course of intervention. Intervention is also key since all forms of intervention will have as part of their goals the reduction of further suicidal behaviour. The PATHOS screening interview (Kingsbury 1993) provides a useful shorthand for the assessment of suicidal adolescents and includes the most important components for making judgements about intent and risk. Assessment also provides an opportunity for the negotiation of a 'no suicide contract', which may be a necessary precursor of therapeutic intervention. The 'contract', which can be written or verbal, is designed to focus attention on positive action rather than negative withdrawal, so that the adolescent can feel free to express recurrent suicidal ideas, or to let people know when motivation is waning. It is a shared responsibility, since it requires not only positive action on the part of the adolescent, but also that others be available consistently so that there is ready access to a sympathetic listener when required.

Intervention

Previous research on the characteristics of adolescents with DSH in the UK has generated important clues about the kinds of factor that might be relevant in designing and delivering interventions. For example, there has been general agreement that children with DSH come from families with disturbed relationships and where there are high levels of interpersonal and social stress (Hawton *et al.* 1982; Taylor and Stansfield 1984; Kerfoot 1988; Hawton and Fagg 1992). The quality of communication within the family is often poor (Richman 1979) and their problem-solving skills may be quite limited (Hawton 1986). It becomes possible, therefore, to target interventions into specific areas of individual and family functioning, and to devise ways in which these interventions can be evaluated. It is known from studies of adults who attempt suicide, as well as from child and adolescent studies, that these individuals are difficult to engage in treatment and follow-up (Morgan 1979; Taylor and Stansfield 1984; Kerfoot and McHugh 1992) and that it is an under-resourced area of work in the UK generally (Black 1992). All of these factors need to be taken into account when planning and designing therapeutic services.

A variety of treatment approaches have been reported in the literature and some of these have been subject to scientific evaluation. For example, a more formalized version of the 'no suicide contract' is the 'green card' system, which was set up within a service for adults with suicidal behaviour (Morgan and Owen 1990). In return for agreeing to a 'no suicide contract' the individual is given a green card, which gives immediate access to professional help and advice in specified clinical settings. The provision of 24-hour access to professional help via the green card has been shown to reduce suicide attempts and threats in an adult population (Morgan *et al.* 1993). A similar study based on readmission to hospital on demand, which was conducted with a younger age group, produced some positive signs, even though the overall treatment results failed to reach statistical significance (Cotgrove *et al.* 1995). Only 6% of the green card group re-attempted during the following year, while 12% of the control group made a further attempt.

Existing studies suggest that treatments that engage the individual in an active and challenging way, and are flexible with regard to timing and setting, are likely to have more success that more traditional approaches. Studies also indicate that treatment programmes that are focused on specific difficulties, such as poor problem-solving, dysfunctional family communications, and negative cognitions, are more likely to increase treatment compliance and to reduce suicidal ideation, than more open-ended, exploratory therapies. Social problem solving therapy (SPST) has been used to good effect with groups of college students scoring significantly for suicidal ideation (Lerner and Clum 1990). Compared with supportive group therapy, SPST proved to be superior in reducing depressive symptoms and hopelessness in a group of 18–24-year-olds but was no more effective in reducing suicidal ideation.

Cognitive behavioural therapy (CBT) is an individual approach that specifically addresses hopelessness, and has been used successfully in the treatment of depression in children and adolescents (Wood *et al.* 1996), and in treating depression and suicidality (Lewinsohn and Clarke 1990). Dialectical behaviour therapy (DBT) is another cognitive behavioural approach that combines CBT with psychotherapy, and group behavioural skills training to treat suicidal young adults who also meet the criteria for borderline personality disorder. In a controlled trial, DBT was successful in reducing both the number and lethality of subsequent attempts but, although there were reduced scores at follow-up on depressive symptomatology, hopelessness, and suicidal ideation, they failed to reach statistical significance (Linehan *et al.* 1991).

A number of family approaches are currently being employed and evaluated, and our own brief family intervention (BFI) used insights from research and practice to develop an approach that is brief, focused, intensive, action-oriented, and home-based (Kerfoot *et al.* 1995). The BFI was evaluated in a randomised controlled trial and results showed significantly greater compliance with BFI than with routine treatment, and significant and sustained improvement for non-depressed suicidal adolescents (Harrington *et al.* 1998).

Outcomes

There have been few long-term follow-up studies and child to adult outcomes are largely unknown. A Swedish study (Otto 1972) found that 4% of his adolescent sample had killed themselves when followed up 10–20 years later. The need for such studies is underlined by the finding from cross-sectional studies that young people who harm themselves have many of the risk factors for adverse outcomes in later life. Information is also needed on the long-term costs associated with deliberate self-harm, so that budgets can be planned on the basis of evidence, thereby maximizing benefits for patients.

Challenges

The complex nature of self-harm and, in particular, the impulsivity associated with its occurrence in adolescence, has meant that few of the treatment studies cited have had a sustained and positive effect. Well-defined studies focusing on the efficacy of after-care, and its outcome, are much needed, not only because of the dangers associated with acts of DSH, but also because these episodes are often markers of severe, social, interpersonal, or psychiatric difficulties. The risk of repetition calls for increased efforts to develop interventions that are geared to the specific needs of young people and their families, and controlled studies to evaluate their effectiveness. Targeted developments of this kind make the most efficient use of scarce resources, are likely to increase compliance among service-users, and give greater cost-effectiveness to purchasers of services.

Bibliography

Adams, D. M., Overholser, J. C., and Spirito, A. (1994) Stressful life events associated with adolescent suicide attempts. *Canadian Journal of Psychiatry, 39*, 43–8.

Andrews, J. A. and Lewinsohn, P. M. (1992) Suicidal attempts among older adolescents: prevalence and co-occurrence with psychiatric disorders. *Journal of the American Academy of Child and Adolescent Psychiatry, 31*, 655–62.

Black D (1992) Mental health services for children. *British Medical Journal*, **24**, 12.

Brent, D., Perper, J. A., Mortiz, G., Liotus, L., Schweers, J., and Cannobio, R. (1994a) Major depression or uncomplicated bereavement? A follow-up of youth exposed to suicide. *Journal of the American Academy of Child and Adolescent Psychiatry*, **33**, 231–9.

Brent, D. A., Perper, J. A., Mortiz, G., Baugher, M., Schweers, J., and Roth, C. (1994b) Suicide in affectively ill adolescents: A case control study. *Journal of Affective Disorders*, 193–202.

Buckstein, O. G., Brent, D. A., Perper, J. A., Mortiz, G., Baugher, M., Schweers, J., *et al.* (1993) Risk factors for completed suicide among adolescents with a lifetime history of substance abuse: a case control study. *Acta Psychiatrica Scandinavica*, **88**, 403–8.

Cotgrove, S., Zirinsky, L., Black, D., and Weston, D. (1995) Secondary prevention of attempted suicide in adolescence. *Journal of Adolescence*, **18**, 569–77.

De Wilde, E. J., Kienhorst, I. C. W. M., Diekstra, R. F. W., and Wolters, W. H. G. (1993) The specificity of psychological characteristics of adolescent suicide attempters. *Journal of the American Academy of Child and Adolescent Psychiatry*, **32**, 51–9.

Harrington, R., Kerfoot, M., Dyer, E., McNiven, F., Gill, J., Harrington, V., *et al.* (1998) Randomized trial of a home-based family intervention for children who have deliberately poisoned themselves. *Journal of the American Academy of Child and Adolescent Psychiatry*, **37**(5), 512–18.

Hawton, K. (1986) *Suicide and attempted suicide among children and adolescents*. Beverley Hills: Sage Publications.

Hawton, K. and Fagg, J. (1992) Deliberate self-poisoning and self-injury in adolescents: a study of characteristics and trends in Oxford 1976–1989. *British Journal of Psychiatry*, **161**, 816–23.

Hawton, K. and Goldacre, M. (1982) Hospital admissions for adverse effects of medicinal agents (mainly self-poisoning) among adolescents in the Oxford region. *British Journal of Psychiatry*, **141**, 166–70.

Hawton, K., Cole, D., O'Grady, J., and Osborn, M. (1982) Adolescents who take overdoses: their characteristics, problems and contacts with helping agencies. *British Journal of Psychiatry*, **140**, 118–23.

Hawton, K., Fagg, J., Simpkin, S., Bale, E., and Bond, A. (1997) Trends in deliberate self-harm in Oxford 1985–1995: implications for clinical services and the prevention of suicide. *British Journal of Psychiatry*, **171**, 556–60.

Hawton, K., Arensman, E., Wasserman, D., Hulten, A., and Bille-Brane, U. (1998) Relation between attempted suicide and suicide rates among young people in Europe. *Journal of Epidemiology and Community Health*, **52**, 191–4.

Kerfoot, M. (1988) Deliberate self-poisoning in childhood and early adolescence. *Journal of Child Psychology and Psychiatry*, **29**, 335–43.

Kerfoot, M. and McHugh, B. (1992) The outcome of childhood suicidal behaviour. *Acta Paedopsychiatrica Scandinavica* **55**, 141–5.

Kerfoot, M., Harrington, R., and Dyer, E. (1995) Brief home-based intervention with young suicide attempters and their families. *Journal of Adolescence*, **18**, 557–68.

Kerfoot, M., Dyer, E., Harrington, V., Woodham, A., and Harrington, R. (1996) Correlates and short-term course of self-poisoning in adolescents. *British Journal of Psychiatry*, **168**, 38–42.

Kingsbury, S. (1993) Parasuicide in adolescence: a message in a bottle. *Association of Child Psychology and Psychiatry Review*, **15**, 253–9.

Lerner, M. S. and Clum, G. A. (1990) Treatment of suicide ideators: a problem-solving approach. *Behavioural Therapy*, **21**, 403–11.

Lewinsohn, P. M. and Clarke, G. N. (1990) Cognitive behavioural treatment for depressed adolescents. *Behavioural Therapy*, **21**, 385–401.

Lewinsohn, P. M., Rohde, P., and Seeley, J. R. (1994) Psychosocial risk factors for future adolescent suicide attempts. *Journal of Consulting and Clinical Psychology*, **62**, 297–305.

Linehan, M. M., Armstrong, H. E., Suarez, A., Allmon, D., and Heard, H. L. (1991) Cognitive behavioural treatment of chronically parasuicidal borderline patients. *Archives of General Psychiatry,* **48**, 1060–4.

Martunnen, M. J., Aro, H. M., Henriksson, M. M., and Lonnqvist, J. K. (1991) Mental disorder in adolescent suicide: DSM-IIIR Axes 1 and II diagnoses in suicides among 13–19-year-olds in Finland. *Archives of General Psychiatry,* **48**, 834–9.

Martunnen, M. M., Aro, H. M., and Lonnqvist, J. K. (1993) Adolescence and suicide: a review of psychological autopsy studies. *European Child and Adolescent Psychiatry,* **2**, 10–18.

McClure, G. M. C. (1994) Suicide in children and adolescents in England and Wales. *British Journal of Psychiatry,* **165**, 510–14.

Morgan, H. G. (1979) *Death wishes? The assessment and management of deliberate self-harm.* London: Wiley.

Morgan, H. G. and Owen, J. H. (1990) *Persons at risk of suicide: guidelines on good clinical practice.* Nottingham: Boots.

Morgan, H. G., Jones, E. M., and Owen, J. H. (1993) Secondary prevention of non-fatal self-harm: the green card study. *British Journal of Psychiatry,* **163**, 111–2.

Office of National Statistics (1999) *Health statistics quarterly.* London. The Stationery Office.

Otto, U. (1972) Suicidal acts by children and adolescents: a follow-up study. *Acta Psychiatrica Scandinavica,* Supplementum 233.

Pfeffer, C. R. (1992) Relationship between depression and suicidal behaviour. In *Clinical guide to depression in children and adolescents* (ed. M. Shafii, and S.L. Shafii). Washington: American Psychiatric Press.

Pfeffer, C. R., Klerman, G. L., Hurt, S. W., Kakuma, T., Peskin, J. R., and Siefker, C. A. (1993) Suicidal children grow up: rates and psychosocial risk factors for suicidal attempts during follow-up. *Journal of the American Academy of Child and Adolescent Psychiatry,* **32**, 106–13.

Richman J (1979) The family therapy of attempted suicide. *Family Process,* **18**, 131–42.

Shaffer, D. (1974) Suicide in childhood and adolescence. *Journal of Child Psychology and Psychiatry,* **15**, 275–91.

Taylor, E. A. and Stansfield, S. A. (1984) Children who poison themselves: a clinical comparison with psychiatric controls. *British Journal of Psychiatry,* **145**, 127–32.

Wood, A., Harrington, R., and Moore, A. (1996) Controlled trial of a brief cognitive behavioural intervention in adolescent patients with depressive disorder. *Journal of Child Psychology and Psychiatry,* **37**, 737–46.

Depressive disorders

Richard Harrington

Introduction

Until recently it was widely believed that depressive disorders were rare in young people. Young children were thought to be incapable of experiencing many of the phenomena that are characteristic of depressive disorders in adults (Harrington 1994). Affective disturbance in adolescents was often dismissed as adolescent 'turmoil'. Over the past twenty years, however, there has been a substantial change in the ways in which mood disturbance among the young has been conceptualized. The use of structured personal interviews has shown that depressive syndromes resembling adult depressive disorders, can and do occur among both pre-pubertal children and adolescents. Indeed, clinical research in the UK has suggested that as many as one in ten referrals to child psychiatrists suffer from a depressive disorder (Kolvin *et al.* 1991). Depression may be becoming more prevalent among young people (Fombonne 1995).

Definition and classification

ICD-10 and DSM-IV criteria

Most clinicians nowadays use one of the major adult schemes for diagnosing depressive disorder in both children and adolescents, DSM-IV (American Psychiatric Association 1994) or ICD-10 (World Health Organization 1993). The schemes differ in many small ways, but at the core of both is the concept of an episodic disorder of varying degrees of severity that is characterized by depressed mood or loss of enjoyment, which persists for several weeks and is associated with certain other symptoms.

Both DSM-IV and ICD-10 distinguish between mild, moderate, and severe episodes of depression. The schemes take different approaches, however, in their definitions of severity. In ICD-10, severity is defined by symptoms; whereas in DSM-IV, severity is defined in terms of symptoms and functional impairment. Classifying depression by severity is useful, as severity is the single best predictor of response to treatment. As a general rule, a depressive episode that leads to complete cessation of functioning in any one domain (e.g. not going to school, complete social withdrawal) can be regarded as severe.

Both diagnostic schemes also distinguish between psychotic and non-psychotic episodes of depression. Psychotic depression, which is characterized by mood congruent delusions and hallucinations, is very uncommon before mid-adolescence. Nevertheless the concept is helpful because psychotic symptoms presage a worse adult prognosis and a greatly increased risk of conversion to bipolar disorder.

Other subtypes are less well-established. DSM-IV and ICD-10 have a category for chronic mild depression lasting one or more years—dysthymia. However, longitudinal studies have shown that in young people there is much overlap of major depression and dysthymia (Kovacs *et al.* 1994) and it is likely, therefore, that they are part of the same problem.

Co-morbidity between depression and other child psychiatric disorders is very common (see below), and DSM-IV and ICD-10 take different approaches to it. In ICD-10, it is assumed that a mixed clinical picture is more likely to be the result of a single disorder with different manifestations, than of two or more disorders that happen to occur in the same individual at the same time. ICD-10, therefore, has a category for mixed disorders, mixed disorders of conduct and emotions (F92), which includes the subcategory depressive-conduct disorder (F92.0). DSM-IV, by contrast, usually allows the investigator to diagnose several supposedly separate disorders, with the result that, in surveys based on DSM, it is quite common to find individuals with three or more diagnoses.

The application of adult diagnostic criteria to children and adolescents has been useful, but there are some limitations. First, adult criteria work less well in younger age groups, where it is often necessary to make assumptions about the meaning of some symptoms (for example, that a child who is negative and difficult to please has depressed mood). Second, current diagnostic systems have not really solved the problem of co-morbidity. Many children and adolescents with depressive disorder have other psychiatric problems, and it is often unclear in clinical practice which problem is primary (see below).

Epidemiology

Recent studies have estimated the 1-year (or less) prevalence of major depressive disorder in adolescence is between 1% and 2% (Simonoff *et al.* 1997), through 3% (Cohen *et al.* 1993; Lewinsohn *et al.* 1998), to 6% (Olsson and von Knorring 1999). The prevalence is much lower in pre-adolescents, at around one per thousand (Meltzer *et al.* 2000). This increase in the incidence of depressive disorder occurs during early adolescence.

Age trends in the incidence of depression are stronger in girls than in boys (Angold *et al.* 1999b). Most studies have found that in pre-pubertal children, there is either no gender difference in the prevalence of depression or there is a small male preponderance. In contrast, by late adolescence the female preponderance found in adult depression is well-established.

Clinical picture

The main features of depressive disorder in young people are emotional changes, cognitive changes, motivational changes, and neuro-vegetative symptoms.

Emotional symptoms

The main emotional symptom is depressed mood. Mood may be described as sad, blue, or down. The child may cry more than usual but in some cases patients report that, although they feel like crying, they are unable to do so. Some children will deny feeling sad but will admit to feeling 'bad'. DSM-IV states that, in children, irritable mood may substitute for depressed mood. The young person no longer derives as much pleasure from life: this anhedonia may sometimes precede depression of mood.

Cognitive changes

These include feelings of low-self esteem with an exaggerated assessment of current life difficulties. Typically, depressed children or adolescents will have nothing to say when asked about their good points. There may be difficulties making decisions, either because of lack of confidence or because of subjective difficulty with thinking. When depression is severe, the patient may feel that they are wicked or feel guilty for minor past misdemeanours, such as stealing. It should be noted, however, that it is normal for older children and adolescents to feel guilty about parental separation. Hopelessness and helplessness may also be prominent. Suicidal ideas are particularly serious in the presence of such symptoms.

Motivational changes

Low energy, apathy, tiredness, and poor concentration are all common in depressive disorder. Failure to complete tasks may make feelings of guilt and lack of confidence worse. School information may be crucial for a proper assessment of poor concentration.

Neuro-vegetative symptoms

These include changes in appetite, weight, sleep rhythm, libido, energy level, and activity. In deciding whether these changes are abnormal, the clinician must take into account the young person's developmental stage. For example, 9-year-olds, on average, sleep one hour more than 14-year-olds. Somatic symptoms are particularly common in adolescents, who may present to the doctor with headache, abdominal pain or other regional pain. The clinician can be so distracted by these symptoms that the depressive syndrome, of which they are a part, goes unrecognized.

Differential diagnosis and co-morbidity

The first diagnostic issue is the differentiation between 'normal' mood and depressive disorder. Defining the boundaries between extremes of normal behaviour and psychopathology is a dilemma that pervades much of child psychiatry. It is especially problematic to establish the limits of depressive disorder in young people because of the cognitive and physical changes that take place during this time. Adolescents tend to feel things particularly deeply and marked mood swings are common during the teens. It can be difficult to distinguish these intense emotional reactions from depressive disorders. By contrast, young children do not find it easy to describe how they are feeling and often confuse emotions such as anger and sadness. They have particular difficulty describing the key cognitive symptoms of depression, such as hopelessness and self-denigration. Depressive disorder should therefore only be diagnosed when there is impairment of social role functioning, when symptoms of unequivocal psychopathological significance are present (such as severe suicidality), or when symptoms lead to significant suffering.

The next diagnostic issue concerns the distinction from other psychiatric disorders. Depression in this age group is associated with almost all the other child psychiatric disorders, including conduct disorder, anxiety states, learning problems, hyperactivity, anorexia nervosa, and school refusal. In clinical samples, co-morbidity with one or more of these disorders usually exceeds 75%. Moreover, some of the symptoms that are part of the depressive constellation may arise as a symptom of other disorders. Thus, restlessness is seen in agitated depression, hypomania, and hyperkinetic disorder. As a general rule, the double diagnosis should be made only when symptoms that are not simply part of another disorder, clearly indicate the separate presence of a depressive disorder.

The final issue is whether the depressive disorder is part of an organic illness or substance abuse. Although it is very uncommon for organic illness to present with depression alone, any physical illness will increase the risk of depressive disorder, especially those that directly affect the brain (e.g. organic brain syndromes, endocrine disorders). Associations have been described with endocrine disorders and organic brain syndromes. There is growing evidence of an association between adolescent depression and substance abuse.

Assessment

Although the accurate diagnosis of depressive disorder is an important part of clinical management, assessment only starts with the diagnosis, it does not stop with it. Depressed young people usually have multiple problems, such as educational failure, impaired psychosocial functioning, suicidal behaviour, and co-morbid learning disorders. Moreover, they tend to come from families with high rates of psychopathology and may have experienced adverse life events. All these problems need to be identified and the causes of each assessed. Depression is a strong risk factor for both attempted and completed suicide, and in high-risk cases, the assessment should also indicate the degree of risk that patient poses to himself.

All patients with depression who are going to have anti-depressants should have a medical history and examination. It is not usually necessary to conduct a physical examination in depressed adolescents, though one should be conducted if the history suggests a physical disorder could account for the depression. Relevant laboratory tests include haematology, biochemistry, urinary drugs screen, and thyroid function tests.

The final part of the assessment involves the evaluation of the young person's personal and social resources. There is evidence that being successful at school or in other areas of life can protect young people from the effects of adverse life experiences (Rutter 2000). The best guide to the child's ability to solve future problems is his or her record in dealing with difficulties in the past. The ability of the family to support the patient should also be evaluated.

Aetiology

Depressive disorder is sometimes a reaction to a single severe stressor. Current aetiological theories suggest, however, that depression in young people more often arises from the accumulation and interaction over years of biological, psychological, and social factors. These factors comprise the combination of (1) genetic influences, (2) the effects of chronic adversity, and (3) precipitating stressful events. They act through psychological and biochemical processes to produce the depressive syndrome. Once established, the syndrome is often prolonged by maintaining factors.

Genetic factors are probably less important in unipolar depressive conditions than in bipolar disorders, accounting for perhaps 50% of the variation in depressive symptomatology in adolescents (Silberg et al. 1999). Recent studies suggest that genetic effects are often indirect, acting through temperamental traits that increase vulnerability to stress (Silberg et al. 2001). They may also act by increasing the risk of psychiatric disorders, such as anxiety and conduct disorders, which are themselves strong risk factors for depression (Angold et al. 1999a).

Chronic adversities include both intra-familial and extra-familial factors (Goodyer 1990). The most important familial factors are parental depression and other psychiatric disorders, family discord, and parenting problems, including abuse (Hammen 1991). The most important extra-familial factors are peer relationship problems (including bullying) and substance abuse.

Precipitating stressful events most commonly arise from the chronic stressors, described in the previous paragraph, and include acute family problems (e.g. parental separation), a breakdown of a relationship with a peer, and parental mental illness (Rutter 2000). The effects of acute stressful events depend to an important extent on their context and the degree of threat that they pose to the child (Rutter and Sandberg 1992). For example, the death of a grand-parent has much more impact on a child if the grandparent was the primary caretaker or an important source of support for that child.

Psychological processes are thought to play an important part in mediating the link between adversity and the development of depression (McCauley *et al.* 1988). For example, in cognitive theory it is suggested that depressed people develop a distorted view of the world (such as the expectation that things will always go wrong), which is caused by earlier adversity. When the child experiences current adversity, these negative cognitions become manifest as automatic negative thoughts (e.g. the thought that 'it is hopeless, I knew I was no good at that') and this then leads to depression.

Biological theories have consisted, for the most part, of downward extensions of models first developed with adults. The best known theory is the amine hypothesis, which proposes that depression is caused by under-activity in cerebral amine systems. Depression in young people may also be related to high levels of cortisol (Goodyer *et al.* 2001).

Maintaining factors can include (1) any of the above risk factors, (2) psychological or biolog-ical 'scarring' arising from the first depressive episode, or (3) the symptoms of depression itself (e.g. sleep disturbance leads to poor concentration, which in turn worsens negative thinking).

Treatment

Clinical management and treatment setting

The general principles of treatment follow from the description of the depressed young per-son's difficulties outlined above. Co-morbidity is frequent and there are many complications such as suicidal behaviour. Other types of adversity are part of the cause and may need inter-vention in their own right. Therefore, attention must be paid to biological, familial, educa-tional, and peer contributions. As with other child psychiatric disorders, it is important not only to treat the presenting problems, but also to foster normal development. A treatment pro-gramme, therefore, has multiple aims: to reduce depression, to treat co-morbid disorders, to promote social and emotional adjustment, to improve self-esteem, to relieve family distress, and prevent relapse.

The initial clinical management of depressed young people depends greatly on the nature of the problems identified during the assessment procedure. The assessment may indicate that the reaction of the child is appropriate for the situation in which he or she finds him- or herself. In such a case, and if the depression is mild, a sensible early approach can consist of the inter-ventions such as regular meetings, sympathetic discussions with the child and the parents, and encouraging support. These simple interventions, especially if they are combined with meas-ures to alleviate stress, are often followed by an improvement in mood. In other cases, particu-larly those with severe depression or suicidal thinking, a more focused form of treatment is indicated.

It is important that the clinician considers a number of key questions early on in the management of depressed young people. The first is whether the depression is severe enough to warrant admission to hospital. Indications for admission of depressed children are similar to those applicable to their adult counterparts and include severe suicidality, psychotic symptoms, or refusal to eat or drink. A related question is whether the child should remain at school. When the disorder is mild, school can be a valuable distraction from depressive thinking. When the disorder is more severe, symptoms such as poor concentration and motor retardation may add to feelings of hopelessness. It is quite common to find in such cases that ensuring that the child obtains tuition in the home, or perhaps in a sheltered school, improves mood considerably.

The second question is whether the depression is complicated by other disorders such as behavioural problems. If it is, then as a general rule it is best to sort out these complications before embarking on treatment for the depression.

The third question concerns the management of the stresses that are found in many cases of major depression. It is sometimes possible to alleviate some of these stresses. However, in the majority of cases, acute stressors are just one of a number of causes of the depression. Moreover, such stressors commonly arise out of chronic difficulties such as family discord, and may therefore be very hard to remedy. Symptomatic treatments for depression can therefore be helpful even when it is obvious that the depressive symptoms occur in the context of chronic family or social adversity that one can do little to change.

Treatment algorithm

Figure 14.1 shows an algorithm for the treatment of moderately severe depression (depressive disorder that has not led to complete cessation of functioning in at least one domain). Findings from the control arms of pharmacological and psychological treatment trials suggest that around one-third of adolescents with major depression will remit given the basic clinical management outlined in the previous section, which should therefore be the first approach in most cases.

The best first-line treatment for moderately severe depressive disorder, which persists despite initial clinical management, has not yet been firmly established in comparative randomized trials. Many authorities suggest, however, that action-orientated psychological treatments, such as cognitive-behaviour therapy or interpersonal psychotherapy, are usually the interventions of first choice. If these fail, or are not available, then a trial of antidepressant medication should be considered (see below).

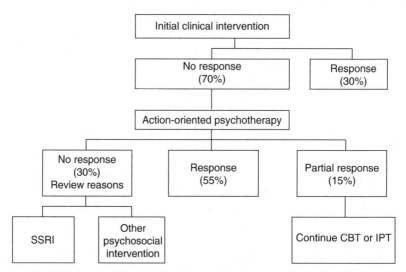

Fig. 14.1 A treatment algorithm for moderately severe depressive disorder.

Severe major depression, in which there is complete inability to function in at least one major social domain (e.g. not going to school or not seeing friends because of depression) is much less likely to respond to psychological treatment than mild or moderate depression (Jayson *et al.* 1998). The first-choice intervention is therefore likely to include anti-depressant medication. Severely depressed youngsters often need intensive support, such as through a day unit or assertive outreach programme.

Psychological interventions

The most widely used psychological interventions with depressed young people are action-orientated here-and-now individual psychological treatments, particularly cognitive-behaviour therapy and interpersonal psychotherapy.

Many slightly different cognitive-behavioural approaches have been developed for depressed children and adolescents (Clarke *et al.* 1990; Stark 1990; Wilkes *et al.* 1994). Most programmes have the following features. First, the therapy often begins with a session or sessions on emotional recognition and self-monitoring. The aim is to help the young person to distinguish between different emotional states (e.g. sadness and anger) and to start linking external events, thoughts and feelings. Second, behavioural tasks may be used to reinforce desired behaviours and thence to help the young person to gain control over symptoms. Self-reinforcement is often combined with activity scheduling, in which the young person is encouraged to engage in a programme of constructive or pleasant activities. Patients are taught to set realistic goals, with small steps towards achieving them, and to reward themselves at each successful step on the way. At this stage, it is quite common to introduce other behavioural techniques to deal with some of the behavioural or vegetative symptoms of depression. For example, many depressed youngsters sleep poorly and will often be helped by simple sleep hygiene measures. Third, various cognitive techniques are used to reduce depressive cognitions. For example, adolescents may be helped to identify cognitive distortions and to challenge them using techniques such as pro-con evaluation. Techniques to reduce negative automatic thoughts, such as 'focus on object', are also employed.

CBT has been used in both school and clinical settings. There have been at least six randomized controlled studies of CBT in samples of children with depressive symptoms recruited through schools and in three of them CBT was significantly superior to no treatment. A meta-analysis of randomized trials with clinically diagnosed cases of depressive disorder found that CBT was significantly superior to comparison conditions such as remaining on a waiting list or having relaxation training (pooled odds ratio of 2.2) (Harrington *et al.* 1998a).

Interpersonal psychotherapy (IPT) is based on the premise that depression occurs in the context of interpersonal relationships. Like CBT, IPT is a brief time-limited therapy. The two main goals are to identify and treat, first, depressive symptoms and, second, the problems associated with the onset of depression. Two randomized trials have shown significant benefits from IPT in depressed adolescents (Rossello and Bernal 1996; Mufson *et al.* 1999).

There have been at least four randomized controlled trials of family therapy in adolescent depressive disorder. Two involved a family intervention only (Brent *et al.* 1997; Harrington *et al.* 1998) and two examined the value of parental sessions given in parallel with individual CBT (Lewinsohn *et al.* 1990; Clarke *et al.* 1999). None of these trials have found significant benefit from using family treatment. It would be premature though to conclude that family interventions have no place in managing juvenile depression. The association between juvenile depression and family dysfunction is so strong that family interventions should sometimes be considered. However, they should not in general be first line treatments.

Other interventions

Depressed patients often have many different kinds of problems and therefore a clinician treating a depressed young person will need access to the full range of child mental health services, including social work and special educational provision.

Pharmacotherapy

The first-line pharmacological treatments are the serotonin-specific reuptake inhibitors (SSRIs), such as fluoxetine and paroxetine. Three recently published randomized trials have produced positive results, with response rates of between 50% and 70% (Emslie *et al.* 1997, 2002; Keller *et al.* 2001). It should be noted, however, that placebo response rates in these studies have usually exceeded a third, which means that four or five patients must be treated with an SSRI to obtain one who has actually benefited from the SSRI. Once again, this underlines the importance of offering non-specific treatments before medication in most cases.

Once the decision is taken to prescribe medication, it is very important that an adequate course is given. This means ensuring not only that the correct dose is prescribed but also that every effort is taken to ensure compliance.

As Table 14.1 shows, there are many different types of anti-depressant. There is little evidence that any one drug is better than another. The main differences between them are their half-lives, their ability to inhibit the cytochrome P_{450} (CYP450) system in the liver, and their active metabolites. These differences can sometimes be important clinically. For example, the long-half life of fluoxetine means that there may have to be a delay of several weeks before an anti-depressant that can interact with it (e.g. a monoamine oxidase inhibitor) can be given. On the other hand, the shorter half-life of paroxetine may account for its greater association with discontinuation reactions than some other anti-depressants. The P_{450} cytochrome is important because many of the SSRIs are inhibitors of one of the enzymes that metabolizes tricyclics and other psychotropic drugs, CYP2D6. This means that potentially toxic levels can occur if the tricyclics and SSRIs are given together.

SSRIs seem to have fewer side-effects than tricyclics and do not usually require specific cardiovascular monitoring (Gutgesell *et al.* 1999). However, symptoms such as dry mouth and gastro-intestinal upset can be a problem, and there has been concern about the so-called 'serotonin syndrome' (Gillman 1999). This 'syndrome', which is probably better regarded as the extreme end of the continuum of toxicity, is characterized by alterations in cognition, behaviour, autonomic and central nervous system function as a result of increased post-synaptic serotonin receptor agonism. Abrupt discontinuation of SSRIs can lead to symptoms such as dizziness, nausea, and lethargy, which may raise parental concerns about addiction. SSRIs

Table 14.1 Anti-depressants

Name	Dose (mg/day)	Half-life	Form	Inhibits P_{450} system
Citalopram	20–60	36 h	Tablet or liquid	2D6—some
Fluoxetine	20–60	9 days[a]	Tablet or liquid	2D6—yes
Paroxetine	20–50	24 h	Tablet or liquid	2D6—much
Sertraline	50–150	26 h	Tablet	2D6—yes
Venlafaxine	75–375	11 h (slow release)	Tablet	2D6—weak

[a]Active metabolite has a very long half-life.

should generally be tapered slowly over 4 weeks (Drug and Therapeutics Bulletin 1999). If the patient still has difficulties coming off SSRIs with a shorter half-life (e.g. paroxetine) then a switch to a longer acting SSRI (e.g. fluoxetine) may be helpful.

Auditing the results of treatment

There are many published studies on the rate of response of depressed young people to both psychological and pharmacological treatments, so it is now possible to compare the performance of a service with external standards. For example, for moderately severe major depression one would normally expect a response rate at 8–10 weeks ('response' being defined as no longer meeting DSM criteria for major depression) to either CBT or an SSRI of between 55% and 65%. Failure to achieve a response rate of more than 50% should trigger a review of referral pathways, treatment protocols and staff training.

Treatment issues

The most important clinical problem is failure to respond to the initial treatment. As a general rule, failure to respond to psychological treatment is an indication for starting an SSRI. In patients who fail to respond to an adequate course of SSRI there should be a review of the possible reasons. Non-compliance can be a major issue in this age group, and blood levels (if available) may help to identify this problem. There should also be a review of the diagnosis, and of any possible co-morbid problems such as abuse, family discord, bipolar disorder, drug dependence, or physical illness.

In patients who fail to respond to one SSRI, the Texas Consensus Conference (Hughes *et al.* 1999) recommended a trial of another (e.g. paroxetine, increasing by 10-mg increments to 50 mg daily), on the grounds that some of the SSRIs are chemically distinct. If the young person fails to respond to a second SSRI, then monotherapy with another anti-depressant should be considered, such as venlafaxine (modified release, up to 225 mg daily). Failure to respond to a third anti-depressant should trigger a review of the clinical state. In many services it would be at this point that other forms of therapy might be considered, such as admission to an in-patient unit. Augmentation with another agent might also be an option, but only if the patient has derived at least some benefit from the first treatment. Combination treatments can, however, be associated with toxicity. For example, SSRIs such as fluoxetine can increase blood levels of other psychotropics such as risperidone.

From time to time the clinician will encounter major depressive conditions in pre-adolescent children. These conditions tend to show more co-morbidity with other psychiatric disorders than adolescent depressive disorders and a stronger association with adversity, particularly family problems. The first-line treatments are usually, therefore, directed at these problems. If these treatments fail then one or more of the treatments outlined above might be considered.

Outcome

In the short-term, major depressive disorder in adolescents has a good prognosis, with about an 80% chance of remission within a year (Harrington and Vostanis 1995). However, among those who recover there is an increased risk of another episode, of around 40%. This increased risk of further depression extends into adult life (Harrington *et al.* 1990). A high proportion of depressed cases show other psychiatric disorders later in life, including anxiety disorder, conduct disorder, and personality disorder (Fombonne *et al.* 2001a, b). In comparison with non-depressed young people, there is a greatly increased risk of suicide, approximately 4% over the following 15 years (Harrington *et al.* 1990; Rao *et al.* 1993; Fombonne *et al.* 2001b). A worse outcome is associated with increased severity of depression, greater impairment at the time of the index episode, family discord, a family history of depression, and co-morbidity with conduct disorder. The prognosis of conduct problems is no different in the presence of depression, so young people with depressive conduct disorder are at risk of all the adverse outcomes of conduct disorder, including criminality and antisocial personality disorder (Harrington *et al.* 1991).

N.B. Readers should note that this chapter was written by Professor Harrington before the Committee on the Safety of Medicines (CSM, 2004) and the Medicines and Healthcare products Regulatory Agency (MHRA, 2004) in the UK issued their statements in 2004 that have offered warnings about and, effectively, placed limitations on prescribing selective serotonin re-uptake inhibitor (SSRI) anti-depressants for children and young people who have major depression or a depressive disorder.

Since then, in November 2004, the National Institute for Clinical Excellence (NICE) has issued the first draft of its guidance on treating depression in young people. Readers are referred to that document and to subsequent confirmed guidance from NICE. They are advised to read those and other relevant and authoritative publications alongside this chapter when considering treatment regimes for children and young people with depression as recent advice updates Professor Harrington's recommendations.

References

American Psychiatric Association (1994) *Diagnostic and statistical manual of mental disorders—DSM-IV* (4th edn). Washington DC: American Psychiatric Association.

Angold, A., Costello, E. J., and Erkanli, A. (1999a) Co-morbidity. *Journal of Child Psychology and Psychiatry*, **40**, 57–87.

Angold, A., Costello, E.J., Erkanli, A., and Worthman, C.M. (1999b) Pubertal changes in hormone levels and depression in girls. *Psychological Medicine*, **29**, 1043–53.

Brent, D., Holder, D., Kolko, D., Birmaher, B., Baugher, M., Roth, C., *et al.* (1997) A clinical psychotherapy trial for adolescent depression comparing cognitive, family, and supportive treatments. *Archives of General Psychiatry*, **54**, 877–85.

Clarke, G., Lewinsohn, P., and Hops, H. (1990) *Leaders manual for adolescent groups. Adolescent coping with depression course.* Eugene, OR: Castalia Publishing Company.

Clarke, G. N., Rohde, P., Lewinsohn, P. M., Hops, H., and Seeley, J.R. (1999) Cognitive-behavioural treatment of adolescent depression: efficacy of acute group treatment and booster sessions. *Journal of the American Academy of Child and Adolescent Psychiatry*, **38**, 272–9.

Cohen, P., Cohen, J., Kasen, S., Valez, C.N., Hartmark, C., Johnson, J., *et al.* (1993) An epidemiological study of disorders in late childhood and adolescence—I. Age- and gender-specific prevalence. *Journal of Child Psychology and Psychiatry*, **34**, 851–67.

Committee on Safety of Medicines (CSM) (2004) Selective serotonin reuptake inhibitors SSRIs: overview of regulatory status and CSM advice in relation to major depressive disorder (MDD) in children and adolescents. Summary of clinical trials. http://medicines.mhra.gov.uk/aboutagency/regframework/csm/csmhome.htm. [Accessed 15 April 2004]

Drug and Therapeutics Bulletin (1999) Withdrawing patients from anti-depressants. *Drug and Therapeutics Bulletin*, **37**, 49–52.

Emslie, G., Rush, A., Weinberg, W., Hoog, S.L., Ernest, D.E., Brown, E.B., *et al.* (1997) A double-blind, randomized placebo-controlled trial of fluoxetine in depressed children and adolescents. *Archives of General Psychiatry*, **54**, 1031–7.

Emslie, G.J., Heiligenstein, J.H., Wagner, K.D., *et al.* (2002) Fluoxetine for acute treatment of depression in children and adolescents: a placebo-controlled randomized clinical trial. *Journal of the American Academy of Child and Adolescent Psychiatry*, **41**, 1205–15.

Fombonne, E. (1995) Depressive disorders: time trends and putative explanatory mechanisms. In *Psychosocial disorders in young people: time trends and their origins* (ed. M. Rutter and D. Smith), pp. 544–615. Chichester: Wiley.

Fombonne, E., Wostear, G., Cooper, V., Harrington, R.C., and Rutter, M. (2001a) The Maudsley long-term follow-up of child and adolescent depression: I. Psychiatric outcomes in adulthood. *British Journal of Psychiatry*, **179**, 210–17.

Fombonne, E., Wostear, G., Cooper, V., Harrington, R.C., and Rutter, M. (2001b) The Maudsley long-term follow-up of child and adolescent depression: II. Suicidality, criminality and social dysfunction in adulthood. *British Journal of Psychiatry*, **179**, 218–23.

Gillman, P.K. (1999) The serotonin syndrome and its treatment. *Journal of Psychopharmacology*, **13**, 100–9.

Goodyer, I.M. (1990) Life experiences, development and childhood psychopathology. Chichester: Wiley.

Goodyer, I.M., Park, R.J., and Herbert, J. (2001) Psychosocial and endocrine features of chronic first-episode major depression in 8–16-year-olds. *Biological Psychiatry*, **50**, 351–7.

Gutgesell, H., Atkins, D., Barst, R., Bruck, M., Franklin, W., Humes, R., *et al.* (1999) AHA scientific statement: cardiovascular monitoring of children and adolescents receiving psychotropic drugs. *Journal of the American Academy of Child and Adolescent Psychiatry*, **38**, 1047–50.

Hammen, C. (1991) *Depression runs in families. The social context of risk and resilience in children of depressed mothers.* New York: Springer Verlag.

Harrington, R. (1994) Affective Disorders. In *Child and adolescent psychiatry: modern approaches* (3rd edn) (ed. M. Rutter, E. Taylor, and L. Hersov), pp. 330–50. Oxford: Blackwell Scientific.

Harrington, R., Whittaker, J., Shoebridge, P., and Campbell, A. (1998a) Systematic review of efficacy of cognitive behaviour therapies in child and adolescent depressive disorder. *British Medical Journal*, **316**, 1559–63.

Harrington, R.C., Fudge, H., Rutter, M., Pickles, A., and Hill, J. (1990) Adult outcomes of childhood and adolescent depression: I. Psychiatric status. *Archives of General Psychiatry*, **47**, 465–73.

Harrington, R.C., Fudge, H., Rutter, M., Pickles, A., and Hill, J. (1991) Adult outcomes of childhood and adolescent depression: II. Risk for antisocial disorders. *Journal of the American Academy of Child and Adolescent Psychiatry*, **30**, 434–9.

Harrington, R.C., Kerfoot, M., Dyer, E., McNiven, F., Gill, J., Harrington, V., *et al.* (1998b) Randomized trial of a home based family intervention for children who have deliberately poisoned themselves. *Journal of the American Academy of Child and Adolescent Psychiatry*, **37**, 512–8.

Harrington, R.C. and Vostanis, P. (1995) Longitudinal perspectives and affective disorder in children and adolescents. In *The Depressed child and adolescent. developmental and clinical perspectives* (ed. I.M. Goodyer), pp. 311–41. Cambridge: Cambridge University Press.

Hughes, C.W., Emslie, G.J., Crimson, M.L. Trivedi, M.H., Toprac, M.G., Sedillo, A., *et al.* (1999) The Texas Children's Medication Algorithm Project: report of the Texas Consensus Conference Panel on Medication Treatment of Childhood Major Depressive Disorder. *Journal of the American Academy of Child and Adolescent Psychiatry*, **38**, 1442–54.

Jayson, D., Wood, A.J., Kroll, L. Fraser, J., and Harrington, R.C. (1998) Which depressed patients respond to cognitive-behavioral treatment? *Journal of the American Academy of Child and Adolescent Psychiatry*, **37**, 35–9.

Keller, M.B., Ryan, N.D., Strober, M., Klein, R.G., Kutcher, S.P., Birmaher, B., *et al.* (2001) Efficacy of paroxetine in the treatment of adolescent major depression: a randomized, controlled trial. *Journal of the American Academy of Child and Adolescent Psychiatry*, **40**, 762–72.

Kolvin, I., Barrett, M.L., Bhate, S.R., Berney, T.P., Famujiwa, O.O., Fundudis, T., *et al.* (1991) The Newcastle Child Depression Project: diagnosis and classification of depression. *British Journal of Psychiatry*, **159** (suppl. 11), 9–21.

Kovacs, M., Akiskal, H.S., Gatsonis, C., and Parrone, P.L. (1994) Childhood-onset dysthymic disorder. Clinical features and prospective naturalistic outcome. *Archives of General Psychiatry*, **51**, 365–74.

Lewinsohn, P.M., Clarke, G.N., Hops, H., and Andrews, J. (1990) Cognitive-behavioural treatment for depressed adolescents. *Behavior Therapy*, **21**, 385–401.

Lewinsohn, P.M., Rohde, P., and Seeley, J.R. (1998) Major depressive disorder in older adolescents: prevalence, risk factors, and clinical implications. *Clinical Psychology Review*, **18**, 765–94.

McCauley, E., Mitchell, J.R., Burke, P., and Moss, S. (1988) Cognitive attributes of depression in children and adolescents. *Journal of Consulting and Clinical Psychology*, **56**, 903–8.

Medicines and Healthcare products Regulatory Agency (MHRA) (2004) Selective Serotonin Reuptake Inhibitors (SSRIs): Overview of regulatory status and CSM advice relating to major depressive disorder (MDD) in children and adolescents including a summary of available safety and efficacy data. Last updated 08/04/04. http://medicines.mhra.gov.uk/ [Accessed 10 December 2004].

Meltzer, H., Gatward, R., Goodman, R., and Ford, T. (2000) *Mental health of children and adolescents in Great Britain.* London: The Stationery Office.

Mufson, L., Weissman, M.M., Moreau, D., and Garfinkal, R. (1999) Efficacy of interpersonal psychotherapy for depressed adolescents. *Archives of General Psychiatry*, **56**, 573–9.

National Collaborating Centre for Mental Health commissioned by the National Institute for Clinical Excellence (NICE) (2004) Depression in Children: identification and management of depression in children and young people in primary, community and secondary care. National Clinical Practice Guideline. Draft for first consultation. http://www.nice.org.uk/pdf/Depn_child_1stcons_Fullguideline.pdf

Olsson, G.I. and von Knorring, A.L. (1999) Adolescent depression: prevalence in Swedish high-school students. *Acta Psychiatrica Scandinavica*, **99**, 324–31.

Rao, U., Weissman, M.M., Martin, J.A., and Hammond, R.W. (1993) Childhood depression and risk of suicide: preliminary report of a longitudinal study. *Journal of the American Academy of Child and Adolescent Psychiatry*, **32**, 21–7.

Rossello, J. and Bernal, G. (1996) Adapting cognitive-behavioural and interpersonal treatments for depressed Puerto Rican adolescents. In *Psychosocial treatments for child and adolescent disorders: empirically based strategies for clinical practice* (ed. E.D. Hibbs and P.S. Jensen), pp. 157–85. Washington DC: American Psychological Association.

Rutter, M. (2000) Negative life events and family negativity: accomplishments and challenges. In *Where inner and outer worlds meet: essays in honour of George W Brown* (ed. T. Harris), pp. 25–40. London: Taylor and Francis.

Rutter, M. and Sandberg, S. (1992) Psychosocial stressors: concepts, causes and effects. *Euro Child Adolesc Psychiatry*, **1**, 3–13.

Silberg, J., Pickles, A., Rutter, M., Hewitt, J., Simonoff, E., Maes, H., *et al.* (1999) The influence of genetic factors and life stress on depression among adolescent girls. *Archives of General Psychiatry*, **56**, 225–32.

Silberg, J., Rutter, M., Neale, M., and Eaves, L. (2001) Genetic moderation of environmental risk for depression and anxiety in adolescent girls. *British Journal of Psychiatry*, **179**, 116–21.

Simonoff, E., Pickles, A., Meyer, J.M., Silberg, J.L., Maes, H.H., Loeber, R., *et al.* (1997) The Virginia twin study of adolescent behavioral development. Influences of age, sex, and impairment on rates of disorder. *Archives of General Psychiatry*, **54**, 801–8.

Stark, K.D. (1990) *Childhood depression: school-based intervention.* New York: Guilford Press.

Wilkes, T.C.R., Belsher, G., Rush, A.J., and Frank, E. (ed.). (1994) *Cognitive therapy for depressed adolescents.* New York: Guilford Press.

World Health Organization (1993) *The ICD-10 classification of mental and behavioural disorders. Diagnostic criteria for research.* Geneva: World Health Organization.

Psychoses, developmental, and neuro-psychiatric disorders in childhood and adolescence

Peter Hill

Introduction

Any child and adolescent mental health service will, from time to time, have to deal with conditions of low frequency but potentially high severity. Some of these will be the result of extreme social adversity, so that enduring patterns of aggressive or callous behaviour have developed as a result of abuse or neglect. Typically these will be known to social and educational authorities in the first instance. Yet there are others in whom exceptionally disturbed behaviour arises on the basis of biological factors, at least in large part. For these, the subject of this chapter, it is often the case that social provision alone will be inadequate, and medical or clinical psychological skills need to be brought into play.

They can be considered under several headings.

Psychoses

As with a number of conditions in medicine, psychotic disorders first occurring in childhood or adolescence are generally more severe than psychoses that begin later in life. Not all psychoses in the young are schizophrenia. Severe distortions of perception, thought, emotion, and behaviour with hallucinations, delusions, and disorganized personal functioning are a feature of several conditions in childhood and adolescence. Although at first sight such a picture resembles that of schizophrenia in adulthood, as development continues over years it becomes clear that it may also be an initial manifestation of a major affective disorder, particularly bipolar disorder. This may account for the finding that the sex ratio for psychosis in general in adolescence is often equal. Whatever the ultimate disorder category, early onset psychoses have a particularly poor prognosis and are hard to treat. The approaches used in adult psychiatry do not always work. Some apparently psychotic conditions, such as the rare Kleine–Levin syndrome, are largely confined to adolescence. Others are associated with other problems such as illicit drug use or types of encephalopathy less usual in adults, such as the PANDAS conditions resulting from immunological cross-reaction to streptococcal infections or the neuro-degenerative conditions such as metachromatic leucodystrophy.

Although the prevalence for psychotic disorder in the age-matched general population is about 1/10 000 at age 13, this has risen to about 18/10 000 by age 18 (Gillberg *et al.* 1986).

Schizophrenia itself, when it occurs in the young, is essentially the same condition as in adults with genetic, psychosocial, and neuro-biological factors involved in its genesis. It appears to be a condition characterized by abnormal adolescent brain development, rather than degeneration (Hollis 2002). Several investigators (e.g. Nopoulos *et al.* 1998) have concluded that the neurological abnormalities are relatively more evident in the young.

Most young people with a psychotic clinical picture will need admission to a child or adolescent psychiatric in-patient unit for close clinical observation, safety, and to reduce the burden of care on their family. The extreme psychological disturbance and safety issues mean that such an admission may need to be carried out urgently, so that the relevant unit must be able to provide this. There may be issues of consent. Relevant adolescent psychiatrists should be approved under Section 12 of the Mental Health Act, since general adult psychiatrists are not always fully conversant with the ethical issues surrounding admission, as far as the young are concerned. In general, it is against national policy to admit children to adult wards, though there are occasional instances in which an extremely disturbed 17-year-old may actually best be managed by nursing staff on an adult psychiatric ward. On the other hand it is hardly ever appropriate for a psychotic teenager to be nursed on an acute paediatric ward.

Forethought is the watchword and it is important for a local service to have drawn up:

agreements about urgent admission procedures to one or more selected child or adolescent psychiatric in-patient units;

ethical protocols to avoid muddle over consent to admission;

rapid tranquillization protocols to avoid the extremes of uncontrolled behaviour and inappropriate sedation.

In many parts of the UK, the volume of provision of in-patient psychiatric care for children and adolescents is inadequate, and young people are admitted to NHS or private units far from their families and community. A longer view may need to be taken to ensure local availability. Not uncommonly, the spend on distant placements is enough to finance the building and staffing of a local unit, but the relatively low frequency of admissions masks this. In the last few years, the Health Advisory Service has carried out costing exercises for a number of health authorities, which have repeatedly illustrated this. In an earlier era, psychiatric in-patient units were largely planned or managed by NHS Regions, who had a broader and more strategic view of the costs and needs, so that the move to more local management of commissioning has lead to a loss of this more general view.

Because the young are, prospectively, likely to have a longer period of their life taking anti-psychotic medication, atypical anti-psychotics are currently favoured as first-line medication. These are appreciably more expensive, at least at first sight, than traditional medication. A local drug budget needs to be able to support this. Similarly, because of the generally greater severity of schizophrenia in the young, there is likely to be a proportionally more frequent recourse to clozapine in order to treat resistant cases, and the cost of blood count monitoring should be allowed for.

Most cases of psychosis will be chronic, so that there will need to be good working links between CAMHS and an adult mental health service, especially to ensure that the age range 16–19 is catered for without factional disputes.

Neuro-developmental disorders

Various specific developmental delays in which a skill (reading, language, interpersonal communication, concentration, etc.) is difficult to acquire, in spite of adequate intelligence, age, and tuition, may present to either developmental paediatric services or CAMHS. These include dyslexia, dyspraxia (motor planning difficulty or developmental co-ordination disorder), and specific developmental disorders of language. Although not necessarily of great clinical severity, it is the more serious cases that present to CAMHS and their assessment can be protracted or complex. The question posed by referrers to CAMHS is often whether a specific disability (such as delayed speech development) is, in part, the result of emotional factors. In order to answer this, the additional services of paediatrics, speech therapy, educational psychology, physiotherapy, and occupational therapy are needed. Usually it is easier to arrange joint assessments with local developmental paediatrics than to attempt total assessment within CAMHS. Access to children's neuro-psychology assessment services is becoming more important because it may lead to treatment tailored to the individual child, rather than resorting to general remediation packages or an unjustified belief in catch-all approaches such as 'counselling'.

Autistic spectrum disorders can reasonably be conceptualized as neuro-developmental. Because they affect behaviour and emotions directly, they are rather more likely to be dealt with by CAMHS staff but, once again, an active link with developmental paediatric services is important. There seems to be an unusually high rate of requests for second diagnostic opinions in this area, and forward planning can ensure this happens smoothly. Matters can become fraught, since the absence of objective tests means that diagnosis is a matter of judgement. Wide dissemination of information about these conditions, particularly Asperger's syndrome, has led to a diagnosis or treatment recommendation being offered by non-specialists on the basis of checklists or media articles, without clinical experience or even basic knowledge of medical classification rules and treatments being applied.

Not uncommonly, education of children with developmental disorders is implemented in mainstream schools and the school staff are dependent on specialist advice. Educational psychology cannot always meet this and it is often the case that CAMHS staff receive a number of requests to attend educational meetings in schools; a time demand that needs budgeting for. Clinical psychologists, in particular, may find themselves being asked to carry out assessments or interventions, such as classroom management programmes, in areas where educational psychology is weak or overburdened with special educational needs administration.

Increasing scientific knowledge has identified biological developmental deviations in the above and a number of other conditions: obsessive-compulsive disorder, Tourette's syndrome, ADHD, schizophrenia, and bipolar disorder. Usually these are genetically based but they may also arise on the basis of brain injury or infection in a few cases. As the anatomical and physiological abnormalities identified have always been in the nervous system, the term neuro-developmental has been increasingly used.

Tourette's syndrome, as currently defined, is not that rare (studies yield different figures ranging from 0.1% to 2.9%) but most cases are mild. So-called 'full-blown' Tourette's is a devastating, chronic condition in which multiple tics, motor and vocal, combine with obsessive repeating of the utterances or behaviour of others, sleep disorders, odd fascinations, obsessive-compulsive symptoms, rage attacks, and an ADHD picture. It is highly likely to result in the affected child being bullied. All this will require detailed medical, social, and educational management, possibly with referral to a tertiary level centre.

Characteristically, neuro-developmental disorders are co-morbid with each other, so that a child with ADHD is also likely to have dyslexia and dyspraxia, for instance (Kaplan et al. 1998). Quite often parents and teachers raise the question as to whether one diagnostic label is more appropriate than another, when in fact both are relevant. To avoid this sort of misunderstanding, a full multidisciplinary assessment should be carried out early in treatment.

Brain injury

Over the last few decades, the widespread use of car seat belts and cycle helmets, as well as improved major injury care, has meant that children with what would previously have been fatal head injuries are surviving. However, they are likely to be considerably impaired, physically and psychologically. There may well be physical injuries to limbs, hearing or visual loss, and epilepsy. The circumstances of the injury (road traffic accidents, etc.) may also have lead to death or injury of other family members.

Traumatic brain injury may be diffuse (generalized, usually following a closed head injury) or focal (localized to a single area of the brain and typically resulting from a penetrating injury, bleed or infection). When it results from injury, it may also be mild (various definitions but for psychiatric purposes, a post-traumatic amnesia of less than one week) or severe, when there has been coma or prolonged interference with memory. Mild brain injury in itself does not usually cause psychiatric disorder, though there may be post-traumatic stress symptoms or issues arising from the death of others in the same incident.

Severe, diffuse, traumatic brain injury can present in a way comparable to frontal lobe injury with social disinhibition, poor motivation, irritability, and extreme self-centredness. Commonly there are also significant problems with fatiguability, poor concentration, slowness, and weak memory. There is usually a fundamental change in personality, which parents understandably find very hard to accept. Affected children may need extensive rehabilitation, sometimes residential, and considerable support from various agencies. They are vulnerable to a range of psychiatric disorders as a consequence of injury to the brain, which is the organ of the mind.

Recovery

Ambulant, reasonably intelligent children with severe, diffuse, traumatic brain injuries may initially be judged to have recovered wonderfully well and medical optimism leads to discharge from neurosurgical follow-up, but as the months pass, emotional, behavioural, and learning problems reveal themselves. It is at this stage that they are likely to present to a CAMHS service. Not uncommonly there are behavioural, educational, and relationship problems of considerable severity and chronicity.

Deaf children

Children with hearing impairments have a high rate of psychiatric disorder (Hindley *et al.* 1994), especially when educated in partial hearing units in mainstream schools where they seem prone to bullying. Readers should see Chapter 21 in which Hindley and Williams deal with the psychiatric impacts of sensory impairments in more detail.

Children with partial hearing loss who use speech present little difficulty to services but markedly deaf children, or parents whose first language is sign language, present major communication problems for hearing staff and a signing interpreter will be needed. For many deaf children, this arrangement will be sufficient but, if there are particular difficulties, consultation with one of the few specialist deaf child and adolescent psychiatric services providing a tertiary level service is indicated.

Challenging behaviour

Markedly aggressive behaviour, whether directed towards the self or others, is commonly described as challenging, if it appears to be irrational, or uncontainable, by ordinary measures within the family, school, or community. From the point of view of a health service it is something that is most likely to be manifested by a child or adolescent with general learning disability or an autistic spectrum disorder. Attacks on parents, teachers, or siblings may, in such children, be precipitated by fear or intolerance of imposed change, as well as by anger or perceived threat. Biting oneself, head-banging, picking at skin, or hitting one's own face may represent a serious threat to physical health.

Aggressive outbursts, which are seen as disproportionate to circumstances and therefore raise a question about the perpetrator's mental health, may also be seen in association with children who have been abused, physically or emotionally, as well as in victims of bullying. Psychosis is a rare cause but rage attacks (episodic dyscontrol) are quite common in children with Tourette's syndrome and in some with ADHD.

Although there has been recent interest in the use of various medications (risperidone, clonidine, stimulants) to control frequent aggressive outbursts and self-injurious behaviour, the use of cognitive-behavioural approaches is central to the management of challenging behaviour and more likely to produce lasting benefit. Because such interventions commonly depend on a functional analysis of provoking and maintaining factors for the individual child's situation, local intervention is generally preferable to placement in a remote, specialist centre. Nevertheless it may be necessary to import consultation from such a centre in order to facilitate local intervention.

A local shortage of appropriate placements for psychotic young people may result in them being placed in inappropriate settings, such as a paediatric ward, and this may provoke challenging behaviour. Protocols for the management of this need to be agreed for staff in such settings who may also require training in appropriate self-defence. Nevertheless, prevention is preferred to cure, and mental health guidelines such as the Royal College of Psychiatrists' Council Report 41 (1995) can be studied and adapted to local circumstances, non-psychiatric settings and for young patients.

Conclusion

There is a reasonably short list of conditions or problems that occur infrequently in any CAMHS but have appreciable resource implications when they do. *Ad hoc* management is likely to be expensive and of poor quality. Forward planning should reduce the cost of intervention and improve the management of the problem for the child or adolescent concerned.

References

Gillberg, C., Wahlstrom, J., Forsman, A., Hellgren, L., and Gillberg, J.C. (1986) Teenage psychoses: epidemiology, classification and reduced optimality in the pre-, peri- and neonatal periods. *Journal of Child Psychology and Psychiatry*, **27**, 87–98.

Hindley, P.A., Hill, P.D., McGuigan, S., and Kitson, N. (1994) Psychiatric disorder in deaf and hearing impaired children: a prevalence study. *Journal of Child and Adolescent Psychiatry*, **35**, 917–34.

Hollis, C. (2002) Scizophrenia and allied disorders. In *Child and Adolescent Psychiatry* (4th edn) (ed. Rutter, M. and Taylor, E.), ch 37, pp. 612–35. Oxford: Blackwell Scientific.

Kaplan, B.J., Wilson, B.N., Dewey, D., and Crawford, S.G. (1998) DCD may not be a discrete disorder. *Human Movement Science*, **17**, 471–90.

Nopoulos, P.C., Giedd, J.N., Andreason, N., and Rapoport, J. (1998) Frequency and severity of enlarged septi pellucidi in childhood-onset schizophrenia. *American Journal of Psychiatry*, **155**, 1074–9.

Royal College of Psychiatrists (1995) *Strategies for the management of disturbed and violent patients in psychiatric units*. London: Council Report 41.

Young people with eating disorders

Greg Richardson and Ian Partridge

Definitions

Eating disorders present in a number of forms: anorexia nervosa, bulimia nervosa, atypical variations of both, feeding problems in children, differentiated by Lask and Bryant-Waugh (2000) as food avoidance emotional disorder, extreme faddiness, restrictive eating, food refusal, food phobia, and one aspect of pervasive refusal syndrome. Obesity is the result of the major eating disorder of our time. Problematic eating patterns may also be a part of other conditions that affect the mental health of children and their families. Anorexia nervosa is a disorder, characterized by fear of fatness, in which reduction of caloric intake and maximum usage of energy results in serious weight loss. Bulimia nervosa, more characterized by fear of loss of control over eating, results in episodes of bingeing and vomiting, and a preoccupation with weight and diet. The childhood-onset eating problems are defined by Fox and Joughin (2002).

Epidemiology

Anorexia nervosa may affect up to 1% of 15–20-year-old girls, although abnormal concerns about eating are considerably higher in that population (Monck *et al.* 1990). Anorexia may commence prior to puberty. About 10% of anorexics are male. Bulimia nervosa is thought to be considerably more common but develops later in adolescence. Picky eating in younger children covers a broad spectrum and is quite common, although rarely interfering with growth and development, the repercussions on vulnerable families of food fads may seriously disrupt their emotional functioning. Pervasive refusal is a rare but severely debilitating condition (Lask *et al.* 1991). Obesity is a disorder to which CAMHS have not really made a contribution.

Causation

Eating disorders appear to be of multi-factorial aetiology with genetic, individual, biological, familial, and socio-cultural factors interacting. Finding causes does not appear to have been helpful in informing helpful interventions, although the avoidance of starvation may improve the pathophysiological and psychological alterations that serve to sustain the disorder (Steinhausen 2002).

Assessment

Although many young people with eating disorders have similar characteristics, the family will only be able to work productively if they consider the individual and family factors affecting their child to have been fully understood. The family should be assessed with particular reference to an over-concerned relationship between parents and child, and its causes (Shoebridge and Gowers 2000), as well as an assessment of the family's motivation for change. A discussion with the parents to understand their concerns and thoughts on their child's difficulties should initiate therapeutic engagement with them. An individual mental state assessment of the young person should be undertaken with the assistance of the completion of a rating scale such as the Eating Attitude Test (Garner and Garfinkel 1979) or the Eating Disorders Inventory (Garner *et al.* 1983). Physical examination should include height and weight measurement of the young person and calculation of body mass index. Heights and weights should be plotted on centile charts. Investigation of biochemical and metabolic functioning may well be indicated. An ECG should be performed, particularly if the usage of drugs is being considered.

Interventions

The management of children and adolescents with eating disorders is one of the more taxing problems presenting to CAMHS. The psychopathology of the condition presenting in bright, articulate young people who waste away in the face of the conflicts they are facing, immobilizes, emotionally and cognitively, those trying to help them. Despite the evidence that professional interventions have little effect on the outcome of eating disorders in adults (Ben-Tovim *et al.* 2001), denying interventions to troubled families and dying young people is not an option. A response from CAMHS is required that entails the development of a strategy for the management of these disorders, which are problematic both in themselves and in their sequelae. Eating disorders generate anxiety in both families and referrers, whereas the identified patient often denies a problem, particularly in the case of anorexia nervosa. Anorexia and bulimia nervosa are often surrounded by secrecy, denial, disingenuity, and dishonesty, particularly by the identified patient, but also by family members and over-involved professionals. These factors are complicated by the pathology of starvation, which affects cognitive and emotional processes (Fichter and Pirke 1990). Physical consequences, in both the short and long term, can be serious (Sharp and Freeman 1993), the young people therefore require both physical and psychological management. As eating disorders originate in, and interact at, the individual, familial, and social levels, the family must be worked with as well as the patient; indeed, in adolescent anorexia nervosa, the family are the main therapeutic tool (Russell *et al.* 1987). In-patient care, which is sometimes considered to be the only treatment option, is expensive and those who are admitted have a worse prognosis (Gowers *et al.* 2000).

The management of a young person with an eating disorder depends upon family agreement on the necessity to maintain a healthy weight without pathological behaviours such as induced vomiting. Weight-monitoring then becomes integral to management. The family and the young person will require educating on the psychobiology of eating disorders, with particular emphasis on developmental influences. It may be helpful to undertake individual work with the young person to address the difficulties they are having in addressing the developmental tasks of adolescence. Motivational interviewing techniques may also be helpful (Treasure and Ward 1997), as may the use of self-help manuals (e.g. Schmidt and Treasure 1993). Parents will require support in addressing their problems as they ensure their child eats properly. Family therapy is the treatment of choice for those under 19 with a history of less than 3 years (Russell *et al.* 1987). It may be helpful to have a relationship and contract with an in-patient facility, so that admission can be arranged when required. Whoever has the responsibility for assessing and managing the young person and their family must be able to undertake all these tasks.

Outcomes

Anorexia and bulimia nervosa are disorders that seriously interfere with the lives and development of those who suffer from them. Anorexia nervosa has a high mortality from starvation initially and from suicide in later life (Emborg 1999). Most intervention studies show little variation in outcome with about half recovering and one-fifth remaining seriously disabled. The outcome for younger patients is considered to be a little better (Steinhausen 2002). The outcome for younger children with eating problems is generally good (Fox and Joughin 2002) apart from pervasive refusal syndrome.

Challenges

Services are cut according to the available cloth of resources and manpower, taking account of the evidence base, in order to provide effective clinical provision. However they are provided, there must be a clear operational policy that details how young people with eating disorders are managed in the wider CAMHS, ensuring referrals are responded to promptly. There must also be a range of therapeutic options available for young people and their families, individually tailored to their needs. Ready access to colleagues in physical and paediatric health, for the management of the physical aspects of eating disorders, should be available.

Tier 2 provision

Work with these young people and their families may occur at Tier 2, as many services will manage eating disorders within their day-to-day provision, with individual members of the service managing cases as allocated, if no one service member has a special interest in this condition. There may be individuals who develop a special interest in this area, but they will not have the support of professionals from other disciplines with differing skills and a full assessment will be time-consuming. The service is therefore unlikely to be comprehensive. Referral on to specialist or in-patient provision may be required for unresponsive problems.

Tier 3 provision

A specialist Tier 3 provision, ensures that the perspectives and skills of a multidisciplinary team, co-ordinated by a senior clinician, are brought to bear in a co-ordinated manner. This will utilize existing resources of personnel with a specialist interest, specialist knowledge, and specialist experience at a designated time to provide a discreet and recognized (e.g. by the Eating Disorders Association) service. In addition, team cohesion within the wider CAMHS ensures that specialist expertise and experience is not hived off, so that it becomes inaccessible to the rest of the service. The development of expertise within team members can then be utilized to meet training needs and requirements for a range of disciplines. Equally, CAMHS members, who are not members of the eating disorders team, may have skills that the team may call upon for advice on the management of certain aspects of a case. Training programmes for those with whom young people with eating disorders first come into contact, such as teachers, school nurses, health visitors, and general practitioners, may be offered. Similarly, consultation services can be offered to Tier 1 professionals who wish to discuss eating disorder related problems. The establishment of links with Tier 1 acts as an educational and consultative resource to ensure early and accurate detection, and to discuss the necessity and method of referral to specialist services. A range and variety of treatment options become available and there is effective use of time, so that young people and their families are seen speedily and regularly within a mutually supportive team. Pressure upon such a small service could lead to the unwelcome lengthening of waiting-lists, but if the team size, and clinics, are geared to the needs of the catchment population, which is overtly defined, this should not be a problem. Supervision is built into the organization of the team and can, if and when necessary, be live. Being part of a wider CAMHS, with a wider mental health perspective, means that practitioners do not become blinkered in outlook by operating entirely within the field of eating disorders. Such specialist provision within an existing CAMHS is labour-intensive and removes resources from existing service provision; however, these young people would still have to be managed by the service. Non-attendance can prove costly in terms of the allocation of team time, but a specific clinic, whose purpose is well-explained, appears to reduce non-attendance rates. From the commissioning point of view, problems of differential funding for different disorders are avoided as the service is funded through the generic CAMHS (Roberts *et al.* 1998).

Tier 4 provision

Eating disorders may require in-patient management due to the severity of the condition and the physical sequelae, which may require close liaison with paediatric, gastro-enterological, or endocrinology colleagues in an acute hospital. Hospital admission may also be requested when the family or referring professional feel they are making no progress, and levels of anxiety generated within the family, the individual, or involved professionals are becoming intolerable. The poorer prognosis of young people admitted to in-patient facilities has to be weighed against the need to ensure that these young people do not starve to death or die from the metabolic complications of starvation. In-patient care will, therefore, be inevitable for a certain number of cases. Mechanisms and working arrangements, financial, contractual, and clinical, with in-patient facilities, must be in place to ensure these young people can be admitted urgently when required. In-patient care must only ever be part of a care pathway that starts in the young person's local community and returns there. It is therefore necessary to ensure that the period of in-patient care has a clearly defined and agreed purpose between the family, the community CAMHS, and the in-patient facility; discharge being agreed when that purpose has been met.

Stand-alone specialist provision

In recent years there has developed both community and residential based services dealing solely with eating disorders. Often operating in the independent sector, they are separated and divorced from generic CAMHS. Their development appears to have been a response to the poor arrangements between NHS community CAMHS and in-patient facilities in which in-patient care has not been speedily available for young people. They are an expensive option and work with local CAMHS is often difficult because of distance. Young people with eating disorders, and their families, often express a preference for care within a specialist resource, as they do not consider they are appropriately placed with other young people with mental disorders. This may have some validity or it may reinforce the psychopathology that perpetuates the condition. There is no evidence that specialist resources have better outcomes than generic Tier 4 CAMHS.

Acknowledgements

This chapter is based on our work and experience with all the past and current members of the Lime Trees Eating Disorders team.

References

Ben-Tovim, D., Walker, K., Gilchrist, P., Freeman, R., Kalucy, R., and Esterman, A. (2001) Outcome in patients with eating disorders: a 5-year study. *Lancet*, **357**, 1254–7.

Emborg, C. (1999) Mortality and causes of death in eating disorders in Denmark 1970–1993: a case register study. *International Journal of Eating Disorders*, **25**, 243–51.

Fichter, M.M. and Pirke, K.M. (1990) Psychobiology of Human Starvation. In *Anorexia nervosa* (ed. H. Remschmidt, and M.H. Schmidt), pp. 13–29. Cambridge, MA: Hogrefe and Huber.

Fox, C. and Joughin, C. (2002) *Childhood-onset eating problems: findings from research*. London: Gaskell.

Garner, D. M. and Garfinkel, P. E. (1979) The eating attitude test: an index of the symptoms of anorexia nervosa. *Psychological Medicine*, **9**, 273–9.

Garner, D.M., Olmsted, M.P., and Polivy, J. (1983) Development and validation of a multidimensional eating disorder inventory for anorexia nervosa and bulimia. *International Journal of Eating Disorders*, **2**, 15–24.

Gowers, S.G., Weetman, J., Shore, A., Hossain, F., and Elvins, R. (2000) Impact of hospitalisation on the outcome of adolescent anorexia nervosa. *British Journal of Psychiatry*, **176**, 138–41.

Lask, B. and Bryant-Waugh, R. (2000) *Anorexia nervosa and related eating disorders in childhood and adolescence*. Hove: Psychology Press.

Lask, B., Britten, C., Kroll, L., Magagna, J., and Tranter, M. (1991) Children with pervasive refusal. *Archives of Disease in Childhood*, **66**, 866–9.

Monck, E., Graham, P., Richman, N., and Dobbs, R. (1990) Eating and weight-control problems in a community population of adolescent girls aged 15–20 years. In *Anorexia nervosa* (ed. H. Remschmidt and M. H. Schmidt), pp. 1–11. Göttingen: Hogrefe and Huber.

Roberts, S., Foxton, T., Partridge, I., and Richardson, G. (1998). Establishing a specialist eating disorders team. *Psychiatric Bulletin*, **22**, 214–16.

Russell, G. F. M., Szmukler, G. I., Dare, C., and Eisler, I. (1987) An evaluation of family therapy in anorexia nervosa and bulimia nervosa. *Archives of General Psychiatry*, **44**, 1047–56.

Sharp, C.W. and Freeman, C.P.L. (1993) The medical complications of anorexia nervosa. *British Journal of Psychiatry*, **162**, 452–62.

Schmidt, U. and Treasure, J. (1993) Getting better bit(e) by bit(e). Hove: Lawrence Erlbaum Associates.

Shoebridge, P. and Gowers, S.G. (2000) Parental High concern and adolescent-onset anorexia nervosa. A case control study to investigate direction of causality. *British Journal of Psychiatry*, **176**, 132–7.

Steinhausen, H-C. (2002) Anorexia and Bulimia Nervosa. In *Child and adolescent psychiatry* (ed. M. Rutter and E. Taylor), pp. 555–70. Oxford: Blackwell.

Treasure, J. and Ward, A. (1997) A practical guide to the use of motivational interviewing in anorexia nervosa. *European Review of Eating Disorders*, **5**, 102–14.

Homeless children and young people

Panos Vostanis

Definition

Homeless families include all adults with dependent children who are statutorily accepted by local authorities (housing departments), and are usually accommodated for a brief period (from few days to several months) in voluntary agency, local authority or housing association hostels. The statutory definition does not include families who have lost their homes and live with friends or relatives, on the streets, in squats, or as travellers. This population, predominantly mothers with pre-adolescent children, is the focus of this section of Chapter 14, with some reference to single young homeless people living in the streets. Many of these young people (at least those under 16 years) are in the care of the local authority, and the challenges of meeting their needs are addressed in another section of this chapter. Homeless families in the UK and Western Europe increasingly include refugees and asylum seekers.

Epidemiology

It is estimated that up to 100, 000 families in the UK fulfil these criteria each year (Vostanis and Cumella 1999), many of whom have several episodes of housing and family breakdown. Homeless children have a variety of health needs in relation to poor children in stable housing, such as lower birth weight, anaemia, dental decay, delayed immunizations, lower height, and a greater degree of nutritional stress. They are also more likely to suffer accidents, injuries, and burns, and a range of developmental delays, such as in receptive and expressive language, visual motor and reading skills (Webb *et al.* 2001). They are particularly likely to have low educational attainment.

Epidemiological research has found high prevalence rates in most child mental health problems and disorders, without any particular trend of specificity. In pre-school and primary school age children, behavioural problems include sleep disturbance, feeding problems, aggression, and hyperactivity. Anxiety and post-traumatic stress disorders are often precipitated by life events such as witnessing domestic violence. About one-third of children admitted to hostels in Birmingham were reported to have mental health problems that required clinical assessment and treatment (Vostanis *et al.* 1997). Without intervention, children's and parents' difficulties were likely to persist after rehousing in the community (Vostanis *et al.* 1998).

Homeless adolescents and street youth are likely to present with depression and suicide attempts, alcohol and drug misuse, and vulnerability to sexually transmitted diseases, including AIDS (Craig *et al.* 1996; Wrate and Blair 1999). A high proportion of homeless mothers also have similar psychiatric disorders, again mainly depression and substance misuse.

Causation

Studies in the UK and North America have shown that homeless families have been exposed to multiple adversities and life-events prior to the episode of homelessness, which are both chronic and acute. Such events include family conflict, violence, and breakdown; limited social support networks; recurrent moves; poverty and unemployment (Bassuk *et al.* 1996). Mothers are more likely to have suffered abuse in their own childhood and adult life, and children have increased rates of placements on the at-risk child protection register, because of neglect, physical and/or sexual abuse (Vostanis *et al.* 1997). The main reasons for family homelessness are domestic violence and neighbourhood harassment (about 50% and 25%, respectively, in our studies), followed by refugee status, financial reasons, or loss of housing.

Assessment

There are several issues to consider in both assessment and treatment. The first is the need for effective screening or referral of appropriate cases to the mental health staff involved with the hostels. Otherwise, they will be overwhelmed by the multiple social, health, and educational needs of these families. Housing staff usually act as the first contact point, and it is important that they receive training in identifying either broad causes for concern (aggressive behaviour, nightmares, withdrawal, self-harm) or risk factors (experiencing domestic or other kinds of violence, history of abuse, previous episodes of homelessness, parental illness, or substance misuse). This is not easy, as most families are admitted when in crisis, without any information from other agencies, while parents may even under-report problems in child protection cases. For this reason, housing and social services departments need to establish an automatic system of exchanging information, particularly on previous placements on the child protection register and the reasons behind them.

This system of identifying appropriate referrals has been applied in an outreach mental health service in Birmingham, based around a community psychiatric nursing post (Tischler *et al.* 2002). In such a model, it is essential to establish links with other appropriate agencies, who will undertake their respective assessments, if appropriate, such as education welfare officers, health visitors, or social workers.

An alternative model adopts a broader base assessment of needs by designated professionals. This has been applied in Leicester, with the appointment of family support workers, who assess all families at the time of admission on their health, educational, and social needs (Tischler *et al.* in press). They then either undertake direct work, mainly parent-training and behavioural therapy, or liaise with appropriate agencies, including the local CAMHS. In this model, the mental health professionals are more likely to be involved in the assessment of appropriate cases (recent examples include post-traumatic stress disorder, depression, self-harm, and autism), while the vast majority of cases will either not be referred by the family support worker or will be managed through consultation. Both models rely heavily on a weekly service liaison meeting, which is a fundamental part of the assessment process.

Interventions

The nature of the interventions needs to be adapted to the characteristics of the child and family population, i.e. their high mobility, difficulties in accessing or engaging with services, and longstanding serious problems that need to be dealt with in parallel, if not as a priority (mainly domestic violence, child protection, and loss of housing). The following types of intervention are appropriate:

1. The assessment and identification of needs can be defined as an intervention in its own right for homeless children as, otherwise, they would not have come to the attention of services.

2. Liaison with, and referral to, appropriate local agencies during the family's stay at the hostel, in preparation for rehousing in the community.

3. Clinical interventions can be compromised by the brief admission period. However, several treatment modalities are appropriate, as long as they are provided at the hostel, and preferably continued after rehousing. Sometimes, families are more likely to engage if the intervention (e.g. parenting group) is part of social activities at the hostel. Despite the constraints, a number of clinical interventions were provided by the CPN outreach service in Birmingham (Tischler *et al.* 2002). Behavioural advice and strategies, solution-focused therapy, and parent-training are the most relevant to the behavioural and parenting difficulties of homeless children and their parents. Brief psychotherapy or cognitive-behavioural therapy are effective for older children or adolescents with post-traumatic stress, anxiety, or depressive disorders. It is also important to involve the local adult mental health service to treat adult mental illness, particularly depression, and the drug and alcohol service, as many parents will present with substance misuse.

4. Training of housing staff and other agencies involved in the assessment and management of homeless children and families is an important objective of a mental health service.

Outcomes

There has been limited research on the multiple outcomes of homelessness in young people. Craig *et al.* found that 50% of young people had poor accommodation outcome at 1-year follow-up, 75% were unemployed, half of those with mental illness or substance misuse at first interview continued to do so after 1 year, with some new episodes occurring during the same period, while 40% of young women had become pregnant.

In a longitudinal study with families also re-assessed 1 year after becoming homeless, we found that mental health problems among children and parents remained, in the absence of intervention (Vostanis *et al.* 1998). In addition, families had difficulty in accessing services or being re-integrated in the community, even after being rehoused.

In a subsequent study, we evaluated the impact of the outreach mental health service, using both quantitative and qualitative methods. Families were re-assessed 4–6 months after their admission to the hostel and the brief clinical intervention. Children who had received the intervention, were found to have significantly improved on behavioural and hyperactivity ratings, while there was less conclusive impact on emotional problems (Tischler *et al.* in press). The input of the community psychiatric nurse was positively perceived by parents at follow-up, who described benefits from both the mental health intervention (individual work with the children and parenting advice) and the support with housing and social benefits, as well as children's education.

Challenges

Challenges for services are similar to those faced by other socially excluded groups. In addition, homeless families experience multiple and complex needs, and frequently move across service boundaries. As most services, including schools and CAMHS, operate on a model of social stability (even in deprived areas), they are unlikely to be accessible to these families either at the time of breakdown, or between different residences. This has been demonstrated by a number of studies, particularly the poor access to primary care services (Brooks *et al.* 1998) and education

(Power *et al.* 1995). Considering the high level of psychiatric morbidity among children and parents, their contacts with mental health services, mainly CAMHS, are limited (Cumella *et al.* 1998).

The first step towards setting up a comprehensive service is to include homeless children and families as a group in need in all related policies and commissioning documents, such as the local Joint Children's Strategy and Health Improvement Plans. This will ensure a strategic allocation of funding, which may come from a variety of sources rather than only from new CAMHS monies, although it is desirable that mental health posts are based at the local CAMHS. This will ensure continuity of treatment for clients, as well as training, supervision, and support for staff otherwise working in isolation.

Possible service models have already been discussed. These include a family support model with close links with CAMHS, an outreach mental health service through a primary mental health worker or community psychiatric nursing post (Tier 2), or designated mental health staff time from the specialist (Tier 3) service, such as psychology, child psychiatry, or psychiatric nursing (also Tier 2 role). A clinical challenge for CAMHS staff is to adapt and apply 'traditional' psychotherapeutic approaches with socially excluded populations and in settings such as hostels or residential units.

Large inner-city geographical areas pose additional problems, with families moving between CAMHS, adult mental health services, primary care groups, schools, and social services boundaries. These should be negotiated in advance between all agencies. Most staff face conflict between their pressurizing generic caseload and the designated time required to work meaningfully with homeless families. This particularly applies to health visitors, education welfare officers, and social workers, but will also affect mental health staff. Hostels are not always popular with services, as they generate high client turnover for general practitioners and schools, for which reason financial incentives should be considered by health and local authorities. Partnership with voluntary agencies such as Women's Aid and parent support groups, community projects, the police, housing associations, and new initiatives such as Sure Start, is also imperative. A multi-agency senior managers forum or steering group can ensure that all these valuable resources are utilized effectively and within common and clear objectives. Policy makers should remain in touch with frontline practitioners and, most importantly, family needs, to be able to meet such a difficult but ultimately extremely gratifying task.

Acknowledgements

The two described posts have been developed by the Birmingham Health Authority (Community Psychiatric Nursing post) and Leicestershire Health Authority (Family Support Team), in partnership with the Birmingham and Leicester Housing Departments respectively. The epidemiological assessment of need of homeless families was supported by the Nuffield Foundation. The outreach mental health service evaluation was funded by a West Midlands NHS Research and Development Grant, and the family support service was evaluated thanks to a research grant by the PPP Healthcare Trust.

Bibliography

Bassuk, E., Weinreb, L., Buckner, J., Browne, A., Salomon, A., and Bassuk, S. (1996). The characteristics and needs of sheltered homeless and low-income housed mothers. *JAMA*, **276**, 640–6.

An assessment of need in family shelters by the main research group in the United States. It highlights the complex health and social needs of these families.

Brooks, R., Ferguson, T., and Webb, E. (1998). Health services to children resident in domestic violence shelters. *Ambulatory Child Health*, **4**, 369-74.

A UK study demonstrating the lack of access to mainstream health services by homeless families in shelters.

Craig, T., Hodson, S., Woodward, S., and Richardson, S. (1996) *Off to a bad start: a longitudinal study of homeless young people in London.* London: The Mental Health Foundation.

A longitudinal epidemiological study of single young homeless people in London. It found a range of complex and persisting mental health needs, histories of residential care, family breakdown, poor educational attainment and unstable accommodation.

Cumella, S., Grattan, E., and Vostanis, P. (1998). The mental health of children in homeless families and their contact with health, education and social services. *Health and Social Care in the Community*, **6**, 331–42.

A study on homeless families' contacts with services. It found a large discrepancy between their level of need and service utilization, particularly CAMHS.

Power, S., Whitty, G., and Youdell, D. (1995). *No place to learn: homelessness and education.* London: Shelter.

A survey among local educational authorities in England, commissioned by Shelter. It established a variety of reasons for homeless children's poor access to education settings.

Tischler, V., Karim, K., Rustall, S., Gregory, P., and Vostanis, P. A family support service for homeless children and parents: users' perspectives and characteristics. *Health and Social Care in the Community*, in press.

Description of an innovative family support service for homeless children and their parents, with quantitative data on their psychosocial characteristics and qualitative interviews on their experiences of the service.

Tischler, V., Vostanis, P., Bellerby, T., and Cumella, S. (2002). Evaluation of a mental health outreach service for homeless families. *Archives of Disease in Childhood*, **86**, 158-63.

A qualitative and quantitative evaluation of an outreach mental health service for homeless families, who were re-assessed after rehousing, and were compared to homeless families without access to the CPN service.

Vostanis, P. and Cumella, S. (ed.) (1999).*Homeless children: problems and needs.* London: Jessica Kingsley.

A text of multiple agency perspectives on the needs of homeless children and families. There are guidelines for commissioning, service development, and clinical practice.

Vostanis, P., Grattan, E., Cumella, S., and Winchester, C. (1997). Psychosocial functioning of homeless children. *Journal of the American Academy of Child and Adolescent Psychiatry*, **36**, 881–9.

An epidemiological study of 113 homeless families with 249 children. It found high psychiatric morbidity in children and parents, but also multiple adversities that precipitated the episode of homelessness.

Vostanis, P., Grattan, E., and Cumella, S. (1998). Mental health problems of homeless children and families: longitudinal study. *British Medical Journal*, **316**, 899–902.

An one-year follow-up of homeless children and families. This demonstrated the continuation of mental health problems among children and adults, without intervention.

Webb, E., Shankleman, J., Evans, M., and Brooks, R. (2001). The health of children in refuges for women victims of domestic violence. *British Medical Journal*, **323**, 210-13.

A health assessment of families victims of domestic violence, highlighting their complex health and psychosocial unmet needs.

Wrate, R. and Blair, C. (1999). Homeless adolescents. In *Homeless children: problems and needs*, (ed. P. Vostanis and S. Cumella), pp. 83–96. London: Jessica Kingsley.

An epidemiological study of mental health and related needs in single young homeless people in the streets of Edinburgh. The study provides important recommendations for service development, particularly the introduction of peers or advocates.

Hyperactive children

Gill Salmon

Definition

Hyperactivity is an attribute of childhood behaviour that occurs as a continuum of severity, crossing the threshold into disorder when it is severe, developmentally inappropriate, and causing functional impairment at home and at school (Overmeyer and Taylor 1999; Curran and Taylor 2000).

There are two diagnostic classifications in common professional use. The ICD-10 category, hyperkinetic disorder (HD) 'is characterized by: early onset (before age six years); a combination of overactive, poorly modulated behaviour with marked inattention and lack of persistent task involvement; and pervasiveness over situations (e.g. home, classroom, clinic) and persistence over time of these behavioural characteristics' (WHO 1992, pp. 262–6). DSM-1V, however, uses the term attention-deficit/hyperactivity disorder (ADHD), the essential features of which are 'a persistent pattern of inattention and/or hyperactivity that is more frequent and severe than is typically observed in individuals at a comparable level of development'. The symptoms causing the impairment must have been present before the age of 7 years and be seen in at least two settings. There are three subtypes of ADHD: predominantly inattentive, predominantly hyperactive-impulsive, and combined type (American Psychiatric Association 1994, pp. 78–85). The latter roughly equates to HD and is probably what is meant by the term 'severe ADHD' referred to in the National Institute for Clinical Excellence Guidance on the use of methylphenidate (NICE 2000). As many UK clinicians in practice use the combined type criteria when making a diagnosis, the term ADHD will be used from here on to refer to all children presenting with hyperactive behaviour.

Overall, perhaps as many as 65% of children with ADHD will have one or more co-morbid psychiatric or other conditions (Beiderman *et al.* 1991). These include oppositional defiant disorder, conduct disorder, anxiety and mood disorders, Tourette's syndrome, as well as specific learning or communication disorders.

Epidemiology

The prevalence rate of ADHD is usually estimated at 3–5% in school-aged children (American Psychiatric Association 1994), although recent systematic reviews report ADHD prevalence estimates as wide as 2–18% (Rowland *et al.* 2002). This compares with a prevalence rate for HD of around 1% of primary school aged boys. The condition occurs three to four times more frequently in boys than girls (Ramchandani, *et al.* 2002). A childhood diagnosis of ADHD has long-term implications with more than 70% continuing to fulfil diagnostic criteria in adolescence, and up to 65% of adolescents still presenting with the disorder as adults (Jadad *et al.* 1999). Toone and Van der Linden (1997) suggest that 0.5–1 % of the young adult population has symptoms associated with ADHD and would benefit from access to psychiatric services. The implications for service provision are immense, as it is likely that most adult services are not currently meeting the needs of this patient group, both in terms of taking over the care of patients who grow too old for children's services, as well as providing help and advice to previously undiagnosed adults who are now presenting (Keen *et al.* 2000).

Causation

The underlying causes of ADHD are not fully understood, although it is likely that both psychosocial and biological factors play a part (Cantwell 1996). Whilst there is evidence to support the role of genetic factors in ADHD (heritability estimates range from between 0.7 to 0.9 of the phenotypic variance in twins), the mode of inheritance is still unclear and is likely to be moderated by factors such as environment and gender. Molecular genetic studies suggest that the dopamine DRD-4 receptor gene and the dopamine transporter gene (DAT) may be involved (Thapar *et al.* 1999; Curran and Taylor 2000). Environmental factors, which also seem to have a causative role, include: adverse events during pregnancy and birth, e.g. drug exposure *in utero*; brain infections, e.g. encephalitis; neurotoxin exposure, e.g. lead poisoning; and some forms of psychosocial adversity, for example, where there is history of child abuse or neglect, or multiple foster placements (Haddad and Garralda 1992; American Psychiatric Association 1994). There is little evidence however that ADHD can arise purely out of social or environmental factors, such as poverty, family chaos, diet, or poor parent management (Barkley 1990). It is thought that the genetic and/or environmental factors which lead to ADHD do so by altering the brain structures and functions associated with cognitive executive functioning.

Assessment

Assessment of children and adolescents with suspected ADHD is multi-modal and multi-agency. It should be comprehensive, so as to exclude alternative explanations for the symptoms and uncover any coexisting disorder, and should make use of standardized diagnostic criteria such as DSM-IV or ICD-10. Where coexisting learning difficulties are suspected, a thorough assessment by an educational or clinical psychologist will also be helpful.

There are no laboratory tests that have been established as diagnostic in the assessment of ADHD; diagnosis is based on the observations and clinical history provided by those carers and professionals who know the child best. A variety of broad- and narrow-range rating scales can be used to gather information from parents, teachers, and young persons (Collett *et al.* 2003). Narrow-band scales, e.g. the Conners Rating Scales-Revised (Conners 1997) are the most helpful when assessing children for ADHD (American Academy of Pediatrics 2000), although broad-band scales e.g. The Child Behaviour Checklist (Achenbach 1991) and the Strengths and Difficulties Questionnaire (Goodman 1997) can usefully be used to screen for co-morbidity (American Academy of Child and Adolescent Psychiatry 1997). The importance of obtaining information on the child from his/her school is evidenced by teacher-rated scales tending to provide a more accurate overview of the child's behaviour than parent-rated scales, and teacher-identified features of ADHD being far more often associated with continued ADHD problems than those of parents' (Klein and Mannuzza 1991; Taylor *et al.* 1996). Additional information can be obtained, often before the first appointment, by requesting school reports that specifically address symptom areas, as well as copies of reports from other involved professionals, e.g. educational psychologists, behaviour support teachers, and speech and language therapists.

Pre-assessment information-gathering, however, is not diagnostic in itself and should only be used in conjunction with a clinical interview with the parenting figures and the child, physical examination, and consideration of more detailed investigations, e.g. EEG, brain scans, neuro-psychological tests, fragile-X test, audiograms, and detailed speech and language assessment, where there is a clinical indication (Taylor *et al.* 1998). Current data does not support the use of laboratory measures such as continuous performance tests (which measure vigilance or distractibility) or measures of activity levels (Baumgaertel and Wolraich 1998; American Academy of Pediatrics 2000).

Interventions

When ADHD is recognized and managed at an early stage, many of the educational and psychosocial difficulties can be addressed (Cantwell 1996). Untreated, however, the prognosis is poor with anti-social behaviour, social and peer problems, substance misuse, criminal activity, and later psychiatric diagnoses commonly occurring, particularly where there is coexistent conduct disorder (Swanson *et al.* 1998; Cantwell 1996).

Conventional treatment options tend to be either behavioural and/or pharmacological, and essentially aim to reduce the core symptoms of inattention, hyperactivity, and impulsivity, as well as targeting the associated effects of these on psychosocial and educational functioning.

Evidence-based behavioural interventions include behavioural parent training and behavioural interventions in the classroom. Evidence to support the use of individual therapies, including cognitive behavioural therapy and play therapy, is lacking (Pelham *et al.* 1998; National Institutes of Health 2000). Parent training programmes utilizing contingency management, as well as standard behavioural techniques, are increasingly being offered in community as well as clinic settings. Benefits may include a reduction in the child's disruptive behaviour across settings and in the level of family stress, as well as an increase in parents' own self-confidence in their parenting ability (Cantwell 1996). Such programmes are also a valuable tool for managing pre-school ADHD (Sonuga-Barke *et al.* 2001). School-based interventions using similar techniques (DuPaul and Eckert 1997), as well as social skills training for children and their carers, have also been found to be of benefit (Frankel *et al.* 1997). Despite the evidence for the benefits of behavioural approaches, the improvements that are made in the short term are typically not as large as those obtained with medication (Pelham *et al.* 1998) and where response is sub-optimal, pharmacological interventions should also be considered.

There is a huge evidence-base to support the use of stimulant medication, at least in the short term, in the management of ADHD, with about 80% of patients having clinically meaningful benefits (Swanson *et al.* 1998; Greenhill *et al.* 1999; Jadad *et al.* 1999; Joughin and Zwi 1999; Lord and Paisley 2000). Stimulant medications available in the UK, such as methylphenidate and dexamphetamine, act by reducing the core symptoms of hyperactivity, inattention, and impulsivity and can also have a beneficial effect on conduct problems, social skills, academic performance, and executive functioning.

The multi-modal treatment study of children with ADHD (MTA) has helped to clarify the efficacy of both pharmacological and behavioural interventions, and their place in the overall management strategy of children with ADHD (Jensen *et al.* 1999a, b). In this study, 597 children with ADHD-combined type were randomly allocated to one of: medication only; an intensive behavioural treatment involving parent, child, and school; a combination of the medication and behavioural intervention; and standard community care. Although sizeable reductions were seen in ADHD symptoms over time in all four groups, there were significant differences between the groups in the degree of the change, with the children in the combined medication and behavioural intervention, and the medication-only groups doing the best of all. Interestingly, the medication-only group achieved a greater reduction of core ADHD symptoms than those receiving standard community care, even though most of these latter children were receiving medication. The difference was put down to the careful titration of medication based on close collaboration between parents, teachers, and clinicians in the medication only group, and is likely to alter clinical practice in this area.

The National Institute of Health consensus statement on ADHD (National Institutes of Health 2000) notes that (consistent with MTA findings) combined treatments may offer some modest advantages over medication treatments alone, in particular that lower total daily doses of methylphenidate seem to be effective and that parent satisfaction is higher. It is now known that patient's co-morbidity profiles can help clinicians to determine the intervention package most likely to be of benefit, but ultimately, the acceptability to the child and family of any particular treatment package on offer will influence their final decision (Jensen *et al.* 2001).

A recently published UK protocol for treating ADHD in secondary care out-patient practice stipulates that medication should only be considered where the patient meets the DSM-1V criteria for ADHD (combined type), psychological treatments are insufficient alone, and parent and school will co-operate with the monitoring process (Hill and Taylor 2001). In practice, the optimum dose of medication is usually identified by starting with low doses, followed by gradual increases guided by clinical effects and side-effects (Greenhill *et al.* 2001). Even after a careful initial titration of medication, which aims at obtaining optimum improvement of clinically significant ADHD symptoms with no significant side-effects, most children will require dose modification in the long term, thus justifying the need for long-term continuous monitoring (Vitiello *et al.* 2001). Once established on medication, assessment of psychological response (e.g. using Conners' 1995, abbreviated scale, completed by parents and school) and physical monitoring (of height, weight, blood pressure, and pulse) is recommended with regular consideration being given to a 'trial without medication' to assess whether there is a continuing need.

Outcomes

To date, there are no long-term studies looking at the efficacy (and safety) of stimulants or psychosocial treatments. In addition, no information is available on long-term educational, psychosocial, or occupational outcomes of individuals who have received treatment (National Institutes of Health 2000). Clinical experience, however, points to the majority of children requiring medication to be continued for many years (Greenhill *et al.* 1999; Overmeyer and Taylor 1999).

Challenges

Over the last ten years or so, ADHD has become a commonly diagnosed childhood disorder in the UK, referrals for which are now overwhelming specialist services. This new demand on services is both due to recent scientific advances, as well as the large increase in parental expectations and knowledge. Purchasing has not yet taken into account this increased workload. Research from the USA indicates that as many as 30–50% of referrals to child and adolescent mental health services are specifically related to ADHD (Popper 1988; Barkley 1996). In addition, there is concern about the large number of unidentified cases of children with ADHD, with the gap between those who could potentially benefit from services and those receiving services growing wider (Sloan *et al.* 1999).

A multi-professional approach to the assessment and treatment of children and adolescents with suspected ADHD should be the basis for a streamlined 'seamless' service and may prevent unnecessary interventions being put in place by one agency where alternatives have been found effective (Keen *et al.* 1997). The drawing up of multi-agency protocols for ADHD management, which offer a single point of entry, accurate and planned assessment and treatment, and referral on to another agency only where problems are not improving or where they are very severe from the outset, may be one way of addressing the problem. The development of specialist ADHD services, which draw on professionals from different agencies (e.g. specialist behaviour teachers, community paediatricians, and/or child and adolescent psychiatrists, school nurses, mental health workers, clinical psychologists) for sessional input, is also likely to help. Specialist ADHD clinics are, however, already close to saturation point and given the necessity for long-term follow-up of children on medication, employment of non-consultant grade doctors or ADHD nurse practitioners needs to be considered. Production of shared care guidelines between general practitioners and local CAMHS, which has already happened in many areas in the UK, should facilitate the provision of long-term prescribing and monitoring. It seems likely that purchasers will need to commission additional services to meet the need and achieve the level of multi-agency co-operation that will be required (Overmeyer and Taylor 1999).

Serious concerns persist regarding the adequacy of the assessment process, the wide variations in current clinical practice, the lack of behaviour management offered prior to, or alongside, prescription of stimulants, the minimal integration of disciplines and agencies to provide comprehensive, multi-modal treatments, as well as poor long-term liaison with schools regarding individual children (Sloan *et al.* 1999). Guidelines and protocols that lend themselves to audit, have now been published in Europe (Taylor *et al.* 1998; NICE 2000; Hill and Taylor 2001), as well as the USA (American Academy of Child and Adolescent Psychiatry 1997; Baumgaertel and Wolraich 1998; American Academy of Pediatrics 2000). It is likely that they, as well as the recently published medication treatment algorithms for children with ADHD and its major co-morbid conditions (e.g. Pliszka *et al.* 2000a, b), will help to reduce variation between practitioners and thus result in enhanced patient outcomes.

There is a wealth of recent research, which should be helpful in highlighting the areas new resources need to target. For example, there is a need for greater access to behavioural interventions, such as parent training in the community, particularly for parents of pre-school children, as well as extension of behavioural treatments past the initial period to prevent loss of treatment gains. Additionally, within schools, learning support assistants can be trained up to provide behavioural support to teachers and school-wide interventions, e.g. social-skills based programmes and student-mediated conflict resolution programmes (Wells *et al.* 2000). Such initiatives, which could involve staff from multiple agencies, would be best planned and/or commissioned jointly, but unfortunately, in some areas of the UK, are currently being established on a rather *ad hoc* basis as monies become available, thus actually increasing the risk of duplication of input and information overload for parents.

References

Achenbach, T.M. (1991) *Integrative guide for the 1991 CBCL/4–18, YSR and TRF profiles.* Burlington: University of Vermont Department of Psychiatry.

American Academy of Child and Adolescent Psychiatry (1997) Practice parameters for the assessment and treatment of children, adolescents and adults with attention-deficit/hyperactivity disorder. *Journal of the American Academy of Child and Adolescent Psychiatry,* **36** (10, supplement), 85S-121S.

American Academy of Pediatrics (2000) Clinical practice guideline: diagnosis and evaluation of the child with attention-deficit hyperactivity disorder. *Pediatrics*, **105**, 1158–70.

American Psychiatric Association (1994) *Diagnostic and statistical manual of mental disorders* (4th edn). (DSM-1V) Washington, DC: American Psychiatric Association.

Barkley, R.A. (1990) *Attention deficit hyperactivity disorder: a handbook for diagnosis and treatment.* New York: Guilford Press.

Barkley, R.A. (1996) Attention-deficit hyperactivity disorder. In *Child psychopathology* (ed. E.J. Mash and R.A. Barkley), pp. 45–58. New York: Guilford Press.

Baumgaertel, A. and Wolraich, M. (1998) Practice guideline for the diagnosis and management of attention deficit hyperactivity disorder. *Ambulatory Child Health*, **4**, 45–58.

Beiderman, J., Newcorn, J., and Sprich, S. (1991) Co-morbidity of attention deficit hyperactivity disorder with conduct, depressive, anxiety and other disorders. *American Journal of Psychiatry*, **148**, 564–77.

Cantwell, D. (1996) Attention deficit disorder: a review of the past 10 years. *Journal of the American Academy of Child and Adolescent Psychiatry*, **35**, 978–87.

Collett, B.R., Ohan, J.L., and Myers, K.M. (2003) Ten-year review of rating scales. V: Scales assessing attention-deficit/hyperactivity disorder. *Journal of the American Academy of Child and Adolescent Psychiatry*, **42**, 1015–37.

Conners, C.K. (1995) *The Conners rating scales: instruments for the assessment of childhood psychopathology.* North Tonawanda, NY: Multi-Health System.

Conners, C.K. (1997) *Conners rating scales—revised.* Windsor, UK: NFER.

Curran, S. and Taylor, E.A. (2000) Attention deficit-hyperactivity disorder: biological causes and treatments. *Current Opinion in Psychiatry*, **13**, 397–402.

DuPaul G. J. and Eckert, T. L. (1997) The effects of school-based interventions for attention deficit hyperactivity disorder: A meta-analysis. *School Psychology Review*, **26**, 5–27.

Frankel, F., Myatt, R., Cantwell, D., and Feinberg, D. (1997) Parent-assisted transfer of social skills training: Effects on children with and without attention-deficit hyperactivity disorder. *Journal of the American Academy of Child and Adolescent Psychiatry*, **36**, 1056–64.

Goodman, R. (1997) The strengths and difficulties questionnaire: a research note. *Journal of Child Psychology and Psychiatry*, **38**, 581–6.

Greenhill, L.L., Halperin, J.M., and Abikoff, H. (1999) Stimulant medications. *Journal of the American Academy of Child and Adolescent Psychiatry*, **38**, 503–12.

Greenhill, L. L., Swanson, J. M., Vitiello, B., et al. (2001) Impairment and deportment responses to different methylphenidate doses in children with ADHD: The MTA titration trial. *Journal of the American Academy of Child and Adolescent Psychiatry*, **40**, 180–7.

Haddad, P.M. and Garralda, M.E. (1992) Hyperkinetic syndrome and disruptive early experiences. *British Journal of Psychiatry*, **161**, 700–3.

Hill, P. and Taylor, E. (2001) An auditable protocol for treating attention deficit/hyperactivity disorder. *Archives of Disease in Childhood*, **84**, 404–9.

Jadad, A.R., Boyle, M., Cunningham, C., et al. (1999) Treatment of Attention-Deficit/Hyperactivity Disorder. *Evidence Report/Technology Assessment*: Number 11(Prepared by McMaster University under contract No.290–97–0017) Agency for Health Care Policy and Research and Quality.

Jensen, P.S., Arnold, L.E., Richters, J.E., et al. (1999a) A 14-month randomized clinical trial of treatment strategies for children with attention-deficit/hyperactivity disorder. *Archives of General Psychiatry*, **56**, 1073–86.

Jensen, P.S., Arnold, L.E., Richters, J.E., et al. (1999b) Moderators and mediators of treatment response for children with attention-deficit/hyperactivity disorder: the multi-modal treatment study of children with attention-deficit/hyperactivity disorder. *Archives of General Psychiatry*, **56**, 1088–96.

Jensen, P.S., Hinshaw, S.P., Kraemer, H.C., *et al.* (2001) ADHD co-morbidity findings from the MTA study: comparing co-morbid subgroups. *Journal of the American Academy of Child and Adolescent Psychiatry*, **40**, 147–58.

Joughin, C. and Zwi, M. (1999) *Focus on the use of stimulants in children with attention deficit hyperactivity disorder.* Primary evidence-base briefing no.1. London: The Royal College of Psychiatrists.

Keen, D.V., Olurin-Lynch, J., and Venables, K. (1997) Getting it all together: developing a forum for a multi-agency approach to assessing and treating ADHD. *Educational and Child Psychology*, **14**, 82–90.

Keen, D., Bramble, D., and Olurin-Lynch, J. (2000) Attention- deficit hyperactivity disorder: How much do we see? *Child Psychology and Psychiatry Review*, **5**, 164–8.

Klein, R. G. and Mannuzza, S. (1991) Long-term outcome of hyperactive children: a review. *Journal of the American Academy of Child and Adolescent Psychiatry*, **30**, 383–7.

Lord, J. and Paisley, S. (2000) *The clinical effectiveness and cost-effectiveness of methylphenidate for hyperactivity in childhood.* Version 2. London: National Institute for Clinical Excellence.

National Institute for Clinical Excellence (2000) Guidance on the use of methylphenidate (Ritalin, Equasym) for attention deficit/hyperactivity disorder (ADHD). In *Childhood Technology Appraisal Guidance-no 13.* London: National Institute for Clinical Excellence.

National Institutes of Health (2000) National Institutes of Health consensus development conference statement: diagnosis and treatment of attention-deficit/hyperactivity disorder (ADHD). *Journal of the American Academy of Child and Adolescent Psychiatry*, **39**, 182–93.

Overmeyer, S. and Taylor, E. (1999) Annotation: principles of treatment for hyperkinetic disorder: practice approaches for the UK. *Journal of Child Psychology and Psychiatry*, **40**, 1147–57.

Pelham, W.E., Wheeler, T., and Chronis, A. (1998) Empirically supported psychosocial treatments for attention deficit hyperactivity disorder. *Journal of Clinical Child Psychology*, **27** 190–205.

Pliszka, S.R., Greenhill, L.L., Crismon, M.L., *et al.* (2000a) The Texas children's medication algorithm project: report of the Texas consensus conference panel on medication treatment of childhood attention-deficit/hyperactivity disorder. Part 1. *Journal of the American Academy of Child and Adolescent Psychiatry*, **39**, 908–19.

Pliszka, S.R., Greenhill, L.L., Crismon, M.L., *et al.* (2000b) The Texas children's medication algorithm project: report of the Texas consensus conference panel on medication treatment of childhood attention-deficit/hyperactivity disorder. Part 11: tactics. *Journal of the American Academy of Child and Adolescent Psychiatry*, **39**, 920–7.

Popper, C.W. (1988) Disorders usually evident in infancy, childhood or adolescence. In *Textbook of psychiatry* (ed. J.A. Talbott, R.E. Hales, and S.C. Yudofsky), pp. 649–735. Washington, DC: American Psychiatric Press.

Ramchandani, P., Joughin, C., and Zwi, M. (2002) Attention deficit hyperactivity disorder in children. *Clinical Evidence*, **7**, 262–71.

Rowland, A.S., Lesesne, C.A., and Abramowitz, A.J. (2002) The epidemiology of attention-deficit/hyperactivity disorder (ADHD): a public health view. *Mental Retardation and Developmental Disabilities Research Reviews*, **8**, 162–70.

Sloan, M.T., Jensen, P., and Kettle, L. (1999) Assessing the services for children with ADHD: Gaps and opportunities. *Journal of Attention Disorders*, **3**, 13–29.

Sonuga-Barke, E., Daley, D., Thompson, M., Laver-Bradbury, C., and Weeks, A. (2001) Parent-based therapies for preschool attention-deficit/hyperactivity disorder: a randomized controlled trial with a community sample. *Journal of the American Academy of Child and Adolescent Psychiatry*, **40**, 402–8.

Swanson, J.M., Sergeant, J.A., Taylor, E., Sonuga-Barke, E.J.S., Jensen, P.S., and Cantwell, D.P. (1998) Attention-deficit hyperactivity disorder and hyperkinetic disorder. *The Lancet*, **351**, 429–33.

Taylor, E., Chadwick, O., Heptinstall, E., and Danckaerts, M. (1996) Hyperactivity and conduct problems as risk factors for adolescent development. *Journal of the American Academy of Child and Adolescent Psychiatry*, **35**, 1213–26.

Taylor, E., Sergeant, J., Doepfner, M. *et al.* (1998) Clinical guidelines for hyperkinetic disorder. *European Child and Adolescent Psychiatry*, **7**, 184–200.

Thapar, A., Holmes, J., Poulton, K., and Harrington, R. (1999) Genetic basis of attention deficit and hyperactivity. *British Journal of Psychiatry*, **174**, 105–11.

Toone, B.K. and Van der Linden, G.J.H. (1997) Attention-deficit hyperactivity disorder or hyperkinetic disorder in adults. *British Journal of Psychiatry*, **170**, 489–91.

Vitiello, B., Severe, J.B., Greenhill, L.L. *et al.* (2001) Methylphenidate dosage for children with ADHD over time under controlled conditions: Lessons from the MTA. *Journal of the American Academy of Child and Adolescent Psychiatry*, **40**, 188–96.

World Health Organization (1992) *The ICD-10 classification of mental and behavioural disorders: Clinical descriptions and diagnostic guidelines.* Geneva: World Health Organization.

Wells, K., Pelham, W., Kotkin, R., *et al.* (2000) Psychosocial treatment strategies in the MTA study: rationale, methods, and critical issues in design and implementation. *Journal of Abnormal Child Psychology*, **28**, 483–505.

Chapter 15

Children and adolescents who have chronic physical illness

Michael Shooter

Introduction

Our picture of childhood is a rosy one—of carefree good health, interrupted occasionally by minor illness; of innocent peer group play and academic achievement. Not for children the degenerative diseases of later life, of shrinking cognitions, restricted mobility, and a world shut down to the ambulance and the hospital bed. Yet some 10–20% of children will now develop a chronic, physical illness by the age of 18, illness that will affect them for long periods of time, waxing and waning through life; illness that can be 'managed' but not cured (Eiser 1990).

True, the increasing ability of doctors to save life has been matched by an increasing recognition of the limitations of what treatment has to offer. The number of deaths in neonatal intensive care units due to withdrawal of treatment increased 5-fold between the mid-seventies and the mid-nineties (Shooter 1998). But advances in medico-surgical technology have converted many erstwhile, short-lived, fatal diseases into long-term disabilities that are survivable but 'life-threatening' in its broadest sense.

Children with such illnesses run twice the risk of developing psychological problems compared to their healthy peers. The cognitive, emotional, behavioural, and social lives of all of them will be affected to some extent. For a substantial minority, their illness will be of such severity that it will interfere with every aspect of daily activity (Behrman and Vaughan 1996). In other words, the question of 'life or death' has been turned into one of 'quality of life.'

The implications are huge, not only for the child and family concerned, but for the skills, attitudes, and organization of the team that is called upon to help them. Consider, for example, the child with acute lymphocytic leukaemia requiring bone-marrow aspirations, courses of chemotherapy, or irradiation; consider the child with end-stage kidney disease or cystic fibrosis, faced with organ transplantation and a life on immuno-supressive drugs; consider the child with diabetes, whose life revolves around injections and diet (Stuber 1996).

Twenty years ago, we were asked to think about how the traditional hierarchical roles of acute medicine can become blurred in such situations (Taylor 1979). The physician may be the ultimate authority in the world of 'disease'—of blood chemistry and organ function that can be examined and measured objectively. He has less control over 'illness'—the symptoms caused by their malfunction: the nausea, breathlessness, pain, or dizziness that vary so much from patient to patient. It is the individual child and family who are the experts in their 'predicament'—the experience of the illness that is unique to each one of them. Understanding predicament requires a multi-dimensional approach in which the child psychiatrist will have much to offer.

Has research kept up with this shift in emphasis? Just a decade ago, exploration of these 'secondary handicaps' was described as a story of 'revision, replication and neglect' (Pless and Nolan 1991). By the end of the decade, research of increasingly sophisticated methodology was said to have given us 'a clearer idea of the complexity of aetiology, interventions and outcomes' (Stuber 1999). This chapter aims to plot a path through the thicket of papers that have sprung up in-between and beyond.

Models

The combination of childhood, illness, and its sequelae can feel overwhelming. What the treatment team need is a framework of understanding and there is no shortage to choose from as the models have developed over time. 'Medicine's own illness, the body–mind split, has begun to heal' (Hardwick and Bigg 1997) as ideas have shifted from a broad division into physical illness and psychological illness, through the recognition of a group of psychosomatic illnesses in between, to the assertion that all illnesses lie somewhere along the psychosomatic spectrum (Lask and Fosson 1989). Nowhere is this more true than in childhood illness that is always a mixture of physical and psychological components, the balance between which moves around from disease to disease, individual to individual, and time to time.

The 'Biosocial Approach' (Serrano 1993) takes the model one stage further. Paediatric illness can be considered as an 'objective reality' (the systematic dysfunction, lesions, or complications), a 'subjective reality' (the psychological experience of not feeling well), and an 'inter-subjective reality' (the social implications for the child, family, medical team, and the social institutions that surround them all). The child 'suffers' his/her illness on every level, to the extent that it may become a way of relating to people within the family and the outside world. This not only indicates the holistic approach needed to treat the illness, but also explains why it may be difficult for the child or family to get back to normal functioning, if and when the illness resolves.

Struggling to understand the variability of depression in chronically ill children, a 'diathesis–stress model' is postulated (Burke and Elliott 1999). The outcome is proportional to interaction between the child's vulnerability (the diathesis), and the illness and life events both caused by it and independent of it (the stressors). The diathesis has biological components (genetic predisposition, temperament, and gender), cognitive/affective components (low self-esteem, negative attributional style, external locus of control, and ineffective coping strategies), and social/behavioural components (insecure attachments and poor peer group relationships). Vulnerabilities might be expected to be uniformly distributed across all childhood illness, but the particular characteristics of individual illness might interact with those vulnerabilities in different ways. Thus illnesses and their treatment that cause bodily disfigurement might be critical for children who already have low self-esteem, negative attributional style, and difficulty making friendships. In general, if the 'strength of the diathesis is low' (i.e. the child has few vulnerabilities), depression is likely to develop only if the illness impinges directly on central nervous systems regulating mood. If the 'strength of the diathesis is high' (i.e. the child has multiple vulnerabilities), then a minor illness might be enough to tip the child into depression, particularly if coupled with a major life event such as change of school or family difficulties.

Building on this, much controversy has centred on whether different illnesses cause different psychosocial reactions in children and families (Gartstein et al. 1999). The 'discrete disease model' focuses on the adaptation to one chronic condition (e.g. cancer, asthma, and diabetes) with the assumption that it will impose unique demands on child and family, which will govern clinical practice. The 'non-categorical model' implies that the challenge of pain, hospitalization, treatment side-effects, school and family disruption, are common to all illnesses. Services might include cross-illness support groups for children and adolescents or their parents, on the assumption that they face common issues, whatever their diagnosis. 'Mixed models' look for similarities and differences, grouping illnesses into clusters imposing common psychological demands proportional to the onset, course, and outcome of the disease and the degree of incapacitation it causes (Rolland 1994). Thus, haemophilia would be characterized as acute, relapsing, possibly fatal, and generally non-incapacitating; many childhood cancers would be characterized as acute, progressive, potentially fatal, and gradually incapacitating; juvenile rheumatoid arthritis would be characterized as of gradual onset, progressive course, non-fatal but occasionally quite severely incapacitating. The assumption is that all children would struggle with the same issues in any disease that fitted the group profile—thus opening the way for cross-fertilization of ideas across diagnoses and services. Units treating kidney disease and cystic fibrosis in children, for example, might learn a lot from each other, if they were not so introspective, and the child psychiatrist might act as liaison officer, not only between child/family and treatment team, but between different treatment teams themselves.

Finally, it has been said, what matters clinically in any childhood illness, is the interplay between risk factors and resilience (Wallander and Varni 1998). Risk factors would include disease characteristics (diagnosis, the severity of handicap, medical complications such as bowel or bladder control, degree of visible disfigurement, and cognitive impairment), the level of their interference in the child's independent life, and psychosocial stresses (everything from major life-events to every day hassles). Resilience might involve intra-personal factors (competence, temperament, motivation, and problem-solving abilities), social-ecological factors (family dynamics, social support, and practical resources), and stress-processing factors (cognitive appraisal and coping strategies). To put it at its most simplistic, the child with a severe handicap might survive psychologically, if blessed with intelligence and equable temperament, extended family support, good friends, a sympathetic school teacher, and the money to make major alterations to the house. A child with none of those advantages might succumb psychologically to a much more minor disability.

In essence, what most of these models are suggesting, is that anyone trying to work with a chronically ill child and family will need to fit together a jigsaw of understanding, each piece of which is crucial to the overall picture (Shooter 1997). The pieces outlined briefly below include the characteristics of the individual child; the illness, and how its particular demands cut across the developmental needs of the child; the family, cultural and peer group dynamics in the child's world; and the skills, supports, and co-ordination within the wider helping systems in which they find themselves. They are illustrated with reference to vignettes, which will be familiar to any child psychiatrist involved in paediatric liaison work, in hypothetical or imaginary long-term or crisis situations.

Vignettes

Lewis (5)

Lewis has neuro-fibromatosis, with granulomatous patches developing in key areas of his body. He has one patch behind his right eye, which is protuberant, cyclops-like, the lid barely able to close around it. The national eye hospital, who have been monitoring him as an out-patient, say that they will consider a prosthesis when he is older and better able to deal with it psychologically. Surgeons have carried out three operations to bypass a patch in his lower left leg with a new blood supply, but he is severely disabled by it.

Lewis has been referred to child psychiatry as 'depressed' because he refuses to go to school or talk to his friends when they call, is tearful, and irritable, and spends most of his time playing on the computer in his bedroom. At his appointment, Lewis will not speak, but draws pictures of one-eyed, weeping monsters being chased by other monsters carrying knives.

Kirsty (15)

Kirsty has been in and out of the specialist unit for most of her life with acute exacerbations of her cystic fibrosis. She has two siblings: one much more mildly affected, the other not at all. The family have been through a roller-coaster of despair and hope as the disease has relapsed and remitted over time. Several of her fellow patients have died during the course of her own illness.

In the process, Kirsty and her family have become very close to the much-loved female consultant who has just retired as head of the unit. Heart and lung transplantation was considered for Kirsty but never actively sought because of the parents' fears of the consequences if it failed. Kirsty is now well enough to be back at school and out clubbing with friends at weekends. She has become a very attractive young woman and is the apple of her father's eye. A young, male consultant has persuaded Kirsty to reconsider transplantation and to begin to think about transition to the adult team. The father demands to see him, complaining angrily that it is unethical to talk to his daughter without her parents being present, and that Kirsty cannot consent to anything without their agreement.

Iqubal (10)

Iqubal is a lad with end-stage renal disease and moderate learning difficulties. He is the youngest son of a strict disciplinarian father who dotes on his older, healthy sons and has little time for anyone too ill to help out with the family market-trading business. Iqubal is close to his mother and sisters, in whose eyes he can do little wrong.

Iqubal has already lost one kidney transplant by failing to keep to his medication properly and is now on the paediatric ward with fluid overload and other complications. It has become clear to the staff that Iqubal's mother is bringing him secret bottles of drink, which she hides under her coat.

The staff are divided in their reaction. The doctors, largely male, feel that the mother should be stopped from visiting and Iqubal put on a strict behavioural regime. The nursing staff, largely female, and in closer day-to-day contact, feel more sympathetic to a few 'treats.'

Anne Marie (17)

Anne-Marie has an inoperable cranio-pharyngioma. She is an only daughter and was academically bright, sporty, and popular. She has been discharged to out-patient monitoring and community support, but has multiple deficits, including obesity, incipient diabetes, left-sided weakness, speech and sleep disturbance, and memory loss that fluctuates on top of her general deterioration. She is emotionally labile, occasionally aggressive, and becoming dangerously impulsive, having once leapt out of a moving car.

Anne Marie has been 'looking depressed' for some time, has withdrawn from her peers and has dropped out of school. She has given away most of her possessions. Admitted to the ward with a sudden worsening of her condition, she tells staff that she has 'had enough' and wants to be left to die in peace. Her father and his new partner, with whom she lives, agree with her wishes. Her estranged mother says she is 'not in her right mind', that her husband just wants to get rid of her because she is a burden, and she will 'bring in the lawyers' if the hospital do not actively treat her.

Rhodri (8)

Was diagnosed as having muscular dystrophy after a long period in which the parents were convinced there was something wrong but the doctors sought to reassure them. He is now wheelchair-bound but still attends his local, mainstream primary school, where he has a special, one-to-one helper in the classroom. His parents now feel he has attention deficit hyperactivity disorder because he spends so much time daydreaming in class, fidgets in his wheelchair, interrupts people when they are trying to watch TV, and is generally irritable. They have read all the literature and have persuaded the paediatrician to refer him to child psychiatry 'for that medication.'

Talking to the other professionals involved, the teacher feels that Rhodri could do far more for himself if allowed to, but the class helper is a friend of the family and tends to over-protect him. She has felt discouraged from talking to him about his illness. The general practitioner, who has had arguments with Rhodri's parents in the past, tells you (confidentially) that he is a special child, born after several miscarriages. The father lost his own father at Rhodri's age and has fallen out of contact with another son from a previous marriage. He does not believe in expressing upset.

Peter (14)

Has diabetes and is on twice daily injections of insulin. His non-compliance has led to repeated hospital admissions and there are growing worries about his long-term prospects. He is in local authority care, his single-parent mother having been unable to cope with his behaviour. The natural father's whereabouts are unknown. Peter's foster mother has a grown-up son of her own still living with her, who is also diabetic, being controlled on diet alone. Peter and he get on very well. Peter's mother has once again broken promises of contact.

The paediatrician has referred Peter to child psychiatry and he has begun to attend the adolescent day unit, to which he is driven by taxi 20 miles each day. On his second day, he presents in an obviously unwell state, having presumably failed to take his insulin. One of the SHOs assesses his mental state and finds him still rational, coherent, orientated, and well aware of the consequences of what he has done. Later that morning, he runs off and the police are informed when staff fail to find him.

Peter turns up in the late afternoon, saying that he feels very sick and wants to go to hospital; he is admitted via the accident and emergency department. As the duty child psychiatry consultant, you are rung up in the mid-evening by the paediatrician. He tells you that Peter is refusing to be treated and may soon be comatose. He wants to know if Peter can be injected against his will under the Mental Health Act—'just like force feeding anorexics'. If not, what can be done? Preliminary enquiries show that no one knows who has parental responsibility for Peter.

The individual child

Children under the stress of chronic illness may show their upset in a bewildering variety of ways. Some become antisocial in attitude and behaviour; some withdraw from relationships, or retreat into a fantasy world inside their head that is more comfortable, and controllable, than the world outside. Some increase the seriousness of their physical symptoms or create new ones by direct self-harm, by indirect non-compliance with treatment, or psychosomatic overtones. Some deteriorate in academic performance with heads so full of worry that they have no room for school learning. A framework is needed for predicting how a child might react or intervention is likely to be a hit-and-miss affair. And to begin with, although the evidence for the general link between chronic illness and psychological problems is overwhelming, it is not axiomatic.

Some studies have failed to show lower school performance (despite high absence rates), damage to self-esteem, or more stress in the lives of ill children (Boekaerts and Roder 1999). Others have pointed out that the experience of illness and the decisions that have to be made, may actually make its sufferers more mature. Survivors of cancer may emerge with a stronger sense of their special status, an enhanced appreciation of life, and a healthier set of priorities (Anholt *et al.* 1993). It is doubtful whether ordinary 15-year-olds would be mature enough to make the decision to have a transplant, like Kirsty, knowing that her current wellness was outweighed by the prospect of future exacerbations of her cystic fibrosis—and to take the risk of it going wrong. Certainly, we need to account for a vast difference in individual reactions even to the same illness where 'some children… are well liked by their peers, excel in school, and appear not to suffer from anxiety and depression. Other children are immature for their age, socially awkward, anxious or depressed' (Kliewer 1997).

One approach has been to look at the meaning of stress in chronic illness for each individual child. This cognitive appraisal can be divided into primary appraisal (how threatening is this to me?), measured by an evaluation of stakes index; and secondary appraisal (what can I do about it?), measured by an evaluation of action index (Thies and Walsh 1999). Such concepts can be seen to mature with developmental level. Young concrete thinkers, like Lewis, with external locus of control and simplistic ideas of a stress doing something to him, could be expected to have the persecutory fantasies and fear of peer-group teasing that he shows, horrible though they may be. An abstract thinking, older adolescent, like Anne Marie, with internal locus of control and complex reasoning, can weigh up issues of life and death and make her decisions accordingly, agonizing though they might be in turn. In other words, the important question is not whether behaviour of a chronically ill child is abnormal *per se*, but whether it is abnormal for the reactions that a child of that developmental level, under that stress, might be expected to have. It will help the child psychiatrist to advise the clinical team on the point of intervention and the balance between practical stress management and more open-ended exploration of feelings.

It is a mistake to assume, however, that 'developmental level' is entirely a matter of age. An intelligent 8-year-old like Rhodri might want to talk about his illness, given the chance, while the 14-year-old Peter is still buried, ostrich-like, in a world he has learnt to see as hostile. The ability to understand the concept of illness, to relate it to oneself, and think about the consequences, is as much dependent on permission to ask questions and receive honest answers. Even young children may have an acute awareness of the seriousness of their condition. The decision is not whether to share things with them but whether to allow them to share what they know. To deny that opportunity to Rhodri might be to lock him into a prison of his feelings; to deny the opportunity for Lewis to talk through his fantasies might be cruel indeed. Unfortunately, the child's immediate family and the wider family of the helping system may be on very different developmental levels of their own.

The behaviour-analytic model has looked at how different children and their helpers react in different 'problem situations' common to chronic illness, and how they rank order them in degrees of difficulty. The adolescents with cystic fibrosis, their parents, peers, and professional carers, all saw clinic visits and hospitalization as causing the greatest anxiety and this was clearly linked, in the adolescents' case, with a perception of their own social competence (Di Girolamo *et al.* 1997). This would allow the child psychiatrist to devise role play exercises to teach coping strategies in those situations that are more positive in approach (problem-solving) rather than negative in avoidance (ignoring the problem, wishful thinking, or blame).

The whole issue of coping strategies has been extensively studied and the case made out for routine screening for positive and negative adaptation (Spirito *et al.* 1995). There have been arguments about whether such strategies are 'trait' based (fixed over time and disease situations by a combination of genetically inherited temperament, family learning, and gender) or 'state' based, (changing over time and disease situations); about the pattern of coping or so-called 'trajectory of adaptation' (Frank *et al.* 1998). The answer is almost certainly a compromise in which each child has a certain coping style but may behave differently in different contexts—wanting a hand holding during a painful injection, for example, and shunning all contact in the face of bad news. It explains the ability of adolescents to switch backwards and forwards between child-like and mature reactions to the consternation of everyone around them, and often themselves.

Finally, in-depth studies of children, using audio-taping, journals, and drawings, have shown how those like Kirsty or Iqubal may become adept (for good or ill) at working the hospital system to cope with repeated admissions. Many coping strategies have been identified, including behavioural distraction, resistance or avoidance, co-operative submission, emotional or verbal outbursts, enlisting the support of staff, taking independent control, and a variety of cognitive ploys (Boyd and Hunsberger 1998). Staff can be trained to spot such strategies and meet them with appropriate skills and structures—talking and listening, explaining and informing, maintaining a positive outlook and empathic support, giving a degree of control to the child and, above all, maintaining a familiar and consistent presence in their life. The closeness of the relationship between Kirsty and her former consultant must have carried her through past crises just as surely as it may be a problem now. And such closeness, of course, is a two-way process. Staff may find it just as hard to let go of patients they have known from early childhood.

The illness

In the shifting balance between resilience and risk factors (Patterson and Blum 1996) the characteristics of the illness itself—the uncertainty of diagnosis and prognosis, sudden or gradual onset, steadily progressive, ameliorating or roller-coaster course, the visibility of its effects, the complexity and implications of treatment, brain involvement, and pain—play an important part. And things can go wrong very early in the journey through the medical system upon which the child and family are about to embark (Mrazec 1994).

There have been few studies on the onset of illness but, in general, it is said that an acquired illness causes less complex reactions than those that are innate. An 'act of God' in childhood and adolescence, and the 'why us?', 'what happens now?', 'how can we live with it?', questions that it invokes, painful though it may be, is better than the guilts and recriminations between parents blaming themselves or each other for passing on illness to their child. Just as important is the certainty or uncertainty of diagnosis at the time of onset. If the diagnosis is clear from the start, the child and family can at least begin to come to grips with the process of management. So often, however, as in Rhodri's case, there is a prolonged period in which the parents are convinced that there is something wrong, while clinicians are struggling to reassure them that there is not. The climate of suspicion that sets in here can colour the whole relationship between the family and the medical system from there on. On the other hand, where clinicians know there is something wrong but the parents do not, the temptation is to invent a certainty rather than be honest about the doubts and enlist the parents in a mutual sharing of the investigatory search.

The course of an illness, its narrative history, is crucial. Many childhood illnesses are steadily progressive from congenital or early-infant onset, and the danger here is that the parents and the child get 'out of phase' in their emotional and practical reactions to it. The parents will grieve again at every point in which the implications of the child's illness are brought home to them by another milestone failed, but most of their upset will occur at the time of diagnosis. For the child, however, their illness is their normality; if they are part of a specialized unit dealing with children of the same illness, they may know no other world. By late-childhood or early-adolescence, the parents may have put the prognosis to the back of their minds and be expecting their child to begin to take charge of some aspects of their lives in as normal a way as possible. But this may be just the point at which the child can begin to comprehend their difference and the implications of their prognosis—the point at which to grieve their lot in life. In this potential clash of perceptions, a child with no room to express their grief may chose the most obvious weapon to hand—treatment compliance. It is here that the child psychiatrist may be brought in with tempers frayed all round.

Most childhood illnesses are a roller-coaster of remission and relapse, of hope and despair. A great deal is known about how families fall apart in such conditions, but little about strengths that hold them together. Research has plotted the challenges facing the family through all the switchback of emotions involved in specific diseases such as epilepsy (Ziegler *et al.* 2000) but cystic fibrosis, such as that of Kirsty, remains the paradigm. The child psychiatrist's role is often to provide the constant support closest to the child and parents throughout, acting as interpreter, advocate, and therapist, enough part of the medical system to be trusted as an expert, but distanced enough to be able to work with angers and miseries that the family may not feel able to off-load onto clinicians, upon whom they depend for treatment; but the task can be hard. The author well remembers working with a young boy through the 8 years of his life and the changing psychological tasks involved, from early deterioration towards death and anticipatory grief; to an unexpected improvement and the hope of a heart–lung transplant; to deterioration again on the transplant list; to the miracle of transplant and immediate improvement; to the bitter disillusionment of the chronic rejection process, abandonment of hopes of a second transplant, and the grief before, at, and long after his death. There is no emotion that the patient goes through that the therapist may not also share. Supports are essential for the 'care givers plight.'

The 'visibility' of the illness and the effects of treatment, depend as much on the perceptions of the sufferer as any objective reality. Thus it is hardly surprising that both Lewis and Anne Marie are frightened and miserable in their incapacity, to the extent that their whole self-image is shaken. Iqubal may well feel himself unfairly marked out by his tiredness and short stature. Peter, outwardly untouched, is so frustrated by the restrictiveness of his insulin regime that, at least in part, he is prepared to risk the consequences by ignoring it. On the other hand, a mature teenager like Kirsty, in remission and a relatively carefree life, is able to make a decision about transplant, knowing that her current normality is only a snap-shot in a video film of evolving illness. A transplant itself, of course, may have dramatic psychological implications. A kidney transplant can be seen as something separate from the identity of the recipient, inserted in a different anatomical position, and even given a name by the child involved. Heart and lungs are often seen as the 'soul' of a person; what it means to absorb this into ones own identity has been little researched.

Children with direct brain involvement in their illness have been proved to have more serious problems—behavioural difficulties, less autonomous functioning, and poorer school performance (Howe *et al.* 1993). But the cognitive aspects of such illness, as Anne Marie is testament to, can be much wider. Dysfunction is a product of the direct pathophysiology of the disease (her craniopharyngioma), the stresses associated with trying to cope with that (constant hospitalization and out-patient attendance, as effects wax and wane, on top of a slowly deteriorating situation), and the generalized physical effects of an illness and its growing complications (blood chemistry and bio-rhythm disturbance, toxicity and tiredness combined). Such factors need detailed, repeated assessment over time, liaison with school as well as family, and secondary preventative services for those at risk. Child psychiatrists may have a key role in these wider issues (Brown 1999).

Just as important is concomitant pain, the chronic pain of tissue damage and the acute pain of investigatory or treatment procedures—injections, lumber punctures, bone marrow aspirations, and the like. Full consultation by the primary physician is essential, of course, but there has often seemed to be a resistance to involving child psychiatrists in the general aspects of pain for the child struggling with it and the pain of the parents and staff watching the child do so (Sifford 1997). Conceptual models have considered pain on four, inter related levels—neural activity; conscious pain sensation; cognitive and affective reactions to that sensation; and behavioural responses to them (Schulz and Masek 1996). Treatment therefore is not just a matter of analgesics but includes helping to develop a degree of self-mastering, honest anticipation of pain, good quality information, help with the anxiety and anger that might be involved, and a variety of psychotherapeutic, biofeedback, relaxation and cognitive behavioural techniques. All this means validating the child's perception of pain and its history without the battles so often fought over whether it is 'real' (has a demonstrable organic origin) or 'imaginary' (does not). For many, 'pain and suffering' are inextricably mixed in a vicious circle of increasing pain and its emotional/behavioural concomitants, mutual markers of the need for help (Varni *et al.* 1996).

All these aspects of illness have some general implications for childhood development, adherence to treatment, and levels of competency. Thus the effects of illness and the requirements of its treatment may cut across the normal developmental tasks for a child or adolescent struggling with them (Shooter 2001). The infant's sense of basic trust, developed through consistent, predictable experiences, may be undermined by frequent hospitalizations, separation from parents (however well the hospital is organized to allow them to remain at the bedside), and painful medical procedures. The toddler's push towards autonomy may be frustrated by physical incapacity and the emotional over-protection that prevents the free manipulation and exploration of objects in the surrounding environment. Confinement to the world of illness and the hospital ward may prevent the older child's healthy notion of self-competence that develops through peer-group relationships in school and community (Kliewer 1997). And nowhere is this more obvious than in adolescence.

There has been much research about the developmental complications of illness in adolescence in general (Boice 1998), and of its impact on specific psychological tasks like separation-individuation (Liakopoulou 1999), and the growth of sexuality in all its aspects (Locke 1998). It may be the task of the liaison child psychiatrist to remind the treatment team of the developmental context in which the adolescent's reaction may be more clearly understood.

How can the adolescent learn to live with uncertainty, as the complications of illness add to the strangeness of the pubertal body and mind? How can independence be established amongst adults, family and staff, who have looked after the adolescent since childhood and upon whom the adolescent may increasingly depend for treatment? How can the adolescent discover an identity that is healthily distinct from his peer group, while at the same time being part of that group, when illness undermines self-confidence and disfigurement is such an unwelcome difference? In such situations, the natural ambivalence of adolescents, as they swing backwards and forwards between opposite pairs of feelings, beliefs, and behaviours, can be accentuated. To handle an adolescent who is demanding an adult say in their own illness one minute and retreats into childish needs for comfort the next, or bursts into tears as the needle punctures the fragile skin of his or her identity, requires special skills. These skills may be best contained in specifically trained staff on adolescent wards (Shooter 2001). There is no more miserable sight than a pubertal adolescent girl surrounded by inquisitive toddlers in the paediatric department or trapped between the dying elderly on an adult ward.

Not surprisingly, the clash between the demands of illness, and the demands of child and adolescent development, often devolve into a battle for control. For Lewis, different bits of whose body belong to different hospital teams, his whole life may seem out of his own control and his sense of self-identity demolished. In such circumstances, his emotional and physical withdrawal may be understandable. For an older child like Iqubal, or an adolescent like Peter, the battle is still on to control whatever bit of their life they can. This is often reflected in problems of treatment-adherence and a complex mixture of health beliefs (do I really believe what will happen if I do not comply?), external or internal self-regulation (who says what I should do about my own body anyway?), and systems theory (what are they going to do about it if I don't do as they say?) (Brown and Macias 2001).

These struggles for control may raise important issues about the competence of children and adolescents to make decisions for themselves, which require skilled assessments of capacity, a strong appreciation of what is in a child's clinical best interests, and the knowledge of how to seek that through all the realities and mythologies of common law, Children Act, and Mental Health legislation. Clearly, Peter may need 'rescuing' from his own refusal of treatment by his doctors proceeding under common law in the immediate crisis or via parental consent if parental responsibility could be determined. A Specific Treatment Order of the Children Act could be used if parental responsibility was unknown and there was time. The Mental Health Act would not be appropriate in what is a primary physical disorder, like diabetes. Kirsty, on the other hand, is Gillik competent to consent to treatment, against her parents' wishes if need be, although it would be clinically sensible to involve the parents in the decision, as soon as possible. In many life or death situations, however, the situation is far more complex. Disentangling the true wishes of Anne Marie amongst all the competing interests around and inside her may tax the whole team on clinical and ethical grounds. The child psychiatrist may well be called on to decide whether she is in her right mind, in every sense.

In the process of all this, between practical battles over treatment and the appropriate acceptance of death as an option, it is easy to miss quite serious psychiatric sequelae of the physical illness. Adolescent girls, who slip more often than boys into frank depression and suicidal ideation, do not seek help more often than ordinary adolescents (Suris et al. 1996), while professionals may overlook the signs before their very eyes (Kashani and Breedlove 1994). Diagnosis may be difficult where distress is somatized and becomes part of the general illness symptoms; ward teams may not be alerted to the needs of children who lie quietly in their own unhappiness. In the end, those children who react to the issue of control by passive submission (Meijer et al. 2000) may be more worrying, if less disturbing, than those who have at least enough spirit left to be non-compliant.

Family and culture

The inner world of the child and the impact the illness and its treatment have upon this inner world, must be seen within the context of family and culture. The picture is not all gloomy.

Some chronic illnesses, such as juvenile arthritis, have been shown to elicit such positive coping mechanisms in families that they have increased their closeness and co-operation compared to controlled groups (Aasland *et al.* 1998). Despite methodological flaws, however, the general finding is that the child's psychological adjustment is proportional to the family's levels of cohesion, conflict, and flexibility, as they struggle to come to terms with illnesses that interfere with every aspect of their daily routines. Vicious circles may be set up between family conflict and the child's acting-out behaviour at home and in school, and between family cohesion and rates of hospitalization and medication (Soliday *et al.* 2001)—such that family interventions have both emotional and practical implications. But it is also clear that clinicians generally underestimate the burden on families of looking after a chronically ill child (Canning *et al.* 1996).

With the help, perhaps, of the child psychiatrist, treatment teams need to be aware of the dynamics of the child's particular family—its relationships, the roles built on those relationships, the mythology the family has about illness and its treatment, and the rule-book handed down from one generation to the next about how they face up to crisis. 'Is this a family that shares information and emotions openly and constructively together, or do they remain aloof from each other in their unhappiness, condemning a child to a lonely illness?' (Shooter 2001). The family will be required to adapt over time to a continually changing pattern of illness and the tasks needed in this family development have been listed—accepting the condition, managing it on a day-to-day basis, coping with stresses and crises, allowing family members to express and manage their feelings, educating others around them, and establishing a wider social network, both emotionally and practically—while simultaneously meeting the normal developmental needs of the ill child and of other family members (Clawson 1996). Surprisingly, many families have the flexibility to achieve this but problems may arise in boundaries (where one parent becomes enmeshed with the ill child), in hierarchies (where the child comes to dominate the family with the threat of illness symptoms), in alliances (where the child and primary caregiver exclude the rest of the family), and symptom induction (where the illness reflects the conflicts around it) (Sein 1999).

Attention has focused on how the family can become 'triangulated', as the ill child and the primary caregiver (usually the mother at the hospital bedside) become over-close, to the exclusion of the rest (the father and siblings at home) (Seiffge-Krenke 1998). The primary caregiver's own emotional health may suffer and influence that of the ill child, in turn (Frankel and Wambold 1998). Parents who are not themselves in conflict, may feel socially isolated and de-skilled by their child's illness and a perceived lack of role in treatment compared to the white-coated 'parents' and their hospital technology. Stronger parents, like those of Rhodri or Kirsty, may enter into a battle for autonomy over their child with the professionals involved.

Methodological flaws (use of co-operative volunteers, small sample sizes across mixed aged groups, and unstandardized questionnaires) have bedevilled studies of the particular needs of the siblings of chronically ill children. Some have shown no more disturbance in these siblings than in controlled groups, and even less than in those of psychiatrically ill children (Fisman *et al.* 2000); but, in general, the rates appear to be double that of general community peer groups. Again it may be under-reported by parents who 'protect' siblings from the implications of the illness and therefore receive no feedback from children who fear to ask questions (Stallard *et al.* 1997). Asked directly about their perceptions, most of these children reveal no differences in positive feelings to their ill sibling, no conflict with them, battles for authority, or feelings of parental favouritism (Weis *et al.* 2001) but stress begins to emerge as the severity of the illness increases. Well siblings begin to worry about their brother's or sister's prognosis, about being shut out of a role in looking after them, or of contact with parents who are absent dealing with it. They may feel guilty about their own magical role in the illness, if they have been secretly angry with the ill child at the centre of it all and about the precariousness of their parents' emotional well-being (Gardner 1998). They may even feel guilty, like Kirsty's less affected siblings perhaps, about their own good health.

What these siblings need is open, honest information, couched in language and in a form that they can understand (especially young boys), an opportunity to ask questions and share feelings with the family, a role in the helping process, some special time for themselves, and an outlet for normal social activities. The implications for the professional helping system are obvious, in attitudes and organization, both at the time of the child's illness and long after death, as siblings may remain haunted by the experience, may become over-protected by parents who have already lost one child, or may be used as the resurrected fulfilment of the hopes and ambitions of their dead siblings, to the loss of their own identity.

Finally, the ill child is trapped within the family history and culture, to the extent that the illness and reactions to it may take on a meaning beyond their face value. They may even come to perform a vital function within the family dynamics. There can be no doubt, for example, that the resistance to allowing Rhodri to explore the feelings about his illness and its prognosis is partly due to the unresolved bereavement issues in his father's life. Talking openly about Rhodri's losses might mean opening up those losses too, and the parents seem happier diverting the issue onto a battle about diagnosis, 'concreting' their son's condition in the process. Parents may become so embroiled in their own needs and the illness that they neglect the ordinary needs, as in Kirsty's case, of the developing child.

The helping system

Children with chronic illnesses do not exist in a vacuum. They live at the centre of a number of overlapping circles of help that individually and in combination, both constructively and destructively, have a major impact on their psychological welfare.

The inter-relationships between education, health, and behaviour have been clear for a quarter of a century or more (Rutter *et al.* 1970). 'Failure in school quickly limits a child's future'; it compounds the undermining influence of the illness itself and further erodes the child's sense of self worth. Thus, 30–40% of ill children have been shown to have school difficulties. The factors involved are both primary (neuro-cognitive changes due to the illness or its treatment) and secondary (school absences, illness induced stress, constraints on physical and social activities, and decreased expectation from the school and the healthcare system, all set in the context of families that are often poor and dysfunctional, without the strength to fight for the best opportunities for their child). Long after the original studies showed how vital it is for such children, despite these difficulties, to participate in an educational programme appropriate to their ability, in as least a restrictive physical setting possible, the message seems to have fallen on deaf ears. 'No current systematic set of procedures ensures that children with chronic illness receive such educational opportunities' (Perrin and MacLean 1988). Has the situation improved now that medical technology has increased the life-expectancy and functional capabilities of the children and guarantees have been written into educational and disability legislation on both sides of the Atlantic? (Sexson and Dingle 1997).

The politics of inclusion in Britain has swung away from special schools to the maintenance of ill children in mainstream education wherever possible, to 'minimise the consequences'

(Department of Health 1996). But there has been little research on how the children themselves feel in this environment (Lightfoot *et al.* 1998). Those interviews that have been carried out with children of all types of severity of illness, show them valuing school and actively managing their condition there, but needing a great deal of support with the practicalities of their disability and its treatment, the disruption of school absences, exclusion from ordinary activities, other people's reaction to their illness, and relationships in general. Much of this support is found informally through parents (especially mothers) who act as go-between, carrying information to the educational and healthcare systems, and from peer groups. Some children wish the illness to remain private but are bullied nonetheless, both verbally and physically, because of their difference. Most seem to relish the open support they get from friends who know a lot about their condition, with whom they are able to discuss their feelings, who give practical help in carrying bags or pushing wheelchairs, act as unofficial advocates for them from day to day, and alert adults in a crisis. The children particularly value the support of any close teacher/confidant who manages to walk the difficult tight-rope between over-playing the disease and its disability (allowing the child to break rules and treating them as a pet), and underemphasis (by failure to make allowances for tiredness, time out to manage medication, or emotional upset).

The same research, however, shows little improvement in a more formal support system. Schools themselves are still built largely for the physically able, with ill children effectively excluded from break-time social activities, by playground safety rules, or being forced to wait at the top or bottom of stairs that have no alternative lifts or ramps. There is often poor inter-agency collaboration between systems working within schools (special educational needs co-ordinators and educational psychology services) and those outside (GPs, community paediatricians, and the hospital-based team) (Larcombe 1995). School-time can be further disrupted by appointments and non-vital procedures, which might easily have been arranged around school hours, and teachers themselves feel uninformed, ill advised, and unsupported (Court 1994). They know little about the illness itself or the treatment side-effects, so that the giving of medication becomes a battle ground and children are often unnecessarily excluded from activities that might have been vital to their relationships. Anxious teachers will naturally play safe and children with chronic illnesses may be sent home so often that they are effectively excluded from mainstream school and drop back into the further isolation of a home-tutor system or chronically under-funded hospital teaching provision. It may well be the child psychiatrist who is in the best position to act as advocate between the educational and healthcare professional systems, as well as working with the individual child or family themselves. The supports needed in cases like that of Lewis, Rhodri, Iqubal, or Anne Marie are obvious, but those pupils with less striking current disabilities, like Peter (with his diabetes) or Kirsty (in cystic fibrosis remission) may benefit from a school liaison approach too.

Liaison services with paediatricians, in contrast, have been extensively studied. There have been major writings on the organization of liaison services as a whole over a decade or more (Mrajek 1994; Morgan and Lask 1996) and in specific settings, including teaching hospitals (Black *et al.* 1990), child development centres (Evered *et al.* 1989), and general practice (Subotsky and Brown 1990).

Such liaison work may take place at many levels, beginning with the referral of individual children like Lewis for assessment and treatment. Care needs to be taken that the referral process does not alienate the child and family by redefining the illness as psychiatric in their eyes. Many is the child who has dropped through the net between the referring paediatrician and a child psychiatric clinic, which is seen as remote in distance, attitude, and implication.

Child psychiatrists have experimented, successfully, with long-term therapeutic groups for children, working on developmental growth, understanding of their illness, and adaptation to it (Stauffer 1998). Family therapy services have attempted to address the impact of the child's illness on family functioning and patterns of interaction between the family and healthcare professionals (Sayger *et al.* 1996).

Indirect help, aimed at the healthcare staff, may be just as valuable. Child psychiatrists have much to offer in: general paediatric teaching programmes on child development and the impact of illness on it; skills based on that understanding; and the handling of clinical and ethical crisis (Seedhouse and Lovett 1992), as paediatricians work their way logically through agonizing situations like that presented by Anne Marie. One-off advice may be given in individual cases, which may contribute to the paediatrician's keener appreciation of general issues, such as an adolescent's noncompliance, both acute (Peter) and chronic (Iqubal) (Shooter 2001), and the handling of distressed and angry parents, like Kirsty's father (Shooter 2002). Such one-off advice may be consolidated into regular joint discussion of the management of 'challenging cases', centred around multidisciplinary meetings that are an accepted and mandatory part of the paediatric programme (Menahem *et al.* 1997). These are often found, on audit by consumer satisfaction questionnaires, to be more of a support for senior staff carrying the burden of responsibility than a learning experience for junior ward staff (North and Eminson 1998). In some instances, such covert support in Balint-like discussions of difficult case decisions, has developed into an openly accepted and welcomed forum for sharing the day-to-day stress of paediatric practice and the heightened emotions that surround a girl like Anne Marie, decisions about her immediate clinical care, and the aftermath as staff struggle to come to terms with what happened.

The outcome of all this work has been subject to meta-analysis of many studies (Kibby *et al.* 1998), and judged by the results of psychiatric intervention in specific disease procedures (McQuaid and Nassau 1999) and by hospital admission rates (Kelly and Hewson 2000)—with generally positive findings. Yet, only around one-quarter of those chronically ill children who could be said to require mental health liaison interventions, actually receive them (Bauman *et al.* 1997). Why is this so? Practical difficulties, of course, can be insurmountable, as generic child psychiatrists, hard-pressed by problems and agencies elsewhere, can spare little time for journeys to the paediatric ward, and senior paediatricians, overwhelmed by clinical crises and rotating on shift work, can spare just as little time for sitting down with specialized child liaison workers to discuss the wider implications of case management. This is not helped where child psychiatry and child health find themselves in different employing trusts, although personal relationships across organizational boundaries may be stronger than those within it.

Often, however, 'the language, attitudes and work practices between medical and psychiatric staff may be so disparate that collaboration, even if attempted, may be resisted and may easily break down' (Menahem *et al.* 1997). A fragile trust set up through the driving force of particular senior members on both sides, disappears with the departure of one or other of them and the old mythologies may emerge—that the mental health of children with chronic physical illnesses does not affect their physical health; that it does not affect the quality of their medical care, health outcomes and functioning; that interventions designed to enhance such children's mental health have no impact on their illness; and that the provision of integrated mental health services is extremely costly and does not reduce overall healthcare expenditure (Walders and Drotar 1999).

In such circumstances, it is not surprising that the emotions of a seriously ill child faced with life and death concerns well beyond his or her years, of parents heartbroken by seeing their child so shackled by illness at a point in their life when they should be carefree; and of professional caregivers 'mired in apparently endless patterns of psychosocial and physical dysfunction and developmental arrest', should sometimes boil over (Wood 1995). What is more, it is easy for different individual staff or staff groups to take on the attitudes, emotions, and behaviours already being displayed within the family, as in Iqubal's case, that may in turn reflect the ambivalent feelings within the child. Thus they may reinforce, rather than resolve, the dynamics involved. At times this may develop into chronic friction between agencies, as in the case of Rhodri, or an acute battle over a critically ill patient, like Anne Marie. This does nothing for the needs of the child at the centre of it all. The child psychiatrist called in to help, may need all their systems therapy skills to avoid becoming part of the same triangulation process.

Unlike Anne Marie, most children with chronic physical illness will now survive through adolescence into adulthood (Viner, personal communication). This has presented paediatric teams with a new and increasingly pressing problem: 'transition'. On the one hand, from a developmental perspective, the older adolescent, like Kirsty, needs to pass on to the adult team just as any adolescent would move into the adult world outside. On the other hand, such transition poses huge difficulties for the adolescent with disabilities (Schultz and Liptak 1998). It may be as difficult for staff to allow those patients that they have nursed from childhood to grow up and leave, as it may be for parents to trust the adult teams on the other side and the adolescent him or herself to summon up the courage to leave those they have relied upon for so long. In the end, whatever the daily ups and downs of illness, and whatever agonizing crises they have all been through, however high the emotions may have run at times, the paediatric staff must learn to 'let go'. It may again be the child psychiatrist who can best help the child across the great divide between paediatric and adult services.

References

Aasland, A., Novik, T., Flato, B., and Vandvik, I. (1998) A multi modal, prospective assessment of outcome in families of children with early onset of juvenile chronic arthritis. *Families, Systems and Health*, **16**, 267–80.

Anholt, U., Fritz, G., and Keener, M. (1993) Self-concept in survivors of childhood and adolescent cancer. *Journal of Psychosocial Oncology*, **11**, 1–16.

Bauman, L., Drotar, D., Leventhal, J., Perrin, E., and Pless, I. (1997) A review of psychosocial interventions for children with chronic health conditions. *Paediatrics*, **100** (2), 244–51.

Behrman, R. and Vaughan, V. (1996) *Nelson text book of Pediatrics*. Philadelphia, PA: Saunders.

Black, D., McFadyen, A., and Broster, G. (1990) Development of a psychiatric liaison service. *Archives of Disease in Childhood*, **65**, 1373–5.

Boekaerts, M. and Roder, I. (1999) Stress, coping and adjustment in children with a chronic disease. A review of the literature. *Disability and Rehabilitation*, **21**, 311–37.

Boice, M. (1998) Chronic illness in adolescence. *Adolescence*, **33**, 927–39.

Boyd, J. and Hunsberger, M. (1998) Chronically ill children coping with repeated hospitalisations: their perceptions and suggested interventions. *Journal of Pediatric Nursing*, **13**, 330–42.

Brown, R. (ed.) (1999) *Cognitive aspects of chronic illness in children*. New York: Guilford Press.

Brown, R. and Macias, M. (2001) Chronically ill children and adolescents. In *Handbook of psychological services for children and adolescents* (ed. J. Hughes and A. La Greca), pp. 353–72. New York: Oxford University Press.

Burke, P. and Elliott, M. (1999) Depression in pediatric chronic illness. A diathesis-stress model. *Psychosomatics*, **40**, 5–17.

Canning, R., Harris, E., and Kelleher, K. (1996) Factors predicting distress among caregivers to children with chronic medical conditions. *Journal of Pediatric Psychology*, 21, 735–49.

Clawson, J. (1996) A child with chronic illness and the process of family adaption. *Journal of Paediatric Nursing*, 11, 52–61.

Court, S. (1994) *The health/education boundary. A study of primary school teachers understanding of childhood illness and its potential to disrupt the educational process.* Unpublished MSc Thesis. Newcastle upon Tyne.

Department of Health (1996) *Child health in the community—a guide to good practice.* London: NHS Executive.

Di Girolamo, A., Quittner, A., Ackerman, V., and Stevens, J. (1997) Identification and assessment of ongoing stressors in adolescents with a chronic illness: an application of the Behaviour-Analytic model. *Journal of Clinical Child Psychology*, 26, 53–66.

Eiser, C. (1990) *Chronic childhood disease.* Cambridge: Cambridge University Press.

Evered, C., Hill, P., Hall, D., and Hollins, S. (1989) Liaison psychiatry in a child development clinic. *Archives of Disease in Childhood*, 64, 754–8.

Frank, R., Thayer, J., Hagglund, K., Vieth, A., Shopp, L., Beck, N., et al. (1998) Trajectories of adaption in pediatric chronic illness: the importance of the individual. *Journal of Consulting and Clinical Psychology*, 66, 521–32.

Frankel, K. and Wamboldt, M. (1998) Chronic childhood illness and maternal mental health—why should we care? *Journal of Asthma*, 35, 621–30.

Fisman, S., Wolf, L., Ellison, D., and Freeman, T. (2000) A longitudinal study of siblings of children with chronic disabilities. *Canadian Journal of Psychiatry*, 45, 369–75.

Gardner, E. (1998) Siblings of chronically ill children: towards an understanding of process. *Clinical Child Psychology and Psychiatry*, 3, 213–27.

Gartstein, M., Short, A., Vannatta, K., and Noll, R (1999) Psychosocial adjustment of children with chronic illness: an evaluation of three models. *Developmental and Behavioural Pediatrics*, 20, 157–63.

Hardwick, P. and Bigg, J. (1997) Psychological aspects of chronic illness in children. *British Journal of Hospital Medicine*, 57, 154–6.

Howe, G., Feinstein, C., Reiss, D., Molock, S., and Berger, K. (1993) Adolescent adjustment to chronic physical disorders—I. Comparing neurological and non-neurological conditions. *Journal of Psychology and Psychiatry*, 34, 1153–71.

Kashani, J. and Breedlove, L. (1994) Depression in medically ill youngsters. In *Handbook of depression in children and adolescents* (ed. W. Reynolds and H. Johnston), pp. 427–42. New York: Plenum Press.

Kelly, A. and Hewson, P. (2000) Factors associated with recurrent hospitalisation in chronically ill children and adolescents. *Journal of Paediatric Child Health*, 36, 13–8.

Kibby, M., Tyc, V., and Mulhern, R. (1998) Effectiveness of psychological intervention for children and adolescents with chronic medical illness: a meta-analysis. *Clinical Psychology Review*, 18, 103–17.

Kliewer, W. (1997) Children's coping with chronic illness. In *Handbook of children's coping: linking theory and intervention* (ed. S. Wolchik and I. Sandler), pp. 275–300. New York: Plenum Press.

Larcombe, I. (1995) *Reintegration into school after hospital treatment.* Aldershot: Avebury.

Lask, B. and Fosson, A. (1989) *Childhood illness: the psychosomatic approach.* Chichester: Wiley.

Liakopoulou, M. (1999) The separation—individuation process in adolescents with chronic physical illness. In *Trauma and adolescence*, vol. 1 (ed. M. Sugar), pp. 93–107. Madison: International University Press.

Lightfoot, J., Wright, S., and Sloper, P. (1999) Supporting pupils in mainstream school with an illness or disability: young people's views. *Child Care, Health and Development*, 25 (4), 267–83.

Locke, J. (1998) Psychosexual development in adolescents with chronic medical illnesses. *Psychosomatics*, **39**, 340–9.

McQuaid, E. and Nassau, J. (1999) Empirically supported treatments of disease related symptoms in pediatric psychology: asthma, diabetes and cancer. *Journal of Pediatric Psychology*, **24**, 305–28.

Meijer, S., Bijstra, J., Mellenbergh, G., and Wolters, W. (2000) Social functioning in children with chronic illness. *Journal of Child Psychology and Psychiatry*, **41**, 309–17.

Menahem, S., Roth, D., and Haramati, S. (1997) Psychiatric collaboration in a paediatric department. *Australian and New Zealand Journal of Psychiatry*, **31**, 214–8.

Morgan, K. and Last, B. (1996) Paediatric liaison psychiatry. In *Seminars in liaison psychiatry* (ed. E. Guthrie and F. Creed), pp. 192–219. London: Gaskell.

Mrazek, D. (1994) Disturbed emotional development in severely asthmatic children. In *Assessment of quality of life in childhood asthma* (ed. M. Christie and D. French), pp. 71–80. Harwood Academic Publishers/Gordon Langhorne, PA, England.

North, C. and Eminson, M. (1998) A review of a psychiatry-nephrology liaison service. *European Child and Adolescent Psychiatry*, **7**, 235–45.

Patterson, J. and Blum, R. (1996) Risk and resilience among children and youth with disabilities. *Archives of Pediatric and Adolescent Medicine*, **150**, 692–8.

Perrin, J. and MacLean, W. (1988) Children with chronic illness. The prevention of dysfunction. *The Pediatric Clinics of North America*, **35**, 1325–37.

Pless, B. and Nolan, T. (1991) Revision, replication and neglect—research on maladjustment in chronic illness. *Journal of Child Psychology and Psychiatry*, **32**, 347–65.

Rolland, J. (1994) *Families, illness and disability: an integrative treatment approach.* New York: Basic Books.

Rutter, M., Tizard, J., and Whitmore, K. (1970) *Education, health and behaviour.* London: Longmans, Green.

Sayger, T., Bowersox, M., and Steinberg, E. (1996) Family therapy and the treatment of chronic illness in a multidisciplinary world. *The Family Journal*, **4**, 12–21.

Schultz, A. and Liptak, C. (1998) Helping adolescents who have disabilities negotiate transitions to adulthood. *Issues in comprehensive paediatric nursing*, **21**, 187–201.

Schulz, M. and Masek, B. (1996) Medical crisis intervention with children and adolescents with chronic pain. *Professional Psychology: Research and Practice*, **27** (2), 121–9.

Seedhouse, D. and Lovett, L. (1992) *Practical medical ethics.* Chichester: John Wiley and Sons.

Seiffge-Krenke, I. (1998) Chronic disease and perceived developmental progression in adolescence. *Developmental Psychology*, **34**, 1073–84.

Sein, E. (1999) Chronic illness: the child and the family. *Current Paediatrics*, **9**, 177–81.

Serrano, J. (1993) Working with chronically disabled children's families. A Biopsychosocial approach. *Child and Adolescent Mental Health Care*, **3**, 157–68.

Sexson, S. and Dingle, A. (1997) Medical problems that might present with academic difficulties. *Child and Adolescent Psychiatric Clinics of North America*, **6**, 509–22.

Shooter, M. (1997) The impact of death, divorce and disaster on young people. *Current Opinion in Psychiatry*, **10**, 268–73.

Shooter, M. (1998) The ethics of withholding and withdrawing therapy in infants and young children. In *CAPD/CCPD in children* (ed. R. Fine, S. Alexander, and B. Warady), pp. 433–50. Boston, MA: Kluwer Academic Publishers.

Shooter, M. (2001) An adult's guide to adolescence. *Current Paediatrics*, **11**, 218–22.

Shooter, M. (2002) Coping with distressed and aggressive parents. *Current Paediatrics*, **12** (1), 67–71.

Sifford, L. (1997) Psychiatric assessment of the child with pain. *Child and Adolescent Psychiatric Clinics of North America*, **6**, 745–81.

Soliday, E., Kool, E., and Lande, M. (2001) Family environment, child behaviours and medical indicators in children with kidney disease. *Child Psychiatry and Human Development*, **31**, 279–95.

Spirito, A., Stark, L., Gil, K., and Tye, V. (1995) Coping with everyday and disease—related stressors by chronically ill children and adolescents. *Journal of the American Academy of Child and Adolescent Psychiatry*, **34**, 283–90.

Stallard, P., Mastroyannopoulou, K., Lewis, M., and Lenton, S. (1997) The siblings of children with life-threatening conditions. *Child Psychology and Psychiatry Review*, **2**, 26–33.

Stauffer, M. (1998) A long term psychotherapy group for children with chronic medical illness. *Bulletin of the Meninger Clinic*, **62**, 15–32.

Stuber, M. (1996) Psychiatric sequelae in seriously ill children and their families. *The Psychiatric Clinics of North America*, **19**, 481–93.

Stuber, M. (1999) Psychiatric considerations for physical illness. *Current Opinion in Psychiatry*, **12**, 399–403.

Subtotsky, F. and Brown, R. (1990) Working alongside the general practitioner: a child psychiatric clinic in the general practice setting. *Childcare, Health and Development*, **16**, 189–96.

Suris, J-C., Parera, N., and Puig, C. (1996) Chronic illness and emotional distress in adolescence. *Journal of Adolescent Health*, **19**, 153–6.

Taylor, D. (1979) The components of sickness: diseases, illnesses and predicaments. *Lancet*, **2**, 1008–10.

Thies, K. and Walsh, M. (1999) A developmental analysis of cognitive appraisal of stress in children and adolescents with chronic illness. *Children's Healthcare*, **28**, 15–32.

Varni, J., Rapoff, M., Waldron, S., Gragg, R., Bernstein, B., and Lindsley, C. (1996) Chronic pain and emotional distress in children and adolescents. *Developmental and Behavioural Pediatrics*, **17**, 154–61.

Walders, N. and Drotar, D. (1999) Integrating health and mental health services in the care of children and adolescents with chronic health conditions: assumptions, challenges and opportunities. *Children's Services: Social Policy, Research and Practice*, **2**, 117–38.

Wallander, J. and Varni, J. (1998) Effects of paediatric chronic physical disorders on child and family adjustment. *Journal of Child Psychology and Psychiatry*, **39**, 29–46.

Weiss, K., Schiaffino, K., and Ilowite, N. (2001) Predictors of sibling relationship characteristics in youth with juvenile chronic arthritis. *Children's Health Care*, **30**, 67–77.

Wood, B. (1995) A developmental biopsychosocial approach to the treatment of chronic illness in children and adolescents. In *Integrating family therapy* (ed. R. Mikesell and D. Lusterman), pp. 437–55. Washington DC: American Psychological Association.

Ziegler, R., Erba, G., Holden, L., and Dennison, H. (2000) The co-ordinated psychosocial and neurologic care of children with seizures and their families. *Epilepsia*, **41**, 732–43.

Chapter 16

Young people with troublesome behaviour

Barbara Maughan

Definitions

Many children show troublesome behaviours at some point in their development. For a minority, defiance, disruptiveness, and aggression become so severe that they impair other aspects of functioning, compromise relationships, and risk conflict with parents, teachers, and peers. Disruptive behaviours of this kind are among the most common reasons for referral to child mental health services; they are also some of the most challenging to treat.

The psychiatric classification systems define two categories of antisocial disorders in childhood: oppositional defiant disorder (ODD), marked by irritability, temper outbursts, disobedience, and negativity; and conduct disorder (CD), characterized by rule-breaking, verbal and physical aggression, lying and stealing, and violation of others' rights. Both categories are recognized to be heterogenous, and also to shade into one another; especially among boys, the oppositional young child often develops more severe conduct problems or delinquent behaviours as time goes on. Several different approaches to sub-typing have been proposed, some based on the particular behaviours that young people display, others on their developmental history. Loeber, for example, has distinguished between overt conduct problems, such as bullying and aggression, covert problems, such as lying and stealing, and authority conflict behaviours, such as truancy and running away, arguing that each may follow a distinct developmental pathway (Loeber *et al.* 1993). A second approach suggests divisions according to age at onset, based on extensive evidence that early childhood conduct problems often persist, show a distinct risk-profile, and have a markedly poorer long-term outlook, than those that develop for the first time in the teens (Moffitt 1993).

CD and ODD are frequently accompanied by other psychosocial and educational difficulties. Poor peer relationships are common, as are poor school achievement and specific learning problems; children with disruptive behaviour problems are also at risk of a range of other psychiatric disorders. In childhood, attention deficit hyperactivity disorder (ADHD) forms a precursor to CD in some children; while in adolescence, problems with alcohol and substance use often develop from a background of antisocial and troublesome behaviours. Less predictably perhaps, children with CD/ODD are also at increased risk of emotional problems, in particular depression and low mood.

Epidemiology

Community studies have consistently shown that CD and ODD are among the most common disorders of childhood and adolescence. Prevalence estimates vary with the exact criteria applied: the most recent UK study, based on a national sample of some 10 000 children, found that over 5% of 5–15-year-olds met criteria for one or other of these disorders (Meltzer *et al.* 2000). This overall figure concealed important variations, both by gender and by age. Like all other studies, the UK data showed that disruptive behaviour problems are much more common in boys than in girls. Age-trends have been less consistently reported; the UK data suggested that rates of oppositionality remain relatively constant across childhood and adolescence, but that conduct problems increase steadily with age, especially in the teens. Taken together, these trends resulted in rates of ODD/CD of 2.7% (girls) and 6.5% (boys) in 5–10-year-olds, rising to 3.8% and 8.6%, respectively, in young people aged 11–15. Although conclusive data on historical trends are still lacking, many commentators now argue that rates of conduct problems have increased in recent decades, and that gender differences may also have narrowed somewhat over time.

Causation

A wide variety of factors, biological, psychological, and social, are now thought to contribute to the development and maintenance of conduct disorders (Hill 2002). How far any individual risk is strictly causal is more difficult to determine. Many well-established correlates overlap, and when children's problems are long-standing, simple unidirectional models of causation almost certainly fail to capture the complex, cumulative nature of the processes involved. The temperamentally difficult child may evoke negative responses from parents, or the trouble-some adolescent seek out similarly delinquent peers. Because so many features of disruptive behaviours involve interactions with others, reciprocal effects of this kind—whereby the child's own behaviour plays a part in 'selecting' adverse environments—may be especially important in understanding the onset and persistence of conduct problems (Scarr and McCartney 1983).

Most models for the aetiology of early onset, aggressive behaviours assume that they arise from the interaction of individually-based vulnerabilities and environmental risks (Rutter *et al.* 1998). Of the numerous individual factors examined, low resting heart rate and lower heart rate variability have shown relatively consistent links with early onset aggressive and dis-ruptive behaviours (Raine *et al.* 1997), suggesting that autonomic under-arousal may form one key component of risk. Neuro-psychological deficits—lower IQ, poor verbal skills, and impair-ments in executive function—have also been proposed as central to vulnerability for early onset conduct problems (Moffitt 1993). Characteristic patterns of social cognition, whereby young people over-attribute hostile intent to others, are among other individual correlates of disrup-tiveness and aggression, though their causal role remains less certain.

Alongside these individual factors, generations of research have shown that troublesome child behaviours are more likely to develop in adverse family and social circumstances. Poverty and social disadvantage, disorganized neighbourhoods, poor schools, family breakdown, parental psychopathology, harsh and ineffective parenting, and inadequate supervision are all strong correlates of conduct disorder (Loeber and Stouthamer-Loeber 1986). Once again, how-ever, interpreting the meaning of these links has proved more challenging. Though less herita-ble than most other childhood disorders, conduct problems do involve a heritable component, most important for early onset difficulties co-morbid with hyperactivity, less salient for delin-quency beginning in the teens (Simonoff 2001). Many apparently 'environmental' effects may thus reflect gene–environment interplay, whereby heritable child characteristics evoke particu-lar responses from parents, or heritable parent characteristics influence the styles of parenting and models of behaviour that parents provide. At present, research is only at the very earliest stages of teasing out how these complex processes arise.

Whatever their more distal origins, particular styles of parenting have consistently been associated with early onset conduct problems. Parents of troublesome children are less likely to anticipate and pre-empt difficult behaviour before it arises, less likely to follow through on instructions, and more likely to become involved in escalating spirals of confrontation with their children when disciplinary conflicts arise (Patterson 1982). In some instances these arbitrary and inconsistent approaches shade into harsh treatment or abuse. In addition, the affective quality of parent–child relationships is often compromised, so that interactions are negative or even hostile rather than positive and harmonious.

These individual and family vulnerabilities are most strongly associated with conduct problems that begin in childhood. Moffitt (1993) and others have argued that adolescent-onset difficulties reflect quite different causal processes, centring most importantly on associations with deviant peers. In adolescence, relatively normative rebellious tendencies are accentuated by the adolescent 'maturity gap'—the limbo years when young people have reached biological maturity but are not yet accorded adult social roles. As models for their behaviour, rebellious adolescents often choose their more delinquent peers. Peer influences play a key role in the genesis of adolescent conduct problems in boys, and also seem important for girls. Here, early puberty has been identified as an additional risk, argued to increase the likelihood that early maturing girls will associate with older peers, and so become involved in behaviours inappropriate for their age (Moffitt *et al.* 2001). Finally, though the mechanisms involved are uncertain, exposure to sexual abuse also appears to contribute to risk for conduct problems in girls.

Assessment

Because conduct problems affect so many aspects of young people's development, assessment also needs to be multi-faceted, involving information-gathering from schools and other agencies, as well as from carers and young people themselves. Of all the parties involved, the young person may be the least concerned about his or her difficulties, and may indeed resent the referral. Yet the child's perspective is crucial, both to a comprehensive account of behaviour and to an understanding of family or other problems that may be exacerbating current difficulties. Establishing a positive working relationship with the young person early in the contact is thus especially important.

Drawing on this range of sources, assessments should establish the nature of the child's behaviour problems (including impulsive behaviour and risk-taking) at home, at school, and in other settings; the extent to which they impair other aspects of functioning; and the history of their development over time. Because co-morbid conditions can affect the course of troublesome behaviours, and may require specific interventions, it is important to enquire about symptoms of ADHD, anxiety, and depression, as well as antisocial behaviours *per se*. The quality of the young person's peer relationships, as well as the types of activities undertaken with peers, are important in formulating treatment plans, as are assessments of his or her interpersonal skills and approaches to conflict negotiation. Ideally, diagnostic interviews should be accompanied by a full psychometric assessment. If that is not possible, a full report should be obtained from the school, covering not only the impact of behaviour problems in the school setting but also strengths and weaknesses in academic attainments, and the presence of any specific learning difficulties.

Assessment of family relationships and parenting styles is crucial. If there is widespread family disharmony, or marked discord between parents, treatment plans may need to address these specifically. Where possible, it is valuable to observe family interactions during a joint task; in addition, it is useful to get a detailed 'blow-by-blow' account of a recent episode of difficult behaviour—what prompted it, how it developed, and how it was eventually resolved. The affective tone of family interactions will also be important: do parents or carers see the young person in a predominantly negative light, or is there also evidence of sensitivity to the child's needs, and of warmth and approval?

Interventions

Antisocial behaviours account for 30–40% of referrals to child mental health services (Audit Commission 1999). As this brief overview suggests, they also pose major challenges for intervention. To be effective, interventions need to address the full range of the young person's difficulties—at home, at school, and in the wider community—in a developmentally appropriate way. Because conduct problems often arise in disadvantaged and troubled families, broader family problems may also need to be targeted, but by the same token families may also be especially hard to engage. And because conduct problems often follow a chronic course, short-term interventions are rarely successful, and treatment may need to be undertaken over extended periods.

Controlled trials have now identified four main types of intervention as most promising— though by no means universally successful—in the treatment of troublesome childhood behaviours (Kazdin 2001). Few studies have tracked treated groups over extended follow-up periods, however, and most have focused exclusively on behavioural outcomes; as a result, very little is known about the extent to which currently-advocated treatments hold long-term benefits or are successful in reducing associated impairments.

For young children, parent management training (Webster-Stratton and Hancock 1998), in which parents are taught (individually, in groups, or even through the use of videos) to pay attention to and reinforce desirable behaviours, and to practice effective strategies for dealing with undesirable ones, have probably the strongest support from evaluative research. Cognitive problem-solving skills training (designed to improve the young person's understanding of interpersonal situations and extend their repertoire of effective responses) and functional family therapy have also shown some positive effects. And finally, for more severe adolescent problems, multi-systemic family therapy (Henggeler *et al.* 1998), drawing on a broad spectrum of techniques to address individual, parental, family, and peer relationship problems, has shown promising outcomes in trials undertaken to date. Where co-morbid psychiatric conditions such as ADHD or depression are present, these may require separate and specific treatments.

Alongside clinic-based approaches, interventions for conduct problems frequently require attention to other aspects of young people's needs. If specific learning difficulties have been identified, or school performance is affected, appropriate educational support should be arranged; teachers may also welcome guidance on the management of behaviour problems in the classroom. For older children and adolescents, links with adult-supervised community resources can prove valuable in reducing associations with deviant peers and enhancing social skills.

Outcomes

There is now little doubt that the long-term outlook for many children with conduct problems is poor (Maughan and Rutter 2001). Longitudinal studies in a number of countries, and in different historical eras, have documented a litany of adverse adult outcomes: persistent antisocial behaviours and offending; problems in employment; difficulties in both social and intimate relationships; high rates of alcohol problems and substance use; increased risks of a range of other adult psychiatric disorders; and compromised physical health. The prognosis is poorest for early onset problems that persist through adolescence, but recent findings suggest that even adolescent-onset difficulties—once thought to be of relatively limited significance for later development—are nonetheless associated with less satisfactory progress in early adult life. Though troublesome children frequently come from disadvantaged backgrounds, these poor outcomes are not simply a function of childhood adversity. Adult development is compromised for boys and for girls, though often in rather different ways: outcomes for boys tend to be characterized by continuing antisocial behaviours, risks of substance abuse, and problems in employment; while for girls, early pregnancy, unsupportive relationships, depression, and parenting difficulties may be more central features (Moffitt *et al.* 2001). Where they arise, positive adult relationships and job involvements can function as 'turning points' out of antisocial trajectories in adult life. All too often, however, troublesome young people seem attracted to one another as partners in early adulthood; as a result, inter-generational continuities in antisocial behaviour are likely to be high.

Challenges

When they persist, troublesome childhood behaviours undoubtedly place a heavy burden on individuals and their families. Economic evaluations are now beginning to highlight the extent of the financial costs they impose on society (Scott *et al.* 2001). Against that background, continuing work on the development of effective prevention and treatment strategies is clearly of the highest priority. How far delivery of those interventions should be seen as solely, or even predominantly, the province of child mental health services has been a matter of debate (see, for example: Goodman and Scott 1997). Childhood conduct problems are common, and child mental health services are scarce; educational, criminal justice, and social services professionals frequently need to be involved in treatment planning for troublesome children, and in many instances play central roles. Ensuring effective patterns of joint working, and the sharing of knowledge and skills between professional groups, constitute further key challenges, if the needs of troubled and troublesome young people are to be appropriately met.

References

Audit Commission (1999) *Children in mind.* London: Audit Commission.

Goodman, R. and Scott, S. (1997) *Child psychiatry.* Oxford: Blackwell Science.

Henggeler, S.W., Schoenwald, S.K., Borduin, M.D., and Cunningham, P.B. (1998) *Multisystems treatment of antisocial behaviour in children and adolescents.* New York: Guilford Press.

Hill, J. (2002) Biological, psychological and social processes in the conduct disorders. *Journal of Child Psychology and Psychiatry*, **43**, 133–64.

Kazdin, A. (2001) Psychosocial treatments. In *Conduct disorders. Cambridge monographs in child and adolescent psychiatry* (ed. J. Hill and B. Maughan), pp. 408–48. Cambridge: Cambridge University Press.

Loeber, R. and Stouthamer-Loeber, M. (1986) Family factors as correlates and predictors of juvenile conduct problems and delinquency. In *Crime and justice: an annual review of research*, vol. 7 (ed. N. Morris, and M. Tonry,), pp. 29–149. Chicago: University of Chicago Press.

Loeber, R. Wung, P. Keenan, K. Giroux, B. Stouthamer-Loeber, M. Van Kammen, W, and Maughan, B. (1993) Developmental pathways in disruptive child behavior. *Development and Psychopathology*, **5**, 101–32.

Maughan, B. and Rutter, M. (2001) Antisocial children grown up. In *Conduct disorders. Cambridge monographs in child and adolescent psychiatry* (ed. J. Hill, and B. Maughan,), pp. 507–52. Cambridge: Cambridge University Press.

Meltzer, H., Gatwood, R., Goodman, R., and Ford, T. (2000) *Mental health of children and adolescents in Great Britain*. London: The Stationery Office.

Moffitt, T.E. (1993) Adolescence-limited and life-course-persistent anti-social behaviour: a developmental taxonomy. *Psychological Review*, **100**, 674–701.

Moffit, T.E., Caspi, A., Rutter, M., and Silva, P.A. (2001) *Sex differences in antisocial behaviour*. Cambridge: Cambridge University Press.

Patterson, G.R. (1982) *Coercive family process*. Eugene Oregon: Castilia Publishing Company.

Raine, A., Brennan, P., and Farrington, D.P. (1997) Biosocial bases of violence, conceptual and theoretical issues. In *Biosocial bases of violence* (ed. A. Raine, P. Brennan, D.P. Farrington, and S.A. Mednick), pp. 1–20. New York: Plenum.

Rutter, M., Giller, H., and Hagell, A. (1998) *Antisocial behaviour by young people*. Cambridge: Cambridge University Press.

Scarr, S. and McCartney, K. (1983) How people make their own environments: a theory of genotype-environment effects. *Child Development*, **54**, 424–35.

Scott, S., Knapp, M., Henderson, J., and Maughan, B. (2001) Financial cost of social exclusion: follow up study of antisocial children into adulthood. *British Medical Journal*, **323**, 191–4.

Simonoff, E. (2001) Genetic influences on conduct disorder. In *Conduct disorders. Cambridge monographs in child and adolescent psychiatry* (ed. J. Hill and B. Maughan), pp. 202–34. Cambridge: Cambridge University Press.

Webster-Stratton, C., and Hancock, L. (1998) Training for parents of young children with conduct problems: content, methods, and therapeutic processes. In *Handbook of parent training* (2nd edn) (ed. J.M. Briesmeister and C.E. Shaefer). pp. 98–152. New York: Wiley.

Chapter 17

Caring for ethnic minority and refugee children

Kedar Nath Dwivedi

It is a supposition of cultural psychology that when people live in the world differently, it may be that they live in different worlds. (Shweder 1991: 23)

Introduction

The population of Great Britain (www.statistics.gov.uk) in 1998 was about 56.7 million, including 53.0 million whites and 3.7 million ethnic minorities. Ethnic minorities include black Caribbean 0.5 million, black African 0.3 million, black-other 0.29 million, Indian 0.94 million, Pakistani 0.56 million, Bangladeshi 0.23 million, Chinese 0.16 million, other Asian (non-mixed) 0.19 million, other-other (including mixed) 0.4 million. The ethnic minority populations are mainly concentrated in the more urbanized parts of the country. Nearly three-fourth of the ethnic minority population live in the metropolitan counties of Greater London, Greater Manchester, West Yorkshire, and West Midlands, compared to less than a quarter of the white population. For example, compared with less than one in ten of all white people of Great Britain, nearly half of ethnic minority people of Great Britain live in Greater London. The majority of the original ethnic minority population in the UK came with the migration of Jewish people from Russia in the late-nineteenth century followed by Afro-Caribbeans, and Southeast Asians in the 1950s and 1960s, when thriving industry in the UK wanted workers; and then there was a political upheaval in Uganda. Since the ending of primary immigration, some people from developing countries have entered the UK as asylum seekers. Many East European refugees, as a result of wars involving 'ethnic cleansing' in their own countries, came to the UK during latter half of the 1990s. The number of refugee children arriving is rising annually. Recently white collar IT workers, mainly from India, nurses from Spain, and teachers from various countries, have also been targeted to make up the shortfall of the UK workforce (Banhatti and Bhate 2002).

In a survey about the mental health of children and adolescents in Great Britain by the Office of National Statistics on behalf of the Department of Health (Meltzer *et al.* 2000) showed a prevalence of ICD-10 mental disorder by ethnicity as: 9.5% in white, 12% in black, 8% in Bangladeshi and Pakistani, 4% in Indian, and 10% in other children. As there are only a few more studies of this nature (e.g. Goodman and Richards 1995; Hackett *et al.* 1991; Kramer *et al.* 2000; Stern *et al.* 1990), there is a need to conduct more studies to explore the impact of ethnicity, culture, and minority status on child mental health, service provision, and uptake.

Vulnerability and protective influences

Just like any other child, ethnic minority children are also exposed to same stresses and are vulnerable to anxiety, depression, conduct disorder, post-traumatic stress, and other mental disorders (Dwivedi 2000; Dwivedi and Varma 1997a, b). In addition, they tend to experience stress related to racism and to their dislocated family background, producing serious consequences. 'Racism is the belief that some races or ethnic groups are superior to others, which is then extended to justify actions that create inequality' (Bhopal 2001). The Policy Studies Institute (Coker 2001) found 20–26% of the 'white' participants admitting to prejudice against ethnic minorities in the national representative survey. The Macpherson Report (Home Office 1999) defined institutional racism as 'the collective failure of an organisation to provide an appropriate and professional service to people because of the colour, culture or ethnic origin'. Racism can lead to direct or indirect racial discrimination, as regards access to health care, welfare, local amenities, environmental quality, and to the undermining of their culture, identity, and self-image. Experience of racial bullying and abuse in schools, play grounds, and other places leaves children and their families feeling hopeless. Racism denigrates and dehumanizes communities, leading to the lowering of their self-esteem, sense of worthlessness, and depression (Fernando 1988).

Banks (2002a) points out that the social perception of children of mixed 'race' origin and, most often their white mothers, in Britain has historically been negative, as they are seen as representing a threat to the purity of white British society. However, there is a growth in the number of mixed 'race' relationships, as the Fourth National Survey of Ethnic Minorities (PSI 1997) found that 20% of married and co-habiting African-Caribbean adults, 17% of Chinese, and 4% of Indians and African-Asians had white partners.

In many ethnic minority cultures, the emotional support from one's extended family, especially in times of stress, is the essential ingredient of any coping strategy and an aspect of healing. Such a fragmentation of social structure also makes them vulnerable to loss of their cultural strength and of traditional arrangements and creation of new ones but, these new arrangements may still not fit in with their new context (Perelberg 1992).

Woodcock (2002) highlights that governments routinely enact legislation to deter asylum seekers. Thus the political climate toward asylum seekers and refugees in host countries is often hostile and xenophobic, and a lack of hospitality permeates every layer of welfare provision, from social security and health to schooling.

Ethnicity and culture

Ethnicity includes culture and McGoldrick (1982) describes the ethnic group as those who perceive themselves as alike by virtue of their common ancestry, real or fictitious, and who are so regarded by others. People from different ethnic groups also tend to experience and express their distress differently (Patel 1994). In fact, culture has an impact on almost all aspects of our lives, family processes, world view, attitudes to self and others, identity, beliefs about health and illness, expectations from others including professionals, help-seeking and help-giving behaviours, attitude to religion, morality, and so on. For example, some cultures promote differentiated family maps containing differentiated or segregated roles, tasks, and activities, and have a socio-centric view of individuals in a role relationship, in contrast to differentiated (symmetrical, egalitarian, or democratic) family maps with the egocentric emphasis on the autonomy of the individual. Thus the impact of culture on child development, coping strategies, personality traits and their disorders, and on pathogenesis are bound to be substantial (Ekblad 1988).

Child rearing

Cultural assumptions and ideologies have an enormous impact on child-rearing practices. For example, Roland (1980) highlighted some major differences as regards early child-rearing practices between the Western and Indian cultures. Accordingly, 'independence' is viewed as the cherished ideal and 'dependence' as a despicable state in the Western culture. The Eastern cultures, in contrast, place more emphasis on 'dependability' and parents are usually at pains to ensure that their children grow up in an atmosphere where parents are a model of dependability. This leads to an atmosphere of immediate gratification of physical and emotional needs, physical closeness, indulgence, common sleeping arrangements, and a rather prolonged babyhood. There is often no need for transitional objects, as separation experiences for very young children are considered traumatic and therefore avoided. Also, the emphasis on self-regulation of emotion, empathy, and avoiding hurting other's feelings requires development of a style that places more value on indirect, hypothetical, and metaphorical communication turning it into an art form (Dwivedi 1997a, 2002).

Acculturation and ethnic identity

It appears that a stronger sense of belonging to one's own ethnic group is associated with more positive attitudes toward out-groups (Romero and Roberts 1998). Such a social-group identity shows the strongest predictive power for psychological well-being, such as: symptoms outcome, life satisfaction, and self-esteem (Sam 2000; Smith *et al.* 1999). However, the transmission of their cultural values to the ethnic-minority children growing up in another culture is much harder, as it can very easily be undermined by other cultural ideologies. The term 'racial identity' or 'ethnic identity' as a part of social identity is used to mean how an individual conceives of themselves in relation to their ethnic group (however they define this group membership) and how they perceive their 'goodness of fit' within their ethnic group (Banks 2002b). Cross (1995) outlines the advantages of a positive black identity, and black children can be helped to overcome the negative images that impact on them by specific techniques (Banks 1992). Similarly, Poston (1990) describes the stages for the development of ethnic identity in mixed-race people.

Public services

The publication of the Macpherson Report (Home Office 1999) has highlighted the systemic and institutional racial inequality and injustice throughout public services.

Education

It is not only children who behave in a racist manner but also some of their teachers as well, as the research looking at the experiences of young ethnic-minority children in nursery and primary schools has clearly highlighted (Wright 1992). They were often aware of the racial harassment but reluctant to deal with it and, in fact, held negative stereotypes themselves. German (2002) points out that African-Caribbean children start school with the best grasp of basic skills and maintain their lead until at least 7 years of age, but by the time they reach 16 years of age, they are among the least successful ethnic groups. Mehra (1998) highlights the alarmingly high rate of exclusion of Asian children, in addition to that of black children, from schools. There is clearly an absence of effective bilingual teaching and progress towards multi-lingual provision in schools. Gurnah (1989) emphasizes the need for multi-lingual studies in schools for the necessary development of children and particularly as a support for ethnic-minority pupils with first languages other than English.

Welfare

The 1989 Children Act recommends giving full consideration to the racial origin and ethnic, cultural, religious, and linguistic background of the child but there seems to be little evidence of cultural pluralism in appropriate and adequate service provision (Association of Directors of Social Services 1983; Commission for Racial Equality 1989). Tizard and Phoenix (1989) have pointed out that black children living in white families fail to develop a positive black identity, suffer from identity confusion, and develop a negative-self concept, believing or wishing they were white. White families, unless they are carefully trained, cannot provide black children with the survival skills that they need for coping with racial prejudice in society; the children will grow up unable to relate to black people and at the same time will experience rejection by white society. Similar issues can arise from residential care. Mehra (2002) has summarized recommendations for good practice for social care and health including residential care. Similarly Zeitlin (2002) has summarized recommendations for good practice as regards the fostering and adoption of ethnic-minority children. Banks (2002a, b) and Rodriguez *et al.* (2002) look at the unfolding of ethnic identity development in different contexts and practical ways of offering help. Gibbs and Moskowitz-Sweet (1991) have suggested that mixed-race adolescents will tend to experience conflicts around major psychosocial developmental tasks.

Woodcock (2002) highlights that asylum-seeking refugee children face numerous practical difficulties as basic as entitlement to housing, schooling, and so on; they have far fewer legal rights than indigenous children and will have been exposed to a range of emotional events, which may include terrifying experiences, massive loss, disruption, fear, and huge unexpected changes. Because of their disturbing nature it will be difficult for them, their carers, and the professionals to hold in mind such experiences. Their practical, legal, and emotional problems are further compounded by this triple jeopardy. Practical approaches of working with refugee children and their families, adopting the human rights perspective, are also elaborated by Woodcock along with a list of helpful resources.

Mental health

Development of culturally sensitive services requires the commitment of the commissioners as well. For example, with a great deal of effort, an outreach child mental health service for a range of ethnic-minority communities was set up in Northampton with the help of joint-funding arrangement. Various culturally sensitive therapeutic groups for mental health promotion, prevention, and treatment were developed for children, adolescents, and their parents. But the local Primary Care Trust in their commissioning role decided to discontinue the service. The users from the ethnic-minority communities were devastated by this decision and made their views known as well. Despite this, a promising and productive service was killed in its very infancy.

Unless a culturally sensitive service is carefully developed, there is usually a poor service uptake of routine child mental health services by the ethnic-minority families. This is often due to a complexity of factors such as a clash of cultural values between the professionals and the families, lack of awareness of the role of professionals in the ethnic minority communities, lack of faith in such services, a sense of alienation, communication difficulties, and so on.

Professional attitudes

Therapists appear to take different positions in their approach to diversity; some believing in the universality of family processes have little use of contextual variables such as race, gender, or ethnicity (Falicov 1995). Dayal (1990) points out that the emotional availability of many professionals to ethnic-minority families is often very limited. Some fail to respond on the grounds that they cannot understand the cultural ways of ethnic-minority families (Fernando 1988), while others look for, and quickly find, a 'cultural-conflict' type of explanation. Professionals who unwittingly conflate cultural differences with psychopathologies can further exacerbate the ethnic-minority children's emotional difficulties. Many Asian youngsters, at times of distress and when needing help, do end up identifying with such projections and present to the professionals with problems in ways that are more likely to elicit a sympathetic response; for example, a complaint of restrictive parenting, fear of arranged marriage, and so on (Ahmed 1986). Goldberg and Hodes (1992) demonstrate how self-poisoning by a number of Asian adolescent girls symbolizes the acting-out of the view of the dominant group that the minority is 'poisonous' or 'harmful'.

Inclusion and sensitivity

The agenda of equality and inclusion needs to incorporate the whole spectrum of concepts ranging from access, opportunity, entitlement, targeting, promotion, positive discrimination, and anti-discrimination. Whether it is parenting, counselling, group therapy, or family therapy it needs to be culturally congruent and sensitive, considering, among other things, value systems, body language, channels of communication, metaphorical, narrative, and indirect communications (Barratt *et al.* 1999; Dwivedi 1993, 1997b). Burnham and Harris (2002) highlight the need for adopting a position of changing position, not only because of therapeutic curiosity but due to the fact that ethnicity and culture are constantly emerging. It requires creating a context in which the needs of ethnic-minority families can be expressed to the services that aim to meet those needs. Otherwise the needs that will be met will be those hypothesized by the professionals. Even if there is a genuine willingness to respect other cultural values, it is difficult to do so without adequate preparation, development, and training.

Lau (2002) points out that family therapists from a Western European ethno-cultural background, working with ethnic-minority families, need to pay attention to the tensions in the interface between them and their client families. In order for the therapists to gain credibility and use culturally generated materials to enhance the family's problem-solving skills, and mobilize strengths derived from traditional values and practices, it is important that the therapist develops an understanding and respect for the cultural and religious differences between them and their client families. Maitra and Miller (2002) have examined the meeting between the psychological therapist and ethnic-minority families as a meeting between two cultures that may contain a conflict between potentially opposing, and possibly irreconcilable, views of childhood. With the help of a number of very informative case examples, they highlight the significance of the process whereby this meeting is negotiated. Fateh *et al.* (2002) point out that talking about culture is like talking about everything else, because talking about culture is talking about being a human being connected to other human beings. Lau (2002) also offers several useful questions to be kept in mind while assessing families.

Conclusion

There is growing recognition of the acute need to improve services by setting up community outreach work, interpreter, and translation services, culturally sensitive therapy and by also giving voice to subjugated narratives. Professional development needs to incorporate the perspective of difference and diversity aiming not only to raise cultural awareness by gaining knowledge but also cultural sensitivity through experiences that challenge one's respective cultural identities and their influence on understanding and acceptance of others.

References

Ahmed, S. (1986) Cultural racism in work with Asian women and girls. In *Social work with black children and their families* (ed. S. Ahmed, J. Cheetham, and J. Small), pp. 140–54. London: Batsford.

Association of Directors of Social Services (1983) *Social services and ethnic minorities, report of a questionnaire survey on social services departments and ethnic minorities.* London: ADDS.

Banhatti, R. and Bhate, S. (2002) *Mental health needs of ethnic minority children.* pp. 66–90. London: Jessica Kingsley.

Banks, N. (1992) Techniques for direct identity work with black children. *Adoption and Fostering, BAAF,* **16**, 19–24.

Banks, N. (2002a) Mixed race children and families. In *Meeting the needs of ethnic minority children* (ed. K.N. Dwivedi). pp. 219–32. London: Jessica Kingsley.

Banks, N. (2002b) What is a positive black identity. In *Meeting the needs of ethnic minority children* (ed. K.N. Dwivedi). pp. 151–69. London: Jessica Kingsley.

Barrat, S., Burck, C., Dwivedi, K., Stedman, M., and Raval, S. (1999) Theoretical Bases in relation to race, ethnicity and culture in family therapy training. *Context,* **44**, 4–12.

Burnham, J. and Harris, Q. (2002) The emergence of ethnicity: a tale of three cultures. In *Meeting the needs of ethnic minority children* (ed. K.N. Dwivedi), pp. 117–99. London: Jessica Kingsley.

Bhopal, R. (2001) Racism in medicine: the spectre must be exorcised. *British Medical Journal,* **322**, 1503–4.

Butler, N. and Golding, J. (1986) *From birth to five: a study of health and behaviour of Britain's five year olds.* Oxford: Pergamon.

Coker, N. (ed.) (2001) *Racism in medicine: an agenda for change.* London: Kings Fund.

Commission for Racial Equality (1989) *Race equality in social services departments, a survey of opportunity policies.* London: CRE.

Cross, W.E. (1995) The psychology of nigrescence: revising the Cross model. In *Handbook of multicultural counselling* (ed. J.G. Ponterotto, J.M. Casas, L.A. Suzuki, and C.M. Alexander), pp. 93–122. London: Sage Publications.

Dayal, N. (1990) Psychotherapy services for minority ethnic communities in the NHS—a psychotherapist's view. *Midland Journal of Psychotherapy,* **11**, 28–37.

Dwivedi, K.N. (ed.) (1993) *Group work with children and adolescents: a handbook.* London: Jessica Kingsley.

Dwivedi, K.N. (1996) Race and the child's perspective. In *The voice of the child: a handbook for professionals* (ed. R. Davie, G. Upton, and V. Varma), pp. 153–69. London: Falmer Press.

Dwivedi, K.N. (ed.) (1997a) *Therapeutic use of stories.* London: Routledge.

Dwivedi, K.N. (ed.) (1997b) *Enhancing parenting skills: a guide for professionals working with parents.* Chichester: Wiley.

Dwivedi, K.N. (ed.) (2000) *Post-traumatic stress disorder in children and adolescents.* London: Whurr.

Dwivedi K.N. (2002) Culture and personality. In *Meeting the needs of ethnic minority children*, 2nd edn (ed. K.N. Dwivedi), pp. 42–65. London: Jessica Kingsley.

Dwivedi, K.N. and Varma, V.P. (ed.) (1997a) *A handbook of childhood anxiety management*. Aldershot: Ashgate.

Dwivedi, K.N. and Varma, V.P. (ed.) (1997b) *Depression in children and adolescents*. London: Whurr.

Ekblad, S. (1988) Influence of child rearing on aggressive behaviour in a transcultural perspective. *Acta Psychiatrica Scandinavica*, **78** (Supplement 344), 133–9.

Falicov, C.J. (1995) Training to think culturally: a multidimensional comparative framework. *Family Process*, **34** (4), 373–88.

Fateh, T., Islam, N. Khan, F., Ko, C., Lee, M., Malik, R., *et al.* (2002) In *Meeting the needs of ethnic minority children*, 2nd edn (ed. K.N. Dwivedi), pp. 130–50. London: Jessica Kingsley.

Fernando, S. (1988) *Race and culture in psychiatry*. London: Croom Helm.

German, G. (2002) Antiracist strategies for educational performance. In *Meeting the needs of ethnic minority children*, 2nd edn (ed. K.N. Dwivedi), pp. 200–18. London: Jessica Kingsley.

Gibbs, J.T. and Moskowitz-Sweet, G. (1991) Clinical and cultural issues in the treatment of bi-racial and bi-cultural adolescents. *Families in Society: The Journal of Contemporary Human Services*, **72** (10), 579–92.

Goldberg, D. and Hodes, M. (1992) The poison of racism and the self poisoning of adolescents. *Journal of Family Therapy*, **14**, 51–67.

Goodman, R. and Richards, H. (1995) Child and Adolescent psychiatric presentations of second generation Afro-Caribbeans. *British Journal of Psychiatry*, **167**, 362–9.

Gurnah, A. (1989) After bilingual support? In *Education for equality: some guidelines for good practice* (ed. M. Cole). London: Routledge.

Hackett, L., Hackett, P., and Taylor, D. (1991) Psychological disturbance and its associations in the children of the Gujarati community. *Journal of Child Psychology and Psychiatry*, **32**, 851–6.

Home Office (1999) *The Stephen Lawrence Inquiry: Report of an Inquiry by Sir William Macpherson of Cluny*. London: The Stationary Office.

Kramer, T., Evans, N., and Garralda, E.M. (2000) Ethnic diversity among child and adolescent psychiatric clinic attenders. *Child Psychology and Psychiatry Review*, **5** (4), 169–75.

Maitra, B. and Miller, A. (2002) Children, families and therapists. In *Meeting the needs of ethnic minority children*, 2nd edn (ed. K.N. Dwivedi), pp. 108–29. London: Jessica Kingsley.

McGoldrick, M. (1982) Ethnicity and Family Therapy. In *Ethnicity and family therapy* (ed. M. McGoldrick, J.K.Pearce, and J. Giardano), pp. 3–29. New York/London: Guilford Press.

Mehra, H. (1998) The permanent exclusion of Asian pupils in secondary schools in central Birmingham. *Multicultural Teaching*, **17** (1), 42–8.

Mehra, H. (2002) Residential care for ethnic minorities children. In *Meeting the needs of ethnic minority children*, 2nd edn (ed. K.N. Dwivedi), pp. 252–63. Jessica Kingsley: London.

Patel, V. (1994). The cross-cultural assessment of depression. *Focus on Depression*, **2** (1), 5–8.

Perelberg, R.J. (1992) Familiar and unfamiliar types of family structure: towards a conceptual framework. In *Intercultural therapy: themes, interpretations and practices* (ed. J. Kareem and R. Littlewood). Oxford: Blackwells Scientific Publications.

Poston, C.W.S. (1990) The bi-racial identity developmental model. A need edition. *Journal of Counselling and Development*, **69**, 153–5.

PSI (Policy Studies Institute) (1997) *Ethnic minorities in Britain*. London: Fourth National Survey, PSI.

Rodriguez, J., Cauce, A.M., and Wilson, L. (2002) A conceptual framework of identity formation in a society of multiple cultures: applying theory to practice. In *Meeting the needs of ethnic minority children*, 2nd edn (ed. K.N. Dwivedi), pp. 299–320. London: Jessica Kingsley.

Roland, A. (1980) Psychoanalytic perspectives on personality development in India. *International Review of Psychoanalysis*, **1**, 73–87.

Romero, A.J. and Roberts, R.E. (1998) Perception of discrimination and ethnocultural variables in a diverse group of adolescents. *Journal of Adolescence*, **21**, 641–56.

Sam, D.L. (2000) Psychological adaptation of adolescents with immigrant backgrounds. *The Journal of Social Psychology*, **140** (1), 5–25.

Shweder, R.A. (1991) *Thinking through cultures: expeditions in cultural psychology*. Cambridge, MA: Harvard University Press.

Smith, E.P., Walker,K., Fields, L., Brookins, C.C., and Seay, R.C. (1999) Ethnic identity and its relationship to self-esteem, perceived efficacy and prosocial attitudes in early adolescence. *Journal of Adolescence*, **22**, 867–80.

Stern, G., Cottrell, D., and Holmes, J. (1990) Patterns of attendance of child psychiatry outpatients with social reference to Asian families. *British Journal of Psychiatry*, **156**, 384–7.

Tizard, B. and Phoenix, A. (1989) Black identity and transracial adoption. *New Community*, **15**, 427–37.

Woodcock, J. (2002) Practical approaches to work with refugee children. In *Meeting the needs of ethnic minority children*, 2nd edn (ed. K.N. Dwivedi), pp. 264–82. London: Jessica Kingsley.

Wright, C. (1992) Early education: multiracial primary school classrooms. In *Racism and education* (ed. D. Gill, *et al.*). London: Sage Publications.

Zeitlin, H. (2002) Adoption of children from minority groups. In *Meeting the needs of ethnic minority children*, 2nd edn (ed. K.N. Dwivedi), pp. 233–51. London: Jessica Kingsley.

Chapter 18

Forensic mental health services for children and adolescents

Susan Bailey and Richard Williams

Introduction

This chapter primarily refers to legislation, service development, and policy in England and Wales but, in so doing, provides core underpinning principles for delivering services throughout the developed world.

Together, children and teenagers make up a quarter of the total population in the UK and this is broadly similar in other European countries. Of the 7.5 million adolescents in the UK, 3.9 million are between the ages of 10 and 14, and a further 3.6 million are between the ages of 15 and 19 (Coleman and Schofield 2003). Of all offenders, 50% are under the age of 21, and between one-quarter and one-third of all those in custody under 21, are on remand (Bailey and Dolan 2004).

Throughout Europe and North America, young people at the interface between the criminal justice system and mental health services are in multiple jeopardy of risk for social exclusion, alienation, and stigmatization (Bailey 1999, 2003). Definition of this interface group varies across and within agencies, but its members' needs are diverse. They require a range of mental health services that can only be effective if services provided by a range of agencies are well-integrated.

Young people account for an estimated 7 million crimes a year. A substantial part of offending happens as young people are maturing as a result of them testing out their boundaries. Some of this behaviour may become entrenched, but only a very small percentage of young people go on to become persistent offenders. The psychosocial and biological factors that place young people at risk of offending and/or of developing mental health problems and disorders are well-established in both the national and international literature (Junger-Tas 1994; Rutter and Smith 1995; Shepherd and Farrington 1996; Rutter *et al.* 1998; Rutter 1999; Kazdin 2000). However, it is still the case that, across Europe, North America, and in the UK, young offenders with specific mental disorders only become the subject of mental health assessments late in their careers, when the focus is often on medico-legal issues in the arena of juvenile court proceedings (Doreleijers *et al.* 2000).

Now mental illness in young offenders is increasingly significant for reasons that span diverse political concerns held by those who are primarily interested in saving the public from young offenders (Grisso and Schwartz 2000), those who are concerned with fundamental fairness in adjudicating of young people, and others who wish to promote public safety or to address mental illness in young people as a simple matter of beneficence. Public health policy has long recognized governments' obligations to attend to the basic health needs of prisoners and the importance of meeting the health and mental health needs of children (Longley *et al.* 2001).

A continuing catalogue of governmental reports in England and Wales, whether emanating from policy and practice relating to childcare, health (e.g. Mental Health Foundation 1999), justice or prison have highlighted the under 18s in the juvenile justice system as the most needy and disadvantaged in respect of their access to healthcare (Audit Commission 1996, 1999; Department of Health 2003).

Research evidence: prevalence rates of mental disorder in young offenders

Studies of the prevalence of mental disorders and mental health problems that lead to serious impairment of young people's social functioning continue to demonstrate high levels of psychopathology and vulnerability (Rolf et al. 1990).

Gunn et al. (1996) found a diagnosis of primary mental disorder in a third of young men aged 16 to 18 who were sentenced by courts. A health needs survey of youth court attenders (Dolan et al. 1999) revealed high levels of medical problems, substance misuse, and psychiatric disorder, including early onset psychosis. These findings were confirmed by a study conducted by, and for, the Office for National Statistics (ONS) in Britain (Lader et al. 2000). A comprehensive study of young people in one region in England who had severe problems (Nicol et al. 2000) showed that they had high levels of unmet mental health needs, including unaddressed early onset psychosis. Recent reviews from the USA, including studies on girls, reveal prevalence rates in juvenile justice youth much higher than for young people in the general population: four times higher for substance misuse, and three to four times higher for affective disorder. These findings were consistent across the studies, despite different geographic locations and methods of measurement (Grisso 2000; Kazdin 2000).

Key questions for researchers remain (Graham 1999, 2000). What do we know about the empirical relationships between mental ill health and delinquency? What proportion of mentally ill youths is delinquent? What proportion of delinquent youths is mentally ill? Once understood and identified, the ongoing challenge remains that of how a trained workforce should deliver 'fit for purpose' services within finite resources.

The statutory and policy frameworks in England and Wales

The Children Act 1989 reformed law by bringing public and practice law under one statutory system. With implementation of the Crime and Disorder Act 1998, the governments in England and Wales began a complete overhaul of the entire youth justice system.

The United Kingdom is a signatory to the United Nations Convention on the Rights of the Child. The Human Rights Act 1998 (which contains what is referred to as the European Convention) establishes general principles that, in any decision involving a child, his/her best interests shall be a primary consideration (Article 3) and that a child has the right to express his/her views in all matters affecting his/her life (Article 12) (Bailey and Harbour 1998). The UN Convention (as distinct from the European Convention) also deals specifically with the youth justice process in its Articles 37 and 40. The United Nations Minimum Standards for the Administration of Juvenile Justice (or Beijing Rules) provide more detailed guidelines.

Article 24 of the UN Convention states that children have the right to 'the enjoyment' of the highest attainable standard of health and to facilities for the treatment of illness, and no child shall be deprived of their right of access to healthcare services. In England, recent case law has established that children in 'prison' should have their full rights recognized under the Children Act 1989 and regimes should be Children Act compliant.

The principle aim of the youth justice system is to prevent offending by children and young persons (Crime and Disorder Act 1998, s.37). A court must also have regard to the welfare of any child or young person who appears before it (Children and Young Persons Act 1933, s.44).

The Youth Justice Board for England and Wales (established in September 1998) monitors the operation of the youth justice system and also manages the juvenile secure estate—institutions that are contracted to provide places of detention for young people aged 10–17: youth offender institutions (YOIs); local authority secure children's homes (LACHs); and detention training centres (DTCs); and older girls are still detained in adult female prisons.

Since April 2000, all local authorities in England and Wales have co-ordinated their work with young offenders in a local multidisciplinary agency, the youth offending teams (YOT), which are required by the Crime and Disorder Act 1998 (s.39(5)) to include at least one of the following:

- social worker;
- probation officer;
- representative of the local education authority;
- police officer; and
- representative of the local health authority.

Each local authority has a duty to safeguard and provide for the welfare of children who are in need (Children Act 1989, s.17). The main agency that discharges this duty is the social services department. When a child is considered to have suffered, or to be at risk of suffering, 'significant harm' and that harm is attributable to the care received from his/her parents, the local authority may institute care proceedings in the family proceedings court.

The Youth Court in England and Wales is the main criminal court that deals with children but, presently, it has no power to refer a child to the Family Proceedings Court, even if there are considerable concerns regarding his/her welfare.

Every criminal jurisdiction should have a minimum age below which children shall be presumed not to have the capacity to infringe the penal law (UN Convention on the Rights of the Child, Article 40.3a). This minimum age 'shall not be fixed at too low an age level, bearing in mind the facts of emotional, mental and intellectual maturity' (Beijing Rules, rule 4.1). In England and Wales, the age of criminal responsibility is set at 10 years (Children and Young People Act 1933, s.50).

Although there is no continuing evidence that the level of youth offending is higher, in England and Wales, Scotland and Ireland, these countries still send a greater proportion of children to prison than other states in the EU. Although criminal offences cannot be sanctioned by the criminal law when committed by someone who is below the minimum age for criminal responsibility, this does not mean that official intervention in the life of those children involved in crime is avoided. Frequently throughout Europe, the civil law and/or social welfare systems are used to provide effective, intense interventions and support.

The Youth Justice Board has established a series of minimum standards for regimes to be produced by prison services, local authorities, and private and voluntary sector provisions to meet the specific needs of under 18 year olds. They include standards for mental healthcare and give priority to ensuring that:

- all young people in the youth justice system have access to health services that are free at the point of delivery;
- the quality of healthcare is on a par with that available for other young people;

any special needs are taken into account when delivering assessments, treatments and health education; and

all services are funded and provided by local health agencies to levels that are comparable with the care for any young people who have not offended.

The YOTs are required to assess each child who has contact with them. The assessments are facilitated through a standardized questionnaire named ASSET. The ASSET, though concentrating on factors seen as likely to influence risk of further offending, contains a supplementary assessment to examine each child's vulnerability while in custody. A specific mental health screen (November 2003) can be found on the Internet at www.youth-justiceboard.gov.uk/ Practitioners portal/Health/Mental Health. It has evolved from the Salford Needs Assessment (Kroll et al. 1999), has been piloted with YOT workers and prison officers and, together with training, is being rolled out as an attachment to ASSET. It should help YOTs to select cases that are appropriate for referral to local generic specialist child and adolescent mental health service (Specialist CAMHS) at Tiers 2 and 3, and other agencies that support young people's emotional well-being (often at Tier 1).

Forensic mental health has been defined by Mullen (2000) as an area of specialization in the criminal sphere that includes assessing and treating those people who are both mentally disordered and whose behaviour has led, or could lead, to offending. However, defining forensic mental health services in terms of assessing and treating mentally abnormal offenders delineates an area of concern that could potentially engulf much of mental healthcare.

A current culture of blame and shame has led to professionals' fears of being held responsible for failing to protect their fellow citizens from the violent behaviour of those who have been in their care (Royal College of Psychiatrists 1999). Of particular importance, Mullen stresses making available mental health expertise to address the mental health component of social problems. He argues this should not conflict with tradition and medical practice if the aim is to identify and relieve disorder in order to benefit, primarily, patients, but also through their more adequate care and management to benefit those they, potentially, threaten. He stresses the importance of rigorous risk assessment and management, especially where there is a combination of substance misuse, mental disorder, and offending. This principle must, surely, also follow in the arena of adolescent forensic mental healthcare.

Traditionally, child and adolescent mental health practitioners have continued to work as generalists. Within their roles, they may include forensic work, not only within childcare proceedings, (Black et al. 1998; Butler-Sloss 1998) but also direct forensic medico-legal work in which young children are the alleged perpetrators, rather than the victims, of crime. Therefore, a strategic approach to commissioning and delivering forensic mental health services for children and adolescents should:

develop effective services in predictable ways that meet actual needs;

ensure delivery of services that are built upon established concepts of service design according to a strategic framework;

through long-term planning, address specifically the requirements of an adequate size and composition of the workforce, which is appropriately trained, supervised, and managed.

Any configuration of child and adolescent forensic mental health services should be developed in the light of:

awareness of the scope of the existing services;

recognition of the nature of current demands;

analysis of the gaps in the capacity of the existing services considered against the potential capability of the professionals who are engaged in delivering engaged in those services and application of the evidence-base:

awareness of the current growth points in professional practice, service developments and research (Williams 2004).

Clinical problem profiles

In their summary for practitioners of the main messages from their review of the research into anti-social behaviour, Rutter *et al.* (1998) stressed the heterogeneity of anti-social behaviour that is related to the pervasiveness, persistence, severity, and pattern of such behaviour. Matters drawn out for particular comment included:

overlaps with attention deficit/hyperactivity disorder;

early onset anti-social behaviour;

violent anti-social behaviour that is associated with features of abnormal personality in adolescence and with serious mental disorders in late childhood and early adolescence;

sexual offences;

juvenile homicide;

drug use and abuse;

medically caused crime; and

crime associated with emotional disorder or post-traumatic stress disorder (PTSD).

These conclusions sit alongside the previously described needs surveys and findings from the long-term follow up studies of young people in secure care (Little and Bullock 2004). Five 'career routes' emerged from the latter:

young people in long-stay care;

those in prolonged special education;

those whose behaviour suddenly deteriorated in adolescence;

one-off grave offenders; and

serious and persistent offenders.

Thus, when looking at service provision for young people with mental health needs who offend (or more extreme instances of co-morbidity), broad, but often overlapping, sets of problems that are associated with current multi-morbidity are identified and have to be addressed in concert (see Fig. 18.1).

Early onset anti-social behaviour

Early onset anti-social behaviours include aggressive, violent, disruptive behaviour, coercive sexual activity, arson, and fluctuation in both mood state and levels of social interaction. In some cases, there is evidence of underlying learning/educational difficulties and attention-deficit/hyperactivity disorder (Scott 1998). Scott stresses the need for CAMHS to offer assessments that are integrated with those of other agencies, and to work with young children with anti-social behaviour in a family context, using parent management training strategies that are combined with individual interventions for young children that are capable of taking into account sub-typing of conduct disorder based on age of onset.

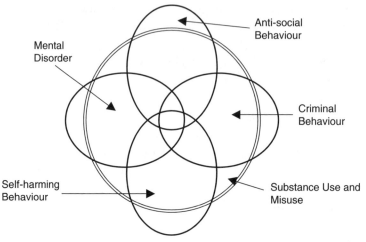

Fig. 18.1 The interacting problems of severely difficult and disruptive children and adolescents.

Criminal behaviour

For those adolescents who display the criminal behaviours of interpersonal violence, arson, and, in particular, sexual offences, there is an increased drive to approach the tasks of assessing the needs and risks presented by, and managing the treatment of, young perpetrators as a specific entity with a focus on developmental issues. This contrasts sharply with past tendencies to apply adult treatment models to young people (Vizard 2004).

Repetitive high-risk behaviours

Female adolescents who make serious attempts at self-harm and suicide and those who self-mutilate, interspersed within a pattern of externalizing destructive behaviours, raise grave anxieties for the staff who work in existing services, but, even so, violent behaviour in girls is underestimated, partly due to the difficulty in applying diagnostic criteria to conduct disorders in girls (Jasper *et al.* 1998). Criteria for conduct disorder in pre-adolescent girls are non-specific and insensitive. At the same time, there is the need to be more alert to the impact of past abuse in the lives of offending boys who go on to harm themselves (Bailey 2004). The risk in their later adult lives, for both girls and boys, is that of developing personality disorder and this must be set against current uncertainty about services for adults with severe personality disorder (Bailey 2002). The full range of psychological therapies should be available to those vulnerable adolescents, particularly those who are leaving care and are at risk of entering custody. The indications are that multi-systemic therapy (MST) is effective with these high-risk children. Combined family and community-based interventions can produce better long-term clinical outcomes for older adolescents and cost savings for society (Henggeler 1999).

Substance misuse

Substance misuse by young people has increased rapidly over the past 10 years. The importance of an integrated health service response to substance misuse by young people was clearly stated in the NHS Health Advisory Report of 1996 and by the Standing Conference on Drug

Abuse (Children's Legal Centre 1998) and is supported by research (Bushell *et al.* 2002). Intensive forms of intervention for young people who misuse substances and who have complex needs should include providing specialist residential services and mental health teams that include child and adolescent psychiatrists and forensic psychiatrists (Ferdinand *et al.* 2001; Grella *et al.* 2001).

Mental illness

A lead-in period of up to 1–7 years to early onset psychosis, during which there is a marked variety in the degree of non-psychotic behaviour, highlights the importance of accurately assessing young offenders who show multiple high-risk episodes and fluctuations in their mental states. Situations of particular vulnerability and risk are homelessness and penal remand detention. Interconnections between homelessness, mental disorders, substance misuse, and offending are complex and remain poorly understood. A flexible approach is required from mental health services that work in court diversion schemes in which there are innovative partnerships with voluntary sector agencies that work with young people. Girls are particularly vulnerable, as are young people from minority ethnic groups. At present, no specialized facilities are available for young girls in prison, and 16 and 17-year-olds are still sent to prisons for adult women (HMPS 1999).

Adolescents with learning disabilities

Lessons learned in practice suggest that adult forensic learning disability services should be stretched to offer services over longer periods of time in ways that match the pace at which the adolescents with a learning disability can cope and change. All the while, these services must balance the inherent vulnerabilities of a very needy group of people with risks to others.

The challenges of collaborative commissioning

In England, the External Working Group set up to make recommendations to the Department of Health for the National Service Framework for Children in England (Department of Health 2003) and, in Wales, the Welsh Assembly Government (National Assembly for Wales 2001) have recommended fundamental shifts in the culture of services, such that they are designed, commissioned and delivered to better reflect the needs and opinions of the young people who use them. On completion and implementation, the separate children's national service frameworks (NSFs) in England and Wales are likely to confirm a real commitment of the government of each country to improve healthcare for children and young people, including those within all youth justice settings.

This priority is based on the principle of life pathways for children, and concern to improve health and reduce offending by young people. The inevitable performance pressures on healthcare, social care, education, and youth justice services reveal the diverse perspectives in dealing with the complex psychological problems of young people who offend.

In any country, high-quality commissioning is vital to developing forensic CAMHS. To succeed, commissioners must be given the executive authority to undertake the task, and their approach must be multi-agency, skilled, and knowledge-based.

In times of considerable and ongoing organizational change and restructuring of commissioning and services in England and Wales, it is important to build on any successful existing arrangements and accept that specific commissioning arrangements might vary in detail across different parts of a country but there remain underpinning core principles to ensure equitable, as well as process-orientated effective evidence-based, outcome delivery of specialist services.

Recent analyses of demand and needs for services, commissioning exercises, and clinical experience in this field have elucidated the nature, breadth, and depth of the task (Kurtz *et al.* 1997; Bailey and Farnworth 1998; Audit Commission 1999; Knapp and Henderson 1999; Knapp *et al.* 1999).

The tasks facing forensic CAMHS

According to Williams (2004), the tasks facing comprehensive forensic CAMHS encompass delivering:

Diagnostic and advisory services:

ambulatory, community, and out-patient assessments;

consultation within and between agencies in care planning;

preparation and presentation of opinions, including report preparation;

attendance at courts to give professional evidence or expert opinion;

advising other professionals in the course of their work.

Therapeutic services:

ambulatory, community, and out-patient therapeutic interventions;

residential and/or in-patient assessments care and treatments;

Teaching, training and support for other professionals.

Research.

The client group requiring NHS-funded secure in-patient care

In an analysis of all information relating to groups of young people referred to established healthcare services offering highly specialized forensic mental health services to adolescents, the Health Services Management Centre (HSMC) in the University of Birmingham drew out the following broad diagnostic categories:

Offenders—those young people who are required by the courts to be cared for and/or treated in a setting of security as a part of their sentence or pending their trial for alleged serious offences.

Adolescents with severe mental illness—adolescents who have a serious and possible enduring mental illness and who require treatment in a secure setting in order to engage them in treatment and/or to protect them from harming themselves or others or from falling prey to serious exploitation.

Mentally disordered offenders—adolescents who fill the criteria for both of the categories above (i.e. they have committed serious offences that require their care in a special, including secure, setting and they have a serious mental disorder that requires they be cared for and treated in a controlled setting). Individuals in this category may have:

committed an offence, including a serious offence as a consequence of pre-existing disorder; or

developed a serious psychiatric disorder subsequent to committing an offence for which they have been sentenced to care in a particular setting including secure settings.

Disordered and chaotic individuals—adolescents in this category are those whose behaviour presents containment, diagnostic and/or remedial challenges of such a marked degree that:

their needs and those of others around them have not been met by less secure settings or placements; and

the possible consequences of failing to restrict their behaviour are potentially very serious risks to the physical health of the individuals themselves or others (in some circumstances, this may include risks arising from substance use or misuse of severe degree).

Adolescents who have serious learning disabilities coupled with problems in the other categories above but who are also considered to:

be at risk of serious exploitation; and/or

require specialized care and treatment in a contained setting, which cannot be provided in less controlled settings.

In particular, arising from this work, HSMC sought to draw attention to the greater frequency than is often recognised, of learning disabilities in the client group and also the very high levels of substance use, findings that were confirmed by Kroll *et al.* (2002) in studies of young people in secure detention.

In a review of the Gardener Unit in Salford, the NHS Health Advisory Service (HAS) (1994) produced a summary of the nature of secure in-patient resources that it saw as required. Its priority client group included:

mentally disordered offenders;

sex offenders and abusers;

severely suicidal and self-harming adolescents;

very severely mentally ill adolescents;

adolescents who need to begin psychiatric rehabilitation in secure circumstances; and

brain-injured adolescents and those with severe organic disorders.

The HAS saw the greatest immediate need as being for an increase in secure NHS-funded provision for those with very severe mental illness, very severely suicidal and self-harming young people, and brain-injured adolescents and those with severe organic disorders, recognizing that some of these services are being developed within the independent sector. Additionally, the HAS stressed the need to develop and evaluate programmes of specialist intervention for adolescents who are sex offenders and abusers, mentally disordered offenders, and young people who are misusers of substances, to offer follow-on from intensive psychiatric in-patient care back out into the community.

Current NHS commissioning arrangements in England and Wales

Generic guidance on commissioning CAMHS was issued by Welsh Assembly Government in 2003. WHC (2003) 63 describes a structure in which Tier 1 services are to be commissioned by Local Health Boards, Tiers 2 and most of Tier 3 by three consortia or CAMHS Commissioning Networks (CCNs), and the remaining elements of Tier 3 and all of Tier 4 by Health Commission Wales (HCW). This advice applies, therefore, to commissioning forensic CAMHS, which are now the responsibility of the three CCNs as recommended and HCW because, as we shall see, we conceive of comprehensive forensic CAMHS as being a combination of Tier 3 and Tier 4 tasks.

In England, from April 2002, adolescent forensic service in-patient services were designated for central funding and to be the responsibility of the National Specialist Commissioning Advisory Group (NSCAG). This subsumed responsibility for commissioning the existing 28 available medium-secure psychiatric in-patient beds in Manchester and Newcastle. NSCAG services provide medium-secure psychiatric care for young people whose severe mental illness contributes to their serious offending. New beds have opened in Birmingham with active planning for beds in London and the South of England. There are 12 identified specific forensic adolescent secure beds in the independent sector. There are no comparable beds in either the public or independent sectors in Northern Ireland, Scotland, or Wales.

NSCAG-commissioned forensic CAMHS are the agencies that are most likely to deal with the most challenging and treatment-resistant individuals. In our opinion these specialist in-patient services should be expected to work only with young people who present the highest risks and, generally, only those who have been assessed as having a mental disorder.

Multi-agency approaches

In addition to further developing of secure adolescent forensic psychiatric in-patient units, other initiatives, including joint Department of Health, Youth Justice Board, and prison health-care plans, are now underway, which should have a direct positive impact on services for young offenders. Many other government initiatives, such as increasing mental health services for children who are looked after by local authorities and at higher risk for offending, together with increasing services for early intervention and prevention, in collaboration with other children's agencies, should also have an indirect but nonetheless positive impact on meeting the mental health needs of young offenders earlier in their life routes. Good health and social care partnerships are emerging in new behaviour resource centres, which aim to prevent vulnerable young offenders who have complex needs entering secure detention.

Getting the environment and care planning right

Nonetheless, entry of young people into secure care presents opportunities that should not be lost but it does require a strategic response to address how custodial environments should actively provide therapeutic, as well as control/reparative, functions (Rose 2002). Within the custodial facilities, there is need for planned environments that are capable of providing individualized psychosocial cultures that support young people's healthy development. But achieving this objective requires expertise and support from Specialist CAMHS.

As in the adult sector, implementing case-management processes, such as that based on the Care Programme Approach (CPA) and Multi-agency Public Protection Panels (MAPPP) for young people who cause the greatest concerns, could begin to provide both improved continuity of interventions over time and encourage multi-agency collaboration to protect against the escalation of high risk. In-reach/out-reach psychological services from Specialist CAMHS to these custodial settings are essential. However, additional resources and detailed workforce planning is essential if this level of collaboration is to be achieved in the medium term.

Developing of mental health screening, need and risk assessment tools that are shared across the agencies, should assist in better integrating delivery of purposeful interventions. There remains an outstanding yet urgent need to model successfully a population-based system that is actively supported by the health, justice, social care, and education agencies, which are accountable for providing effective practices.

Workforce and training

Harding (1999), representing the view of agencies outside the health services, stressed the importance of an approach to young offenders that is not dependant on adult mental health services, together with an emphasis on delivering mental health training to non-mental health professionals. Inter-agency training is the best way of ensuring that a balance is struck between overloading Specialist CAMHS with inappropriate referrals and vulnerable young people being missed in the system, with the risk that they present in crisis and with severe mental health problems late in their offending careers.

Key success features for future training and development include:

flexible training (including distance learning);

team training;

accreditation that is acceptable to all the professional bodies;

bridging the theory-into-practice divide;

producing credible competent practitioners who are fit to work at every link in the chain;

training adequate numbers of specialist practitioners;

raising the knowledge and skills of selected practitioners relevant to forensic CAMHS;

developing a language and philosophy that is shared across the disciplines;

training practitioners to shared understandings of each other's roles; and

articulating the roles and values of each discipline within the context of a system that is able to offer best care.

The approach to developing the workforce should encompass the educational needs of staff in delivering the activities and functions of each tier of CAMHS. The general components of high-quality education and training include providing adequate opportunities for:

supervision;

life-long learning;

reflective practice;

critical application of practice;

appreciation of models of risk and resilience;

learning that is based on:

developmental concepts

work with families

work with human systems

understanding how to cope with complexity and uncertainty

learning about:

evidence-based interventions

values-based practice (Fulford and Williams 2003)

understanding how to manage substance misuse in forensic CAMHS settings and practice.

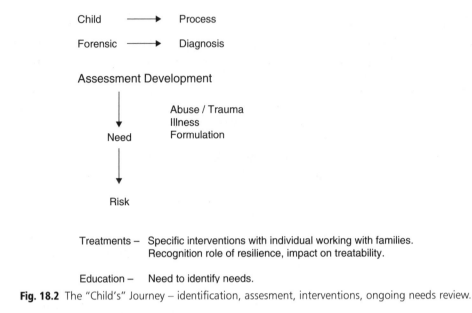

Fig. 18.2 The "Child's" Journey – identification, assesment, interventions, ongoing needs review.

A strategic framework for forensic mental health services for children and adolescents

Now that we have presented a range of background information and analysis of the evidence, we next provide a strategic framework for forensic CAMHS with the intention of aiding development of comprehensive services. We have developed our approach with awareness that any attempt made to apply strategic approaches to one component of comprehensive CAMHS, in this instance forensic CAMHS, must link well with the ways in which the wider realm of CAMHS is developing. If not, there is a substantial risk of creating more, rather than fewer, fault lines in service delivery. Therefore, we propose a conceptual model that augments and develops the original Four-tier CAMHS Strategic Framework (NHS Health Advisory Service 1995) to include forensic CAMHS (Williams 2004). We are grateful to Arnold Publishing for permission to reproduce a new version of part of a chapter that appears in a recent text (Bailey and Dolan 2004).

In summary, the forensic CAMHS we propose should deliver three main functions: specialist services provided locally by Tier 3 of the Specialist CAMHS; centres of special forensic expertise at Tier 4, which include in-patient services; and peripatetic teams outreaching from the centres of special forensic expertise to provide advisory, educational, and clinical services in locations distant from the centre and in close conjunction with Tier 3 forensic teams in local areas.

Tier 3: services provided by generic Specialist CAMHS

Our approach envisages that forensic CAMHS for most young people should be provided by the local generic Specialist CAMHS. Currently, a huge amount of 'forensic' work is done by local specialist services, though it does not come close to meeting the needs of individuals or of the agencies for advice and intervention. Current forensic services, broadly conceived to reflect all circumstances in which there is an interface between clinical practice and application of the

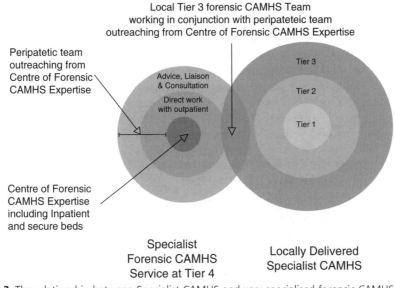

Fig. 18.3 The relationship between Specialist CAMHS and very specialised forensic CAMHS at Tiers 3 and 4.

various legislations bearing on minors, appear to be provided on a substantially *ad hoc* basis in which the level of particular experience, interest, and time available to particular practitioners plays a large part. Also, much of the expert evidence that is provided to the courts relies upon individual relationships between particular legal and mental health practitioners. Thus, currently, services are not the subject of planning or deliberate endeavours to match them with established need. All too often, there is imprecise or extremely limited co-operation between the agencies (i.e. mainly when particularly difficult cases arise) in planning, commissioning, and delivering forensic services or advice, and there are big gaps in the multidisciplinary contributions required to deliver effective expert assessments, interventions, advisory and reporting services that many consider to be important.

Yet, if the career routes of young people with forensic problems are to become more rational, the process decisions made by the agencies need to be put onto a more predictable basis. Establishing local specialist forensic CAMHS requires specific and focused activity by commissioners, working with service providers, to develop multi-agency services of appropriate capability and with effective inter-agency communications. Ideally, we recommend that each local Specialist CAMHS should develop to have at least one identified team that has greater expertise in the forensic arena. These teams should not, and could not, conduct all the forensic work but should provide a focus of capability and advice, and should lead for the local Specialist CAMHS on forensic matters.

Tier 4: peripatetic advisory services provided by outreach teams based in centres of special expertise

Our approach also envisages that the response of local specialist forensic CAMHS teams at Tier 3 is augmented by advice, training, and consultation offered by identified peripatetic outreach teams (at Tier 4) that are based in, and work from, a discrete number of centres of special expertise in forensic CAMHS (also at Tier 4).

This aspect of the work of the peripatetic teams should be indirect, consultative, advisory, educational, and supportive. In such a scenario, responsibility for managing individual cases would continue to be with the staff of local services at Tier 3. Already, there are examples of this kind of relationship but the present level of resources and the volume of highly specialized services are nowhere near sufficient to meet the demand for an adequate number of outreach teams.

Thus, our recommendation requires relationships between the centres of special expertise and local Specialist CAMHS to be moved from their current *ad hoc* nature to a planned framework in which each local Specialist CAMHS has defined links with an identified specialist centre. Much planning, training, and new resources will be required to arrive at this position.

Tier 4: peripatetic clinical services provided by outreach teams based at centres of special expertise

Our framework envisages that the outreach services (also at Tier 4), as provided by members of staff from a centre of special expertise, also see clients directly, by deliberate agreement, and, relatively, close to their homes, rather than at the centre. Our idea is that the staff of the outreach service should work in conjunction with the staff of the local agencies at Tier 3. In these cases, the peripatetic team shares with Tier 3 locally responsibility for the direct work with young people and their families.

Tier 4: services provided at centres of special expertise

In our framework, Tier 4 functions also include those services that are delivered directly to patients and their families at the centres of special expertise in forensic CAMHS. Currently, there are few of them in the UK. Therefore, they will need to be developed in a planned way to provide sufficient in-patient care at a variety of levels of security and dependency to cover a sufficiently wide range of psychiatric disorders and the complexity of problems experienced by the young people who require them.

We think that, separately, each centre of special expertise should offer core competencies and discharge certain common functions. However, the analyses summarized in this chapter show that none singly can focus on the whole of the potential client group. Therefore, our plan envisages that there should be co-ordination in the way in which the centres of special forensic expertise are developed, so that, taken together in the UK, the range of services that they offer is complementary. Put another way, these centres should, together, be able to offer interventions at very specialized levels for all the major components of the client group in acknowledged and planned ways.

The levels of in-patient and day-patient care provided by the specialist centres should include:

Open units (where the special expertise and training of the staff is the key factor that differentiates them from more local psychiatric, social and education services);

high-dependency units;

intensive assessment, and care intervention units; and

units that can offer psychiatric assessment, care, and treatment at medium levels of security.

An agenda for future planning and commissioning activity

Core issues—lessons from existing services

The core of the position taken in this chapter is that there is need for substantial action to develop rational forensic CAMHS that will contribute positively to the career routes followed by young people who need them. These services should become more predictable, purposeful, and better matched with the needs of the potential client group. Application of the strategic framework presented here should enable more focused and much better co-ordinated development work to be undertaken and would, thereby, contribute significantly to achieving the goal.

This chapter has identified the major shortage of expertise if services are to respond appropriately to the great range of mental health needs of young people generally and, particularly, young people who require forensic CAMHS. It seems highly probable that current gaps in the workforce contribute powerfully to inadequate responses to the alienation, marginalization, and exclusion that may arise in part from mental disorder in the most challenging young people. A more organized framework of better commissioning and provision might prevent some young people from moving inappropriately towards the extremes of provision.

Currently, the availability of specialist forensic services at all of the tiers conceived here is low and poorly planned. Strategic vision, planning, leadership, and management (see chapters 2 and 3), new resources, and greater numbers of better trained staff are required to deliver all of the three components at Tiers 3 and 4.

Nonetheless, elements of a more mature service do exist, mainly in England, but, as identified, they have no unifying or predictive framework. This leaves individual services and the care and case management of individuals to be guided by:

local professional opinion and experience, and the nature and quality of commissioner–provider relationships;

local inter-agency and intra-agency dynamics and pressures; and

what is presently available.

It is also plain that this situation and the poverty of the present arrangements for commissioning and managing forensic CAMHS results in:

poor planning and execution of care for individuals; and

poor continuity of very specialized care for this client group.

Many of the individuals who receive very specialized care do so as a result of:

determined advocacy by particular members of service staff;

the turbulence they create;

the endurance of commissioners and/or service providers;

lack of proper external quality assurance and performance management of the kinds that might be required by an experienced commissioner for those services that do exist, due to:

commissioner inexperience;

high rates of out-of-area-treatments (OATs) and out-of-county placements;

long distances between the location of specialist services and many patients' homes;

lack of performance-management mechanisms for the existing services; and

inadequate mechanisms to enable local referrers to review their cases when admitted to more distant, very specialized services and, thereby, continue to contribute to high-quality care and case management.

The way ahead

Alternatively, the approach suggested here is one in which the agencies combine to collaboratively plan, fund, deliver, and manage the performance of forensic CAMHS that are based on:

multi-agency concepts;

cross-sector approaches and close working relationships between sectors and agencies;

expansion of NHS-funded local and outreach assessment and treatment capacity; and

expansion of NHS-funded secure and other in-patient services.

One of the critical issues is that of how to determine or predict which of the young people exhibiting characteristics that bring them into the potential client group, should follow each of the avenues described by Little and Bullock (2004). This indicates the need to build up much better data in order to define more precisely which of the young people who are in the broad category of 'troublesome youth' will need input from forensic CAMHS.

While the number of young people who require the most specialized services is relatively small, their accurate prediction based on the analysis of risk factors is difficult. Therefore, the primary purpose of comprehensive assessment should be to ensure appropriate early intervention. This might, in turn, prevent placement breakdowns, which is one of the routes that can lead, inexorably and over long periods in some cases, towards referral for secure psychiatric in-patient placement. Thus, comprehensive assessment is needed for young people who are considered to come within the broad categories defined by the characteristics that have been referred to earlier in this chapter. This includes some young people who are presently referred to Specialist CAMHS, a proportion of those who are clients of the social and/or education support services, and young people referred to the YOTs, and the other youth justice, probation and penal services.

The commissioning agenda

Moving forward is likely to be aided by an agenda for commissioning that is shared between individual healthcare agencies and local authorities exercising their responsibilities jointly, together with more concentrated patterns of regional and national commissioning for some of the most expert services and especially those at Tier 4. The model described for Wales has many of the features that we think are required (Welsh Assembly Government 2003).

We recommend that development of similar strategic templates for children and adolescents and its co-ordination with the work of Strategic Health Authorities and Primary Care Trusts (in England) and Local Health Boards and Health Commission Wales (in Wales) could produce an appropriate commissioning mechanism. Within this vision, PCTs (in England) and CAMHS Commissioning Networks (CCNs) in Wales would be responsible for commissioning Tier 3 services in a way that is harmonized with Tier 4 services that are commissioned nationally in Wales and regionally in England. Similar mechanisms are required in Northern Ireland and Scotland.

In order to respond to this ambitious agenda, work is necessary at all tiers, supported by improved resources, staffing, and staff training. In particular, a programme of commissioner training and development is vital. Our agenda cannot be achieved unless particular commissioners are identified, and given continuing and sustained responsibilities for forensic CAMHS. In addition, there is a need for a series of activities of a more general nature that will require collaboration and debate on a wide basis, including:

work on better defining the client group(s);

more cross-agency comprehensive-needs assessments conducted against agreed common protocols;

mapping of the present array of services across all agencies;

agreement and implementation of a comprehensive plan for individual case assessment based on the best of present expertise;

a programme of targeted research and service evaluation;

collection of a more substantial database based on agreed cross-agency assessment criteria; and

a programme of organizational development for service planners and providers.

Tier 3

At Tier 3, there is much to be done. Achieving an expanded capability in the forensic arena cannot be achieved easily or quickly, especially given the other demands on generic Specialist CAMHS, and the existing staff and resource shortages. Nonetheless, the plan we envisage in this chapter is that of moving towards each local Specialist CAMHS as being the first port of call for requests for specialized forensic mental health service opinions delivered by teams of staff with identified responsibilities and training in this area. Each team should work in conjunction with the other local agencies to make recommendations as to the use of the other tiers of expertise guided by sustained relationships with the specialized centres of expertise. In this way, a local forensic CAMHS could provide specialist back-up to the YOTs (through outposted staff and access to generic Tier 3 services) and gateways to the more specialized tiers.

Our plan requires considerable multidisciplinary expansion of the forensic capability of local CAMHS in order that they are able to develop good local linkages between the peripatetic teams outreaching from the centres of special forensic expertise for young people with:

the specialist CAMHS in identified local areas;

services for young people who use and misuse substances;

child-care agencies;

Youth Offending Teams;

local authority services of all types;

secure units for children and adolescents in the area; and

medium-secure units for adults.

Children and adolescents who fall into the client group appropriate to a forensic CAMHS are often highly mobile and frequently known to more than one agency. Sometimes their moves between agencies and sectors of care are planned, but, all too often, referrals are made by the processes of exclusion, result from exhaustion of the capabilities of particular services, or are made in desperation as a last-ditch attempt to help. All too rarely does it seem that the care of individuals is subject to rigorously planned integrated care pathways. Therefore, a focus on analysing patient flows (patients' journeys) and the design of appropriate care pathways are important matters for appropriate R&D. The objective should be planned care, initiated at the local level, being the basis on which integrated services are delivered.

Tier 4

The outreach or peripatetic teams (working from centres of special forensic CAMHS expertise) should have the ability to cascade an increased volume of very specialized out-patient and educational services in support of local services and, particularly, local Tier 3 forensic CAMHS teams in developing their knowledge and skill through teaching and consultation with local practitioners.

Application of information technology, including tele-medicine and video-conferencing, would bring the centres of special expertise into much closer contact with the more distant local Specialist CAMHS. In this way, the present informal network of relationships between local services and a judiciously expanded number of specialist centres could be developed into an established and recognized pattern of planned care.

Currently, there is lack of mental health liaison services for consultation between the NHS and services provided by other sectors of care for children and adolescents who are very difficult to manage and hard-to-place. However, the accumulating evidence of the high level of psychiatric symptoms and/or disorders in these groups of young people, makes the case for much improved liaison and consultative services provided not only to Tier 3 forensic CAMHS but also to probation services, YOTs, secure units, and young offender institutions. Also, there is a lack of targeted remedial, therapeutic, and care programmes of tested efficacy for adolescent sexual offenders and for the victims of abuse. Thus, there is need for the peripatetic teams to develop effective programmes of care, in conjunction with local services, and to teach and consult with practitioners in all sectors of care as well as the local Specialist CAMHS.

It is inherent in this proposal, that development of peripatetic outreach teams requires prior developments, locally, at Tier 3 and, nationally, at Tier 4. Each local service would need to be at an enhanced level of capability and each of the very specialized centres would need to have identified responsibilities for committing resources to the peripatetic teams. Each outreach team could then develop an awareness of services in all sectors of care so as to act as an information exchange.

Centres of special forensic expertise and the role of secure in-patient services

There is clear opinion held by many professionals and managers in the field that there is a need to expand the number of centres of special expertise for adolescents who have severe mental illness and who require treatment in settings that offer security. The strategic framework presented here indicates that each should be capable of providing:

> very specialized in-patient care;

> outreach clinical services; and

> teaching and research.

As identified earlier, we believe that these centres of expertise should be developed into a complementary network. Thus, planning future services requires development of harmonised and equally comprehensive commissioning expertise.

The reviews summarized in this chapter indicate that there is a small yet definable group of young people within the overall client group of forensic CAMHS which might benefit from secure in-patient treatment in the healthcare system. Current evidence indicates that their problems cover the full range of psychiatric disorders. In addition, there are five other key matters:

> the need to recognize the high levels of substance use and misuse in the client group;

> the special needs of learning disabled clients;

> the challenges of differentiating those clients who require NHS-funded secure in-patient care within the overall client group, given the high prevalence of symptoms and disorders in the client group as a whole;

awareness that it is unlikely that each individual secure in-patient unit could deliver assessment, care, and treatment effectively and appropriately to all of those who might benefit from such intervention and care (a matter of case-mix and specialization); and

the need to distinguish those young people who require secure in-patient care from those likely to benefit from lower levels of security.

While each of these matters needs further work, there appears to be a general consensus among those involved in this field that there is a need to increase the number of in-patient beds within very specialized forensic CAMHS, including those in secure settings, for a range of young people from the diverse potential client group.

The young people who appear to have the greatest immediate needs for increased secure NHS-funded provision include those with:

very severe mental illnesses (reflected in current NSCAG in-patient developments);

recurrent very severe self-harming behaviours; and

serious brain injury and some with other severe organic disorders.

Additionally, there is the need to develop and evaluate focused programmes of specialist intervention for adolescents who are:

sex offenders and abusers;

mentally disordered offenders;

users and, particularly, misusers of substances;

in need of a secure setting in which to begin psychiatric rehabilitation; and

learning disabled, as well as having other characteristics of the client group.

Given the profile of use of existing facilities, there is also a requirement for further research into the needs of both boys and girls, and for young people from minority ethnic origins for the most specialized resources in all sectors of care. Another important area for future development is the need to ensure liaison between secure in-patient facilities funded by the NHS and the secure residential facilities offered by other sectors.

Bridging across all these needs and activities is better and safer identification of that small group of adolescents who, by virtue of their prodromal anti-social personalities, are without appropriate intervention and likely to place others at serious risk.

Training professionals and managers for the future

Such an ambitious programme cannot be delivered rapidly, but, unless deliberate planned action is taken, it is arguable that nothing coherent is likely to result and, despite their good intentions, local services will be left to react inadequately to crises. We recognize the contemporary pressures and provide a workforce framework through which to plan developments rationally. A key feature that has emerged several times is the current lack of both the volume, and the levels, of specialist expertise to deliver the kinds of services that could be supported by current capabilities, or by those that are likely to emerge through continuing professional development and research.

Several themes have run close beneath the surface. Arguably, the most powerful of those relates to the agendas for recruitment and training that will be necessary to underpin any service advancements. Our strategic framework cannot be delivered without a longer term workforce-development plan.

The augmented Four-Tier Strategic Framework identified in this chapter indicates that different levels of specialist expertise are required. Our opinion is that it is not feasible to base service planning around the provision of the full spectrum of forensic CAMHS by, and from, the most specialized centres. Nonetheless, they are critically important. We must build on the current circumstances in which it appears that the most common and frequent demands for expert forensic CAMHS-capability are likely to require a defined level of expertise made available through local Specialist CAMHS. Equally, this chapter substantiates the notion that it is unlikely that this expertise can be developed or sustained without considerable training, additional recruitment, and backing delivered by an expanded number of centres of special forensic expertise each with strong academic connections.

Our framework envisages that patients could be moved through a more comprehensive and rational system according to need and negotiated, purposeful, and evaluated care programmes. Knowledge, expertise, and skill should also be key commodities that are moved purposely through the proposed network of forensic CAMHS; they are not simply a by-product of work with patients/clients, service users and carers. Thus, training and academic support, research, and development should also be major matters for planning. They are required, not only by professionals working within the various service tiers but, also, by those staff who manage service delivery and those who plan and commission services. Therefore, in parallel with the strategic framework offered here, this chapter also offers a four-level outline framework for training. We provide an initial list of topics for training in Appendix 18.1.

Level 1: general specialist training

Basic knowledge about forensic mental health matters, and the skills to assess and manage children and adolescents who might fall into the client group for forensic CAMHS should form part of the training for many professions. They include professionals who work within local generic Specialist CAMHS (including psychiatrists, nurses, social workers, psychologists, AHPs, and teachers), the staff of YOTs, certain education service support staff, and children's teams in local authority social services departments.

In addition, workers in non-statutory sector projects, which have a remit for work with young people, police officers, and prison staff require familiarity, at least, with the concepts that are inherent in the work of forensic CAMHS.

Level 2: advanced training

Each local Specialist CAMHS should move in the direction of appointing a multidisciplinary team of professionals that leads on providing forensic CAMHS at Tier 3. Its members should be more than averagely skilled in assessment techniques, report writing, and in presenting themselves before courts, as well as in the construction of programmes of care with a forensic focus. Additionally, many probation officers on the staff of YOTs need advanced training that goes beyond that required on a day-by-day basis by the staff of the generic elements of Specialist CAMHS. We describe this level of training and expertise as level 2.

Level 3: very specialized training required by the staff of day-patient and in-patient services offered by the centres of special forensic expertise

Staff who work at the centres of expertise, and particularly those who work with day-patients and in-patients, require a particularly high level of training, in order to discharge their responsibilities.

They should have thorough working knowledge of the law and be trained in techniques of control and restraint appropriate to young people, as well as in more focused assessment and therapeutic techniques relevant to discharging particular programmes of care for, and intervention with, some of the most troubled young people. Previous sections in this chapter have identified aspects of the client group and particular programmes that require staff to develop special expertise.

Level 4: very specialized training required by the peripatetic staff of the centres of special expertise

Our strategic framework places particular responsibilities upon staff who offer outreach services. They require full training at all of the levels identified so far (1 to 3). Additionally, they should have advanced communication skills, the most effective of self-presentation skills, particular experience in mental health case (indirect) consultation, and a high level of skills in teaching. Some of them should also be skilled in the techniques of service evaluation and in quantitative and qualitative research methodologies (Williams 1999, 2000).

Concluding comments

This chapter began by identifying the high rates of involvement of young people in offending and the researched evidence of the associations for young people between offending, mental disorder, substance misuse, and learning difficulties and disabilities. We have recognised the challenges that still remain to be faced in effectively designing, planning, commissioning and delivering comprehensive forensic CAMHS for the UK. We recommend moving from the present *ad hoc* system in which services have developed around the, often charismatic, advocacy of individuals, usually service providers, to a more rational commissioning and performance managed system that is led by policy, driven by strategy and based on need. In this chapter, we provide a rational, evidence-based and partially tested strategic framework and the outlines of a workforce training plan.

The challenge of more purposefully managing the professional process decisions and, thereby, influencing the career routes of the young people involved according to their needs lies at the heart of the strategic intent and direction that we propose.

While the number of young people requiring the most specialized services is relatively small, their accurate prediction based on the analysis of risk factors is difficult. Therefore, the primary purpose of comprehensive assessment (Kroll *et al.* 2002) should be to ensure appropriate early intervention. This might, in turn, prevent placement breakdown, which is one of the routes that can lead, inexorably in some cases, to referral to what will continue to be specialist, oversubscribed, secure psychiatric in-patient placements (Bailey 2003).

We identify the advantages of strategic framework in support of this task. The strategic framework we present is capable of:

- containing an appropriately wide range of service activities that should enable the healthcare contribution to forensic CAMHS to be developed in conjunction with the roles of other agencies;

- identifying the roles of centres of special forensic expertise; and

- clarifying the functions of health-provided secure and community-based care.

Unapologetically, we focus on improving the NHS-funded contribution to wider multisector services. Similar work is needed to identify the parallel service developments that are required within each of the other sectors. The result that has emerged from our analyses and proposals sets an ambitious agenda for service development. While services are currently thin and the volume of of expertise required to move rapidly to delivering such a comprehensive array of services is missing now, this and other books (e.g. Bailey and Dolan 1004) ably demonstrate that the skills and knowledge do exist from which more effective services might be developed. Recruiting capable staff, training them and providing resources to support their work will be vital elements in moving forward. This calls for a coherent and long-term workforce development plan.

References

Audit Commission (1996) *Misspent youth—young people and crime.* London: Audit Commission.

Audit Commission (1999) *Children in mind—report on child and adolescent mental health services.* London: Audit Commission.

Bailey, S. (1999) The interface between mental health, criminal justice and forensic mental health services for children and adolescents. *Current Opinion in Psychiatry,* **12,** 425–32.

Bailey, S. (2002) Expert paper: antisocial personality disorder: children and adolescents. Liverpool: NHS national programme on forensic mental health research and development.

Bailey, S. (2003) Young Offenders and Mental Health. *Current Opinion in Psychiatry* **16,** 581–91.

Bailey, S. and Dolan, M. (2004) *Textbook of adolescent forensic psychiatry.* London: Arnold.

Bailey, S. and Farnworth, P. (1998) Forensic mental health services. *Young Minds,* **34,** 12–3.

Bailey, S. and Harbour, A. (1998) The law and a child's consent to treatment (England and Wales). *Child Psychology Psychiatry Review,* **4,** 1–5.

Black, D., Harris, H., and Wolkind, S. (ed.) (1998) *Child psychiatry and the law.* London: Gaskell.

Brown, S.A., Amico, A.J.D., McCarthy, D.M., and Tapert, S.F. (2001) Four-year outcomes from adolescent alcohol and drug treatment. *Journal of Studies on Alcohol,* **62,** 381–8.

Bushell, H.D., Crome, I., and Williams, R.J.W. (2002) How can risk be related to interventions for young people who misuse substances? *Current Opinion in Psychiatry,* **15,** 355–60.

Butler-Sloss, E. (1998) In *Child psychiatry and the law* (ed. Black D, Harris, H., and Wolkind S), pp. iii–ix. London: Gaskell.

Children's Legal Centre (1998) Standing conference on drug abuse.

Coleman, J. and Schofield, J. (2003) *Key data on adolescence trust for study of adolescence.* Brighton: TSA Publishing.

Department of Health, Social Services Inspectorate of the Department of Health and the Department for Education (1995) *A handbook of mental health—a text in the Health of the Nation series.* London: Department of Health.

Department of Health (2003) *Getting the right start: national service framework for children—emerging findings.* London: Department of Health. www.doh.gov.uk/nsf/children/gettingtherightstart

Dolan, M., Holloway, J., Bailey, S., and Smith, C. (1999) Health status of young offenders appearing before juvenile courts. *Journal of Adolescence,* **22,** 137–44.

Doreleiyers, T.A.H., Moser, F., Thys, P., Van England, H., and Beyaert, F.H.L. (2000) Forensic assessment of juvenile deliquents: prevalence of psychopathology and decision making at court in the Netherlands. *Journal of Adolescence,* **23,** 263–75.

Ferdinand, R.F., Blum, M., and Verhulst, F.C. (2001) Psychopathology in adolescence predicts substance use in young adulthood. *Addiction,* **96,** 861–70.

Fulford, K.W.M. and Williams, R. (2003) Value-based child and adolescent mental health services? *Current Opinion in Psychiatry,* **16**(4), 369–76.

Graham, P. (1999) *Research and therapeutic interventions: bridging the chasm.* The 1999 Rutter Lecture, given at the Faculty of Child and Adolescent Psychiatry of the Royal College of Psychiatrists Annual Residential Meeting, Manchester, UK, 22 April 1999.

Graham, P. (2000) Treatment interventions and findings from research: bridging the chasm in child psychiatry. *British Journal of Psychiatry,* **176,** 414–9.

Grella, C.E., Hser, Y-I., Joshi, V., and Rounds-Bryant, J. (2001) Drug Treatment Outcomes for Adolescents with Comorbid Mental and Substance Use Disorders. *The Journal of Nervous and Mental Disease,* **189,** 384–92.

Grisso, T. (2000) Law and psychiatry: the changing face of juvenile justice. *Psychiatric Services,* **51** (4), 425–6.

Grisso, T. and Schwartz, R.G. (2000) *Youth of Trial.* A Developmental Perspective on Juvenile Justice 1–7, Chicago and London: University of Chicago Press.

Gunn, J., Madden, A., and Swinton, M . (1996) Treatment needs of prisoners with psychiatric disorders. *British Medical Journal,* **31,** 1521–4.

Harding, J. (1999) *Providing better services for mentally disordered offenders: pitfalls and prospects.* Probation Journal Special Issue—Working with Mentally Disordered Offenders 83–8.

Hengeller, S.W. (1999) Multi-systemic therapy: an overview of clinical procedures, outcomes and policy indications. *Child Psychology Psychiatry Review,* **4,** 2–10.

Jasper, A., Smith, C., and Bailey, S. (1998) 100 girls in care referred to an adolescent forensic mental health service. *Journal of Adolescence,* **21,** 555–68.

Joint Prison Service/NHS Executive Working Party (1999) *The future organisation of prison health care.* London: HM Prison Service.

Junger-Tas, J. (1994) *delinquent behaviour among young people in the Western World.* Amsterdam: Kugler.

Kazdin, A.E. (2000) Adolescent development, mental disorders and decision making of delinquent youths. In *Youth On Trial A Developmental Perspective on Juvenile Justice 2* (ed. T. Grisso and R.G. Schwartz), pp. 33–65. Chicago and London: University of Chicago Press.

Knapp, M. and Henderson, J. (1999) Health economic perspectives and evaluation of child and adolescent mental health services. *Current Opinions in Psychiatry,* **12,** 393–7.

Knapp, M., Scott, S., and Davies, J. (1999) The cost of anti-social behaviour in younger children. *Clinical Child Psychology Psychiatry,* **4** (4), 457–73.

Kroll, L., Rothwell, Bradley, D., Shah, P., Bailey, S., and Harrington, R.C. (2002) Mental health needs of boys in secure care for serious or persistent offending a prospective longitudinal study. *Lancet,* **259,** 1975–9.

Kroll, L., Woodham, A., Rothwell, J., Bailey, S., Tobias, C., Marshall, M., *et al.* (1999) Reliability of the Salford Needs Assessment Schedule for Adolescents. *Psychological Medicine,* **29** (4), 891–902.

Kuperman, S., Schlosser, S.S., Kramer, J.R., Bucholz, K., Hesselbrock, V., Reich, T., *et al.* (2001) Risk domains associated with an adolescent alcohol dependence diagnosis. *Addiction,* **96,** 629–36.

Kurtz, Z., Thorne, R., and Bailey, S. (1997) *Study of the demands and needs for forensic child and adolescent mental services in England and Wales report to the Department of Health.* London: Department of Health.

Kurtz, Z. (1996) *Treating children well—A guide to using the evidence base in commissioning and managing services for the mental health of children and young people.* London: The Mental Health Foundation.

Lader, D., Singleton, N., and Meltzer, H. (2000) *Psychiatric morbidity among young offenders in England and Wales.* London: Office for National Statistics.

Little, M. and Bullock, R. (2004) Administrative frameworks for very difficult children and adolescents. In *Adolescent forensic psychiatry* (ed. S. Bailey and M. Dolan), ch. 24. pp. 336–44. London: Arnold.

Longley, M., Williams, R., Furnish, S., and Warner, M. (2001). *Promoting mental health in a civil society: towards a strategic approach.* London: The Nuffield Trust.

Maziade, M. and Bouchard, S. (1997) Long term stability of diagnosis and symptom dimensions in a systematic sample of patients with onset of schizophrenia in childhood and early adolescence, positive/negative distinction in childhood predictors of adult outcome. *British Journal of Psychiatry,* **169**, 371–8.

Mental Health Foundation (1999) *Bright futures.* London: Mental Health Foundation.

Mullen, P.E. (2000) Forensic mental health. *British Journal of Psychiatry,* **176**, 307–11.

National Assembly for Wales (2000a) *Everybody's business—a consultation document.* Cardiff: National Assembly for Wales.

National Assembly for Wales (2000b) *Everybody's business—strategy document—child and adolescent mental health services.* Cardiff: National Assembly for Wales.

NHS Health Advisory Service, Mental Health Act Commission, Department of Health Social services Inspectorate (1994) *A review of the adolescent forensic psychiatry service based on the Gardener Unit, Prestwich Hospital, Salford, Manchester.* London: NHS Health Advisory Service.

NHS Health Advisory Service (1995) *Together we stand—the commissioning, role and management of child and adolescent mental health services.* London: HMSO.

NHS Health Advisory Service (1996) *The substance of young needs—commissioning and providing services for children and young people who use and misuse substances.* London: HMSO.

Nicol, R., Stretch, D., Whitney, J., Jones, K., Garfield, P., Turner, K., *et al.* (2000) Mental health needs and services for severely troubled and troubling young offenders in a NHS region. *Journal of Adolescence,* **23**, 243–61.

Office for National Statistics (1999) *Mental health of children and adolescents.* ONS (99) 409. London: Government Statistical Service.

Rolf, J., Masten, A., Cicchetti, D., Nuechterlein, K., and Weintraub, S. (ed.) (1990) *Risk and protective factors in the development of psychopathology.* Cambridge: Cambridge University Press.

Rose, J. (2002) *Working with young people in secure accommodation from chaos to culture.* Hove and New York: Brunner-Routlerg L.

Royal College of psychiatrists (1999) *The Royal College of Psychiatry's council report—CR71. Offenders with personality disorder.* London: Gaskell Publications.

Rutter, M. (1999) Psychosocial adversity and child psychopathology. *British Journal of Psychiatry* **174**, 480–93.

Rutter, M., Giller, H., and Hagell, A. (1998) *Anti-social behaviour by young people.* Cambridge: Cambridge University Press.

Rutter, M. and Smith, D.J. (1995) *Psychosocial disorders in young people. Time trends and their causes.* Chichester: Wiley.

Salmon, G. and Williams, R. (2001) *A strategic model for co-operation, partnership and teamwork.* Welsh Institute for Health and Social Care—The First Five Years, pp. 18–22. Pontypridd: University of Glamorgan.

Scott, S. (1998) Aggressive behaviour in childhood. *British Medical Journal,* **316**, 202–6.

Shepherd, J.P. and Farrington, B.P. (1996) The prevention of delinquency with particular reference to violent crime. *Medicine Science and the Law* **36**, 331–6.

Vizard, E. (2004) Assessment and treatment of children who are sexually abusive. In *Text book of adolescent forensic psychiatry* (ed. S. Bailey and M. Dolan). London: Arnold.

Welsh Assembly Government (2003) *WHC (2003) 63 NHS planning and commissioning guidance.* Cardiff: Welsh Assembly Government.

Williams, R. (1999) Managing mental health care: risk and evidence-based practice. *Current Opinion in Psychiatry,* **12**, 385–91.

Williams, R. (2000) A cunning plan—the role of research is evidenced in translating policy into effective child and adolescent mental health services. *Current Opinion Psychiatry,* **13**, 361–8.

Williams, R. (2004) A strategic approach to commissioning and delivering forensic child and adolescent mental health services. In *Text book of adolescent forensic psychiatry* (ed. S. Bailey and M. Dolan). London: Arnold.

Williams, R. (ed.) (2004) *Safeguards for young minds.* 2nd edn. London: Gaskell.

Williams, R. and Richardson, G. (1995) *Together we stand—the commissioning, role and management of child and adolescent mental health services.* London: HMSO.

Appendix 18.1

Post-basic multi-disciplinary training for the staff of child and adolescent forensic mental health services

Knowledge base

Normal child development

Developmental stages

Parent–child relationship: nurture and growth

Attachment theory

Autonomy and separation

Family as context of development

Systems theory

Family life-cycle

Family scripts: intergenerational processes

Family within wider social systems

Cross-cultural issues

Impacts of adversity on development

Concepts and definitions of abuse and neglect

Consequences of childhood abuse trauma

Dysfunctional family-cycles of abuse

Psychology of victimization

Pathways from dysfunctional attachment to disturbed behaviour

Gender differences

Developmental psychopathology

Classification of child and adolescent mental disorders

Multi-axial classification system

Adolescent disturbance in family and social context

Adaptation, accommodation and motivational crisis

Dissociation, PTSD and 'avoidance behaviours'

Borderline states and personality disorders

Deliberate self harm: suicidal and self-injuring behaviour

Depression, self-esteem, and disorders of mood

Psychosis

Anorexia and bulimia

Forensic presentations and mental disorder

Conduct disorder

Psychotic mentally disordered offender

Disorders of sexual development and offending behaviour

Substance abuse and offending behaviour

Prodromal personality disorder and offending behaviour

Learning disability and offending behaviour

PTSD in relation to offences

Legal frameworks

Mental Health Act 1983

Crime and Disorder Act 1998

Children Act 1989

Education Act 1996

European Human Rights Act 1998

Policy and practice frameworks

Child protection procedures

CPA

Clinical practice

Risk assessment/risk management

Definitions: risk, harm, dangerousness

Risk assessment

Risk minimisation strategies

Managing imminent violence

Child and adolescent risk assessment tools
(Ear120B, HCR20)

Therapeutic environments

Providing emotional containment

The safe adult role

Maintaining limits, boundaries and
authority

Native and care

Stimulation and education

Anti-bullying policy and practice

Feedback and confrontation
techniques

Basic group dynamics

Assessment

Application of multi-axial concept

From network through family to
adolescent

Mental state assessment

Use of instruments (SNASA)

Responding to disclosure of abuse

Assessment of needs; use of check-lists

Care planning

Developing a care plan

Integrated and co-ordinated treatment
elements

Key worker role

Review process

Unmet needs

*Working with courts, report writing, giving
evidence*

Basic interview and counselling skills

Motivational interviewing

Integrated therapeutic approaches:

Cognitive behavioural therapy applications

Working with families, e.g. maximizing
family strengths

Offence related therapy

Basic group work concepts of experience

Special secondary modules

Forensic psychotherapy for adolescents

Working with adolescent sex offenders

Trauma focused individual therapy

Cognitive therapy training

Art therapy applications

DBT (dialectical behavioural therapy)/MST
(multi-systemic therapy)

Family therapy applications

Clinical governance

Setting, monitoring standards for practice

Outcomes for health and offence reduction

Applying research knowledge to practice

Chapter 19

Young people and substance misuse

Ilana B. Crome and Eilish Gilvarry

Terminology, description, classification, and diagnosis

Introduction

In this chapter, we survey briefly issues impacting on need, design, and delivery of services and clinical practice regarding substance use and misuse by young people. Because this is a complex series of topics in which it is easy to use terms without clear regard to their meaning, we begin with a survey of current definitions.

Definitions

For professional clinical purposes the International Classification of Diseases (ICD10) (World Health Organization 1992) is the most commonly used diagnostic classification in the United Kingdom. This system outlines two categories: 'harmful use' and 'dependence syndrome' (Edwards and Gross 1976). 'Harmful use' refers to 'a pattern of psychoactive drug use that causes damage to health either mental or physical'.

The 'dependence syndrome' is diagnosed according to three of the following criteria:

a strong desire or sense of compulsion to use substances;

impaired capacity to control substance use;

a physiological withdrawal state with withdrawal relief and avoidance;

tolerance;

a pre-occupation with substance use;

persistent use despite clear evidence of harmful consequences.

ICD10 has much in common with DSM-IV (American Psychiatric Association 1994). However, DSM-IV uses the term 'abuse' (instead of harmful use), which is defined as a maladaptive pattern of substance use leading to clinically significant impairment or distress, as manifest by recurrent use resulting in:

failure to fulfil obligations at work, school, or home;

legal problems;

use in situations in which use is physically hazardous;

continued use despite persistent or recurrent social or interpersonal problems caused or exacerbated by the effects of the substance.

The criteria for dependence are similar in both classifications, though DSM-IV does not include compulsive use.

In the United Kingdom, the NHS Health Advisory Service (HAS) Report (1996) on young people and substance misuse utilized the terms 'use' and 'misuse'. It recognized that drug use often styled as experimental or recreational may also be illegal, and some experimental use may lead to intoxication with associated (occasionally even fatal) consequences. 'Misuse' was defined as 'use that is harmful, dependent use, or use of substances as part of a wider spectrum of problematic or harmful behaviour'. There are, however, more restrictive definitions as follows:

Use: legal use, acceptable socially, medically approved, and non-hazardous, i.e. without impairment of social, psychological or physical functioning. It should, however, be noted that, very rarely, just one dose of a drug can cause serious harm, and even death.

Misuse: unlawful use (illegal or illicit), which is not socially or medically approved, with the potential to cause harm. The term 'hazardous use' is also applied to potentially harmful use.

Harmful use: 'there must be clear evidence that the substance use was responsible for or substantially contributed to physical or psychological harm' (World Health Organization 1992).

Dependence: the criteria are described above. Recent research indicates that a significant minority of young people do develop dependence, especially on alcohol, nicotine, and opiates, and, more recently, cannabis (Stewart and Brown 1995; Rosenberg and Anthony 2001). This diagnosis has important treatment implications.

Terms such as 'normal', the 'norm', 'normative', or 'normalization' have often been applied to young people's drug use. These descriptions have both quantitative (regularity, frequency) and qualitative (social acceptability) elements. None of these terms should be equated to 'safe' use. A framework that links the differing definitions with epidemiological methods, survey types, and the four tier strategic framework is provided by Table 19.1.

Complex spectra and combinations of psychological, psychiatric, physical, and social problems may be present whether young people are described as 'misusers', 'harmful users', or 'dependent users'. We have developed a framework that provides the best fit with clinical decisions, intervention, models of treatment, prevention, and policy (see Table 19.1).

Prevalence and trends

How 'normal', i.e. typical, is substance use in young people? The fact is that more than half of all teenagers do not use substances regularly, and, apart from alcohol, half have not tried potentially addictive substances.

Internationally, numerous epidemiological studies have reported on the prevalence of, and trends in, young people's substance use. These are in school populations, clinical populations, and vulnerable young people, i.e. truants or those involved with the criminal justice system. While different methodologies have been used, some studies, e.g. the Monitoring the Future study in the United States (O'Malley and Johnstone 1999) and the British Crime Survey (Ramsey and Percy 1997; Ramsey and Spiller 1997; Ramsey et al. 2001), have reported at regular intervals on trends. The overall trend is of increasing misuse of substances by young people over the last decade.

Alcohol use

The European School Survey Project on Alcohol and Drugs (ESPAD) study (Hibell et al. 1999), a prevalence study carried out on 15–16-year-olds in 30 countries across Europe, examined their use of alcohol and other substances. It showed that British young people had the highest rate of alcohol use, drunkenness, intoxication, and binge-drinking in Europe.

This is substantiated by the General Household Survey (Office for National Statistics 1998). Thirty-five per cent of young men (aged 16–24 years) were drinking more than 8 units daily and 12% were drinking between 4 and 8 units daily. In this study, about 17% of young women

Table 19.1 Framework for integration of epidemiological methods and provision of services

Definitions	Estimates of consumption and/or criteria	Population on which estimates are likely to be based	Types of survey	Service framework
Use/misuse	Quantity/frequency	General population; school surveys	Office of National Statistics (ONS); General Household Survey (GHS); British Crime Survey (BCS); European ESPAD	Tier 1
Use/misuse	Quantity/frequency – 'regular' use	General population; school surveys	Office of National Statistics (ONS); General Household Survey (GHS); British Crime Survey (BCS); European ESPAD	Tier 2
Harmful use	Harmful use, dependence criteria according to ICD–10	General medical, criminal justice and social services	Home Office Addicts Index (HOAI); Regional Drug Misuse Databases (RDMDs)	Tier 3 – specialist multi-disciplinary services
Dependence	Dependence criteria according to ICD–10	Clinical treatment populations attending specialist services	Treatment populations attending specialist services	Tier 4 – intensive, very specialised services

From Fisher *et al.* 2004.

drank 3–6 units daily and 23% drank more than 6 units daily. Thus, at least 40% of young people drink above 'safe' limits for adults, especially young men. The high rate of female binge-drinking may result in teenage pregnancy and developmental problems for foetuses.

Cigarette smoking

In the United Kingdom, lifetime use of nicotine by 15–16-year-olds was estimated at 69% in ESPAD. Lifetime use of 40 times or more was reported at 26% and use in the last 30 days was estimated at 34%. Daily use at age 13 was 20%: this was the highest in Europe. On all indicators, girls are now using nicotine more frequently than boys.

Illicit drugs

In 1998, one-quarter of 16–29-year-olds admitted using cannabis during the previous year, and 15% during the previous month (Mirrlees-Black *et al* 1998; Kershaw *et al* 2000). While there have been increases since 1998 in the 16–24-year-old group in cocaine and heroin use, these changes were not statistically significant. Cannabis remains the most frequently used drug, with 45% of 16–24-year-olds reporting having tried cannabis. This was confirmed in the ESPAD study (Hibell *et al.* 1999), which indicated that one-third of teenagers had 'ever used' any illicit drug and a similar number had 'ever used' cannabis.

This increase is manifest in attendees at drug treatment agencies, which now number about 145 000 per annum, a rate that is increasing by 20% per annum. One in seven attendees is twenty years old. The trend in young people is to use multiple substances at an earlier age, which is more likely to lead to young people becoming dependent users. Hence the need for an emphasis on preventive programmes, and recognition that epidemiology cannot provide answers as to why or how substance misuse develops.

Prevention programmes

The UN Convention on the Rights of the Child emphasizes the need to protect children from illicit drug use and to prevent use of children in illicit production and trafficking. While the main goal of primary prevention is to prevent onset of substance use, the principal aim of secondary prevention is to reduce the level of use or misuse. Despite numerous initiatives, the net sum of interventions has failed to impact on rising trends since the early 1990s (Bauman and Phongsavan 1999). Indeed, it may be said that these efforts are providing too little, too late.

Prevention programmes are of two types: universal and targeted. The universal approach, aimed at the general population, schools, or identified communities, focuses on awareness raising, drugs education, or community initiatives. One advantage is the lack of 'labelling' of individuals. The major disadvantage is that the intervention may be of greatest benefit to those at lowest risk. This approach may also be unnecessarily expensive.

'Targeted' programmes are aimed at high-risk groups, e.g. school excludees and children with behaviour difficulties, or who offend. This approach offers early intervention, multidisciplinary working and more efficient use of scarce, but costly, resources.

Research is beginning to show which components of educational programmes are most valuable. These include programmes that enhance parental and family functioning, interactive teacher–pupil sessions and group social competence interventions. They should be sustainable over the longer term (with booster sessions over two years), and modified to be applicable to the needs of local communities. Awareness of cultural diversity, with discussions about values, moral and ethical issues is also important.

The focus is on both the short-term and long-term impact of substances. It should be noted that there is a lack of evidence to support peer education, didactic teaching, and media campaigns. Additional but specific prevention programmes may need to be targeted at high-risk groups.

Thus specific knowledge about attitudes to, and skills in, managing resistance to substances is central and should be linked to classroom activities (e.g. literacy), leisure (entertainment), extra-curricular activities (e.g. drama, sports), community activities (e.g. voluntary work), and life skills (e.g. job preparation). While most prevention programmes are designed to reduce risk factors, it is recognized that it is necessary to enhance protective factors as well (see Appendix 19.1).

Risk, resilience, and associations

Predisposition to substance use in young people is multi-factorial, and awareness of potential antecedents is essential when designing either public health prevention programmes or individual treatment plans (Swadi 1999).

Environmental, familial, individual, personality, and educational vulnerabilities may co-exist with availability, social deprivation, and affiliation with drug-using peers and those involved in criminal activity (Hawkins *et al.* 1992; Fergusson *et al.* 1995).

Home environments may be instrumental in young people developing problems. Parental substance use, or approval of substance use, family disruption, poor supervision, and parent–child conflict, as well as low parental aspirations, are linked as risk factors (Catalano *et al.* 1999; Hops *et al.* 1999). Some risk factors, e.g. drug use by peers, are very difficult to modify.

The later a young person is initiated into substance use, the less likely it is that they will develop problems. It should be noted that age of onset in itself is not inevitably predictive of misuse and dependence, but changes in intensity and regularity in the patterns of use do need to be examined.

Statistically, early onset of smoking is associated with substance misuse later on, dependence, and psychiatric disorders, such as conduct disorder (Fergusson 1995; Lewinsohn *et al.* 1999; Riggs *et al.* 1999). Distress, low self-esteem, and mental disorder (e.g. depression, anxiety) increase vulnerability, as does a history of aggression, impulsivity, hyperactivity, and sensation seeking (Sibthorpe *et al.* 1995; Shaffer *et al.* 1996; Zeitlin 1999). These experiences are especially significant because they may mask substance misuse or precipitate problems arising with, or from, use of substances. Furthermore, low educational expectations, attainment, and achievement, as demonstrated by poor school attendance, are associated with substance misuse.

There is extensive literature on the issue of co-morbidity of mental disorder and substance use in both adults and adolescents (Zeitlin 1999; Gilvarry 2000). Longitudinal studies indicate that early severe behaviour problems often characterize the history of those young people who later misuse substances. The combination of conduct disorder and persistent attention deficit hyperactivity disorder (ADHD) has been shown to predict and co-occur with later and persistent substance misuse. Predictably, because this is what the term implies, children with co-morbidity report higher rates of family problems, anti-social behaviour, truancy, and scholastic failure. Young people with these problems, especially if associated with deliberate self-harm or mood disorders, are at increased risk of suicide. Those children with co-morbid disorders show increased use of services, worsened clinical courses and outcomes, and higher rates of deliberate self-harm and suicide.

Factors that are protective, and which may mitigate or inhibit the development of substance misuse, include high self-esteem, high socio-economic status, parental disapproval of substance misuse, family cohesion, and attachments with close supervision (Costa *et al.* 1999). Religious involvement, leisure activities, and higher educational aspirations, abilities, and achievements are also protective.

The role of healthcare professionals in relation to prevention requires more attention: certainly understanding the psychological mechanisms that precipitate initiation into substance misuse and dependence is key.

It is vital to recognize that risk factors include adverse psychosocial problems, and the consequences of substance misuse. Without long-term prospective studies it is almost impossible to know which problems are risk factors, and which result from substance misuse. This suggests circular and interactive associations between cause and effect. Detailed knowledge of these complex interactions may be used to make services attractive. Prevention programmes must be carefully considered, implemented, and evaluated, both as part of a national substance misuse strategy and a broader child health strategy.

Important issues in assessing adolescents who may be using or misusing substances

Systematic assessment is crucial, so that each young person is helped to make the most appropriate decisions. Comprehensive assessment is critical to formulation and subsequent implementation of care plans. The objectives of practitioners should be to elicit sufficient information to form a picture of the current clinical, social, and personal life of each child, and the place of substance use within this framework. This may then need to be communicated to professional colleagues.

The main issue is engagement. Very rarely is one appointment for assessment sufficient to achieve this. Very rarely is substance misuse the only problem. Indeed, more often than not, professionals need to be persistent in their attempts at engagement. Assessment must include identification of goals, strengths, and problems. Despite the fact that there is a range of instruments that have specifically been developed for use with young people, a comprehensive, sensitive history is likely to yield significant information. The place of standardized instruments is to provide confirmations and is collateral to that derived from clinical expertise.

In order to capture the essence of how substance use affects each young person's emotional, cognitive, physical, and social development, practitioners need to be skilled and assertive, but also appealing, astute, and reassuring. Evidence suggests that a less mechanistic, more interactive style, in which each child is encouraged to participate, is more successful. Differentiation between substance use and misuse, and of any associated problems, will assist in offering the most apposite combination of evidence-based interventions, programmes, and settings.

Information about those risk factors that are likely to place a child in immediate danger; about the development of substance misuse; factors that might impinge on choice of a suitable treatment package are vital in order to sustain the care plan. The risk assessment should include inquiry into child protection issues, suicidal risk, extent of chaotic use, and accommodation issues.

The wishes of each child, and how they may, or more fundamentally may not, accept professional opinion are paramount. Assessment of maturity, in relation to consent and refusal, is imperative. The detail and depth of each assessment will be determined in part by the developmental stage of the child, the influence of substances during the interview, practitioner confidence in dealing with unpredictability, and the philosophy of the agency under the auspices of which the initial assessment or subsequent appointments are carried out.

It should be noted that substance use, though clearly potentially a serious problem for young people, need not necessarily be the most worrying cause for concern. In the process of assessing each young person, a keen eye should be kept on the relationships with their family (including siblings), peers, significant others, and on the potential for intervention or prevention for both the young person and their companions, siblings, and parents. The management plan should be based on a balanced interpretation of consistency between the systematic history, clinical condition, and results of any investigations.

Treatment interventions

Advice, information, and education are basic components of interventions. Acknowledgement of problems and motivation is of the essence. The positive effect of motivational interviewing and the value of brief interventions are also emphasized (Wagner et al. 1999). Assistance in recognizing that substance misuse is connected to current problems is another dimension of these programmes. The use of behaviour techniques is appropriate for more extensive substance misuse. These include monitoring use, identification of triggers and high risk situations, stress-reduction techniques, which are alternatives to substance misuse, social skills training, assertiveness skills regarding resistance and refusal, self-esteem enhancement, conflict resolution, and relapse prevention, in addition, social support from groups and individuals is seen as beneficial (e.g. peers, family support, and structured activities [recreation, volunteer, religion]) (Henggeler et al. 1992; Joanning et al. 1992; Kumpfer et al. 1996; Lewis et al. 1990).

Other specific psychological therapies that we suggest, in keeping with the evidence to date, include cognitive and behavioural approaches, 12-step and family therapy (Project MATCH

Research Group 1997a; 1997b). However, these interventions must be combined with other interventions for other complex needs, such as the treatment of conduct or mood disorder, and liaison with school and family, as well as consideration of the need for protection of the child.

Pharmacology and adolescent addiction

Pharmacotherapy is directed at a number of specific areas: treatment of overdose in emergencies, detoxification, substitution or maintenance therapy, and as adjuncts to relapse prevention, as well as treatment of co-morbid disorders.

Treatment of substance misuse

There is little research on the short- or long-term effects of pharmacological therapies for addiction that has been conducted in respect of adolescents. Almost all medications have not been licensed for use in under 18-year-olds. The exception is buprenorphine. Thus decisions to use pharmacological treatment are based on clinical acumen, and extremely careful supervision and monitoring by trained staff, in conjunction with carers in community settings.

Emergency treatment

Both opiates and benzodiazepines have specific pharmacological antagonists, naloxone and flumazenil, respectively, which are useful in emergency settings. General practitioners and paramedics should have naloxone available for the immediate reversal of intoxication.

Detoxification

The majority of adolescents are not dependent and do not usually require detoxification (Department of Health 1999), but some symptomatic treatment may be useful if there are mild withdrawal symptoms. While the same principles apply as for adults, particular care may need to be taken with dosage, depending on body build and age.

The effectiveness of detoxification is limited without further psychological and social support. In-patient detoxification is quicker and more effective than when conducted in the community. But community detoxification is far more widespread, especially as very few suitable and appropriate in-patient facilities (Tier 4) exist for adolescent addicts, even though 1–2% have severe dependence, sufficient to require medically supervised detoxification.

Alcohol withdrawal

For detoxification from alcohol, benzodiazepines, particularly chlordiazepoxide, are the usual treatment of choice. The possibility of misuse of these drugs requires that their use be monitored. It is advisable to consider vitamin supplements during in-patient alcohol detoxification.

Opiate withdrawal

Methadone, lofexidine, and buprenorphine are the most commonly used drugs (Carnwath and Hardman 1998).

If stabilization and reduction is the treatment goal, it should be stressed that treatment may need to persist for some time, with the philosophy of retention in treatment as a key short-to medium-term objective.

Methadone maintenance as the primary treatment for adolescents is not generally advocated (Ball and Ross 1991; Ward et al. 1998). However, although there is no research on maintenance prescribing for young people, there is a small but significant number of injecting dependent heroin users who present to services in England. This group does require intervention, and some young people have derived benefit from methadone stabilization and slow reduction over 3–9 months (Crome *et al.* 1999).

Cessation of smoking

Nicotine replacement and bupropion are routinely available for adults, and the scrutiny of the value of this medication in adolescents by NICE was timely (NICE 2002). The recommendation is that NRT be prescribed by a medical practitioner for young people who smoke more than 10 cigarettes per day.

Relapse prevention

Generally, disulfiram and acamprosate in alcohol misuse, naltrexone for opiate misuse, and bupropion in smokers, aid relapse prevention, but there is no consensus on their application in clinical practice with young people. Thus these interventions should only be undertaken with caution by practitioners who work in specialized services, and the most exacting vigilance is needed before these treatments should be administered.

Treatment of psychiatric disorders

Many young people with complex problems that co-occur with substance use have conditions that can be ameliorated by pharmacological means, often as an adjunct to other interventions, or sometimes as the main intervention. Occasionally, children and young people present to services with psychotic conditions that require appropriate pharmacological management. However, many of the young people with complex problems have underlying neuro-cognitive deficits that manifest through an impaired ability to relate and communicate. This may be linked with marked attentional problems and hyperkinetic behaviours. Therefore there is a role for central nervous stimulants in treating these young people. Stimulant treatment is associated with subsequently reduced illicit drug use (Biederman *et al.* 1999). We think that this probably occurs because young people are helped to adopt more normal and adaptive patterns of behaviour at home and, particularly, in school.

Outcome research

United Kingdom

There have been only two descriptive outcome studies on adolescent substance misuse in the United Kingdom. One has been on adolescent alcohol dependence, the other on young heroin dependent people treated with methadone in an innovative community service setting (Doyle *et al.* 1994; Crome *et al.* 1998, 1999). Initial indications are that, despite multiple disadvantages, the majority of these young people were retained in treatment. This group demonstrates different degrees of success in multiple outcome domains (psychosocial functioning, substance misuse, physical health, methadone reduction) over a range of follow-up periods. However, a sizeable minority, 40%, make substantial improvements on psychosocial function, including attainment and maintenance of abstinence.

United States of America

Catalano *et al.* (1990/91) reviewed 29 studies of treatment outcomes. The diversity of treatment modalities and programmes was immense (Rush 1979; Sells and Simpson 1979).

Research design varied as well, with few controlled studies. However, despite these important limitations, the overall conclusion was that 'some treatment' was superior to 'no treatment'.

More recently, Williams and Chang (2000) comprehensively reviewed the literature evaluating 8 multi-programme, multi-site studies and 45 single-programme studies. Average sustained abstinence rates at 6 months were reported in 38%, and at 12 months in 32%. Of note is the finding that 66.6% of relapse in adolescents occurred in the first 3 months post-treatment. Though only a minority of adolescents actually achieve abstinence by the end of a treatment programme, 12 of the 13 studies in which change was recorded showed that up to 50–60% of young people reduced their use of substances. Treatment also impacts on mental health, family function, schooling, and criminality.

The research showed that the majority of adolescents who entered treatment, improved in terms of substance use and general functioning. In view of the lack of treatment control groups, it is not possible to attribute this improvement either to natural recovery or to treatment. Also there was no demonstrable advantage of one treatment over another. Catalano et al. (1990/91) have previously indicated that there is little evidence to suggest that particular interventions are more effective, but conclusive controlled studies have not yet been undertaken.

Deas and Thomas (2001) do provide an overview of ten controlled studies undertaken since 1990. These studies evaluate family therapy, behaviour therapy, cognitive behaviour therapy, pharmacological interventions, and 12-step approaches. In general, family therapy produced improvements in drug use, crime, and family functioning when compared with family education, counselling and group therapy.

Two studies examined behaviour therapy (Azrin et al. 1994) and cognitive behaviour therapy (Kaminer et al. 1998) with supportive counselling and inter-actional group therapy, respectively. Behaviour therapy was associated with improvement in drug use, school and work attendance, and behaviour.

When sertraline and CBT were compared to placebo and CBT, both treated and placebo groups showed reductions in substance use (Deas-Nesmith et al. 1998). When 12-step therapy was compared to CBT, alcohol reduction was in evidence with 12-step but there were no other differences.

The findings do not consistently indicate the superiority of particular intervention modalities, although there appears to be a trend towards effectiveness of behaviour and family therapies. This provides some limited confirmation of the work of Target and Fonagy (1996), which showed the effectiveness of behaviour treatments for adults and adolescents. This lack of evidence of effectiveness of particular interventions is due in part to the paucity of designated services for teenagers who misuse substances.

The implications of the findings of a recently reported study by Brown et al. (2001) are striking. This study assessed 4-year outcomes from adolescent drug and alcohol treatment centres that focused on 12-step abstinence programmes. Although there was an overall reduction in substance misuse, variability in patterns of substance misuse following treatment was found. First, the greatest reduction was found in stimulant use, with some reduction in alcohol and marijuana use, but nicotine use continued in 75% of cases. Second, the researchers described five groups of young people: abstainers (7%), users (8%), slow improvers (8%), worse with time (25%), and continuous heavy users (48%). This points to substantial diversity of outcome. Not surprisingly, better functioning in multiple domains was found in abstainers compared to those who were worse with time and heavy users. Third, despite their improvement, evaluation showed that subjects still used substances more than the general population.

To conclude, the multiple, individual, and developmental needs of a young person must be recognized by practitioners who provide services for young people. Since substance misuse in young people is best viewed as a symptom of complex dysfunction involving young people and their families, their schools, and environment, it should be stressed that any interventions provided will impact on the complex web constituted by each person's familial, cultural, and environmental background. Collaborative working with other professionals to provide broadly based multi-component approaches is therefore essential. Current treatment approaches adapt evidence-based techniques from the adult addiction field, and child and adolescent mental health fields. Cognitive and behavioural approaches, family based approaches, motivational enhancement, and relapse-prevention therapies have empirical support from the adult literature, and much in common with other cognitive behavioural therapies for young people with behavioural problems (Bien *et al.* 1993). Overall, the evidence indicates that treatment is effective, but since young people are a very heterogeneous group, no single approach can be universally effective.

Models of service delivery

The report of the NHS Health Advisory Service (1996) identified a four-tier framework similar to that used in child and adolescent mental health services. This was confirmed by a subsequent report by the Health Advisory Service (2001). The model is best viewed as a flexible and dynamic strategic tool for service design and commissioning, and a framework to conceptualize the service components of an integrated and comprehensive service for children and adolescents who use or misuse substances. This framework emphasizes the service functions, rather than the disciplines involved in delivering care.

Children and young people may need a range of services from a number of tiers at different times. Tiers 1 and 2 are key to the development of a broad base of services, based on a comprehensive approach and achieving of credibility. Continuity of care from Tier 1, particularly in health and education, is crucial. Where and when possible, the interventions should be co-ordinated and managed within Tier 1. This should reduce stigmatization and attempt to 'normalize' young people and their families. Tiers 3 and 4 act as a base for very specialized and focused service functions interventions.

Tier 1: universal, generic, and primary services

This is the frontline of service delivery and targets all young people. The objective is to ensure universal access and continuity of care for all young people, identify and screen those with vulnerability, identify risks and child protection issues, and embed advice and support on tobacco, alcohol, and drug issues into mainstream services. Functions include providing accurate information and advice, health promotion, support to parents, continued care, and work with other disciplines. Information in many formats should be easily available to children and adolescents, their families, and to all staff in Tier 1. All staff who work in generic services should acquire basic skills in recognizing when young people need help as a consequence of their use of substances and basic styles of intervention. In order to do so, they require support from staff of more specialized services.

Tier 2: the first line of specialist services

Tier 2 describes the frontline of specialist services and includes many of the services for children, such as specialist CAMHS, voluntary youth services, paediatrics, child psychology services, and youth justice teams. The principal aim of these more specialist services is to reduce risks and vulnerabilities, and ensure re-integration and/or maintenance of young children in mainstream services. This tier should target young people who are more vulnerable. Interventions include comprehensive assessments, outreach services, crisis management, advice and counselling, family and child therapy, school-liaison, and pharmacological interventions such as non-addiction based treatments (e.g. methylphenidate for hyperactivity disorder). Parental involvement is key.

It is crucial that a comprehensive approach is adopted; care plans require responses to mental and physical health, education, social and youth offending problems to be integrated. Practitioners with skills in providing addiction services should not be employed in isolation but in parallel to other services for children and adolescents.

Training needs in addition to those of Tier 1 practitioners, are to develop and sustain competence in assessment, child development and protection, and relevant therapies, particularly motivational work, brief interventions, and collaboration with child agencies.

Tier 3: specialist substance misuse and addiction services

The functions of this tier are based on the work of a multidisciplinary team trained to deliver services for young people who are engaged in harmful substance misuse. Teams must be capable of comprehensive assessments and able to design complex care plans. In the UK, teams are varied and early in their development.

Thus in practice they may be delivered by the collaborative work of the youth, mental health, paediatric, addiction, youth justice, and voluntary sectors in varying forms. Teams should target young people with specific drug and alcohol problems. Interventions are multi-component and multi-agency to ensure that the complex needs of these young people are met. It is considered that these services are, at the very least, closely linked with all other services for children, and are not simply addiction services delivered to an adult model. The HAS report of 2001 suggested that specialist drug and alcohol services should be fully integrated into young people's services.

Tier 4: very specialized services

Services at Tier 4 are seen as adjuncts to Tier 3 and used for particular interventions, or focused work for short periods. In the UK there is minimal development of residential rehabilitation for children and young people with severe substance misuse problems, though some older adolescents are able to gain access to services for adults. The way forward might, therefore, include augmenting other existing units such as adolescent and forensic psychiatric in-patients, paediatric units (for complicated detoxification), specialized crises placements, specialized housing, and fostering placements. Formal multi-component or highly intensive therapies may require a residential or intensive day capability.

Models of delivery may vary depending on location, local prevalence of substance use and misuse, the local profile of needs of young people, and the nature of services already present. Young people require the addition of skills in managing addictions integrated with, and embedded into, existing services or the development of new services.

Thus service design should be evidence-based. Strategic leadership and management, the clinical realities, the views of carers and users, policy, and researched evidence should inform the function and structure of services. Services should be multidisciplinary and multi-agency, so that they can be responsive to the real needs and preferences of children, young people, and their families. Equally important is the creation of the right organizational culture, therapeutic environment, collaboration, and workforce recruitment, development and retention (Children and Young People's Unit 2001).

A research agenda

The development of a research strategy relating to substance use and misuse by children and young people is central to the implementation of specific interventions and delivery of services of high quality. Research must be prioritized because of the dearth of available information (Crome 1999).

The experience, expertise, and findings from other countries (e.g. North America and Australia) may usefully point to pertinent issues, areas, or aspects of work. However, they cannot substitute for local knowledge. This will avoid unnecessary duplication, where resources are scarce, and point to where extension, expansion, or innovation are required.

The research strategy should be multidisciplinary, multi-site and multi-levelled. Research groups may consist of a variety of people who bring a range of expertise drawn from addiction psychiatry, child and adolescent mental health services, forensic mental health services, the range of paediatric specialties, the social sciences, criminology, health economics, obstetrics and gynaecology, psychology, education, social services, and management. Co-ordination and collaboration between centres is the most logical way to proceed. Research into policy, commissioning, models of delivery, pharmacological treatment, social care, psychological interventions, training, and settings of services are all important, but under-researched, areas.

Mapping the precise nature of specialist services and reviewing research that has been, or is in the process of being, undertaken is a necessary first step. In the UK, monitoring and evaluation of the few pilot Tier 3 and 4 services that serve young people who misuse substances is fundamental. If possible, every effort should be made, so that the same baseline and outcome measures are used to achieve comparability.

Prior to national implementation of prevention or interventions or other initiatives, pilot projects should be encouraged and evaluated. When services have been successfully established they should be used as action research, so that different short-term, medium-term, and long-term projects can be developed. As well as cross-sectional projects, both prospective longitudinal studies and randomized interventions should be developed. Strategic decisions by funding bodies, policymakers, and researchers revolve around the case for a limited number of costly studies, rather than short-term projects. Prioritization of key areas may emerge.

Increasing concern about the rising rate of substance misuse by young people has not been matched by empirical data relating to causation, consequences, complications, associated problems, and care. Thus there is a pressing need to systematically assess those interventions that have been adapted from other situations, settings, or specialties, to modify and adopt them where appropriate, and to innovate, if possible. This process requires training in research competence and in service design. Protected time for clinicians whose expertise is extensive, but in short supply, is mandatory if we are to undertake such complex tasks. Developments must be integrally linked with active workforce planning.

This is an ambitious agenda. It can only be achieved with the assimilation of available data and extensive collaboration in defining the next steps.

The policy context

There have been many policy changes in the last five years in the United Kingdom. Their main thrust is to maximize the inclusion of vulnerable young people in mainstream services. The principle is that of a child-centred, integrative, and comprehensive approach to facilitate inclusion, improve quality of life, and enhance life's opportunities for all children and young people.

In November 2000, the Children and Young People's Unit (CYPU) was established, with its aim to eradicate child poverty and deprivation, as well as youth social exclusion (Children and Young People's Unit 2001). More recent guidance, 'Co-ordinated Service Planning for Vulnerable Children and Young People in England' (Department of Health 2001) suggests that planning services for all children and young people should be undertaken through one co-ordinated exercise.

The National Drugs Strategy (1998), a 10-year drug strategy for England and Wales, adopts young people as a particular target 'to help young people to resist drug misuse in order to achieve their full potential'. Its underlying principles are integration and joint action anchored in an evidence base, effective communication, and accountability.

Within this strategy, the Young People's Substance Misuse Plans (Department of Health 2001) contain impressive objectives, such as the provision of drugs education to all, and provision of information, advice, and support to all vulnerable young people. These plans recommend joint planning and commissioning within all children's systems of services for young people who use or misuse substances.

Further policy advice is contained in documents from the Standing Conference on Drug Abuse (now Drugscope) (1999, 2000). During 2001 there were additional developments that may impact on the way in which services for young people are provided (NHS Health Advisory Service 2001). The National Treatment Agency was established to set standards for the delivery of services for drug misusers in England (Substance Misuse Advisory Service 1999). As we write in 2003, the English and Welsh governments are designing their separate National Service Frameworks for Children and Young People, both of which are likely to recognize the significance of substance use and misuse by children and young people.

References

Azrin, N.H., Donohue, B., Besalel, V.A., Kogan, E.S., and Acierno, R. (1994) Youth drug abuse treatment: a controlled outcome study. *Journal of Child and Adolescent Substance Abuse, 3*, 1–6.

American Psychiatric Association (1994) *Diagnostic and statistical manual of mental disorders* (4th edn). Washington, DC: American Psychiatric Association.

Ball, J.C. and Ross, A. (1991) *The effectiveness of methadone maintenance treatment.* New York: Springer.

Bauman, A. and Phongsavan, P. (1999) Epidemiology of substance use in adolescence: prevalence, trends and policy implications. *Drug and Alcohol Dependence, 55* (3), 187–207.

Bien, T.H., Miller, W.R., and Tonigan, J.S. (1993) Brief interventions for alcohol problems: a review. *Addiction, 88*, 315–36.

Biederman, J., Wilens, T., Mick, E., Spencer, T., and Faraone, S.V. (1999) Pharmacotherapy of attention-deficit/hyperactivity disorder reduces risk of substance use disorder. *Pediatrics, 104* (2), e20.

Botvin, G.J., Baker, E., Dusenbury, L., Botvin, E.M., and Diaz, T. (1995). Long term follow-up results of a randomized pro-drug abuse prevention trial in 9 white middle class population. *Journal of the American Medical Association, 273*, 1106–12.

Brown, S.A., D'Amico, E.J., McCarthy, D.M., and Tapert, S.F. (2001) Four year outcomes from adolescent alcohol and drug treatment. *Journal of Studies on Alcohol, 62*, 381–8.

Carnwath, T. and Hardman, J. (1998). Randomised double-blind comparison of lofexidine and clonidine in the out-patient treatment of opiate withdrawal. *Drug and Alcohol Dependence 30*, 251–4.

Catalano, R.F., Hawkins, J.D., Wells, E.A., Miller, J., and Brewer, D. (1990/91) Evaluation of the effectiveness of adolescent drug abuse treatment, assessment of risks for relapse and promising approaches for relapse prevention. *International Journal of the Addictions, 25* (9A and 10A), 1085–140.

Catalano, R.F., Gainey, R.R., Fleming, C.B., Haggerty, K.P., and Johnson, N.O. (1999) An experimental intervention with families of substance abuses: one year following of the focus on families project. *Addiction, 94*, 241-54.

Children and Young People's Unit (2001) *Tomorrow's future: Building a strategy for children and young people.* London: Children and Young People's Unit.

Chou, C.P., Montgomery, S., Pentz, M.A., Rohrbach, L.A., Johnson, C.A., Flay, B.R., *et al.* (1998) Effects of a community based prevention program on decreasing drug use in high-risk adolescents. *American Journal of Public Health,* **88** (6), 944–8.

Costa, F., Jessor, R., and Turbin, M. (1999). Transition into adolescent problem drinking: the role of psychosocial and protective factors. *Journal of Studies on Alcohol,* **690**, 480–90.

Crome, I.B. (1999) Treatment interventions – looking towards the millennium. *Drug and Alcohol Dependence,* **55**, 247–63.

Crome, I.B., Christian, J., and Green, C. (1998) Tip of the national iceberg ?: profile of adolescent patients prescribed methadone in an innovative community drug service. *Drugs: education, prevention and policy,* **5**, 195–7.

Crome, I.B., Christian, J., and Green, C. (2000) A unique designated community service for adolescents: policy, prevention and education implications. *Drugs: education, prevention and policy,* **7**, 87–108.

Deas, D. and Thomas, S.E. (2001) An overview of controlled studies of adolescent substance abuse treatment. *American Journal of Addictions,* **10**, 178–89.

Deas-Nesmith, D., Randall, C., Roberts, J., *et al.* (1998) Setraline treatment of depressed adolescent alcoholics: a pilot study. *Alcoholism: Clinical and Experimental Research,* **22**, 74A.

Department of Health (1999) *Guidelines on clinical management. Drug misuse and dependence.* Department of Health Norwich: The Stationery Office.

Department of Health (2001) *Coordinated service planning for vulnerable children and young people in England.* London: Department of Health.

Doyle, H., Delaney, W., and Tobin, J. (1994) Follow-up study of young attenders at an alcohol unit. *Addiction,* **89**, 183–9.

Edwards, G. and Gross, M.M. (1976) The alcohol dependence syndrome: provisional description of a clinical syndrome. *British Medical Journal,* **1**, 1058–61.

Ellickson, P.L., Bell, R.M., and McGuigan, K. (1993) Preventing adolescent drug use: long term results of a junior high program. *American Journal of Public Health,* **83**, 856–61.

Ennett, S., Rosenbaum, D.R., Flewelling, R.L., Bieler, G.S., Ringwalt, C.L., and Bailey, S.L. (1994) Long term evaluation of drug abuse resistance education. *Addictive Behaviours,* **19**, 113–25.

Fergusson, D., Lynskey, M., and Horwood, L.J. (1995) The role of peer affiliations, social family and individual factors in continuities in cigarette smoking between childhood and adolescence. *Addiction,* **90**, 647–59.

Flay, B.R., Koepke, D., Thomson, S.J., Santi, S., Best, J.A., and Brown, K.S. (1989) Six-year follow up of the first Waterloo school smoking prevention trial. *American Journal of Public Health,* **79**, 1371–6.

Friedman, A.S., Schwartz, R., and Utada, A. (1989) Outcome of a unique youth drug abuse programme: a follow up study of clients of Straights Inc. *Journal of Substance Abuse Treatment,* **6**, 259–68.

Frischer, M., McArdle, P., and Crome, I.B. (2004) The epidemiology of substance misuse in young people. In *Young People and Substance Misuse* (ed. I. Crome, H. Glodse, E. Gilvarry, and P. McArdle), pp. 31–50. London: Gaskell.

Gilvarry, E. (2000) Substance abuse in young people. *Journal of Child Psychology and Psychiatry,* **41**, 55–80.

Hawkins, J.D., Catalano, R., and Miller, J. (1992) Risk and protective for alcohol and other drug problems in adolescence and early adulthood: implications for substance abuse prevention. *Psychological Bulletin,* **1212**, 64–105.

Hawthorne, G. (1995) Life education's failure to face the facts. *Addiction,* **90,** 1404–6.

Health Advisory Service (2001) *The substance of young needs.* London: Health Advisory Service.

Henggeler, S.W., Melton, G.B., and Smith, L.A. (1992) Family preservation using multi-systemic therapy: an effective alternative to incarcerating serious juvenile offenders. *Journal of Consulting and Clinical Psychology,* **60**, 953–61.

Hibell, B., Andersson, B., Ahlstrom, S., Balakirevao Bjarnason, T., Kokkevi, A., and Morgan, M. (1999) *The ESPAD (European School Project on Alcohol and other Drugs).* Stockholm: Swedish Council for Information on Alcohol and Other Drugs.

Hops, H., Davies, B., and Lewin, I. (1999) The development of alcohol and other substance use: a gender study of family and peer context. *Journal of Studies on Alcohol,* 1999 (suppl 13), 22–31.

Hurry, J. and Lloyd, C. (1997) *A follow-up evaluation of project CHARLIE: a life skills drug education programme for primary schools.* London: Home Office Drugs Prevention.

Joanning, H., Quinn, T., and Mullen, R. (1992) Treating adolescent drug abuse: comparison of family systems therapy, group therapy and family drug education. *Journal of Marital and Family Therapy,* **18**, 345–56.

Kaminer, Y., Burleson, J., Blitz, C., Sussman, J., and Rounsaville, B. (1998) Psychotherapies for adolescent substance abusers, a pilot study. *Journal of Nervous and Mental Diseases,* **186**, 684–90.

Kershaw, C., Budd, T., Kinshott, G., Mattinson, J., Mayhew, P., and Myhill, A. (2000) *The 2000 British Crime Survey.* London: Home Office.

Kumpfer, K.L., Molgaard, V., and Spoth, R. (1996) The 'Strengthening Families Programme' for the prevention of delinquency and drug use In *Preventing childhood disorders substance misuse and delinquency* (ed. R. Peters and R. McMahon), pp. 241–67. Thousand Oaks, CA: Sage Publications.

Lewinsohn, P., Rohde, P., and Brown, R. (1999) Level of current and past cigarette smoking as predictors of future substance use disorders in young adulthood. *Addiction,* **94**, 913–21.

Lewis, R., Piercy, F., Sprenkle, D., and Trepper, T. (1990) Family-based interventions and community networking for helping drug abusing adolescents. The impact of near and far environments. *Journal of Adolescence Research,* **50**, 82–95.

McBride, N., Midford, R., Farringdon, F., and Phillips, M. (2000). Early results form a school alcohol harm minimisation study: the school and early harm reduction project. *Addiction,* **95**, 1021–42.

Mirrlees-Black, C., Budd, T., Partridge, S., and Mayhew, P. (1998) *The 1998 British Crime Survey: England and Wales.* London: Home Office.

National Drugs Strategy (1998) *Tackling drugs together to build a better Britain. The government's ten-year strategy for tackling drug misuse.* Cm3945. London: The Stationary Office.

NHS Health Advisory Service (1996) *Children and young people. substance misuse services. The substance of young needs.* London: HMSO.

National Institute for Clinical Excellence (2002) *Technology Appraisal Guidance No. 38: Nicotine replacement therapy (NRT) and Bupropion for smoking cessation.* London: National Institute for Clinical Excellence.

Office for National Statistics (ONS) (1998) *General Household Survey.* London: HMSO.

O'Malley, P. and Johnstone, L. (1999) Drinking and driving among US high school seniors 1984–1997. *American Journal of Public Health,* **89**, 678–84.

Perry, C.L., Kelder, S.H., Murray, D.M., and Kleep, K.I. (1992) Community wide smoking prevention: long term outcomes of the Minnesota heart health program and the class of 1989 study. *American Journal of Public Health,* **9**, 1210–6.

Project MATCH Research Group (1997a) Matching alcoholism treatments to client heterogeneity: Project MATCH post treatment drinking outcomes. *Journal of Studies on Alcohol,* **58**, 7–29.

Project MATCH Research Group (1997b) Project MATCH secondary a priority hypothesis. *Addiction,* **92**, 1671–98.

Ramsey, M. and Percy, A. (1997) A national household survey of drug misuse in Britain: a decade of development. *Addiction,* **92**, 931–7.

Ramsey, M. and Spiller, J. (1997) *Drug misuse declared in 1996: latest results from the British Crime Survey Home Office Research Study 127.* London: HMSO.

Ramsey, M., Baker, P., Goulden, C., Sharp, C., and Sondhi, A. (2001) *Drug misuse declared in 2000: results from the British Crime Survey Home Office Research Study No. 224.* London: HMSO.

Riggs, P., Mikulich, S., Whitmore, E., and Crowley, T. (1999). Relationship of ADHD, depression and non-tobacco substance use disorders to nicotine dependence in substance-dependant delinquents. *Drug and Alcohol Dependence*, **54**, 195–205.

Rosenberg, M.F. and Anthony, J.C. (2001) Early clinical manifestations of cannabis dependence in a community sample. *Drug and Alcohol Dependence*, **64** (2), 123–31.

Rush, T.V. (1979) Predicting treatment outcomes for juvenile and young adult clients in the Pennsylvania substance abuse system. In *Youth drug abuse* (ed. G.M. Beschner and A.S. Friedman), pp. 629–56. Lexington MA: Lexington Books.

Sells, S.B. and Simpson, D.D. (1979) Evaluation of treatment outcome for youths in the drug abuse reporting programme (DARP): a follow up study. In *Youth drug abuse* (ed. G.M. Beschner and A.S. Friedman), pp. 571–628. Lexington MA: Lexington Books.

Shope, J.T., Kloska, D.D., Dielman, T.E., and Maharg, R. (1994) Longitudinal evaluation of an enhanced alcohol misuse prevention study (AMPS) curriculum for grades six-eight. *Journal of School Health*, **64** (4), 160–6.

Sibthorpe, B., Drinkwater, J., Gardner, K., and Bammer, G. (1995) Drug use, binge drinking and attempted suicide among homeless and potentially homeless youth. *Australia and New Zealand Journal of Psychiatry*, **29**, 248–56.

Shaffer, D., Gould, M., Fisher, P., Trautman, P., Moreau, D., Kleinman, M., *et al.* (1996) Psychiatric diagnosis in child and adolescent suicides. *Archives of General Psychiatry*, **53**, 339–48.

Standing Conference on Drug Abuse (SCODA) (1999) *Young People and Drugs: Policy Guidance in Drug Interventions.* London: Standing Conference on Drug Abuse & Children's Legal Centre.

Standing Conference on Drug Abuse SCODA (2000) *Vulnerable young people and drugs Opportunities to tackle inequalities.* London: Drugscope.

Stewart, D.G. and Brown, S. (1995) Withdrawal and dependency symptoms among adolescent alcohol and drug abusers. *Addiction*, **9**, 627–35.

Substance Misuse Advisory Service (1999) *Commissioning standards—drug and alcohol treatment and care.* London: HAS.

Target, M. and Fonagy, P. (1996) The psychological treatment of child and adolescent psychiatric disorders. In *What works for whom? A critical review of psychotherapy research* (ed. A. Roth and P. Fonagy), pp. 263–320. New York: Guilford Press.

Vartiainen, E., Fallonen, U., McAlister, A.L., and Puska, P. (1990) Eight year follow up results of adolescent smoking prevention programme: the North Karelia Youth Project. *American Journal of Public Health*, **80**, 78–9.

Swadi, H. (1999) Individual risk factors for adolescent substance use. *Drug and Alcohol Dependence*, **55**, 209–24.

Wagner, E.F., Brown, S.A., Monti, P.M., Myers, M.G., and Waldron, H.B. (1999) Innovations in adolescent substance abuse intervention. *Alcoholism: Clinical and Experimental Research*, **23**, 236–49.

Ward, J., Mattick, P.D., and Hall, W. (1998). *Methadone maintenance treatment and other opiate replacement therapies.* Australia: Harwood Academic Publishers.

Williams, R. and Chang, S. (2000) A comprehensive and comparative review of adolescent substance abuse treatment outcome. *Clinical Psychology: Science and Practice Summary*, **7**, 138–66.

World Health Organization (1992) *International classification of mental and behavioural disorders (ICD)* (10th edn). Geneva: World Health Organization.

Young People's Substance Misuse Plans (2001) *Guidance for drug action teams.* London: UKADCU.

Zeitlin H (1999) Psychiatric co-morbidity with substance misuse in children and teenagers. *Drug and Alcohol Dependence*, **55**, 225–34.

Examples of prevention programmes are described

Smoking prevention

The 1989 Waterloo School Smoking Prevention Trial (Flay *et al.* 1989) used social influences to raise awareness in sixth-grade students. By twelfth grade, programme effects were no longer evident.

The North Karelia Youth Project (Vartiainen *et al.* 1990) used project leaders to enhance refusal skills for smoking. At a 15-year follow up the authors concluded that the intervention delayed smoking uptake but did not prevent it.

The Minnesota Smoking Prevention Project (Perry *et al.* 1992), an intensive school-based behavioural intervention programme, concluded that multiple-intervention components, such as behavioural education in schools, booster programmes to sustain training, and community wide strategies may all be needed to sustain lasting reductions in adolescent tobacco use.

Alcohol prevention

The Alcohol Misuse Prevention Study (AMPS) (Shope *et al.* 1994) focused on reduction by social resistance skills in a high risk student group. Although knowledge increased, alcohol misuse did not change.

The Western Australia Schools Health and Harm Reduction Project (SHAHRP) aimed to reduce harm rather than preventing and delaying use. Dealing with high risk drinking situations was the focus, and positive effects were found (McBride *et al.* 2000).

Drugs, alcohol, and tobacco

Drug Abuse Resistance Education (Ennett *et al.* 1994)—this widely used programme, which is curriculum based and includes resistance and personal skills training, has yielded inconsistent results.

Project ALERT also utilized social resistance skills (Ellickson *et al.* 1993). However, initial positive changes were not sustained. Project STAR (Students Taught Awareness and Resistance) was a 2-year multi-component intervention (family, community, media, health policy, school) with booster sessions. Follow-up demonstrated about 25% less use of cannabis, alcohol and smoking (Chou *et al.* 1998).

Life Skills Training (Botvin 1995) adopted broader personal and social skills to prevent tobacco, alcohol and marijuana use among students. This comprised a 3-year programme including booster sessions.

Life Education Centres (LECs) target young children using mobile classrooms and eclectic techniques. Though popular in some areas, effectiveness has yet to be established (Hawthorne 1995).

The Illiwara Drugs Education Project included teaching, group work, peer and parental influence at primary school. Although fewer children tried nicotine and cannabis there was no change in alcohol use.

Project CHARLIE, evaluated with controls (Hurry and Lloyd 1997) in the UK, used information and life-skills to equip primary school children to resist offers of drugs. Use of tobacco and illegal drug use appeared to be reduced though numbers were small.

Assessment Protocol

Demographics

Age
Gender
Stage of education/training
Employment
Social circumstances: living conditions (homelessness)
Referral details

Drug Use

General

Attitudes to substance misuse
Experimentation/recreational use
Coping mechanisms

Substance used

Tobacco, alcohol, over the counter and prescribed, all illicit
Age of first use/context of use
Current use/last use—quantity/frequency
Use in past week, month and year and previous pattern
Dependence and withdrawal features
Tolerance
Periods of abstinence or reduction
Associated problems: psychosocial and physical
Treatment history including detoxification and
      medication

Past Developmental History

Parental

Parenting relationships including supervision
Parental substance use, mental and physical illness
Employment
Socio-economic status
Developmental issues including competence to consent
Illnesses unrelated to substance misuse

Childhood

Social activities e.g leisure, hobbies, sport, religion
Schooling: attendance, ability and attainment
Behavioural problems/consequences

Social Environment

Living environment: parental home, violence, deprivation
Peer group affiliation/attitudes
Criminality—history/offences/sentences

Psychological Health

Psychological distress
Self image/self esteem
History of depression, ADHD, DSH, psychosis
Recent bereavement or separation
Neglect/abuse
Involvement of Social Services/Care Issues/Criminal Justice System
Treatment agencies involved

Physical Health	Infections e.g. HIV, Hepatitis B & C
	History of STD
	Consequences of route of use

Further Issues	
Collateral information and informants	Parental interview/other agencies/school record
	Toxicology, biochemistry and haematology
Investigations	Mental state
	Legal issues
	Diagnoses, formulation and care plan

Chapter 20

Children and adolescents who have a learning disability: the challenges to services

William Fraser

The extent of needs of younger people and their families

Families of children with learning disabilities (LD) face increased financial, physical, and mental hardship. The parents of young people with learning disabilities have almost invariably the following preoccupations: the search for causes, the need for early assessment and reliable diagnosis, the problem of access to advice on behaviour problems and to respite, the frustrations of statementing (the statement of a child's educational needs), the complexities of transition to adult life and what will become of him/her when 'we are too old to be there for him'.

The cycle of disadvantage for children with learning disabilities is often profound compared to that which is generally found in child psychiatry. First, the causes of learning disability, genetic and acquired, enter into the equation. Greenough *et al.* (1990) comment that disruptive early brain development may jeopardize later experience-dependent systems. Rutter (1989) describes pathways from child to adult life, where a chain of constraining environmental effects are set in motion by a single negative event—a compounded cycle of deprivation. Families with children with learning disability face decreased recognition by teachers of multiple disorders in their children.

The frustrations of the search for causes often exhaust families and are exemplified by the way the MMR scare has clouded the field of Autism (Medicines Control Agency 2001). Autistic disorders are also often not assessed and detected at an early stage, but commonly 1–2 years after the diagnosis is suspected. There is also decreased service utilization when parents are of limited intellect, are unemployed, or in other ways socially disadvantaged.

Fifty per cent of children with learning disabilities have significant behaviour problems. These tend to decrease through childhood in children with severe learning disabilities, but as regards the mildly learning disabled, we do not have longitudinal studies. Children with autistic disorder tend to show rather less aggression and self-aggression in adolescence, although their size may make them harder to manage. Down's children similarly often become calmer, even sluggish, in early adult life. Adults with learning disability have a lower rate of contact with professionals than they had in childhood.

Learning disability affects 2–3% of the population (Rolleveld *et al.* 1997). The higher overall rates of psychological disturbance in children with learning disabilities (Dykens 2000) persist into adult life, with the additional effects of low self-esteem, problems with peers, and long-term effects of co-morbid neuro-psychiatric deficits such as autistic disorder, epilepsy, and attention deficit disorder.

Children with learning disability are often dysmorphic; this may compound self-consciousness in social encounters and low self-esteem. Bullying is more common where there are no stigmata. Bullying is an almost inevitable part of the life of a child with high-functioning autism or Asperger syndrome.

Boys with mild learning disability are twice as likely to offend and in early adult life, four times as likely (Hodgkins 1992). Smoking, alcohol, or substance abuse are not, however, common in this group. There is often a background of considerable social disadvantage in their families, with poor education, housing, and employment. Teenage pregnancy is increased (Rauch-Elnekave 1994).

Sleep problems in children with learning disability are more likely than in ordinary children. They are common, with prevalence rates of at least 35%. They are more severe at a younger age and in the more severely intellectually disabled (Quine 1991), the most problematic being night wakening and settling. They are particularly associated with parental stress.

A confused response

Services for people with learning disabilities have for the last 30 years been based on a well-articulated set of values based on normalization (Box 20.1). This unassailable philosophy has been incorporated into legislation, refined, and modified by the practicalities of public acceptance and funding. As expectations have risen, we have seen increased responsibilities cast on to the educational and social services in respect of children with learning disabilities, and uncovered a dearth of adequate training. As regards the health services, when the traditional mental deficiency institutions closed and specialist nurse training in mental handicap dissolved, a cadre of experienced professionals and their knowledge and skills were lost. We were left with a range of attitudes. As Bullock and Little (1999) pointed out, the sharp differences in theoretical basis and organizational structures that divide our agencies and the different perceptions between, for example, education, social services, and health of what services are for, make communication difficult. We even have difficulty in agreeing definitions on nomenclature. The British term 'learning disability'[1] is confusing and has a different meaning in most other countries. Even in the UK, what does it mean? The assessment of intellectual functioning through reliance on IQ tests is fraught with the possibility of misuse, yet services do demarcate their services' rigidity using IQ tests that have a zone of uncertainty of 3–5 points. Low IQ scores are not sufficient for diagnosis. Community support teams vary in their acceptance criteria geographically throughout Britain. Some address only severe learning disability, some include mild learning disability. Some disagree on what is challenging behaviour.

Only 10–25% of children of normal intelligence who have mental health problems receive mental health help. More than 50% of children with severe learning disabilities have significant mental health problems but only a small percentage receive/d services (Chadwick *et al.* 1998).

----

[1] Learning disability (US = mental retardation) refers to substantial limitations in present functioning. It is characterized by significantly sub-average intellectual functioning, existing concomitantly with related limitations in two or more of the following applicable adaptive skill areas: communication, self-care, home living social skills, community use, self-direction, health and safety, functional academics, leisure, and work manifest before the age of 18 years (AAMR 1992).

Box 20.1 Normalization (Wolfensberger 1972)

* rights
* individuality
* development
* social integration
* culture appropriateness
* age appropriateness
* access to generic services

The procedure of statementing special needs is bureaucratic and for professionals and parents exasperating. It is currently accepted wisdom and government policy to try to fit children with learning disabilities into mainstream environments, if possible. Parents, too, invest too much of their hope on attaining for their child a mainstream education, which may mean simply much larger classes and less special teaching. The mainstream philosophy aspires to creating opportunities for peer-group integration (and accordingly better transition into employment), but special classes have staff who have additional experience or programmes, for example, staff trained in autistic disorders and TEACCH programmes (Schopler 1998). We know that children with low self-esteem and unhappy educational experience are more likely to develop conduct problems. Thus children with mild to moderate learning disabilities are more vulnerable to conduct disorder. The presentation of psychiatric problems in children with learning disability will often be different from those in the intellectually normal. There will also be more attention deficit disorder, more self-injurious behaviour stemming from additional stress, communication difficulties, and low self-esteem, and a higher incidence of disturbances stemming from autistic disorder and specific language disorders. It has also to be explained to the parents of children with autism that rearing such children needs a different set of rules. Approaches to parenting autistic children 'do not come naturally'.

Expectations have also understandably been raised by the accelerating knowledge, skills, and enlightenment of staff across a range of professions involved in developmental medicine. This far exceeds the ability of purchasers to fund gold standard services. Confusion is magnified by ineffective strategic planning and commissioning. For the most challenging children, too many health, education, and social services have resorted to 'out of county' placements, after often unseemly skirmishes over funding with each other and with the parents. 'Out of area' placements are particularly common for young people with severe challenging behaviour. While all children with low-functioning autism will require special education, 60% of children with high-functioning autism also attend a special school; 20% have special education on a part-time basis and extra support in mainstream schools; and 20% attend mainstream schools without extra support; 15% of all children with autism attending special schools are in residential school. The annual average cost for residential care for people with autism and additional learning disability was estimated in 1999 as £29 378 (Jarbrink and Knapp 2001). This increases the procrastination of health/education and social services about doing the right thing. Commissioners may go sightseeing for the best service and return naïvely expecting that hard-pressed local clinicians can emulate standards of tertiary services at a national level.

In theory, the strategic intent of child and adolescent mental health services ought to be to prevent mental health problems and promote young people's well-being and social inclusion across the range of intellect, but many current child and adolescent services in the United Kingdom, and in many other parts of the world, do not have the knowledge, skills, or experience (or if they have, cannot deploy such skills) to take on the care of children with learning disabilities or children on the autistic spectrum.

The adolescent offender who is mildly learning disabled presents a particular problem to services and often there is neither the readiness of CAMHs nor of LD services to plan or provide premises or treat such children. Often their experience of emotional and physical child abuse has kindled problems of sexuality for which there are seldom experienced professionals available. They do not fit easily into forensic services.

Such pressures to rationalize psychiatry services in respect of children come from the Royal Colleges (paediatrics and psychiatry), NICE, local authorities, and children's commissioners (*vide* Wales), and child health service commissioners. The English 2001 White Paper 'Valuing people' identifies the need for CAMHS for learning disabilities, and there are plans to move children (LD services) into an all-purpose children's team. We have to fit our services to children's needs rather than professionals' traditional interests and bailliewicks. Child LD services belong in CAMHS, but need mental health staff experienced in LD services.

There are as many children in the population who are failing to receive services, as those that get them (Rutter cited by Williams 2000), and in the case of children with learning disabilities, research by Angold *et al.* (1987) shows that it is the burden, as experienced by adults in dealing with problematic children, that indicates who gets referred. So also for those with learning disabilities: the ones referred are those in whom families have been unable to get round the burden by their informal arrangements. Gallimore *et al.* (1989) employ the term ecocultural niche, 'econiche' (Super and Harkness 1986) to refer to the family's collective action to accommodate to a handicapped child, based on parental beliefs and attitudes, and visible in routines 'to get through the day'. Knapp and Henderson (1999) have shown the importance of looking at the links between child problems and the impact in adults. Just as child psychiatry is evolving, so is the specialty of learning disability but in a different way from in child psychiatry; learning disability has been a hospital-based service and then a community service; and both child and learning disability services now make demands on the private sector, particularly for offenders and people with autistic disorder.

The diagnoses of learning disability and of autism are usually complex. Even specialists experienced in autism can miss it in some individuals. However, for the pervasive developmental difficulties, there are now a range of screening tests, developmental surveillance, and diagnostic instruments. The problems, however, often really start after diagnosis.

The search for effective interventions is particularly frenetic in autistic spectrum disorders. Two behavioural approaches are the only ones with some evidential basis.

Applied behavioural analysis and contingent positive and negative reinforcement are used in the Lovaas technique (Lovaas 1981). This approach requires over 40 hours per week individual attention and costs exceeding £16 000 p.a. TEACCH recognizes autistic children's needs for environmental stability and predictability, and prominently employs visual cues.

To summarize the strength of scientific evidence of therapeutic approaches to young children with autism, there is strong evidence for intensive behavioural and educational programmes and moderate evidence for psycho-active medications for behaviour disorders; some limited evidence for auditory integration, music therapy, and vitamin therapies; but no evidence for anti-yeast therapy, developmental individual differences relationships (DIR), diet therapies, facilitated communication, hormone therapies, immunological therapies, parent training, and sensory integration therapy (Jacobson and Mulick 2000). Parents search the Web for the latest cures and diets, and websites have been created to help them avoid charlatans (e.g. www.quackwatch.com).

Transition issues

Policies vary in CAMHS at 16 years for children with learning disabilities. Some services declare abruptly that on their sixteenth birthday such children become the responsibility of learning disability services. For children with autistic disorders, responsibilities are even more complex. As 75% of such children have IQs < 70, they will come under learning disability teams (and this amounts to a prevalence of 5 per 10 000—Fombonne 1998) but for the high-functioning autistic or Asperger syndrome adolescent (even commoner, perhaps 1–2 per 1000), there are no clear lines of responsibility.

The confusion can get worse for learning disabled children at transition, which involves moves to further education, vocational and residential placements. It is not only a time of change for the young person but also for their family (Box 20.2; McIntosh and Whittaker 1998). Transition planning includes the young person in decision-making; giving parents their place in the process; attending to cultural issues; improving the opportunities after school; inter-agency collaboration, and recognition that transition is an ongoing process.

Early in 2000 the government launched the Connexions Strategy document (Department for Education and Employment 2000). This described a new youth support service for all young people aged 13–19 to be developed over 2–3 years, to ensure that all young people have the opportunity to learn the skills they need to make a success of their adult lives by providing a high-quality pathway with effective systems of support.

Moving on—late adolescence and beyond

Behaviour problems add to the difficulties of young people with learning disability on entering and holding open employment. Adults with autism and additional learning disabilities exemplify the situation, approximately 15% of whom are in sheltered employment. Of autistic people without learning disability, 35% are in sheltered employment and 50% are sometimes in open employment, and perhaps 10–20% attend day centres.

Box 20.2 Transition issues

Service transition can cover moves to further education, vocational, and residential placements. It is not only a time of change for the young person but also for their family.
(McIntosh and Whitaker 1998)

Concluding remarks

Most of the care for people with learning disability comes from the families, and this greatly increases opportunity costs for parents earning perhaps 20% less than comparable families (Fujiura *et al.* 1994; Office of National Statistics 1998). Family costs for extra expenditure for a child with autism and additional learning disability is at least £2000 p.a., but we need more exact studies. The average lifetime costs for a person with autism and additional learning disability has been estimated as £2.94 million (Jarbrink and Knapp 2001).

Psychiatric services for children with learning disabilities are still geographically haphazard and varied, and the templates for a better deal for families of young people with mental disabilities are slow in being formed. The speed of improvement has not been what was expected three decades ago when 'normalization' was enunciated. We did not then, however, have the knowledge, skills, techniques, or funds to permit inclusion. We now know that some early interventions significantly reduce the likelihood of behaviour problems, and, in the case of autistic disorder, can produce significant IQ gain.

We also are coming to know which interventions are based on evidence, which is now readily accessible from health evidence bulletins—Wales. http://hebw.uwcm.ac.uk and from the National Electronic Library.

References

American Association on Mental Retardation (AAMR) (1992) *Definitions and classification* (9th edn). Washington, DC: AAMR.

Angold, A., Weissman, M.M., John, K., Merikangas, K.R., Prusoff, B.A., Wickramaratne, P. *et al.* (1987) Parent and child reports of depressive symptoms in children at low and high risk of depression. *Journal of Child Psychology and Psychiatry*, **28**, 901–15.

Bullock, R. and Little, M. (1999) The interface between Social and Health Services for child and adolescent persons—unit status. *Current Opinion in Psychiatry*, **12**, 421–34.

Chadwick, O., Taylor, E., and Bernard, S. (1998) *The prevention of behaviour disorders in children with severe learning disability.* Final Report to the NHS Executive. London: Institute of Psychiatry.

Department of Education and Employment (2000) *Connexions the best start in life for every young person.* London: Department of Education and Employment.

Dykens, E.M. (2000) Psychopathology in children with intellectual disability. *Journal of Child Psychology and Psychiatry*, **41**, 407–18.

Fombonne, E. (1998) Epidemiological surveys of autism. In *Autism and pervasive developmental disorders* (ed. F.R. Volkmar), pp. 32–63. Cambridge: Cambridge University Press.

Fujiura, G.T., Roccoforte, J.A., and Braddock, D. (1994) Costs of family care for adults with mental retardation and related developmental disabilities. *American Journal of Mental Retardation*, **3**, 250–61.

Gallimore, R., Weisner, T., Kaufman, S., and Bernheimer, L. (1989) The social construction of the eco-cultural niches: family accommodation of developmentally delayed children. *American Journal of Mental Retardation*, **94**, 216–30.

Greenough, W.T., Black, J.R., Chang, F-L.F., and Sirevaag, A.M. (1990) Might different brain information storage processes operating at different developmental ages affect compensation for early developmental disabilities? In *Key issues in mental retardation* (ed. W. Fraser), pp. 46–56. London: Routledge.

Hodgins, S. (1992) Mental disorder, intellectual deficiency and crime—evidence from a birth cohort. *Archives of General Psychiatry*, **49**, 476–83.

Jacobson, J. and Mulick, J. (2000) System and cost research issues in treatments for people with Autistic Disorders. *Journal of Autism and Developmental Disorders*, **30**, 585.

Jarbrink, K. and Knapp, M. (2001) The economic impact of autism in Britain. *Autism*, 5, 7–22.

Knapp, M.K. and Henderson, J. (1999) Health economic perspectives and evaluation of child and adolescent mental health services. *Current Opinion in Psychiatry*, 12, 393–7.

Lovaas, O.I. (1981) *Teaching developmentally disabled children. The ME book.* Austin, TX: Pro-Ed.

McIntosh, B. and Whittaker, A. (1998) (ed.) *Days of change—a parental guide to developing better day opportunities with people with learning difficulties.* London: King's Fund.

Medicines Control Agency (2001) MMR vaccine: the facts. *Current Problems*, 27, 1–3.

Office for National Statistics (1998a) *New Earnings Survey 1998.* The Stationery Office, London.

Quine, L. (1991) Sleep problems in children with severe learning difficulties. *JMDR*, 35, 269–90.

Rauch-Elnekave, H. (1994) Teenage motherhood: its relationship to undetected learning problems. *Adolescence*, 29, 91–103.

Roeleveld, N., Zeilheis, G.A., and Gabreels, F. (1997) The prevalence of mental retardation: a critical review of recent literature. *Developmental Medicine and Child Neurology*, 39, 125–32.

Rutter, M. (1989) Pathways from childhood to adult life. *Journal of Child Psychology and Psychiatry*, 30, 25–53.

Schopler, E. (1998) *Implementation of TEACCH philosophy. Handbook of autism and pervasive developmental disorders* (2nd edn), pp. 767–95. Chichester: Wiley.

Super, C. and Harkness, S. (1986) The developmental niche: a conceptualisation at the interface of child and culture. *International Journal of Behavioral Development*, 9, 1–25.

Williams, R. (2000) *A cunning plan: integrating evidence, judgment and passion in mental health strategy.* Inaugural lecture, University of Glamorgan, 13 March 2000.

Wolfensberger, W. (1972) *The principle of normalization in human services.* Toronto, ON: National Institute on Mental Retardation.

Chapter 21

Services for children who are hearing or visually impaired

Peter Hindley and Richard Williams

Introduction

The terms hearing impairment and visual impairment cover large groups of children, from children with intermittent hearing impairments due to glue ear or well-managed severe myopia, to deaf children who use sign language or blind children. This section of the chapter on disability is concerned with children who have severe to profound, bilateral, and permanent sensory impairments. In addition, this chapter considers children with combined visual and hearing impairment. It touches briefly on services for hearing children of deaf adults (or CODAs) who often present challenges to generic services.

The prevalence and aetiology of sensory impairment

It is not possible to make a definitive statement about the size of the population of deaf children in the UK. In 1998, The NHS Health Advisory Service (HAS) reported that the National Deaf Children's Society's estimate of 20 000 deaf children being educated in settings that use some form of sign language (from British Sign Language to SSE). However, there is still a substantial number of children being educated in purely aural/oral systems who are likely to become British sign language users when they grow up. In a longitudinal study of deaf children educated in the 1970s and 1980s (Gregory *et al.* 1995) when aural/oral systems were far more prevalent, 70% identified themselves as using either British Sign Language or SSE when they entered adulthood. The outcomes for deaf children are likely to continue changing with the introduction of universal neonatal screening and the use of cochlear implants.

The term 'severe hearing impairment' means children with hearing losses of 70 dB or more, and for severe visual impairment this means children with less than 3/60 Snellen visual acuity or a visual field of 20 degrees or less at maximum diameter. Table 21.1 gives the prevalence of these impairments in childhood populations.

Children with severe to profound hearing impairment are referred to as deaf, and severe visual impairment is shortened to SVI from this point on in this summary. Hindley and van Gent (2002) provide a summary of the epidemiology of hearing and visual impairment.

The majority of deaf children are now deaf as a result of recessive genetic deafness affecting the cochlea or auditory nerve and not causing pervasive brain abnormalities. The minority are deaf as a result of the complications of severe prematurity and intra-uterine (e.g. CMV) or neonatal infections (e.g. meningitis), or complex syndromes, such as CHARGE, many with associated brain and central nervous system abnormalities. These include intra-uterine infections such as CMV and Rubella, perinatal birth trauma and illness, craniofacial abnormalities

Table 21.1 Prevalence of hearing and visual impairments in childhood

Type of impairment	Prevalence
Severe – profound hearing impairment	1/1000
Severe visual impairment	1/10000
Deafness / blindness	1/100,000

and bacterial meningitis. Thus, for the majority of deaf children, developing effective communication and language is their major potential hurdle, and only a minority will have additional impairments, if this is managed effectively.

By contrast, the majority of children with SVI have associated pervasive brain abnormalities and so additional impairments are more common. Even in children with SVI who do not have gross signs of neurological disorders, serious developmental disorders are common (Cass 1998). However, failure to provide deaf children with adequate communication and language, whether British sign language or a spoken language, can lead to significant secondary disabilities of thinking and emotional and social functioning.

The consequences and nature of sensory impairment

Hearing and visual impairment are both low-incidence conditions. However the developmental consequences of hearing and visual impairment are substantially different, and planning and delivery of child and adolescent mental health services (CAMHS) for these two groups of children needs to be substantially different. These two groups share one fundamental feature: that is that the vast majority of deaf children (95%) and children with SVI (more than 99%) are born to parents who are sighted and hearing. The process of parental adjustment to a child with impairment is central to the child's health development and influences CAMHS clinical work profoundly.

Language use in deaf children is a central feature of deafness. The vast majority are born into hearing families but, historically, a majority of deaf children have grown up to use British Sign Language (BSL). Thus, those children who grow up to join the deaf community make a transition from their hearing families, in which spoken language predominates, to a community in which BSL predominates.

BSL is a visuo-spatial language; its grammar and lexicon is wholly different from English. Support for parents and other family members to develop BSL is very variable across the UK and some families are reluctant to do so. Many deaf BSL users identify with a specific deaf culture within which experiencing the world visually, and belonging to an oppressed minority, are central features (Meadow-Orlans and Erting 2000). Thus, for CAMHS, deaf children who use BSL share many experiences with children from cultural minorities but come from families who do not necessarily share the same cultural identity and may have great difficulty in communicating with their deaf child.

When children are born in parts of the country in which BSL is seen as central to deaf children's development, parents are likely to be offered opportunities to learn BSL as soon as their child's deafness is confirmed. There is experience suggesting that, in other areas, oral-aural language is encouraged and parents are, in effect, discouraged from using BSL. As a result, language development in deaf children in the UK is highly idiosyncratic. The HAS (1998) expressed its observation that, 'Some children acquire BSL and have families that have supported and encouraged them to do so, while others acquire BSL as if by default. Yet again, others acquire almost no language, whether spoken or signed, at all'.

The mental health needs of deaf children and children with SVI

The body of knowledge about the mental health needs of deaf children is more substantial than that of children with SVI.

Deaf children are known to be approximately one-and-one-half to two times more vulnerable to mental health problems than hearing children. Thus, my group (Hindley *et al.* 1994) estimated the likely prevalence of child mental health problems (ranging from emotional and behavioural disorders to major mental illnesses) in deaf children and adolescents to be around 40%. However, the majority of these children will, theoretically, not require a specialist service. The NHS Health Advisory Service (HAS) report on CAMHS, *Together we stand* (1995), points out that, in hearing populations with an overall prevalence rate of disorders of up to 25%, 7–10% of children and adolescents have severe problems that meet the criteria for 'caseness' in international classifications and 2.1% have disabling problems. If these figures are adjusted pro rata for a higher overall prevalence of mental health problems, the prevalence of severe problems in deaf children would lie in the range 11–16% and 3.4% for disabling problems.

Twenty thousand is likely to be a conservative estimate of the number of deaf children who could potentially need a specialist mental health service though, if services for deaf children were working at their optimum, this would suggest an annual caseload in the range of 650–3200 for the UK.

Children who have a hearing impairment appear to be vulnerable to both emotional and behavioural problems though, as in the hearing population, more children with behavioural problems are presented to the specialist services. There is no record of proven increased vulnerability to psychotic disorders but deaf children do appear to have a significantly increased vulnerability to autism and related disorders (Hindley 2000).

Children with SVI are also more vulnerable to mental health problems but the epidemiological data is more limited. The only general population study comes from the 1970s and that suggested that approximately 60% of children with SVI have either psychiatric or cognitive problems. It is very difficult to say how this translates into contemporary practice. More recent studies are inconsistent, with some suggesting raised rates of mental health problems in children with VI and others the converse (Hindley and Gent 2002).

Why deaf children and children with SVI are more vulnerable to mental health problems and disorders

Once again, more is known about the mechanisms that link hearing impairment to mental disorder than the equivalent for children with SVI. However, there seems to be an increase in all types of disorder amongst children with SVI, but particularly autism and related disorders (Cass 1998). Primarily, this appears to be as a result of pervasive brain abnormalities, though delays in social development, arising from a lack of visual interaction, may also contribute.

Deaf children's increased vulnerability to emotional and behavioural disorders primarily relates to experiential deprivation as a result of limited communication, and distorted parental attitudes. Experience shows that many children with hearing impairment also have low self-esteem. Their increased vulnerability to autism relates primarily to pervasive brain abnormalities, but limitations in their communication environment may compound communication and social difficulties arising from the autism.

Difficulties and differences in communication clearly have a profound impact on the mental health of children with a sensory impairment (Hindley 2000). Language plays a central role in social and emotional development. Thus, a wide range of related developmental processes are affected in deaf children, whose early language development has been markedly delayed. These processes include:

affect recognition and affect control (Gray *et al.* 2002);

development of meta-cognitive skills (Remmel *et al.* 2002);

impulse control;

self-reflection;

development of interpersonal problem-solving skills;

adverse affects on cognitive development with language deprived deaf children being more likely to have difficulty in de-centring and thinking abstractly (Greenberg and Calderon 2003).

These delays in social, emotional, and cognitive development may be compounded by other factors. The HAS (1998) recounted how children who are deaf may:

be marginalized within their families and hearing peer groups (Lederberg 1993);

encounter linguistic over-protection (parents and teachers simplifying their language to ensure understanding) and emotional over-protection (restriction of age-appropriate experiences); and

be at greater risk of adverse experiences such as bullying (Smith and Sharp 1994) and child abuse (Kennedy 1990; Ridgeway 1993).

A growing majority of deaf children are now educated in local mainstream schools, either in attached units or fully integrated. Research conducted by my group (Hindley *et al.* 1994) has suggested that children in mainstream settings are more vulnerable to mental health problems than children educated in schools for deaf children.

The specific implications of sensory impairment in childhood for services provided for them

Given the incidence of deafness and SVI, CAMHS are more likely to encounter deaf children with additional mental health problems. Nonetheless, in both communities of children, there is a tendency for specialized educational and social services to manage children without involving 'outside' agencies. Also, professionals working with children with specific sensory impairments have legitimate, and sometimes less legitimate, concerns about how much professionals, who are unfamiliar with these children, will be able to accurately assess and manage them. Staff in CAMHS should regard these agencies as essential partners in service delivery.

The HAS report (1998), *Forging new channels*, provides advice about policy, service design, and practice in commissioning and delivering mental health services for people of all ages who are deaf. It provides a strategic framework.

For children with hearing impairment, major concerns relate to:

communication and language;

understanding the developmental consequences of deafness;

understanding the cultural aspects of deafness; and

avoiding the trap of attributing all phenomenology to the deafness.

In addition to specialist agencies, the voluntary organizations and, especially, the National Deaf Children's Society (NDCS) and the specialist mental health services for deaf people are useful resources.

Rooms used by staff to see deaf children need to be uncluttered, and clinicians should avoid sitting with their backs to bright light sources, as this makes both receiving BSL and lip-reading difficult.

Deaf-blind children may need to use hands-on sign interpretation. Deaf children with additional learning difficulties may benefit from a deaf-relay interpreter. Individual clinicians need to consider whether or not to engage a BSL interpreter and to investigate ways of working with interpreters. Clinicians should not, for example, presume that parents' have good levels of competency in BSL, and should avoid using parents as interpreters, since this compromises both the parents and the children. The HAS report, published in 1998, provides relevant information in more depth about BSL and training in it. But, as the HAS report said:

> Clearly, good communication skills are essential for mental health professionals who work with deaf children but the provision of an interpreter is not an adequate solution. The idiosyncratic nature of many deaf children's language development presents a challenge to most BSL interpreters, particularly those for whom BSL is a second language. Because eye contact, and so rapport, is established between the interpreter and the child, a child mental health professional is passing substantial clinical responsibility to the interpreter. Even in the best of circumstances, an interpreter will be expected to carry multiple functions and this can adversely affect the quality of interpretation....

Deaf children's teachers may offer to act as interpreters. Clinicians will need to weigh up the advantages and disadvantages in these situations. Teachers will be familiar with a child's language use and developmental level, and the child may well feel comfortable with them. On the other hand, a teacher is unlikely to be a trained interpreter, may or may not have good sign language skills, and their presence may inhibit the child for a variety of reasons. In the majority of situations we would discourage clinicians from using teachers in this role.

Again the HAS points out the consequences of the matters of prevalence that I recorded earlier when it says:

> However because most families who are seen contain both deaf and hearing people, services require both deaf and hearing staff. In addition to good communication skills, child mental health professionals should have good understanding of deaf culture, links to the adult deaf community and a detailed understanding of the psychosocial consequences of deafness. As with hearing children, parents, siblings and extended family are often key players in maintaining and resolving a deaf child's difficulties. In clinical groups, parents and siblings are more likely to have limited signing skills and an interpreter is essential to allow both deaf and hearing staff to carry out therapeutic work with families. Partly as a result of communication differences, assessment and therapy with deaf children and their families takes longer than similar work with hearing families.

Children with SVI do not necessarily need communication support but similarly need uncluttered rooms that they can explore easily. Clinicians may need to adjust to greater use of touch to explore their environment when working with children who have no light perception or minimal light perception.

Hearing children of deaf adults

Hearing children of deaf parents (CODAs) are an unrecognized group of children in need. The majority of parents who are deaf raise their children successfully, but the minority who experience greater difficulties have major problems in gaining access to mainstream services. A variety of contextual factors need to be born in mind when working with these families. These factors include accessing information, belonging to a cultural minority, and a common experience of disempowerment (Singleton and Tittle 2000). It is important to recognize the cultural discontinuities in many of these families: 95% of deaf adults were born into hearing families and 90% of the children of deaf adults are hearing. Common problems include the 'parentification' of children, parents experiencing difficulty in providing effective limit-setting and managing over-intrusive hearing grandparents. For a small minority of deaf parents, significant difficulties in empathizing with their children contribute to significant problems in parenting their children. There is no reliable, research-based information about the mental health needs of CODAs.

References

Cass, H. (1998) Visual impairment and autism: current questions and future research questions. *Autism*, **2**, 117–38.

Gray, C.D., Hosie, J.A., Russell, P.A., and Ormel, E.A. (2002) Emotional development in deaf children: facial expressions, display rules and theory of mind. In *Context, cognition and deafness* (ed. M.D. Clark, M. Marschark, and M. Karchmer). pp. 135–60. Washington DC: Gallaudet University Press.

Greenberg, M. and Calderon, R. (2003) Social and emotional development of deaf children: family, school and program effects. In *Oxford handbook of deaf studies, language and education* (ed. M. Marschark and P.E. Spencer). pp. 177–89. Oxford: Oxford University Press.

Gregory, S., Sheldon, L., and Bishop, J. (1995) *Deaf young people and their families: developing understanding*. Cambridge: Cambridge University Press.

Hindley, P. (2000). Child and adolescent psychiatry. In *Mental health and deafness* (ed. P. Hindley and N. Kitson). pp. 75–98. London: Whurr's.

Hindley, P.A. and van Gent, T. (2002) Psychiatric aspects of specific sensory impairment. In: *Child and adolescent psychiatry* (4th edn) (ed. M. Rutter and T. Taylor). pp. 842–57. Oxford: Blackwells.

Hindley, P., Hill, P., McGuigan, S., and Kitson, N. (1994) Psychiatric disorder in deaf and hearing impaired children and young people: a prevalence study. *Journal of Child Psychology and Psychiatry and Allied Disciplines*, **55**, 917–34.

Kennedy, N. (1990) *The abused deaf child: the role of the social worker with deaf people*. Report on Conference of National Deaf Children's Society 'Keep Children Safe Project', (September 1990).

Lederberg, A. (1993) The impact of deafness on mother-child and peer relationships. In *Psychological Perspectives on Deafness* (ed. M. Marschark and M.D. Clark). Hillsdale, NJ: Lawrence Earlbaum.

Meadow-Orlans, K. and Erting, C. (2000) Deaf people in society. In *Mental health and deafness* (ed. P. Hindley and N. Kitson). pp. 3–24. London: Whurr's.

NHS Health Advisory Service. (1995) *Child and adolescent mental health services: together we stand*. London: HMSO.

NHS Health Advisory Service. (1998) *Forging new channels—commissioning and delivering mental health services for people who are deaf*. Beaconsfield: British Society for Mental Health and Deafness and SIGN.

Remmel, E., Bettger, J.G., and Weinberg, A.M. (2002) Theory of mind development in deaf children. In *Context, cognition and deafness* (ed. M.D. Clark, M. Marschark, and M. Karchmer). pp. 113–34. Washington DC: Gallaudet University Press.

Ridgeway, S.M. (1993) Abuse and deaf children—some factors to consider. *Child Abuse Review*, **2**, 166–73.

Singleton, J.L. and Tittle, M.D. (2000) Deaf parents and their hearing children. *Journal of Deaf Studies and Deaf Education*, **5**, 221–36.

Smith, P.K. and Sharp, S. (1994) School bullying: insights and perspectives. London: Routledge.

Chapter 22

Children 'looked after' by the state

Michael Kerfoot

Introduction

The Children Act 1989 was arguably the most comprehensive and far-reaching piece of legislation that Parliament had ever enacted in relation to children. Its effects on the future organization, planning, provision, and delivery of services for children and their families was profound, as were its effects upon other agencies having responsibilities towards children. For example, the Act has had important implications for the organization of child and adolescent mental health services, and for the work of child psychiatrists (Harris-Hendricks and Black 1996). The recent publication of a resource book entitled *The mental health needs of looked-after children* (The Royal College of Psychiatrists 2000) is evidence of the growing importance to mental health professionals of activity in this sector of care.

Definitions

Local authority social services departments have an obvious interface with child and adolescent mental health problems through the daily client contacts of social workers that have professional involvement with troubled children and their families in the community. Social workers also have responsibility for children and young people who are 'looked after' by the authority, and who are placed away from their families, either with foster parents or in a residential unit. The interface then becomes broader, encompassing foster parents who need advice and support in caring for a child who has emotional or behavioural problems, or the needs of residential care staff for advice and support in caring for small groups of young people in self-contained units where, because of the strains of communal living, problems may escalate. This does not always involve the social worker in direct client contact. Increasingly, with the growth in family centres, direct work may be 'sub-contracted' to other workers, with the social worker assuming an overall co-ordination role. Children with emotional and behavioural problems carry a higher risk of later difficulties in adult life (Health Advisory Service 1995) and it is particularly important that these are responded to efficiently and effectively.

Epidemiology

In the year ending 31 March 2000, there were 58 100 children 'looked after' by local authorities in England (Department of Health 2001) and this represents around 0.5% of the total child population. The figure represents an increase of 5% on the previous year, and is an increase of 18% on figures published in 1994 (Wolkind and Rushton 1994). Around 65% of children looked after are placed with foster families and this proportion has changed little in recent years, while around 11% are in residential provision. The statistics for children leaving care during 1999–2000 show that 5400 left care during that period, and were equally divided between those leaving at age 16 (2700) and those leaving at 18 (2700). Interestingly, this reflected a decrease compared with the previous year for those leaving at 16, and an increase for those leaving at 18.

Children who are looked after by local authorities have some of the highest rates of mental disorder when compared with young people in the general population. A study of children in care in Oxfordshire (McCann *et al.* 1996) gave a total prevalence of psychiatric disorder of 67% compared with 15% in a matched control sample derived from the same schools. Of those who scored for psychiatric disorder, 79% scored for major disorder. The study also showed that the distribution of disorders is different for those children placed in residential units (96%) and those placed in foster care (57%). The most common disorders were conduct disorder (28%), over-anxious disorder (26%), and depressive disorder (23%). A study from Glasgow of children entering the care system (Dimigen *et al.* 1999) also found significant levels of mental disorder that was largely untreated, since many were not being referred for psychological interventions. The study highlighted a need for early-intervention policies to help these vulnerable children and effective assessment through multidisciplinary discussion and strategic planning. The health needs and provision of healthcare to school age children in local authority care were compared, in a recent study, to those of children living at home (Williams *et al.* 2001). The study concluded that the overall healthcare of children who had been established in care for more than six months was significantly worse than for those living in their own homes, particularly with regard to emotional and behavioural health. The study highlighted the difficulty of gaining access to CAMHS once a problem had been identified, but also the high mobility in some social services that may mean a child is moved on while still waiting to be seen by CAMHS. It is an inevitable consequence, in some cases, that disturbed behaviour left untreated is very likely to contribute to placement breakdown and further disruption to the child.

A recent study undertaken in Leeds (Nicholas *et al.* 2003) explored the current and past contacts of children being looked after, with child and adolescent mental health services. Of the 177 children in the study, 64% had been in contact with these services during the past five years, and 27% had current contact with child mental health services. The authors concluded that the pattern of service delivery locally was changing from one of direct contact between users and services, to one of CAMHS consultation with, and training of, staff in residential children's homes.

Causation

The reasons that bring children into local authority 'care' are also the kinds of reason that contribute to psychiatric vulnerability and risk of developing a disorder. Risk factors may be intrinsic to the child through, for example, developmental delay, communication difficulties, or learning disabilities and may, therefore, generate a number of problems in behaviour, or educational performance, in the school setting. These difficulties will also affect peer-group friendships and may result in alienation and isolation for the child, or perhaps the drift towards children with similar problems, or other disaffected pupil groups. Not surprisingly, family problems often loom large in the backgrounds of 'looked after' children. Serious parental conflict and family breakdown may bring a child into care or there may have been episodes of neglect, physical or sexual abuse, or emotional rejection in the family. Many parents have health worries of their own, some of these relating perhaps to drug or alcohol misuse, but some will also have mental illness. There may, therefore, be a genetic predisposition in the child towards the development of mental health problems (Graham 1991). Environmental factors also take their toll, particularly for those children living in deprived and disadvantaged areas where delinquency, violence, and vagrancy are commonplace. High unemployment leading to socio-economic disadvantage and poverty, poor housing or homelessness, and experiences of discrimination or oppression are familiar to many of these children, and those from black or ethnic minorities in particular are over-represented in the care system (Rowe *et al.* 1989).

Assessment

Assessment for children who are 'looked after' assumes special importance because the child is not living with natural parents and planning therefore has to address both long-term and short-term needs. Introduction of the 'looking after children assessment and action records' was aimed at facilitating planning, decision-making, review, and monitoring. However, information from a number of individuals or agencies may need to be pooled in order to achieve a comprehensive assessment and issues about professional judgement and opinion, and confidentiality of information, may restrict the availability of information to other parties. Joint working, even within the different parts of an organization, rather than between organizations, can become impossible when key information is not shared. Street (1999) highlighted concerns about the quality and quantity of information on children referred to residential provision. The reality for many residential providers appears to be one in which they are frequently asked to provide 24-hour specialist care and/or treatment for highly damaged children and young people with often only the barest of background details or assessment of what is needed. The study raised the concern that many referring professionals did not appear to appreciate the significance of such information. Poor structure, fragmentation, confusing terminology, and inconsistency in the details supplied by different sectors was common, and there was little evidence of inter-agency dialogue or joint assessment.

Intervention

The kinds of intervention needed from CAMHS for looked-after children are no different to those provided for other children, except that the high rate of disorder in the former indicates a high level of unmet need. It is generally acknowledged that the majority of children and young people referred to residential provision present with the most challenging and complex difficulties, where the potential for self-harm or harm to others is often high. A recent study of residential provision provided by the National Health Service and by Social Services Departments indicated a marked shift towards the majority of those referred showing more overtly out of control and aggressive behaviours, both verbally and physically (Street 1999). Accompanying this was an almost total disappearance of those children and young people showing withdrawn and internalized difficulties. Interventions would need to target these specific features of the population, perhaps through a violence-perpetrators group, or through a programme of anger-management training.

Various pieces of legislation, regulations, and guidance followed the implementation of the Children Act 1989, and some of these relate either directly or indirectly to concerns about the assessment and treatment of mental health problems in young people who are accommodated or looked after by local authorities. Much of the 'guidance' points to the need for joint working between health services and local authority services and the Strategic Planning Framework Support Force for Children's Residential Care was formed in 1993 to produce a framework to try and assist local authorities in their strategic planning of residential provision. Throughout, the work of the Support Force stresses a commitment to '... joint strategies and plans ... to be led at the highest level both locally and nationally' (SFCRC Final Report, DoH 1995). This approach has been complemented by recent work from the NHS Executive on joint commissioning of children's services, and subsequent work by the Department of Health, Social Services Inspectorate, and National Children's Bureau on joint service plans (Flood 1996). Among other things, *Modernising social services* (DoH 1998a) contains a number of key proposals for improving multi-agency working, while the Quality Protects Initiative (DoH 1998b) considers how educational opportunities, healthcare, and social care can help looked-after children derive maximum life chance benefits.

Joint working can take a number of forms and a recent survey (Kerfoot *et al.* 2002) explored some of the options for social services departments. Although there was fairly unanimous agreement about the value of the multidisciplinary approach in CAMHS, considerable misgivings were expressed in the survey about the availability, appropriateness, and effectiveness of the approaches on offer for looked-after children. In fairness to CAMHS, however, it was also clear that when social services departments were asking for help, it was usually for their most difficult and complex cases, where the turbulent and complicated case history and continuing difficulties would seriously challenge the effectiveness of any intervention. On the other hand, the survey produced very positive examples of innovative working practices, some involving direct work with children and their carers, and others offering staff development through regular 'teaching' consultations with workers. The use of clinical psychologists, either directly employed by social services or seconded to them, was much in evidence and was regarded by some as a more accessible alternative to mainstream CAMHS. The picture was balanced, however, by examples of CAMHS input to social services through regular, dedicated consultation time, and through dedicated clinic sessions for social services cases. The survey also highlighted examples of more user-friendly mental health services for young people, such as drop-in centres on local estates, and special support services for vulnerable young people leaving care. Pivotal to some of these developments was the creation of primary mental health workers' posts, which acted as a source of consultation in their own right, but also linked CAMHS through the primary care sector to front-line social services workers.

Outcomes

There have been surprisingly few outcome studies of children raised in care, but what there are do indicate better outcomes for those children who are adopted or fostered, than for those raised in residential care (Quinton *et al.* 1984; Triseliotis and Russell 1984; St Clair and Osborn 1987; Cheung and Buchanan 1997). Studies of young people leaving care at 16 indicate considerable vulnerability and disadvantage among those moving into independent living. More than 75% have no academic qualification, over 50% are unemployed, and those leaving care are over-represented among the populations of youth offending institutions, and among the young homeless and those living in poverty (Barnardos 1996; Stein 1997).

Challenges

It is important for social workers to be able to access child and adolescent mental health services when necessary, either as a direct referrer or as the agent for foster carers or residential care staff. There is much anecdotal evidence to suggest that this is a difficult process, even at the best of times. The need for CAMHS input to social services is often acute, yet referral processes are rarely designed to cope with acute or urgent referrals because, even when a 'fast track' referral route exists, this is rarely open to social services. The report from the Audit Commission (1999) suggests that social workers make few referrals to CAMHS because of having to route these through a GP, and then to a waiting-list. There is also difficulty in getting an already vulnerable child to attend a CAMHS setting, where the context is unfamiliar and where the clinical elements may appear threatening or disturbing. Looked-after children may not be encouraged or welcomed as referrals into CAMHS for a number of reasons. First, the problems that have brought these children into care will stem from a complicated and complex array of personal, family, and environmental factors, and may well appear intractable. Second, in addition to a complex personal history, these children often have a complex service history in which referrals may have been made to a number of other child or family services, where psychosocial interventions of various kinds have been tried in the past, but without success. Finally, children with an erratic and disruptive placement history may find it difficult to stay connected to a 'treatment' service because of changes of placement and also changes of social worker. Many of these problems call for better communication between the various sectors of care but also for an expansion in CAMHS provision, so that different models of care or service initiatives can be developed for use with looked-after children. Some of the recent government initiatives such as Quality Protects, and the NHS Modernization Fund and Mental Health Grant for CAMHS (Department of Health 1999) are supporting a number of initiatives aimed at facilitating joint planning and working, and improving access to appropriate services.

The NHS Health Advisory Service review of CAMHS (1995) recommended the creation of primary mental health workers to improve communication and service-delivery between the primary care interface and the different tiers of service within CAMHS. These posts would have a direct relevance for social workers wanting to make referrals and would be a source of advice and guidance since, from the CAMHS viewpoint, it may be difficult to identify what social services' expectations are in making a referral. Alternatively, investing in social worker posts for CAMHS would also provide a point for referral consultation, as well as complex assessments and therapeutic work for looked-after children. Investment of this kind can reduce costs in other sectors for social services departments. A recent study (Byford *et al.* 1999) demonstrated considerable savings for social services in a randomized trial of brief, home-based social work intervention provided by CAMHS, compared with routine care, for suicidal adolescents. Initiatives such as these go some way towards meeting the challenges for social services departments in gaining access to CAHMS, and in creating a climate in which joint planning and working can take place.

Bibliography

Audit Commission (1999) *Children in Mind.* London: Audit Commission.

Barnardos (1996) *Too much—too young: the failure of social policy in meeting the needs of care leavers.* London: Action on Aftercare Consortium.

Byford, S., Harrington, R., Torgeson, D., Kerfoot, M., Dyer, E., Harrington, V., Woodham, A., Gill, J., and McNiven, F. (1999) Cost-effectiveness analysis of a home-based social work intervention for children and adolescents who have deliberately poisoned themselves. *British Journal of Psychiatry,* 174, 56–62.

Cheung, S.Y. and Buchanan, A. (1997) Malaise scores in adulthood of children and young people who have been in care. *Journal of Child Psychology and Psychiatry,* 38, 575–80.

Department of Health (1995) *Residential care for young people—a positive choice?* London: Support Force for Children's Residential Care/Department of Health.

Department of Health (1998a) *Modernising social services.* London: The Stationery Office.

Department of Health (1998b) *Quality protects: transforming children's services.* London: Department of Health.

Department of Health (1999) *NHS Modernisation Fund and Mental Health Grant for child and adolescent mental health services 1999/2002.* London: Department of Health.

Department of Health (2001) *Statistical press notice—children looked after.* www.doh.gov.uk/public/20010094.htm

Dimigen, G., Del Priore, C., Butler, S., Evans, S., Ferguson, L., and Swan, M. (1999) Psychiatric disorder among children at time of entering local authority care: questionnaire survey. *British Medical Journal,* **319,** 675.

Flood, S. (1996) Children's Service Plans. *Young Minds Magazine,* **24,** 24.

Graham, P. (1991) *Child psychiatry: a developmental approach.* Oxford: Oxford University Press.

Harris-Hendricks, J. and Black, M. (ed.) (1996) *Child and adolescent psychiatry—a new century.* (Occasional Paper No: 33). London: Royal College of Psychiatrists.

Kerfoot, M. and Panayiotopoulos, C., and Harrington, R. Social services links with CAMHS: a national survey. *Child and Adolescent Mental Health,* (in press).

McCann, J., James, A., Wilson, S., and Dunn, G. (1996) Prevalence of psychiatric disorders in young people in the care system. *British Medical Journal,* **313,** 1529–30.

NHS Health Advisory Service (1995) *Together we stand: the commissioning, role and management of child and adolescent mental health services.* London: HMSO.

Nicholas, B., Roberts, S., and Wurr, C. (2003) Looked-after children in residential homes. *Child and Adolescent Mental Health,* **8,** 78–83.

Quinton, D., Rutter, M., and Liddle, C. (1984) Institutional rearing, parenting difficulties, and marital support. *Psychological Medicine,* **14,** 107–24.

Rowe, J., Hundelby, M., and Garnett, L. (1989) *Child care now.* London: Batsford/BAAF.

St Clair, L. and Osborn, A.F. (1987) The ability and behaviour of children who have been 'in care' or separated from their parents. *Early Child Development and Care,* **28,** 3. (Special Issue).

Stein, M. (1997) *What works in leaving care?* London: Barnardos.

Street, C. (1999) *Providing residential services for children and young people: a multidisciplinary perspective.* Aldershot: Ashgate.

The Royal College of Psychiatrists (2000) *The mental health needs of looked-after children.* London: Gaskell.

Williams, J., Jackson, S., Maddocks, A., Cheung, W-Y., and Hutchings, H. (2001) Case-control study of the health of those looked after by local authorities. *Archives of Diseases in Childhood,* **85,** 280–5.

Triseliotis, J. and Russell, J. (1984) Hard to place. London: Heinemann.

Wolkind, S. and Rushton, A. (1994) Residential and foster family care. In *Child and adolescent psychiatry: modern approaches* (3rd edn) (ed. M. Rutter, E. Taylor, and L. Hersov). Oxford: Blackwell.

Part 3

Lessons from international perspectives—comparative analyses

Chapter 23

European psychiatry: construction, destruction, and reconstruction

Michael Shooter

Introduction

Despite a tendency for national isolationism, child and adolescent psychiatry has slowly developed a European perspective. Its history has been traced from the first signs of medical work with the 'mental disorders of children' in the second-half of the nineteenth century, through the expansion of the child guidance clinics in the 1920s, the first coining of the words 'child psychiatry' in 1933, the establishment of the first Chair, in Stockholm in 1958, the achievement of speciality or sub-speciality status in most Western European Countries by the end of the 1970s, to the foundation of the UEMS Specialist Section for Child and Adolescent Psychiatry in 1992/93. At this point, it has been said, it could finally be acknowledged as an 'independent, main medical speciality on a European level' (Piha 1997). Issues like diagnosis and training could be standardized, and even relatively new services could fit rapidly into what they saw as the accepted pattern (Hannesdottir 1993).

However, to focus on such unity would be to ignore some major discrepancies. Even within Western Europe, the workforce ranges from 12.5 child psychiatrists per 100 000 in Sweden down to 1.2 in Spain, according to the 'gross national product'. As ever, the poorer a country is, the greater the need of its children, and the less the resources there are to satisfy their needs. Within any one country, there are immigrants, adoptees, refugees, and ethnic minority groups who may be even more disadvantaged in situation and service. In most of Eastern Europe, the newly independent countries of the old Soviet Block are still struggling to throw off the suffocating blanket of hospital-based, medical model, pharmacologically dominated Russian psychiatry, with all its attendant taboos. In great swathes of Central Europe, the Eastern Mediterranean, and, closer to home, in Northern Ireland, child and adolescent psychiatrists are coming to terms with the horrors of man-made and natural disaster. It is these issues that this chapter addresses in a climate in which, all too easily, 'a nation's politics becomes a child's everyday psychology' (Coles 1986).

The Western European context

Following the pioneering work of Rutter, the epidemiology of child and adolescent disorders, their prevalence and age/gender profiles, has been studied in many countries (Moilanen *et al.* 1988). Long-term follow-up of the consequences of untreated problems has proved the necessity for child and adolescent services in terms of adult admission rates and suicide figures (Thomsen 1996) or the general 'accumulated psychosocial burden' (Mellbin *et al.* 1992). The development of such services has been bedevilled by grandiose aims, twin-track health and welfare systems and a troubled political history (Hoger and Rothenberger 1998). Collaboration between child psychiatrists and paediatricians has been poor, even within one helping system (Vandvik 1994), where there is no 'common language' in the perception of children's problems. The particular difficulties of coping with serious disturbance in adolescence with insufficient in-patient beds (Marttunen and Aalberg 1998) will have political echoes everywhere! Changing trends in individual diagnostic categories, such as personality disorder (Steinhausen 1997), or patterns of co-morbidity (Cederblad 1996), represent the unwillingness of child psychiatrists to pin fixed labels on fluid development, as much as their actual prevalence rates. Despite evidence that child psychiatrists are getting younger, are more often female, and are more independent of their adult colleagues, the typical psychiatrist in most countries remains resolutely a male, of middle age, combining adult and child responsibilities (Boer 1999). Worrying numbers of both training and substantive consultant posts remain unfilled. Anxieties about the current state of in-patient adolescent psychiatry (NICAPS Study 2001) have been counterbalanced by the emergence of other treatment modalities, including multidisciplinary day units (Verheij and Sanders-Woudstra 1988; Lucas and Talan 1998).

Attempts have been made to compare problem scores, as defined by check-lists and self-report across many cultures within Western Europe (Fitzpatrick and Deehan 1999) but are often undermined by skewed sampling in social class or mainstream schooling, by poor response rates, and by differences between those cultures that wish to paint as bright a picture as possible and those where 'self praise is no praise'. Others, with a more robust methodology, claim 'a cost effective way to identify problems for which children from diverse cultural backgrounds may need help' not only within Europe, but in comparison to the Far East, the Americas, and Australasia (Crijnen et al. 1997)—but the reliability of culture-bound concepts like 'abnormal psychosocial situations' is still questionable (Goor-Lambo et al. 1994). There have been far too few comparisons between services in different countries, such as Glasgow (Scotland) and Szeged (Hungary) (VanBeinum et al. 1998). Despite the growing confidence of the speciality, Child Psychiatrists, even in Western Europe, have been too wrapped up in their own problems for a true cross fertilisation of ideas.

Disadvantaged groups

We should not always interpret a lower referral rate of some ethnic minorities, such as the Gujarati community in Manchester (Hackett et al. 1990), as a problem. A more integrated family structure with stricter parenting, an expectation of obedience, encouragement of sharing, and an intolerance of childhood tantrums and adolescent aggression, may reduce the need for service intervention. For most, however, like the Bangladeshi community in East London (Hillier et al. 1994) or the Somali community in South East Wales (Davies and Webb 2000), the picture is one of disadvantage within services that struggle to engage them in ways that are culturally sensitive enough in attitude and structure. Even in old-established groups, there may be huge clashes in aims between therapists looking for emotional changes based on in-depth investigation of family function, and parents who come for simple explanation and advice, medication, and symptom-relief in their children. Referral rates are bound to be low where Dutch teachers simply do not spot the problems in their Turkish immigrant pupils (Crijnen et al. 2000) and drop-out rates are high where written information is available only in English and no interpreters are on hand (Hillier et al. 1994). Problems in communication can have dangerous implications where Somali refugees, fresh from defending the lives of themselves and their families from armed attack, react aggressively to school bullies. Yet even there, the skilled use of community leaders can help sort out 'ordinary' psychiatric disorder from the stress of inappropriate placement and handling (Davies and Webb 2000).

The deprivation inherent in the background of refugee groups can cause severe attachment disorders, typified by 'an eager approach, an unawareness of social boundaries, combined with a superficial interest in others, marked deficits in social understanding and interpretation of social cues' in Romanian children adopted into the stablest of families (O'Connor and Rutter 2000). There are now more than 120 000 refugee children in Inner London, for example, with high rates of psychiatric disorder brought with them from their former lives, compounded by the trauma they have been through, and by attempts to assimilate into an alien environment at home and in school. They are under-referred to child and adolescent mental health services by adults unaware of their distress (Hodes 1998), that might be expressed in physical rather than emotional symptoms, and who may be ignorant or afraid of what they see as stigmatizing help, especially where their legal status is questioned by a harsh asylum system. Circumstances are often too chaotic to make sense of a clinic-based service that is bewildering in its practical implications and remote in every sense of the word. Western services will need to be far more flexible to provide the safe emotional haven, backed up by regular health check-ups and Children Act Legislation, where necessary, for such disadvantaged groups.

Post-Soviet Eastern Europe

The old Soviet system, both in Russia and its satellite countries, relied on a network of regional out-patient and in-patient clinics under 'district child psychiatrists', who built up a knowledge of families over generations, who offered free help to even the most disadvantaged, and who could 'summon' them into treatment where necessary (Severny and Smirnov 1997). Such a system, however, was isolated from the educational and social security structures, was directed almost entirely at hospital-based, severe disorder with little community backup before or after-wards, contained nothing for the under 4-year-olds, had no legislative framework to deal with abuse in the family or the institutions designed to help, and was all based on a controlling, organic, and pharmacological view of children's problems. Since it was not permissible to admit to the existence of social problems, all disturbances must therefore have an organic explanation and be treated with medication. The statistics made awful reading.

Even within Russia, there are signs of major changes of attitude and a more psycho-therapeutic approach with the establishment of the Independent Association of Child Psychiatrists and Psychologists in 1993 and a Research Institute for Preventative Psychiatry as part of the Mental Health Research Centre of the Russian Academy of Medical Sciences. But this struggles against a background of insufficient resources, poor training, a lack of confidence that has been called a 'post totalitarian stress syndrome' (Kagan 1998), and an idiosyncratic government decision that in November 1995, 'deleted' child and adolescent psychiatry from the list of medical professions. There have been a growing number of schemes to help structure that change from outside, such as the partnership between Leicester University Medical School and the St Petersburg Child and Adolescent Psychiatric Service, based on lecture courses and two-way exchange programmes (Nicol 1996). Such work has needed skilled attention to differences in terminology and perception, respect for hierarchical conventions, and a very specific focus around local needs, with practical demonstrations. The basic needs may be so great that 'the idea of psychotherapy or analysis suddenly seems an outrageous luxury' (Essenhigh and Vasilyeva 1998). Without a conceptual structure, change has no direction; but new concepts need to be very sensitively implanted.

Meanwhile, services in countries emerging from the Soviet Block have begun more whole-heartedly to embrace the 'exciting process of change approaches' (Puras 1994). In Lithuania, a Centre of Excellence was established at the Vilnius University Children's Mental Health Centre (1991) and the Ministries of Health, Culture/Education and Social Welfare collaborated in the foundation of a National Child Mental Health Programme (1994) to oversee the development of community work, training, research, and links with other countries in Europe. But the services remained, at that time, hospital and medically orientated with heavy overtones of the Russian 'sluggish schizophrenia model'. In Estonia, four years after independence, the number of in-patient beds had been halved, staff–patient ratios improved, the average length of stay dramatically cut, the use of pharmaco-therapy decreased and shifted in emphasis from multiple nootropics (from the Moscow School of Psychiatry's 'neurometabolic cerebroprotectors') to single anti-depressants, and the practice of individual and family psychotherapy expanded reciprocally (Sourander and Piha 1998). Everywhere, it was asserted, further progress was dependent on changes in public and political attitudes rather than finances. But in the realities of a harsh economic climate, practitioners within the new services would need to hold onto the watch word of the Lithuanian Society of Families with Mentally Handicapped Children, called Viltris—'Hope'.

Ironically, in Lithuania itself, as public and professional confidence has broken down with the old social structure, suicide rates have climbed dramatically and psychiatrists have tended to retreat into the old traditional ways. Government money has dried up and child psychiatry has suffered most, inevitably, as medicine has switched wholesale to private insurance schemes. Already that 'hope' seems fragile (Puras 2001).

Child and adolescent psychiatry in countries ravaged by disaster

Reconstructive psychiatry, following man-made or natural disaster, raises controversial issues of definition, of the models used to understand their impact on children, adolescents and families, and of the delivery of services to help them.

Definitions

How can disaster be defined? In one year (1995) there were 200 000 child soldiers between the ages of 6 and 16, 27 million refugees, and 26 million people displaced within their own coun-tries. The stress of exodus and disease killed twenty times as many as the wars did. Altogether $790 000 million was spent on military activities and $120 000 million on developing coun-tries, 110 million land mines in 64 countries killed 800 people per month and mutilated many more (UNICEF 1996). The Armenian Earthquake killed 20 000 people, almost two-thirds of whom were children. At its epicentre, nearly all the schools in Spitak were destroyed, and in some, nearly half the pupils died. Such bald statistics fill us with horror, but tell us little more.

Some authors have tried to standardize and compare the experience of children in 20 differ-ent types of trauma across six countries, each involving some form of threat to personal secu-rity—from death down to the birth of a sibling (Yamamoto et al. 1996). Others have drawn a distinction between 'public' and 'private' wars—between children trapped in armed conflict (whose suffering took place within loving relationships, lying awake in fear but with their fam-ily and peers around them, with a reservoir of peaceful memories to draw upon and a need to recount their stories afterwards), and those in violent households (where suffering took place alone, lying awake listening to their parents' rows, where tension pervaded the whole of their lives and the children went to great lengths to keep it secret from others) (Berman 2000). There is no hierarchy of atrocity for those involved, but most authors have reserved 'disaster' for more massed events that 'overwhelm, at least temporarily, the coping resources of individuals and the community. They scar the memory of the individuals and communities they touch, they have the capacity to forever change the character and life style of individuals and communities, and they confront one's perceptions of the world and individual and collective vulnerability and strength' (Pfefferbaum 1998).

The components of disaster have been divided into 'direct' and 'indirect' aggression (Tomkiewicz 1997). There has certainly been no ethical progress in conflicts within which children are deliberately targeted by snipers, girls are raped, boys conscripted and forced to kill their own families, girls and boys are tortured, and thousands have died on land mines long after the conflict, ostensibly, has ended (Kozaric-Kovacic *et al.* 1997). Indirect effects, in which the social structures surrounding children are destroyed, schools and hospitals shelled, water contaminated, and farm and forest devastated, can be just as great—and separation from their family is perhaps most painful of all. Whether by forced, ethnic cleansing or by well-meaning help in refugee camps (Brunvatne *et al.* 1995), orphanages (Wolff and Fesseha 1998), or fostering schemes (Bilanakis *et al.* 1999), displacement seems to be a particularly distressing aspect of modern warfare. All this suffering, direct and indirect, has been calculated according to its 'intensity' (the proportion of civilian casualties and the barbarity meted out to them) and its 'duration' (Tomkiewicz 1997).

Models of impact

The concept of 'trauma' and its emotional and behavioural consequences, 'post-traumatic stress disorder,' have gained international currency in literature and academic conferences (Shalev *et al.* 2000). It offers one model by which to understand the impact of disaster. Researchers have drawn on the results of individual events over a decade (Yule and Williams 1990; Green *et al.* 1991; Vogel and Vernberg 1993; Parry-Jones and Barton 1995; Putman 1996) to categorize its general affects on children and adolescents. Its application has been studied in massed disasters throughout Europe and the Eastern Meditarranean—in survivors of the Holocaust (Kestenberg 1992; Sigal 1999); adolescents displaced in Bosnia (Becker *et al.* 1999) and under siege in Sarajevo (Husain *et al.* 1998); in Kosovo (Spiegel and Salama 2000), where 90% of the casualties were civilian; in war-time Beirut (Deeb *et al.* 1997) and the 'troubles' of Northern Ireland (Daly 1999); under scud missile attacks during the Gulf War in Israel (Laor *et al.* 2001; Ayalon 1998); the children of the Gaza Strip (Thabet and Vostanis 2000); and in the after-affects of the Armenian earthquake (Miller *et al.* 1993), where families have been condemned to living in tents, on the site of their destroyed homes, in a state of learned helplessness for years after the event.

In contrast to the typical adult presentation of PTSD, a developmental view of symptomatology has been postulated for children and adolescents (Shaw 2000). Pre-school children are said to be less aware of the nature and meaning of threat, rely on 'parental-referencing', and may become disorganized in their emotions and behaviour, and lose some of their developmental capacities, such as bowel and bladder control. School-aged children have greater cognitive appreciation of the dangers, may be disrupted in their sleep, appetite, and academic performance, and lapse into a variety of anxiety, depressive, and somatic disorders. Adolescents may show more adult-like responses, with an open fear of death, or a hedonistic resort to impulsive, delinquent, sexual, substance misusing, acting-out behaviours that add to the danger in themselves. They are less willing to share their feelings than younger children and are particularly dependent on their peer-group reaction. They may lose faith in all adult security and sink, ultimately, into an apathetic or angry rejection of authority (Sugar 1997).

Risk factors include, not only the developmental level of the children, their pre-existing personality, and coping styles, but their proximity to the centre of the disaster and the nature of the trauma involved (Pynoos *et al.* 1993), surrounding community supports in general, the family environment in particular, and, in young children especially, the mental state of their mother. Parents can be both a buffer and a source of distress (Wolmer *et al.* 2000). As always in disaster, from the children of Beirut (Deeb *et al.* 1997) to those of Belfast, it is particular religious and social groups that are most vulnerable. 'The poor, or those who belong to the so-called working class, always live closer to the law, closer to the whims and fancies of political authority...' and closer to destruction (Coles 1986).

All this can be reliably and validly measured, it is claimed, by standard interviews with children and parents (CAPA Life Events and PTSD Module) at various stages of the trauma and its aftermath (Costello *et al.* 1998). Long-term consequences can be identified into adulthood and the treatments designed to prevent those consequences are well worked out. Once physical safety has been established, the child should be encouraged to explore the experience (at his own pace), inaccurate assumptions challenged (with sensitivity), and an assessment of the child's needs carried out (as holistically as possible), stress-management techniques taught (appropriate to the child's age), parents included wherever possible (for their own and the child's benefit), and any of a range of specific therapies considered—individual psychotherapy, cognitive behavioural techniques (Cohen *et al.* 2000), anxiety management, exposure therapy, play therapy, psycho-education, griefwork, group programmes, and medication, where appropriate (Shaw 2000). The literature is full of individual case studies (Oclander-Goldie 1999) and massed experience (Deering 2000). Yet there are major problems with the model, its application to children in these circumstances, and therefore the delivery of help and services based on it.

Helping services

There are core questions to be faced by mental health professionals working with the trauma of childhood, war, and displacement (Summerfield 2000), and the first is one of priorities. 'There is no point in trying to counsel children who are hungry, ill or unsafe' (Deering 2000). Whilst such needs are unlikely to be met in hospitals that have been targeted by shell fire and from which staff may have fled (Mandic *et al.* 1996), the children's basic welfare is paramount. Many is the NGO scheme that has concentrated too early on higher psychiatric interventions while the bullets are still flying or the dust not settled from natural disaster. Part of any emergency 'comfort' must be emotional. Speaking from his own emergence from the death camps of the Second World War, one author describes a mixed state of physical and psychological shock (Tomkiewicz 1997):

> The need for smiles and cuddles should not be overlooked. If you want to save a child who is a victim of war, medical treatment, feeding and vaccination are not enough; physical signs of kindness are needed, and words, which do not always come easily.

In such circumstances, the last thing a child needs to meet, is a mental health worker holding a PTSD check-list; but at some stage an assessment does need to be made of those children whose trauma will resolve spontaneously with support, and those more seriously disturbed and in need of specialized help. Here there have been serious doubts raised about the value of the PTSD model itself. Despite all the research, the application of PTSD to children in disaster, its longitudinal course in childhood, the long-term consequences, and the effectiveness of treatment remain uncertain. More pertinently, it is often seen as a Westernized concept based on an attempt to standardize individual experience into broad categories that simply cannot do justice to the huge discrepancies in the suffering of children, even within the same event, especially where no end may be in sight (Berman 2000):

> For many of these young people, trauma is not an isolated event, but is more chronic in nature, pervading every component of daily life. For them there is no post trauma period. The challenge they face is to find ways of making sense of events which seem quite senseless, not to get over a single bad experience.

Rather than be plunged back into their experience in pursuit of so-called 'narrative therapy' for a 'disease' process, it is argued, what these children need is help to ask very angry and justifiable questions of the adults around them. Why did they do this to us? Why did we lose everything? Why is so little being done to help us? Why haven't the perpetrators been punished? Mental health workers may find such political questions uncomfortable.

Furthermore, the combined assumption of UNICEF, WHO, the NGOs, and the ranks of mental health professionals in their employ, that disaster must have traumatized children and that trauma must be diagnosed and treated, is called into question (Summerfield 2000). An approach based on children as passive recipients of check-lists drawn up by Western psychiatrists and inappropriate to complex, still-evolving situations, and children whose own development is itself maturing, even under the shadow of disaster, should be abandoned. The question is how children can be empowered, in themselves, in their peer group, family, and community, rather than be seen as disordered and in need of individual treatment. The focus shifts from the individual to the group, from identifying weaknesses to building on strengths—and it begins with keeping the family together wherever possible, restoring the normal structure of children's lives at the first opportunity, and working through whatever local networks are available. For all of this, 'neither scientific analysis nor warm hearted concern' are enough (Tomkiewicz 1997).

Such an approach demands, first of all, a proper management of the 'response environment' (Pfefferbaum 1998). Children and families may need protection from the more malign influences of the media that can spread alarm and exploit those under its spotlight in the cause of the public's 'need-to-know'. Firm-handed co-ordination is needed for the increased help the media undoubtedly engenders, lest it descend into a chaos in which NGOs undermine each other's best efforts in competition for the same financial pot and conflict with government priorities (Joshi 1998). International response may be needed to establish a more 'safe, secure and predictable environment' within which the human rights of the children can be protected (Declaration of Amsterdam. Rights of Children in Armed Conflict 1994).

Within this envelope, once the basic needs for shelter, and physical and emotional comfort are satisfied, children will come to rely on as much sense of continuity as possible. Families will need to be kept together, often against the natural wishes of parents to send their children away to a place of greater safety. Familiar objects such as toys and photographs become important things to hold on to in the whirlpool of losses. Good quality information, honestly but sensitively given, is needed to correct misunderstanding and give children a rough outline of what is going to happen in the short- and medium-term future. Routines need to be established early on with spontaneous play and more formal peer-group activities. The 'structure' of school life should be re-established, in every sense of the word, even where buildings have been shattered and staff, like the children, have been killed or scattered. Assessment will be needed of those groups who will manage with the support of front-line, indigenous contacts (such as the general run of teachers in school), and those who would need more specialized help, initially perhaps from outside mental health personnel but 'cascading' training through local workers (particular teachers in schools or community nursing networks). Examples of such 'developmental' schemes, evolving as priority shifts over time, can be seen across Eastern Europe from the post-Dayton agreement years in Bosnia (Yule 2000), to the still ravaged townships of Armenia, a decade after the earthquake. Given the qualities required of them, preparedness, pragmatism, flexibility, sensitivity, endurance, high ethical values, cultural awareness, humility, and emotional and physical bravery—quite apart from their skills, it is small wonder that the helpers may themselves need regular support (Stein 1996). Encouragingly, workers who may feel 'overwhelmed, traumatized, and victimized' have been shown to benefit from the help of fellow mental health professionals, even with totally different religious, ethnic, and cultural values (Gal 1998)—a good model for those children and families they are helping in turn.

The future

It would be good to report that such reconstructive psychiatry is a thing of the past, but the regularity with which disasters continue to occur, both natural and man-made, suggests that the model is vital to the future of child and family work in Europe. At least we have had enough experience of it to have learnt some lessons. We must beware of any colonialist imposition of services from outside, albeit in the name of help. Just as that help should work towards the empowerment of children and families, so it should empower local services and leave the children in their care as soon as possible. Well-meaning training schemes should avoid asset-stripping local services by bringing key personnel to Western Europe on open-ended contracts from which they are unlikely to return to their own countries to put that training into practice. We should work sensitively through a minefield of cultural issues, including different perceptions of problems, different presentations of distress, different attitudes to the stigma of help, and suspicions of non-hierarchical, multidisciplinary working and flexibility of professional roles.

There are a few examples, now, of psychiatric services for adults that have emerged from disaster and are taking control of their own organization under local leadership. The old Yugoslav system in Bosnia/Herzegovenia focused on secondary care through twelve regional hospital psychiatric wards, two clinical centres, and two university hospitals, in Sarajevo and Tuzla. Primary psychiatric care, through the '*domzdravlzas*' and '*ambulantai*' local, community centres, was fairly basic. From 1992 to 1996, this system was destroyed as some 300 000 were killed (16 000 of them children), one million (a quarter of the population) fled the country (650 000 of them children), one million were internally displaced (42 000 of them children), 30% of all health centres and hospitals were destroyed, and most of the psychiatric facilities were bombed or turned into refugee centres. After the Dayton Peace Accord, this was complicated by vast numbers of people returning, many not by choice, to communities in which they are a minority group, whether Bosnjat, Croatian, or Serb (Maglajlic 2001). With WHO help, a scheme was developed for the establishment of community mental health centres with multidisciplinary staff teams to ease the transition of patients from hospital out into the communities in the Cantons. They ran into big problems. Some never secured the staff or the premises to open; staff were often confused about their new roles and stuck instead to the safety of the old, hierarchical, and pharmacological models; the social worker members of the teams, if they existed at all, remained subservient in status, and the divisions between healthcare and social care seemed as wide as ever; there was a lack of CPNs and home-based outreach services; and standards were extremely variable. However, the system is beginning to find its feet in an atmosphere that is moving from demoralization and shame to one of growing self confidence, and in which the user and carer movement is already voicing its strong demands.

It is difficult to find parallel post-disaster examples of child and adolescent mental health services consolidating pilot projects into anything like a national service. When that does happen, further questions will arise in the continued 'chronology of care'. At which point can a scheme dedicated to reconstruction, with all its emergency and short-term goals in the treatment of traumatized communities, be said to have progressed into a generic child and adolescent mental health service, with the usual, long-term strategies for the whole panoply of psychiatric diagnosis? Even more problematically, will that service be 'allowed' to recognize and help with all the Western style social ills that (re-)emerge, ironically, with a more settled existence—suicide, delinquency, teenage pregnancy, school drop-out, domestic violence, child abuse, alcoholism, drug misuse, and child prostitution? Anyone who has worked with the NGOs in the countries of Eastern Europe will know how difficult it is to break the taboos on even mentioning problems that are evident in every public park. To walk away and leave that home culture intact, to the detriment of children and adolescents who live there, is very difficult.

Over large-scale, natural disaster, we have little control; whether we have any greater ability to prevent 'generational cycles of ethnic hatred' (Taylor 1998) is open to debate. But the hope remains in the natural resilience of children and adolescents, even in the most appalling of circumstances, and a greater insight they might carry with them into their own adulthood. On the one hand, every totalitarian regime is aware that children can become fervently nationalistic, if encouraged, and that such fervour can be exploited. How much more so in a climate of fear where children 'chronically malnourished and with little hope of even a minimally secure life, worry that a government seemingly indifferent to them, would turn actively hostile, and send out the Police with orders to shoot and shoot and shoot' (Coles 1986). On the other hand, we know that school-aged children have a sophisticated set of values in which they may support the cause of their country, religious or ethnic group, and yet abhor war (Jagodic 2000). They will, as always, surprise us.

The author has vivid recollections of entering the main square of a small town in the Bihac Pocket at the tail-end of the Bosnian conflict—a town that had changed hands many times as Muslim, Croat, and Serb front-lines fought each other through its streets or shelled it from rival vantage points, to the extent where nearly every building had been reduced to rubble and those families that were left were living in fox-holes. Far from being similarly 'destroyed', the children emerged to ask about the fate of Manchester United and demand an impromptu football game. Of such spirit is reconstructive psychiatry born.

References

Ayalon, O. (1998) Community healing for children traumatized by war. *International Review of Psychiatry*, **10**, 224–33.

Becker, D.F., Werne, S.M., Vojvoda, D., and McGlashan, T.H. (1999) Case Series: PTSD symptoms in adolescent survivors of 'ethnic cleansing' Results from a one-year follow up study. *Journal of the American Academy of Child and Adolescent Psychiatry*, **38**, 775–81.

Berman, H. (2000) The relevance of narrative research with children who witness war and children who witness woman abuse. *Journal of Aggression, Maltreatment and Trauma*, **3**, 107–25.

Bilanakis, N.D., Pappas, E.E., Lecre-Tosevski, D., and Alexiou, D.B. (1999) Children of war fostered by Greek families for six months. The effect of the programme on children and foster mothers. *European Journal of Psychiatry*, **13**, 215–22.

Boer, F. (1999) Child and Adolescent Psychiatry in the Netherlands: patterns of practice. *European Child and Adolescent Psychiatry*, **8**, 57–60.

Brunvatne, R., Lysgard, K.H., and Hjortdahl, P. (1995) Psychosocial preventative work among war refugees. A task for primary health care? *Tidsskrift-for-den-Norske-laegeforening*, **115**, 23–6.

Cederblad, M. (1996) Fifty years of epidemiological studies in child and adolescent psychiatry in Sweden. *Nordic Journal of Psychiatry* (Supplement) **36**, 55–66.

Cohen, J.A., Manmarino, A.P., Berliner, L., and Deblinger, E. (2000) Trauma focused cognitive behavioural therapy for children and adolescents. An empirical update. *Journal of Interpersonal Violence*, **15**, 1202–23.

Coles, R. (1986) *The political life of children.* Boston, MA: Houghton Mifflin Co.

Costello, E.J., Angold, A., March, J., and Fairbank, J. (1998). Life events and post-traumatic stress: the development of a new measure for children and adolescents. *Psychological Medicine*, **28**, 1275–88.

Crijnen, A.A., Achenbach, T.M., and Verhulst, F.C. (1997) Comparisons of problems reported by parents of children in 12 cultures: total problems, externalizing and internalizing. *Journal of American Academy of Child and Adolescent Psychiatry*, **36**, 1269–77.

Crijnen, A.A., Bengi-Arslan, L., and Verhulst, F.C. (2000) Teacher reported problem behaviour in Turkish immigrant and Dutch children: a cross cultural comparison. *Acta Psychiatrica Scandinavica*, **102**, 439–44.

Daly, O. (1999) Northern Ireland: the victims. *British Journal of Psychiatry*, **175**, 201–4.

Davies, M. and Webb, E. (2000) Promoting the psychological well being of refugee children. *Clinical Child Psychology and Psychiatry*, **5**, 541–54.

Deeb, M., Khlat, M., and Courbagi, Y. (1997) Child survival in Beirut during wartime: time-trends and socio-religious differentials. *International Journal of Epidemiology*, **26**, 110–9.

Deering, C.G. (2000) A cognitive developmental approach to understanding how children cope with disasters. *Journal of Child and Adolescent Psychiatric Nursing*, **13**, 7–16.

Essenhigh, C. and Vasilyeva, N. (1998) The partnership between the Early Intervention Institute, St Petersburg, and the Anna Freud Centre, London. *Journal of Child Psychology*, **24**, 153–65.

Fitzpatrick, C. and Deehan, A. (1998) Competencies and problems of Irish children and adolescents. *European Child and Adolescent Psychiatry*, **8**, 17–23.

Gal, R. (1998) Colleagues in distress: Helping the helpers. *International Review of Psychiatry*, **10**, 234–8.

Goor-Lambo, G.V., Orley, J., Poustka, F., and Rutter, M. (1994) Abnormal Psychosocial situations. Preliminary results of a WHO and a German Multicentre Study. *European Child and Adolescent Psychiatry*, **3**, 229–41.

Green, B.L., Korol, M., Grace, M., Vary, M.G., Leonard, A., Gleser, G. *et al.* (1991) Children and disaster, age gender, and parental effects on PTSD symptoms. *Journal of the American Academy of Child and Adolescent Psychiatry*, **30**, 945–51.

Hackett, L., Hackett, R., and Taylor, D.C. (1990) Psychological disturbance and its associations in the children of the Gujurati community. *Journal of Child Psycholgy and Psychiatry*, **32**, 851–6.

Hannesdottir, H. (1993) Child and Adolescent Psychiatry in Iceland. The state of the art, past, present, and future. *Nordic Journal of Psychiatry*, **47**, 9–13.

Hillier, S., Loshak, R., Rahman, S., and Marks, F. (1994) An evaluation of Child Psychiatric Services for Bangladeshi parents. *Journal of Mental Health*, **3**, 327–37.

Hodes, M. (1998) Refugee children. Editorial. *British Medical Journal*, **316**, 793–4.

Hoger, C. and Rothenberger, A. (1998) Provision of child and adolescent psychiatric services in the Federal Republic of Germany. *European Child and Adolescent Psychiatry*, **7**, 176–80.

Husain, S.A., Nair, J., Holcomb, W., Reid, J.C., Vargas, V., and Nair, S. (1998) Stress reactions of children and adolescents in war and siege conditions. *American Journal of Psychiatry*, **155**, 1718–9.

Jagodic, G.K. (2000) Is war a good or bad thing? The attitudes of Croatian, Israeli, and Palestinian children toward war. *International Journal of Psychology*, **35**, 241–57.

Joshi, P.T. (1998) Guidelines for International trauma work. *International Review of Psychiatry*, **10**, 179–85.

Kagan, V. (1998) Child Psychotherapy in Russia. Historical and current review. *Journal of Child Psychotherapy*, **24**, 135–51.

Kesternberg, J.S. (1992) Children under the Nazi yoke. *British Journal of Psychotherapy*, **8**, 374–90.

Kozaric-Kovacic, D., Grubisic-Ilic, M., Bakic-Tomic, L., and Rutic, L. (1997) Children's awareness of danger from fire-arms, land mines, and other explosive devices in Croatia 1996. *Croatian Medical Journal* **38**, 355–64.

Laor, N., Wolmer, L., and Cohen, D.J. (2001) Mother's functioning and children's symptoms 5 years after scud missile attack. *American Journal of Psychiatry*, **158**, 1020–6.

Lucas, G. and Talan, I. (1988) French day hospitals for children: an overview. *International Journal of Partial Hospitalisation*, **5**, 169–83.

Maglajlic, R.A. (2001) A new dawn: the changing face of mental health services in Bosnia and Herzegovina. *Mental Health Care*, **4**, 401–4.

Mandic, Z., Malcic, I., Virovkic-Zunec, B., Krucaj, Z., and Baraban, D. (1996) Paediatrics in Osijek during the war in Croatia 1991–92. *Paediatrica Croatica*, **40**, 175–8.

Marttunen, M. and Aalberg, V. (1998) Adolescent Psychiatry for the specific needs of youth. *Psychiatria Fennica*, **29**, 9–11.

Mellbin, T., Sundelin, C., and Vuille, J-C. (1992) Growing up in Upsala. The role of public services in identification and treatment of health and adjustment problems. *Acta Paediatrica*, **81**, 417–23.

Miller, T.W., Kraus, R.F., Tatevosyan, A.S., and Kamenchenko, P. (1993) Post traumatic stress disorder in children and adolescents of the Armenian earthquake. *Child Psychiatry and Human Development*, **24**, 115–23.

Moilanen, I., Almquist, F., Piha, J., Rasonen, E., and Tamminen, T. (1988) An epidemiological survey of child psychiatry in Finland. *Nordic Journal of Psychiatry*, **42** (Supplement), 9–11.

NICAPS (2001). O'Herlihy, A., Worrall, A., Bannerjee, S., Jaffa, T., Hill, P., Mears, A., *et al.* National In-patient Child and Adolescent Psychiatry Study. Final report to the Department of Health. London: Royal College of Psychiatrists Research Unit.

Nicol, R. (1996) The British approach to child and adolescent psychiatry. A course for Russian post graduates. *European Child and Adolescent Psychiatry*, **5**, 212–5.

Oclander-Goldie, S.S. (1999) The impact of a war experience on the inner world of a young child. *International Journal of Psychoanalysis*, **80**, 1147–64.

O'Connor, T.G. and Rutter, M. (2000) Attachment disorder behaviour following early severe deprivation. Extension and longitudinal follow up. *Journal of the American Academy of Child and Adolescent Psychiatry*, **39**, 703–12.

Parry-Jones, W. and Barton, J. (1995) Post traumatic stress disorder in children and adolescents. *Current Opinion in Psychiatry*, **8**, 227–30.

Pfefferbaum, B. (1998) Caring for children affected by disaster. *Child and Adolescent Clinics of North America*, **7**, 579–97.

Piha, J. (1997) The status of child and adolescent psychiatry in EU and EFTA countries. *European Child and Adolescent Psychiatry*, **6**, 116–8.

Puras, D. (1994) Treatment approaches in Lithuanian Child Psychiatry. Changing the attitudes. *Nordic Journal of Psychiatry*, **48**, 397–400.

Puras, D. (2001) Unpublished communication to conference on 'Coping with Stress and Depression related problems in Europe'. Brussels.

Putnam, F.W. (1996) Post traumatic stress disorder in children and adolescents. *American Psychiatric Press Review of Psychiatry*, **15**, 447–67.

Pynoos, R.S., Goenjian, A., Tashjian, M., Karakashian, M., Manjikian, R., Mandukian, G., *et al.* (1993) Post-traumatic stress reactions in children after the 1988 Armenian earthquake. *British Journal of Psychiatry*, **163**, 239–47.

Severny, A.A. and Smirnov, A.Y. (1997) Current situations in mental health care for children in Russia. *European Child and Adolescent Psychiatry*, **6**, 50–2.

Shalev, A.Y., Yehuda, R., and McFarlane, A.C. (ed.) (2000) *International handbook of human response to trauma*. New York: Kluwer Academic/Plenum Publishers.

Shaw, J.A. (2000) Children, adolescents and trauma. *Psychiatric Quarterly*, **71**, 227–43.

Sigal, J. (1999) Post traumatic stress disorder in children of holocaust survivors (letter). *American Journal of Psychiatry*, **156**, 1295.

Sourander, A. and Piha, J. (1998) Child psychiatry in Estonia (letter). *Journal of the American Academy of Child and Adolescent Psychiatry*, **37**, 250–1.

Spiegel, P.B. and Salama, P. (2000) War and mortality in Kosovo 1998–1999. An epidemiological testimony. *Lancet*, **355**, 2204–9.

Stein, B.D. (1996) Working in a war zone. A child psychiatrist's experience. *Clinical Child Psychology and Psychiatry*, **1**, 337–46.

Steinhausen, H.Ch. (1997) Child and adolescent psychiatric disorders in a public service over seventy years. *European Child and Adolescent Psychiatry*, **6**, 42–8.

Sugar, M. (1997) Adolescents and disaster. *Journal of Adolescent Psychiatry*, **21**, 67–81.

Summerfield, D. (2000) Childhood, war, refugeedom and trauma. Three core questions for mental health professionals. *Transcultural Psychiatry* **37**, 417–33.

Taylor, C.E. (1998) How care for childhood psychological trauma in wartime may contribute to peace. *International Review of Psychiatry*, **10**, 175–8.

Thabet, A.A. and Vostanis, P. (2000) Post traumatic stress disorder reactions in children of war. A longitudinal study. *Child Abuse and Neglect*, **24**, 291–8.

Thomsen, P.H. (1996) A 22–25 year follow up study of former child psychiatric patients. A register based investigation of the course of psychiatric disorder and mortality in 546 Danish child psychiatric patients. *Acta Psychiatrica Scandinavica*, **94**, 397–403.

Tomkiewicz, S. (1997). Children and War. *World Health Forum*, **18**, 295–304.

UNICEF (1996) *The state of the world's children*. New York: Oxford University Press.

Van Beinum, M.E., McGuiness, D., Csik, V., Kalman, J., Parry-Jones, W., and Vetro, A. (1998) Contrasting child and adolescent psychiatry services in Szeged, Hungary, and Glasgow, Scotland. *European Child and Adolescent Psychiatry*, **7**, 105–13.

Vandvik, I.H. (1994) Collaboration between child psychiatry and paediatrics. The state of the relationship in Norway. *Acta Paediatrica*, **83**, 884–7.

Verheij, F. and Sanders-Woudstra, J.A.R. (1988) The history and current status of child and adolescent psychiatric day treatment programs in the Netherlands. *International Journal of Partial Hospitalisation*, **5**, 113–23.

Vogel, J.M. and Vernberg, E.M. (1993) Children's psychological responses to disasters. *Journal of Clinical Child Psychology*, **22**, 464–84.

Wolff, P.H. and Fesseha, G. (1998) Are orphanages part of the problem or part of the solution? *American Journal of Psychiatry*, **155**, 1319–24.

Wolmer, L., Laor, N., Gershon, A., Mayes, L.C., and Cohen, D.J. (2000) The mother-child dyad facing trauma . *Journal of Nervous and Mental Diseases*, **188**, 409–15.

Yamamoto, K., Davis, OL., Dylak, S., Whittaker, J., Marsh, C., and Van der Westhuizen, P.C. (1996) Across six nations. Stressful events in the lives of children. *Child Psychiatry and Human Development,* **26**, 139–50.

Yule, W. and Williams, R.M. (1990) Post traumatic stress reactions in children. *Journal of Traumatic Stress,* **3** (2), 279–95.

Yule, W. (2000) Emmanuel Miller Lecture. From pogroms to ethnic cleansing. Meeting the needs of war affected children. *Journal of Child Psychiatry,* **41**, 695–702.

Chapter 24

Child and adolescent mental health services in Australia and New Zealand: policy and development

Philip Hazell

Background

The populations of Australia (19 million) and New Zealand (3.8 million) are spread across a distance equivalent to a trip from London to Kazakhstan. While both modern societies were shaped by colonization from the United Kingdom and Ireland from the early nineteenth century onward, Australia is presently most influenced by migration from Central Europe, the Middle East, and South East Asia, while New Zealand is a major Polynesian centre. One in five Australians has a non-Anglo-Irish background, while one in five New Zealanders has Maori or Pacific Island heritage. Children and adolescents make up approximately 26–28% of the population in both countries. The Maori and Pacific Islander populations are growing at a faster rate than the Pakeha (European) population in New Zealand, so that in some regions of the country more than half the children are of Maori or Pacific Islander origin. Nevertheless, Australia and New Zealand look predominantly towards the United Kingdom and the United States of America for directions in health service delivery, with adaptations to fit the local context. Both Australia and New Zealand have enjoyed relatively high standards of living, although in recent years there has been some slippage.

The governments of Australia and New Zealand are structured somewhat differently, resulting in variation in the way policy is formulated and legislated. Responsibility in Australia is divided between the federal government that funds a national medical insurance system and sets national policy, such as the National Mental Health Plan, and the state and territory governments that are responsible for hospital and community health services, as well as education and welfare. In effect, 'private' psychiatrists are funded through the federal government, while 'public' psychiatrists are funded through the states and territories. There is an unfortunate tendency for both tiers of government to blame each other for shortfalls in resources for service. In contrast, New Zealand has only one tier of centralized government that interacts directly with local health service providers. In the past fifteen years New Zealand has endured experiments with a number of models for health service administration, which came at one point close to the United Kingdom system of local bodies bidding against each other to provide service at lowest cost. More recently, the New Zealand system has reverted to one similar to Australia in which health services are administered by district health boards.

Mapping mental health and mental health service utilization in Australia and New Zealand

Within Australia a cross-sectional survey has recently been completed of mental health and well-being, involving a national probability sample of 4500 participants aged 4–17 years (Sawyer et al. 2000). The study gives a coarse overview of mental health problems, since only three specific disorders were surveyed (attention-deficit/hyperactivity disorder, conduct disorder, and depression) while the child behaviour checklist was used to provide a global measure of mental health problems. Impact on functioning was measured by the child health questionnaire. Service utilization was also examined.

In overview, 14% of children and adolescents met criteria for at least one of the three mental disorders studied in the previous 12 months. Only 3% of the children and adolescents with a mental disorder had attended a mental health clinic, and only 2% had attended a hospital-based department of psychiatry. Of those meeting criteria for disorder, 4% had attended a private psychiatrist. Children and adolescents with mental disorders were more likely to have received counselling at school (14%), assessment and/or treatment by the family doctor (13%), or treatment from a paediatrician (11%). The authors of the survey also reported data on children and adolescents attending services who had a mental disorder, who scored in the clinical range on the child and behaviour checklist, and whose parents reported that they needed professional help. Of this group, who had more severe problems and perceived need, still only 17% had attended a psychiatrist, mental health clinic, or hospital-based department of psychiatry.

The most common barriers to accessing services were: lack of knowledge about where to obtain help, a perception that the problem could be dealt with without professional assistance, help was requested but not forthcoming, and waiting times that were too long.

New Zealand has contributed two birth cohort studies based in Dunedin and Christchurch, respectively, each of which has contributed around 1000 participants. These studies have reported on a range of child health concerns. Rates of mental disorder reported in successive waves of the studies have been comparable to those conducted in other Westernized countries.

An overview of services

Specialist child and adolescent mental health services in Australia generally cover individuals up to their eighteenth birthday (Birleson et al. 1995); while in New Zealand, child and adolescent mental health services have been contracted to provide service up to their twentieth birthday (Mental Health Commission 1998). In both countries there is a deliberate overlap of two years in services offered by child and adolescent mental health services and adult mental health services. Service providers are expected to collaborate in 'getting the right mix of services appropriate for the mental age of the child or the young person, their mental health needs and their level of family support' (Health Funding Authority 2000). New Zealand child and adolescent mental health services are further subdivided into services for children 0–14 years and services for youth aged 15–19 years (Mental Health Commission 1998). Within Australia the age cut-off between child and youth services ranges from 13 to 15 years. In some regions of both Australia and New Zealand a large bulk of the mental health services for children are delivered by non-specialist services, such as community health and child health services. However, within these teams there may be individuals with extensive experience and training in child and adolescent mental health. Psychologists and social workers, in particular, are often able to move between specialist mental health services and generic services.

Most public sector specialist child and adolescent mental health service is provided through community teams, followed by the psychiatry out-patient departments of children's hospitals, in-patient care in paediatric or adult psychiatric beds, and in-patient care in specialized child and adolescent psychiatric in-patient units. Psychiatric in-patient units for children and adolescents exist in only the mainland capital cities of Australia and in two centres in New Zealand. Owing to a pressure for beds, few if any of these units have been able to offer emergency care. Psychiatric emergencies involving children and adolescents are more likely to be managed in paediatric or adult general psychiatric units. In the state of New South Wales (NSW) there is presently a strong push to redress this problem. Dedicated in-patient units are being built outside the Sydney metropolitan area (NSW Health Department 1999), and there are plans to establish acute psychiatric units within the two major metropolitan paediatric hospitals.

While children and adolescents make up 26–28% of the population in Australia, no state or territory dedicates more than 10% of it's mental health budget on this age group (Birleson *et al.* 2000). Some of the disparity is due to the limited number of expensive in-patient services in the child and adolescent sector, but even taking this into account, there remain inequities. Similar inequities have been identified in New Zealand and have received mention in recent policy documents (Health Funding Authority 2000)

A typical community child and adolescent mental health service within Australia and New Zealand will have up to a dozen clinicians, most of whom are likely to be psychologists or social workers. A psychiatrist may not head the team. The service is likely to be specific to children or youth. The community service may not have a specialized in-patient unit to refer to. Referrals will be received from general practitioners, paediatricians, welfare services, and educational and juvenile justice professionals. Some units may accept self-referral or referral from parents. These services will usually adopt a family focus for the initial assessment interviews. Assessment may take up to three hours and may be spread across three or more appointments (Luk *et al.* 1999) The unit will have developed, or will be developing, a standardized data collection system. The unit will have developed, or will be developing, mental health promotion and prevention activities. The unit may provide outreach to a rural or remote area. This is most likely to take the form of clinicians travelling to remote regions to provide direct service, but in some centres, telemedicine is now operative. The unit may have waiting times of several months, and it can be expected that 20–30% of appointments will default. The unit may have only sessional access to a psychiatrist, and the presence of trainee psychiatrists will depend largely on proximity to a centralized training programme.

Policy

The organization and delivery of child and adolescent mental health services has been influenced by broad policies affecting the health welfare and education sector, and specific policies directed to mental health or even more specifically to child and adolescent mental health services.

Medicare

Medicare is the national health insurance plan introduced to Australia in 1983. Under the system, a significant portion of the fee for any medical consultation (primary care or specialist care) is reimbursed by the federal government. The government sets scheduled fees. Practitioners are encouraged to charge only a small amount above the scheduled fee. The consequence, in theory at least, is that a visit to a specialist medical practitioner is affordable to most families, even though they may not carry private health insurance. A practitioner willing to accept the base fee may bill the government directly, thus avoiding administration costs. More child psychiatrists work in the private sector than the public sector, although there is some overlap. The 'cost' is that these individuals are lost to the supervision of non-psychiatrists, tend not to engage in the planning of clinical services, and are less involved in research and teaching. In contrast, nearly all child psychiatrists in New Zealand work within the public sector and are salaried by their health services.

The Treaty of Waitangi (Te Tiriti o Waitangi)

In recent years within New Zealand there has been significant effort to enact the spirit of the Treaty of Waitangi, which was signed in 1840 by representatives of the crown and Maori, and in which the rights and needs of the Maori would be protected. The process has seen New Zealand move to being officially a bilingual and bicultural nation. The relationship between the Maori and the crown, in the health and disability sector, has formed around three key principles, namely partnership, participation, and protection. Partnership refers to a relationship between the Maori and the crown characterized by good faith, mutual respect, and understanding, and shared decision-making. Participation implies the crown and the Maori will work together to ensure that the Maori participate at all levels of the health and disability sector. Protection indicates that the crown will actively contribute to improving the health status of the Maori and to ensure equal access to mental health services. In a recent document *A national workplan for child and youth mental health services'* (*He Nuka Mo Nga Taitamariki*) (Health Funding Authority 2000), inequalities and access to child and adolescent mental health services were identified between Pakeha on one hand, and Maori and Pacific Islanders on the other. Regions of New Zealand with the highest concentration of Maori and Pacific Island children and youth were found to receive the lowest per capita funding for child and adolescent mental health services. Specific strategies to redress these inequalities will be discussed below under national mental health plans. In Australia, a less explicit process has occurred known as 'reconciliation', which has enjoyed less support from central government than does the Treaty of Waitangi in New Zealand. However, within the spirit of reconciliation, specialist services to Aboriginal children and youth have developed in some states.

Inquiries into social and equality and the needs of the mentally ill

Inquiries have been held under the chairmanship of Burdekin (cited in Whiteford 1995) in Australia, and Mason (cited in Wilson 1997) in New Zealand, examining the needs of the mentally ill. Both inquiries concluded that services were, in general, inadequate, and both highlighted the particular needs of children and youth and of indigenous people. Funding has flowed on from these inquiries, often directed to specific purposes, such as the improvement of Aboriginal mental health, the prevention of suicide, and the treatment of conduct problems, drug and alcohol dependence, and mood disorder.

National mental health strategies

1992 saw the introduction of the first Australian national mental health policy and 5-year plan directed to reforming Australia's mental health services (Whiteford 1995). The national mental health plan was formulated to address inequalities identified in the Burdekin Inquiry. While the needs of children and adolescents were acknowledged, the first national mental health plan was not specifically directed to child psychiatric disorders. In contrast, the second national mental health plan introduced in 1998 (Commonwealth Department of Health and Aged Care 2000) has included a greater focus on the mental health needs of the young and, in particular, has directed attention to promotion, prevention, and early intervention (Raphael 2000). These principles have been written into statewide plans such as the *NSW strategy: making mental health better for children and adolescents* (NSW Health Department 1999). As part of a wider planning process in mental health, a NSW mental health care and prevention plan (unpublished) has been formulated that specifies 'care packages' for children and adolescents categorized according to the severity of their problems. An adolescent, for example, considered to have severe problems not requiring hospitalization, would be expected to receive one 90-minute family-oriented mental health assessment followed by six 45-minute family-oriented community contacts. The authors of the plan emphasize that the care packages are designed, not to dictate clinical practice, but to inform the planning of services.

New Zealand introduced a national mental health plan in 1994 that led to the publication of the *blueprint for mental health services in New Zealand* (Mental Health Commission 1998). This plan articulated in some detail a service model for younger people that divides the service components for children into in-patient services, community based day and residential services, and community based mental health teams. Each form of service receives an indicative number of 'care packages' per 100 000 total population. For youth aged 15–19 years, additional service components include community support services, advice and support for consumers and families, access to newer anti-psychotic medications, alcohol and drug detoxification services, alcohol and drug residential treatment services, alcohol and drug community based teams, and methadone treatment. There is an explicit directive in the Blueprint that resources should be allocated to Maori and to Pacific Islanders proportional to their representation within the population of each health region. The Blueprint has been followed up by a national work plan for child and youth mental health services (Health Funding Authority 2000), which in particular addresses a redistribution of services to meet the needs of Maori and Pacific Islanders, and workforce issues.

Outcome measurement

The use of standardized outcome measures in mental health has become a requirement in the states of Victoria and New South Wales. Other states and territories, and New Zealand, are likely to follow suit. Within New South Wales, standardized outcome measures will be linked with standardized documentation of assessment. While the assessment documentation has not been finalized, the standardized outcome measures will include the health of the nation outcome scale for children and adolescents and the children's global assessment scale. The federal government in Australia has been interested in sponsoring the introduction of standardized outcome measures across Australia. A report prepared by Bickman *et al.* (1999) concluded that no existing measure was ideally suited to the Australian context, and recommended the development of baseline follow-up measures, background measures, and measures of process. At the time of writing, progress on the development of national outcome measures has stalled.

Workforce issues

Australia has one child and adolescent psychiatrist per 23 400 population less than 20 years, compared to one per 27 500 in the United Kingdom (Remschmidt *et al.* 1999) . The ratio is less favourable in New Zealand, but estimates are unreliable because the lower population based rate means that a shift of two or three psychiatrists in or out of the country significantly alters the ratio. Most Australian child and adolescent psychiatrists were locally trained. Up to a half of child and adolescent psychiatrists working in New Zealand were trained elsewhere, most commonly in the United States of America, Canada, or the United Kingdom. It is generally acknowledged that there is a shortage of child and adolescent psychiatrists in all regions. Training in child and adolescent psychiatry in Australia and New Zealand is conducted under the auspices of the Royal Australian and New Zealand College of Psychiatrists. A committee of the college accredits training programmes and accredits the training experience of individual trainees. The capital cities of Australia, and Auckland and Christchurch in New Zealand, offer training programmes. In all but the largest training centres, the directorship position is unpaid. Training in child and adolescent psychiatry has usually been undertaken over 2 full-time years following the completion of 4 years training in general adult psychiatry. The mandatory period of training in general adult psychiatry is soon to be reduced from 4 to 3 years, meaning that the total length of training will reduce from a minimum of 6 years to a minimum of 5 years. There has been a recent trend towards greater co-operation between individual training programs and the sharing of learning resources.

The bulk of the specialist child and adolescent mental health workforce is made up of psychologists, social workers, and mental health nurses. These disciplines do not have specific training in child and adolescent mental health that might parallel the training of psychiatrists. However, some universities and some institutions, such as the NSW Institute of Psychiatry, are now offering generic courses in child and adolescent mental health. Specific therapeutic skills are generally learnt through supervision 'on the job', although increasingly courses are being made available on a fee-for-service basis. Workforce training has been a particular focus in New Zealand and has been embodied in the national workplan for child and youth mental health services (Health Funding Authority 2000). Challenges to workforce development in New Zealand include a lack of national co-ordination and leadership, limited capacity for child and youth sector to provide training opportunities, a shortage of experienced clinicians across all professional groups, and a critical shortage of Maori and Pacific Islanders within the workforce. Future Maori child and mental health staff are likely to come through the Te Rau Puawai professional development course at Massey University. The New Zealand Government is considering the promotion of the training of the child and youth mental health sector through the purchase of child and youth streams in graduate mental health nursing, advanced mental health nursing, and Maori mental health multidisciplinary programmes.

Inter-agency collaboration

As in the United Kingdom, an important component of child and adolescent mental health service delivery in Australia and New Zealand is collaboration with key agencies such as child health services, family welfare, education, juvenile justice, youth services, drug and alcohol services, and a range of non-government organizations. Some of these relationships have been mandated. By way of example, memoranda of understanding have been drawn up in NSW between health and education, and health and community services (welfare). With respect to education, 'school link' positions have been funded in each of the area health services to facilitate the roll-out of mental health promotion and prevention programmes within schools, and to identify pathways to care from education services to specialist mental health services. Also in NSW, recent changes to child protection legislation have placed greater responsibility on health professionals to recognize and report child abuse, and also to monitor the safety of children in the longer term. Compulsory training programmes have been held for health staff throughout the state to educate them about their roles and responsibilities. The children's court of NSW has recently established clinics to assess and advise on the management of children and adolescents brought before the court. These clinics are 'virtual', as most assessments are to be conducted by clinicians working out of their own offices.

Other influences

The Faculty of Child and Adolescent Psychiatry of the Royal Australian and New Zealand College of Psychiatrists was established in its present form in 1988. The faculty membership contributes to the formulation of college position statements on a range of issues. Faculty members also represent the college and speak to the media on a range of issues. The faculty, however, remains small with a total membership of only approximately 250 across Australia and New Zealand. Faculty contributions include comment about the plight of refugee children affected by Australia's current policy towards illegal immigrants. In recent years, Australia and New Zealand have seen the establishment of infant child and adolescent mental health associations that advocate for the needs of children and adolescents affected by mental disorder. These associations have a much wider membership than the specific professional organizations, and there has been a substantial effort to secure the participation of consumers. As such, these associations are proving to be more effective than professional organizations in advocating for the mental health of children and adolescents.

The Australian early intervention network for mental health in young people (AusEinet) was established to co-ordinate a national approach to early intervention for mental health in young people. AusEinet was funded by the Commonwealth Department of Health and Aged Care under the National Mental Health Strategy and the National Youth Suicide Prevention Strategy. The project had three streams, which were: the development of maintenance for national early intervention network for mental health in young people, the identification of promotion of good practice in early intervention, and the re-orientation of service delivery towards early intervention (O'Hanlon *et al.* 2000). AusEinet has produced a range of books including *The national stocktake of prevention and early intervention programs* and a series of booklets entitled *Clinical approaches to early intervention and child and adolescent mental health*, which focus on attention-deficit/hyperactivity disorder, anxiety disorders, conduct problems, the psychological adjustment of children with chronic conditions, and the perinatal period. Model projects that have been described by O'Hanlon *et al.* (2000) include a collaboration between mental health and community services concerning children of parents suffering mental illness, an improvement in mental health literacy among child and youth welfare workers, and interventions directed to children young people with a parent in prison.

The Australian National Youth Suicide Prevention Strategy has also evolved from the National Mental Health Plan and is a response to the recognition that Australia and New Zealand have some of the highest rates of youth suicide in the Westernized world. The goals of the National Youth Suicide Prevention Strategy have been to prevent premature death due to suicide among young people, to reduce the rates of injury in self-harm arising from suicidal behaviour, to reduce the incidence and prevalence of suicidal behaviour, and to enhance resilience, resourcefulness, respect, and an inter-connectedness for young people in families and communities in Australia (Australian Institute of Family Studies 1998). An important flow-on from the concern about youth suicide has been an injection of funds into the child and adolescent mental health sector, particularly services directed to youth. This has enabled the appointment of project officers in some regions, who have worked to improve collaboration between agencies who may see youth at risk, and the development of youth crisis teams, who provide brief ambulatory interventions to young people at risk as an alternative to hospitalization.

A further consequence of the National Mental Health Plan in Australia has been a focus on improved intervention for young people experiencing a first episode of psychosis. In some regions, these individuals are the responsibility of child and adolescent mental health services; in others, they are the responsibility of adult services; and in yet others, there are specific youth health services. A group in the state of Victoria has been particularly influential, and has been responsible for the publication of clinical guidelines (Early Psychosis Prevention and Intervention Centre 1998).

Conclusions

Australia and New Zealand are characterized by ethnic diversity, and by the isolation of rural communities. Within Australia this isolation can be extreme. Inequities in the allocation of mental health resources to children and adolescents have been acknowledged in both countries, as have inequities in the allocation of resources to indigenous people. There have been serious attempts to model mental health services for children and adolescents, with an emphasis on early intervention, and on the development of 'care packages' based on the severity of problems. Such principles are only now being written in to statewide mental health service plans, so that it may be several years before the rhetoric is translated into services. At present there are many initiatives coming from central government, and it is difficult at times to see how these initiatives may inter-relate. Nevertheless, there is considerable momentum for improving child and adolescent mental health services, which has been driven by a number of influential psychiatrists who occupy senior management roles within government departments, and by other mental health professionals who are advocating for change.

References

Australian Institute of Family Studies (1998) *Youth Suicide Prevention Programs and Activities. National Stocktake March 1998.* Melbourne: Australian Institute of Family Studies.

Bickman, L., Nurcombe, B., Townsend, C., Belle, M., Schut, J., and Karver, M. (1999) *Consumer measurement systems for child and adolescent mental health.* Canberra: Department of Health and Family Services.

Birleson, P., Stripp, A., and Wilder, J. (1995) Victoria's Child and Adolescent Mental Health Services: the framework for service delivery. *Australasian Psychiatry,* 3, 420–2.

Birleson, P., Sawyer, M., and Storm, V. (2000) The mental health of young people in Australia: child and adolescent component of the national survey- a commentary. *Australasian Psychiatry,* 8, 358–62.

Commonwealth Department of Health and Aged Care (2000) *Promotion, prevention and early intervention for mental health. A monograph.* Mental Health and Special Programs Branch, Commonwealth Department of Health and Aged Care, Canberra.

Early Psychosis Prevention and Intervention Centre (1998) *The Australian Clinical Guidelines for Early Psychosis.* Melbourne: Early Psychosis Prevention and Intervention Centre.

Health Funding Authority (2000) *A national workplan for child and youth mental health services.* Wellington: Health Funding Authority.

Luk, E.S.L., Robinson, P., Birleson, P., and Cooper, H. (1999) Assessment in child and adolescent psychiatry: Interstate differences. *Australasian Psychiatry,* 7, 141–2.

Mental Health Commission (1998) *Blueprint for mental health services in New Zealand,* pp. 42–5. Wellington: Mental Health Commission.

NSW Health Department (1999) *NSW strategy: making mental health better for children and adolescents,* p. 18. Sydney: NSW Health Department.

O'Hanlon, A., Kosky, Martin, G., Dundas, P., and Davis, C. (2000) *Model projects for early intervention and the mental health of young people. Reorientation of services.* Canberra: Commonwealth of Australia.

Raphael, B. (2000) *A population model for the provision of mental health care.* Canberra: Commonwealth of Australia.

Remscmhidt, H., van Engeland, H., and Piha, J. (1999) Introduction. In *Child and adolescent psychiatry in Europe* (ed. H. Remschmidt, and H. van Engeland,), pp. XIII–XVI. New York: Springer.

Sawyer, M.G., Arney, F.M., Baghurst, P.A., Clark, J.J., Graetz, B.W., Kosky, R.J. *et al.* (2000) *The mental health of young people in Australia. The child and adolescent component of the National Survey of Mental Health and Well-being.* Canberra: Mental Health and Special Programs Branch, Commonwealth Department of Health and Aged Care.

Whiteford, H. (1995) The implications of the national mental health strategy for child and adolescent psychiatry: Twelve key questions. *Australasian Psychiatry,* 3, 246–9.

Wilson, J. (1997) New Zealand mental health strategy: is it making any difference? *Australasian Psychiatry,* 5, 111–4.

Chapter 25

Comparative analyses: challenges facing CAMHS in North America

David R. Offord

Introduction

This chapter covers the major challenges facing the delivery of child and adolescent mental health services in North America. The situation in the United States is covered first, and then this is compared with the circumstances in Canada. The chapter ends with a consideration of some lessons from the North American experience that may be helpful in other jurisdictions.

United States

Unmet need

In the United States, the majority of children and adolescents with a diagnosable mental disorder do not receive any mental health services (Burns *et al.* 1995; Leaf *et al.* 1996). For example, in the study by Burns and colleagues (Burns *et al.* 1995), of those children with a diagnosis plus impairment (seriously emotionally disturbed), only about 1 in 5 (21.6%) had used specialty mental health services in the past three months, and less than half (40.3%) had received any services at all in that time period. These results were in agreement with an earlier report, which indicated that approximately 70% of children and adolescents in need of treatment do not receive any mental health services (US Office of Technology Assessment 1986).

Both the studies by Burns and colleagues (Burns *et al.* 1995) and Leaf and his group (Leaf *et al.* 1996) showed that the targeting of specialty mental health services is, for the most part, appropriate. For instance, in the Burns study, the percentage of children who used specialty mental health services in the past three months varied by diagnosis and impairment as follows: no diagnosis/no impairment—1.6%; diagnosis/no impairment—3.3%; no diagnosis/ impairment—6.0%; and diagnosis/impairment—21.6%. Similarly, in the Leaf study, children with a diagnosis and impaired functioning were 6.8 times more likely to be seen by a specialist compared to those with no diagnosis and a high level of functioning. Lastly, it should be noted that the study by Burns and colleagues presents important data on who provided the services for children who were seriously emotionally disturbed (diagnosis plus impairment). In about 70% of cases, the children received services from the schools, 40% from the specialty mental health sector, 16% from the child welfare sector, 11% from the health sector, and 4% from the juvenile justice sector. Further, for almost half the children with serious emotional disturbances, the public school system was the sole provider of services.

The rate of service use varied by age group. Among pre-schoolers, only 1–2% used any service, in 6–11-year-olds the rate rose to 6–8%, and for adolescents, 12–17, the rate was 8–9%

(Sturm *et al.* 2000). Lastly, while it is not clear whether utilization of specialized mental health services varies by race or ethnicity, there is evidence that the type of service does (US Department of Health and Human Services 1999). For example, most studies have found that African-Americans use in-patient services more than would be expected, based on their numbers in the population. A major problem in determining utilization rates in different racial and ethnic segments of the population is the lack of data on the prevalence of child mental disorder for these subgroups (Attkisson *et al.* 1995; Friedman *et al.* 1996; McCabe *et al.* 1998; Roberts *et al.* 1998).

Barriers to treatment

The obstacles to obtaining specialized mental health assessment and treatment services for children and adolescents are several (Pavuluri *et al.* 1996; Kazdin *et al.* 1997). They include the cost of treatment and the unwillingness of children and their families to seek care. Contributing to the latter are the perceptions that treatments will be demanding and will be ineffective, and will bring with them labelling and stigmatization of the child and the family. Further, a sizeable proportion of families who begin treatment, terminate prematurely. This has been reported to be as high as 40–60% (Kazdin 1996), and one study found that most of the children who begin out-patient treatment attend for only one or two sessions (Armbruster and Fallon 1994). There is evidence too that unawareness of mental health professionals to relevant issues of culture of minority children and families contribute to high premature termination rates (Woodward *et al.* 1992). In addition, children who live in poverty have higher rates of dropping out and shorter lengths of treatment than their middle-class peers (Hoberman 1992). This finding is especially relevant for minority children and their families, since, for example, it has been reported that 90% of African-American youths entering the mental health system live in poverty (Hoberman 1992).

Mix of services

There is a wide range of mental health services for children and adolescents. The most common type is out-patient treatment, and it is estimated that 5–10% of US children and their families make use of this service annually (Burns *et al.* 1998). Out-patient treatment has by far the strongest research base (Weisz *et al.* 1998). At the other end of the spectrum is in-patient hospitalization. An issue of concern for the past two decades is the inappropriate use of in-patient care with rising rates of utilization, without evidence of increased need for such treatment (Knitzer 1982; Weller *et al.* 1995). Not only is in-patient care the clinical intervention with the weakest evidence of effectiveness, but it devours about half the available child mental health resources (Burns 1991). Between the non-restrictive and restrictive environments of out-patient and in-patient treatments, respectively, are partial hospitalization or day treatment and residential treatment centers. While the latter serve only 8% of treated children, they consume almost one-fourth of the child mental health budget (Burns *et al.* 1998). Lastly, there are a growing number of community-based interventions primarily for children with serious emotional disturbances including case management, where the aim is to co-ordinate the provision of services for children and their families who require interventions from multiple providers, home-based services, which focus on providing intensive services in the homes for children and adolescents with serious emotional and behavioural disturbances, therapeutic foster care, therapeutic group homes, and crisis services (US Department of Health and Human Services 1999).

Organization and financing of services

It has been noted that 'the system for delivering mental health services to children and their families is complex, sometimes to the point of inscrutability—a patchwork of providers, interventions, and payers' (US Department of Health and Human Services 1999). There are two service systems delivering mental health services to children and their families—private and public. They are not as distinct as they once were, with some public services being delivered by private organizations.

The private sector, using a health insurance model, provides mental health coverage for children and their families, but the insurance plans usually do not cover required services for complex long-term problems. In these cases, the families have to pay for the services themselves or, in some instances, they give up custody of their children to the state child welfare system to obtain appropriate residential treatment services (Cohen *et al.* 1991; US Department of Health and Human Services 1999). Managed care is now part of the private sector delivery system and it has as a major aim, reducing mental health service costs by limiting both hospital stays and number of out-patient visits (Stroul *et al.* 1998).

The mental health services to children provided by the public sector have Medicaid as a major source of funding. An important issue is that there are a sizeable group of children and families who have no private insurance, cannot afford to pay for services themselves, and do not qualify for the public sector programmes. It is estimated that in 2001 there were in the US 11 million uninsured children, and over 3 million of them did not qualify for existing public programmes (American Academy of Pediatrics website www.aap.org).

Children needing mental health services funded by the public sector are in five distinct service sectors: general health and mental health agencies, schools, juvenile justice, and child welfare (US Department of Health and Human Services 1999). The schools and these agencies have original mandates that did not include the provision of mental health services. However, it has become apparent that children with psychiatric disturbance are an important part of their populations (Friedman *et al.* 1996). For example, in the 1996–97 school year, 1% of the school population, ages 6–17, received some type of special education services because of emotional disturbance (US Department of Education 1997). Further, it is well recognized that children served by the child welfare and juvenile justice systems have much higher rates of emotional and behavioural disorders compared to their peers in the general population, and thus have an increased need for mental health services (Cohen *et al.* 1990; Otto *et al.* 1992; Claussen *et al.* 1998; Duchnowski *et al.* 1998; Quinn and Epstein 1998). Lastly, it should be noted that managed care has begun to infiltrate the public sector (Essock and Goldman 2002). However, this may result in little or no cost savings, with the costs being shifted from one agency to another, for example, from hospitals to child welfare and juvenile justice agencies (Stroul *et al.* 1998).

Effectiveness of services

Important progress has been made over the past decade in establishing efficacious interventions for children and their families with mental health problems (US Department of Health and Human Services 1999). These interventions do more good than harm when delivered in a research setting. For example, around two dozen efficacious treatments have been identified for various disorders in children including ADHD, anxiety disorders, depression, oppositional defiant disorder, and conduct disorder (Chambless *et al.* 1998; Lonigan *et al.* 1998).

However, most of the services delivered in communities have no empirical support behind them and thus are unlikely to be effective; that is, do not do more good than harm in the real world (English 2001). This has led to a re-evaluation of the so-called Clinic-Based Treatment Development Model. In this model, efficacious treatments are developed under laboratory conditions and then deployed to community settings. An alternative strategy being explored is to develop interventions in real-life settings, where variables, usually excluded by researchers, are dealt with up-front (Weisz 1997). Examples of such variables are parental psychopathology, co-morbidity, factors leading to early termination, and providers not having the time to learn new extensive treatment protocols. One last point. Although systems of care, where attempts are made to have an integrated service delivery system providing a continuum of care, result in increased parental satisfaction, there is no evidence that they result in better clinical outcomes than services delivered in the usual way (Hamner *et al.* 1997; Bickman *et al.* 1999).

Two additional areas of major concern in the US in the treatment domain are psychopharmacology and the cultural relevance of interventions. Both have been identified as needing major research initiatives. It has been stated that the gaps in knowledge in psychopharmacologic therapies for children and youth cover three areas: for most prescribed medications, there are no data on safety and efficacy, there is limited information on pharmacokinetics, and there are few studies on the effectiveness of combined medication and psychosocial interventions (Jensen *et al.* 1999). In the cultural domain, there is documentation that racial and ethnic minority groups under-utilize treatment, and exhibit less help-seeking behaviour (US Department of Health and Human Services 1999). There is evidence that culturally appropriate services are helpful to patients because they are in concert with the cultural community and family context in which the patient lives (Szapocznik *et al.* 1988; Hernandez and Isaacs 1998).

Canada

Description

The provision of the bulk of health services, including mental health services for children, in Canada is a provincial responsibility with a major portion of the funding coming from the federal government through various federal-provincial transfer agreements (Federal/Provincial/Territorial committee on Mental Health 1990). Private practice clinicians (e.g. social workers, psychologists) and private-for-profit organizations make relatively little contribution to overall service delivery. All physicians, including child psychiatrists in private practice, are paid by the provincial government usually on a fee-for-service or contract basis. As in the United States, the service delivery system involves multiple sectors and government departments including health, social or community services, education, and justice. The services delivered by these sectors provide the system of care in Canada for children and adolescents with mental health problems.

Challenges and initiatives

The removal of the financial barrier to receiving children's mental health services does not mean that all children who are in need of services are receiving them. For example, the 90 children's mental health centres in Ontario estimated in 1998–99 that there were almost 9000 children waiting for services at any one time (Children's Mental Health Ontario 2000a, b). The average waiting period was estimated to be 5 months. As in the United States, there is great concern in Canada about delivering evidence-based interventions (Children's Mental Health

Ontario 2001, 2002), and for service delivery strategies that provide meaningful rewards and incentives for improved outcomes (Junek and Thompson 1999). Lastly, it should be noted that there is a movement in Canada towards government-sponsored large-scale prevention efforts in the child mental health field. For example, the Ontario Government has funded a large-scale prevention project for young children and their families living in eight disadvantaged neighbourhoods throughout the province (Peters *et al.* 2000). Further, the government has established the Healthy Babies, Healthy Children's program, a service that contacts new mothers within 48 hours of discharge from hospital and offers a home visit by a public health nurse (Ministry of Community and Social Services 2001).

Comment

There are many challenges facing the delivery of mental health services for children and adolescents in North America. However, two stand out, and they are closely intertwined. First, many children, and certainly in the United States the majority, who require specialized mental health services do not receive them. Second, there is a paucity of effective interventions delivered in everyday front-line practice. Taking up the second issue first, it is clear that progress in providing effective interventions for children with mental health problems will highlight the urgency of having a delivery system that reaches all children in need. This will be especially difficult in the United States with their lack of a universal health insurance plan. However, removal of the financial barrier will not ensure that all children who need services will receive them. There is a requirement to know more about how to remove other obstacles to care ranging all the way from instrumental issues, such as location of services, to the perceived stigma of mental illness.

Further, there is an increasing awareness in North America, especially in Canada, that specialized mental health services alone cannot markedly reduce the tremendous burden of suffering from emotional and behavioural problems in children and adolescents (Offord and Bennett 2002). What will be needed, in addition to effective specialized services, will be effective services provided by family physicians and paediatricians, and a combination of effective universal programmes (where all children are offered the interventions) and targeted programmes (where children at increased risk for emotional and behavioural problems are offered the interventions)(Offord *et al.* 1998). These and other strategies will be essential to reduce the size of the population of children in need of specialized mental health services.

Lastly, in both the United States and Canada, there is a need to have a national monitoring system in place to provide data on the extent to which children and youth with mental health problems, not only are receiving services, but appear to be receiving appropriate ones. Such a system could monitor the extent of unmet needs, describe the characteristics of the children and their families in need of services who are not receiving them, identify the barriers to receiving care, and point the way towards reducing the size of the population of children with unmet needs for mental health services.

References

Armbruster, P. and Fallon, T. (1994) Clinical, sociodemographic, and systems risk factors for attrition in a children's mental health clinic. *American Journal of Orthopsychiatry*, **64**, 577–85.

Attkisson, C.C., Dresser, K.L., and Rosenblatt, A. (1995) Service systems for youth with severe emotional disorders: System-of-care research in California. In *Children's Mental Health Services: Research, Policy, and Evaluation* (ed. L. Bickman, and D.J. Rog), pp. 236–80. Thousand Oaks, CA: Sage Publications.

Bickman, L., Noser, K., and Summerfelt, W.T. (1999) Long-term effects of a system of care on children and adolescents. *Journal of Behavioral Health Services and Research*, **26**, 185–202.

Burns, B.J. (1991) Mental health service use by adolescents in the 1970s and 1980s. *Journal of the American Academy of Child and Adolescent Psychiatry*, **30**, 144–50.

Burns, B.J., Costello, E.J., Angold, A., Tweed, D., Stangle, D., Farmer, E.M.Z., and Erkanli, A. (1995) Children's mental health service use across service sectors. *Health Affairs*, **14**, 147–59.

Burns, B.J., Hoagwood, K., and Maultsby, L.T. (1998) Improving outcomes for children and adolescents with serious emotional and behavioral disorders: current and future directions. In *Outcomes for children and youth with emotional and behavioral disorders and their families: programs and evaluation best practices* (ed. M.H. Epstein, K. Kutash, and A.J. Duchnowski), pp. 686–707. Austin, TX: Pro-Ed.

Chambless, D.L., Baker, M.J., Baucom, D.H., Beutler, L.E., Calhoun, K.S., Crits-Christoph, P. *et al.* (1998) Update on empirically validated therapies, II. *Clinical Psychology*, **27**, 138–45.

Children's Mental Health Ontario (2000a) *Children's mental health survey report 1998/99.* Toronto: Children's Mental Health, Ontario.

Children's Mental Health Ontario (2000b) *Guide to children's mental health programs and services.* Toronto: Children's Mental Health, Ontario.

Children's Mental Health Ontario (2001a) *Evidence based practices for depression in children and adolescents.* Toronto: Children's Mental Health, Ontario.

Children's Mental Health Ontario (2001b) *Evidence based practices for conduct disorder in children and adolescents.* Toronto: Children's Mental Health, Ontario.

Claussen, J.M., Landsverk, J., Ganger, W., Chadwick, D., and Litronic, A. (1998) Mental health problems of children in foster care. *Journal of Child and Family Studies*, **7**, 283–96.

Cohen, R., Parmelee, D.X., Irwin, L., Weisz, J.R., Howard, P., Purcell, P., and Best, A.M. (1990) Characteristics of children and adolescents in a psychiatric hospital and a corrections facility. *Journal of the American Academy of Child and Adolescent Psychiatry*, **29**, 909–13.

Cohen, R., Harris, R., Gottlieb, S., and Best, A.M. (1991) States' use of transfer of custody as a require-ment for providing services to emotionally distrubed children. *Hospital and Community Psychiatry*, **42**, 526–30.

Duchnowski, A.J., Hall, K.W., Kutash, K., and Friedman, R.M. (1998) The alternatives to residential treatment studies. In *Outcomes for children and youth with behavioral and emotional disorders and their families* (ed. M.H. Epstein, K. Kutash, and A.J. Duchnowski), pp. 55–80. Austin, TX: Pro-Ed.

English, M. (2001) Policy implications relevant to implementing evidence-based treatment. In *Evidence-based community interventions for youth with severe emotional and beahvioral disorders* (ed. B.J. Burns, and K. Hoagwood). New York: Oxford University Press.

Essock, S.M. and Goldman, H.H. (2002) States' embrace of managed mental health care. *Health Affairs*, **14**, 34–44.

Federal/Provincial/Territorial committee on Mental Health, wGoCaYMH (1990) *Foundation for the Future.* Ottawa, ON: Health Canada.

Friedman, R.M., Kutash, K., and Duchnowski, A.J. (1996) The population of concern: defining the issues. In *Children's mental health: creating systems for care in a changing society* (ed. B.A. Stroul), pp. 69–96. Baltimore, PA: Paul H. Brookes.

Hamner, K.M., Lambert, E.W., and Bickman, L. (1997) Children's mental health in a continuum of care: clinical outcomes at 18 months for the Fort Bragg demonstration. *Journal for Mental Health Administration*, **24**, 465–71.

Hernandez, M. and Isaacs, M.R. (1998) *Promoting cultural competence in children's mental health services.* Baltimore, PA: Paul H. Brookes.

Hoberman, H.M. (1992) Ethnic and minority status and adolescent mental health services utilization. *Journal of Mental Health Administration*, **19**, 246–67.

Jensen, P.S., Bhatara, V.S., Vitiello, B., Hoagwood, K., Feil, M., and Burke, L. (1999) Psychoactive medication prescribing practices for US children: gaps between research and clinical practice. *Journal of the American Academy of Child and Adolescent Psychiatry*, **38**, 557–65.

Junek, W. and Thompson, A.G. (1999) Self-regulating service delivery systems: a model for children and youth at risk. *Journal of Behavioral Health Services and Research*, **26**, 64–79.

Kazdin, A.E. (1996) Dropping out of child psychotherapy: issues for research and implications for practice. *Clinical Child Psychology and Psychiatry*, **1**, 133–56.

Kazdin, A.E., Holland, L., and Crowley, M. (1997) Family experience of barriers to treatment and premature termination from child therapy. *Journal of Consulting and Clinical Psychology*, **65**, 453–63.

Knitzer, J. (1982) *Unclaimed children: The failure of public responsibility to children and adolescents in need of mental health services.* Washington, DC: Children's Defense Fund.

Leaf, P.J., Alegria, M., Cohen, P., Goodman, S.H., Horwitz, and Regier, D.A. (1996) Mental health service use in the community and schools: Results from the four-community MECA Study. Methods for the Epidemiology of Child and Adolescent Mental Disorders Study. *Journal of the American Academy of Child and Adolescent Psychiatry*, **35**, 889–97.

Lonigan, C.J., Elbert, J.C., and Johnson, S.B. (1998) Empirically supported psychosocial interventions for children: an overview. *Journal of Clinical Child Psychology*, **27**, 138–45.

McCabe, K., Yeh, M., Hough, R., Landsverk, J., Hurlburt, M., Culver, S., *et al.* (1998) *Racial/ethnic representation across five public sectors of care for youth.* San Diego: Centre for Research on Child and Adolescent Mental Health Services.

Ministry of Community and Social Services, Ontario (2001) *Reaching every child: Ontario's early years vision.* Toronto: Ministry of Community and Social Services, Toronto, Ontario, Canada.

Offord, D.R. and Bennett, K.J. (2002) Prevention. In *Child and adolescent psychiatry: modern approaches* (4th edn) (ed. M. Rutter, and E. Taylor) pp. 881–99. Oxford: Blackwell Scientific Publications.

Offord, D.R., Kraemer, H.C., Kazdin, A.E., Jensen, P.S., and Harrington, R. (1998). Lowering the burden of suffering from child psychiatric disorder: Trade-offs among clinical, targeted, and universal interventions. *Journal of American Academy of Child and Adolescent Psychiatry*, **37**, 686–94.

Otto, R., Greenstein, J.J., Johnson, M.K., and Friedman, R.M. (1992) Prevalence of mental disorders among youth in the juvenile justice system. In *Responding to the Mental Health Needs of Youth in the Juvenile Justice System* (ed. J.J. Cocozza), pp. 7–48. Seattle, WA: National Coalition for the Mentally Ill in the Criminal Justice System.

Pavuluri, M.N., Luk, S.L., and McGee, R. (1996) Help-seeking for behavior problems by parents of preschool children: A community study. *Journal of the American Academy of Child and Adolescent Psychiatry*, **35**, 215–22.

Peters, R.D., Arnold, R., Petrunka, K., Angus, D.E., Brophy, K., Burke, S.O. *et al.* (2000). *Developing capacity and competence in the Better Beginnings, Better Futures Communities: short-term findings report.* Better Beginnings, Better Futures Research Coordination Unit, Technical Report, Kingston, ON.

Quinn, K.P. and Epstein, M.H. (1998) Characteristics of children, youth, and families served by local interagency systems of care. In *Outcomes for children and youth with behavioral and emotional disorders and their families* (ed. M.H. Epstein, K. Kutash, and A. Duchnowski), pp. 81–114. Austin, TX: Pro-Ed.

Roberts, R.E., Attkisson, C.C., and Rosenblatt, A. (1998) Prevalence of psychopathology among children and adolescents. *American Journal of Psychiatry*, **155**, 715–25.

Stroul, B.A., Pires, S.A., and Armstrong, M.A. (1998) *Health care reform tracking project: tracking state managed care reforms as they affect children and adolescents with behavioral disorders and their families—1997 impact analysis.* Tampa, FL: Florida Mental Health Institute.

Sturm, R., Ringel, J., Bao, C., Stein, B., Kapur, K., Zhang, W., *et al.* (2000) *National estimates of mental health utilization and expenditures for children in 1998.* Department of Health and Human Services, Public Health Service National Institutes of Health Working Paper No. 205.

Szapocznik, J., Perez-Vidal, A., Brickman, A.L., Foote, F.H., Santisteban, D., Hervis, O., *et al.* (1988) Engaging adolescent drug abusers and their families in treatment: A strategic structural systems approach. *Journal of Consulting and Clinical Psychology,* **56,** 552–7.

US Department of Education (1997) *To assure the free appropriate public education of all children with disabilities.* Washington, DC: Nineteenth Annual Report to Congress on the Implementation of the Individuals With Disabilities Education Act.

US Department of Health and Human Services (1999) *Mental health: a report of the surgeon general.* Rockville, MD.

US Office of Technology Assessment (1986) *Children's mental health: Problems and service— a background paper.* Washington, DC: US Government Printing Office.

Weisz, J.R. (1997) *Community clinic test of youth anxiety and depression treatments.* Bethesda, MD: National Institutes of Health, National Institute of Mental Health.

Weisz, J.R., Huey, S.J., and Weersing, V.R. (1998) Psychotherapy outcome research with children and adolescents. *Advances in Clinical Child Psychology,* **20,** 49–91.

Weller, E.B., Cook, S.C., Hendren, R.L., and Woolston, J.L. (1995) *On the use of mental health services by minors.* Report to the American Psychiatric Association Task Force to Study the Use of Psychiatric Hospitalization of Minors: A review of statistical data on the use of mental health services by minors. Washington, DC: American Psychiatric Association.

Woodward, A.M., Dwinell, A.D., and Arons, B.S. (1992) Barriers to mental health care for Hispanic Americans: A literature review and discussion. *Journal of Mental Health Administration,* **19,** 224–36.

Chapter 26

Comparative analyses: CAMHS in developing countries

Atif Rahman, Richard Harrington, and Richard Gater

Introduction

The last three decades have seen significant achievements in child health worldwide. Although problems such as the HIV epidemic in parts of Africa continue to pose new challenges, overall, there has been a decline of about 15% in mortality and disability from malnutrition and infectious diseases (UNICEF 1996). Attention, therefore, has been turning to ways of enhancing the mental development of the majority of children who survive infancy. As Meyers (1992) put it, 'one in 13 children die, but the 12 who survive also need care'.

Several international policy initiatives promote the mental health of children in developing countries. In 1977, for instance, a World Health Organization expert committee on child mental health and psychosocial development (WHO 1977) stressed that governments should be encouraged to devise policies that aid the mental health of children. Such policies should be formulated in co-operation with those involved in juvenile justice, education, and social welfare. More recently, the 1989 Convention on the Rights of the Child (UNICEF 1989) committed signatories to ensuring that all children had the right to develop physically and mentally to their full potential, and to be protected from abuse and exploitation.

This chapter gives an overview of needs, priorities, and service development in developing countries, illustrated with examples of relevant activities undertaken in the last three decades. Many developed countries have 'pockets' of under-development, especially in inner cities, where problems like poverty, poor health, abuse, and violence are common. Knowledge from developing countries can help them to provide better policies, services, and prevention programmes for their own populations.

Scope of child mental health in developing countries

In developed countries, specialized professional groups have evolved that tend to concern themselves with different aspects of child mental health. For instance, child psychiatrists or psychologists deal with mental or behavioural disorders, paediatricians or paediatric neurologists with physical or neurological problems such as epilepsy, community child health services and educational psychologists with the recognition of intellectual disability, and so on. However, in developing countries the scarcity of trained manpower has prevented such specialization from emerging. All manifestations of disturbed functioning of mind and brain tend to be dealt with to a much greater degree by a single group of professionals. For professionals in developing countries the term child mental health, therefore, covers a broad range of problems, including neurological and developmental disorders, mental retardation, educational difficulties, and psychiatric disorders (Graham 1981).

Assessment of needs for mental health services

The emphasis placed on one or other of these mental health problems will depend on local needs and demands. These differ from country to country. For example, in some countries there will be concern about child labour, while in others there will be more concern about street children. Assessment of the specific mental health needs of each community is therefore central to the planning of services.

Several different ways of assessing the mental health needs of children have been proposed (NHS Health Advisory Service 1995; Wallace *et al.* 1997). The most widely used methods are epidemiological, comparative, and corporate (Harrington *et al.* 1999). Variations of these methods have been used in planning CAMHS in developing countries.

Epidemiology of mental health problems and their risk factors

There are many methodological issues to be overcome in the design of epidemiological studies in developing countries (Bird 1996; Hackett and Hackett 1999). For example, information is often lacking on the numbers of individuals in the population. Even when a representative sample is identified, it can be difficult to measure mental disorders accurately. There may be under-reporting of problems that do not lead to medical attention or that are not regarded by the local community as health problems (Kroeger 1983). In many developing countries, high rates of illiteracy limit the utility of questionnaire surveys (though this problem can be partly overcome by using local people to read questionnaires to illiterate adults; Rahman *et al.* 1998).

In spite of these methodological problems, over the past thirty years several epidemiological studies of mental disorders among children in developing countries have been conducted. Early community surveys carried out in Sudan (Cederblad 1968) and Ethiopia (Giel *et al.* 1969) gave prevalence rates of 3–10%. These studies used broad clinical criteria for diagnosis. More recent studies in Nigeria (Abiodun 1993) and India (Hackett *et al.* 1999) report rates of 15% and 9.4%, respectively. The former used the ICD-9 and the latter ICD-10 criteria for mental disorders. Studies on school children conducted in the United Arab Emirates (Eapen *et al.* 1998), yielded DSM IV prevalence rates of 10.4%.

Of interest to health planners may be studies that have looked at rates of mental disorders in children presenting at primary care facilities. For example, a four-country study done in Sudan, Columbia, India, and the Philippines (Giel *et al.* 1981) gave prevalence rates of 12–29% for child psychiatric disorders. Only 10–22% of these cases were recognized by primary health workers. A similar study by Gureje *et al.* (1994) in Nigeria reported DSM-III-R rates of 19.6% for such disorders.

The range of disorders seen in children in developing countries is not too different from that in the West, and includes emotional disorders (anxiety, depression, phobias), behavioural disorders (conduct disorders, hyperkinesis), intellectual disorders (mental retardation, specific learning disabilities), and pervasive developmental disorders (autism, Asperger's syndrome, etc.). Neuropsychiatric disorders such as epilepsy are also very prominent. There may be cross-cultural differences, however, in the presentation of these disorders to healthcare facilities. The somatization of emotional and behavioural disorders is a particularly important phenomenon to recognize.

Studies have also provided information on risk factors for child mental health and development. These include poverty (Duncan *et al.* 1994; Pollitt 1994), malnutrition (Grantham-McGregor and Fernald 1997), urbanization and social change (Rahim and Cederbled 1984; Guiness 1992; Minde 1988), political oppression, war, and displacement (Punamaki 1989; Richmann 1993; Mollica *et al.* 1997; Walton *et al.* 1997) and child labour (WHO 1987).

Knowledge about rates of mental disorders can be essential to convince politicians and fellow professionals that these disorders are an important public health problem. Information on risk factors can also help to prioritize high-risk groups. However, there is a growing realization that epidemiological surveys are of only limited value in planning child mental health services for a community in a developing country. There are three main reasons for this. First, because it is seldom feasible to carry out such surveys specifically for the task of needs assessment in local populations, it is usually necessary to make some kind of extrapolation from studies in other areas. The problem here is that, since rates of mental disorder are likely to vary between areas (e.g. urban versus rural), there can be no guarantee that the findings will be relevant to the community in question. Second, it is unclear how rates of disorder ascertained by traditional epidemiological approaches translate into needs for services or interventions (Harrington *et al.* 1999). Third, such approaches tell us little about what the local community regards as a significant problem and might wish to prioritize. This issue is important because it is certain that in most developing countries the need for services are much greater than supply. It is therefore essential that the priorities of the local community are clearly established at an early point in the needs assessment.

Comparative needs assessment

Comparative approaches involve comparisons between areas of information on indices of morbidity, service use and provision, costs, and outcomes. For example, WHO (Sartorius and Graham 1984) carried out national case studies on child mental health services in eight countries. They used direct (where available) and indirect measures of morbidity to gauge child mental health needs in these countries. Indirect measures included birth weight, prematurity, healthcare utilization data in children, and age-specific suicide rates (there may be underreporting). Other proxy measures such as indices of social deprivation, the number of children in employment, juvenile delinquency rates, or the rate of school non-attendance may provide useful pointers about differences between areas. The basic premise is that certain constellations of health and social characteristics can pinpoint areas whose individuals have increased vulnerability for a wide array of psychosocial and mental health problems. The information on service use and provision can be compared with other districts, or with national estimates of the need for certain kinds of services. It will be appreciated that low levels of service provision in comparison with other areas or with national norms do not necessarily mean that there are high levels of unmet need. However, significant discrepancies can highlight inequalities in access to services and thereby act as a catalyst for change.

Comparative approaches to needs assessment require that adequate records are available. Unfortunately, in some developing countries records are inadequate or out of date. Moreover, it should be borne in mind that population-level risk factors are at best an indirect method for describing mental health needs. For example, while the juvenile delinquency rate may be an indicator that the population in general is at risk of mental disorder, it does not indicate *who* is at risk—the delinquents, children known to delinquents, or all children.

Corporate needs assessment

Corporate approaches to needs assessment involve the synthesis of views about the mental health needs of children from those people and agencies involved in their care. These include mental health services, primary care physicians, social services, education departments, nongovernmental organizations, teachers, parents, and children. It will be appreciated that each of these sources of information will bring different perspectives. For instance, schoolteachers are likely to view mental health needs, not only from the child's perspective, but also from the perspective of the impact that the child's problems may have on the school or other pupils, or both.

One of the most widely used corporate methods is the key-informant technique. This entails interviewing individuals whose social positions make them influential and bring them into contact with a large number of people. Although primarily an ethnographic research method, which was originally used in the field of anthropology, it is now being used more widely in other branches of social and medical investigation. For example, Wig et al. (1980) carried out a key-informant study in three developing countries to study the perceptions of mental illness and their consequences in the community. The results were used to select priorities and design interventions to promote community involvement. The approach has also been used in a study to identify disabled persons in the community by school-children (Saeed et al. 1999). This small study shows that schoolchildren are effective identifiers of disabled children within their home communities and may be a useful resource when there are no trained primary care workers to conduct surveys. The children's ability to identify within the five major disability groups, was relatively robust when compared with medical diagnosis. Similar methods can be used to identify children with mental disorders in local communities. An advantage in using this method, especially in rural areas, is that most communities are close-knit, and children are in close contact with, not just their extended family, but many other community members. It would be possible to select key informants whose cumulative information would represent the whole community under study. These key informants can be asked to identify and provide information about children with mental disorders in their community. Culturally relevant vignettes based on major categories of mental disorders could be used to make the task of identification easier. The interviews could include questions related to the community's attitude and knowledge about the disorders, and the burden of the disorders on the child, family, and community, thus providing information about community concern and seriousness. Informants provide new insights and suggestions, and their support can be essential in implementing the service. The other advantages of this method are that it is conceptually simple and can be done quickly and cheaply. The technique has been described in more detail by Trembley (1989).

Setting priorities

The needs assessment procedures described above help to describe the likely pattern of problems in the local population, the priorities of professionals and parents, and the areas of greatest unmet need. This is likely to identify a multitude of needs for services and care that will exceed the available resources. It will therefore be necessary to set priorities.

Experience in developing countries strongly suggests that setting priorities should be a local affair. Priorities in one country or culture cannot be transplanted to another. Even within one country, there may be variations between different regions or communities. It is also our experience that prioritization should not be carried out in isolation. The collaboration of local health departments and other sectors will be important in the development of CAMHSs, and their commitment will depend on shared priorities. There may be an element of opportunism and timing to respond to current events and political interests. It is often useful to enlist the support of voluntary organizations or well-placed individuals, who may have a vested interest in child mental health. It is also important to ensure that the key players are properly informed of the importance of child mental health problems, and the available interventions. Thus prioritization is often a negotiation that takes account of, and attempts to influence the priorities of other sectors or government policy.

Based on the work of Morley (1973) and Giel and Harding (1971), the WHO have described seven criteria to identify priority problems in their Guidelines for the Elaboration and Management of National Mental Health Programmes (1996). The WHO suggest that, in order to determine priority among a group of different problems, weights can be given to each criterion according to local needs. The seven criteria are based on the following questions:

What is the magnitude of the problem? Either incidence or prevalence rates, which should take account of uneven distributions in the general population (e.g. geographical, urban/ rural, or age variations).

What is the severity of the problem measured in terms of mortality, disability, quality of life, burden on families, or economic loss?

What is the importance attached to the problem by those directly affected by the problem, their families, the technical sector, the public and policy makers? A programme is unlikely to succeed without the interest and participation of the community.

What is the controllability of the problem? In other words, is there evidence that there are effective interventions to prevent, treat or provide rehabilitation for the problem?

What are the available resources to tackle the problem? Are the human, technical, administrative and infrastructure resources available locally, and if not, what is needed to achieve and sustain them?

How much will the programme cost, including premises, salaries, equipment, and ongoing expenses?

What are the institutional commitments? Does this development integrate with other programmes, or does it have knock-on effects that increase or offset the costs or burden on other services. This highlights the importance of prioritizing the sequence of development within a programme. For example, a successful community educational programme may well stimulate a substantial increase in demand for services—the appropriate response should be developed before the demand is induced.

To these seven, can be added: is the programme sustainable? To some extent this is related to the questions on existing resources and costs. Projects that utilize existing resources are more likely to succeed in the long-term than those that require extra ongoing costs. An example of mobilizing existing resources, where there is a shared interest but a need for training or support to carry out an effective intervention, is supporting professional groups who work with children in educational or social services settings. Finally, sustainability may be an issue, where there is a block gift or grant, for example, to fund a research project, which will only support the programme for a limited period of time. After the grant is exhausted, the programme will collapse unless the resources, skills, and organizational capacity to sustain it have been developed (Garner *et al.* 1994).

Models of service

General considerations

For any model of mental health service to succeed, its usefulness must be demonstrated to policy-makers, health planners, professional colleagues, and the general public. While carefully conducted needs assessment exercises are an essential step towards this objective, a systematic approach has to be taken to implement the service at the local and national levels. Constraints such as stigma attached to mental disorders, lack of resources and manpower, lack of political will, and the inertia of planners and co-professionals have to be taken into account. Alliances would have to be made, and resources identified.

Misconceptions about mental disorders are widespread, not just among the lay public, but also among health planners and professionals. It is commonly believed that mental disorders are not 'real' disorders. They are thought to be rare in developing countries, or are considered to be largely untreatable. Some believe that they can be managed only after many years of specialized training, or that mental health is a very specialized and limited field that is separate from mainstream medicine and public health.

There is a substantial body of evidence that indicates otherwise (see subsequent sections). CAMHS can be integrated into the primary care network, and the public health aspects of CAMHS have important relationships with general health. Nevertheless, to obtain local support, it remains important to demonstrate these at the local level.

The models of service delivery described below are not mutually exclusive. In fact, they complement each other and should be integrated (in varying degrees, depending upon needs) to develop a comprehensive child mental health service.

Community and primary healthcare models

The community movement grew out of dissatisfaction with centralized hospital-based models of healthcare. In developing countries, trained mental health professionals often number less than one per million of the population, and the vast majority of people with mental health problems cannot be reached through centralized care. The primary care model brings mental healthcare within the reach of the mass of the population by integrating mental healthcare into the primary care network with support from specialized mental health personnel. This calls for changes in the roles and training of both general health workers and mental health professionals, emphasizes the preventive and promotive aspects of mental healthcare, and encourages community involvement. Empirical evidence of the feasibility of this approach has been provided by the WHO Collaborative Study on Strategies for Extending Mental Healthcare into Primary Healthcare (WHO 1981; Sartorius and Harding 1983), and through successful demonstration projects.

For example, Nikapota (1984) in Sri Lanka began by collecting data to demonstrate the presence of treatable child mental health problems in the community. This was used to convince health planners to include child mental health in the agenda of primary healthcare. A multidisciplinary workshop, consisting of professionals from the health, social, and education sectors, formulated a national policy for child mental health and formed a core group on child mental health, whose function was to implement and monitor service development. Teachers, childcare workers, and all grades of primary care staff were trained, using manuals developed by the WHO. Defined tasks relating to the promotion of healthy development and identification of children with mental health problems were introduced into primary care services. This programme was well-received by policy makers and planners, and became an integral part of the child health services (De Silva *et al.* 1988).

De Jong (1996) in Guinea-Bissau has described the development and evaluation of a comprehensive mental health programme for all age groups. This included two-stage screening of 100 consecutive children attending primary healthcare (PHC) facilities in an urban and rural area, which identified 13% with neuro-psychiatric disturbances. The assessment of the primary care workers' knowledge of mental health revealed that it was very poor. Epilepsy, acute psychosis, depression, psychiatric emergencies, and functional complaints were selected as priority disorders for intervention, based on criteria of point prevalence, community concern, seriousness, susceptibility to management, sustainability of the programme, and the knowledge and skills of PHC workers. Following training and supervision of 850 primary healthcare workers, their diagnostic sensitivity for priority disorders increased from 31% to 85%, and 82% of the patients received appropriate treatment. These improvements were most marked for epilepsy: diagnostic sensitivity increased from 0 to 95%, 90% received correct treatment, and seizure frequency dropped from 16 to 0.34 a month. More than half the patients regained reasonable or full functional capacity. This remarkable programme has been shown to be sustainable over a 10-year period, and shows a viable cost-benefit ratio.

On a smaller scale, in a previously under-served rural area of South Africa, Pillay and Lockhat (1997) engaged local resources by training local primary care nurses and other workers to identify and manage children with uncomplicated psychological problems. The authors, both clinical psychologists, supported the primary care staff through their own clinics, and gave consultations to psychologically disturbed children in communities at a distance of up to 200 kilometres from their hospital base. In one year they helped over 200 children, including a substantial number with post-traumatic stress disorder.

School-based mental health programmes

Schools have an important role to play in the health of children (WHO 1997). Most children attend school at some time during their lives. Schools can have a profound influence on children, their families, and the community. School-based mental health services also have the potential for bridging the gap between need and utilization by reaching disadvantaged children who would otherwise not have access to these services (Armbruster *et al.* 1997).

School-based interventions may be environment-centred or child-centred (Hendren *et al.* 1994). Environment-centred approaches aim to improve the educational climate and provide healthy programmes and role models for the child. These programmes also attempt to enhance the abilities of administrators, teachers, and support staff to deal with the specific areas of emotional or behavioural disturbance they encounter and, when necessary, to liase with mental health professionals and other agencies (e.g. Yale child study center prevention model; Comer 1980).

Child-centred approaches involve individual mental health interventions for children in need, alongside more general classroom programmes to improve coping skills, social support, and self-esteem. Consultations may involve recommendations being given to parents, the teacher, and in some cases, referral to outside agencies (e.g. Primary Mental Health Project in the United States; Cowen *et al.* 1975).

In one such programme in a developing country, these two approaches have been combined. Rahman *et al* (1998) report on a school mental health programme developed in rural areas of Pakistan with the aims of introducing mental health principles to improve the learning environment in the schools, increasing awareness of mental health problems among children, and training teachers and primary healthcare professionals in managing such problems. With the permission and co-operation of the local education authority, a mental health team was formed consisting of a psychiatrist and psychiatric social worker. The team familiarized themselves with the existing educational facilities, and assessed the teacher's knowledge and attitudes to mental health by carrying out focused group discussions. The teachers were given a short training course on common mental health problems in children and adolescents, using a specially designed teachers training manual. A variety of educational methods were devised in collaboration with the teachers, and throughout the programme, the teams made weekly visits to support the programme. Parts of the programme have been evaluated and significant improvements in knowledge and attitude of the school children and community have been demonstrated.

Kapur (1997) reports on similar programmes undertaken in India. Various approaches have been employed. These include direct consultancy in collaboration with parents and teachers through school mental health clinics; training teachers to identify mental problems and provide counselling to problem children; and helping teachers to enhance the school environment. The author discusses the implications of these programmes for other developing countries.

Public health and preventive models

The systematic, population-wide application of preventive measures based on what is known about the causes and outcomes of psychiatric disorders can markedly reduce morbidity from mental ill health among children (Eisenberg 1992). Primary prevention aims to prevent the development of disease. Secondary prevention shortens its duration after it has occurred; and tertiary prevention aims to preserve function when no effective treatment for the disease itself is available. In elaborating the wide scope of prevention, Eisenberg cites the example of pellagra, which at the start of the twentieth century, was the cause of considerable mental morbidity in the US, until its eradication by dietary improvements. He stated that:

> ... this preventive measure was not 'psychiatric' in the narrow sense of the term. However, what matters is not the mode of action of the agent, the venue in which it is applied, or the discipline of the practitioner, but the effectiveness of the measure in preventing, diseases manifested by disturbances in mental function.

Eisenberg identified the components of public health programmes for child mental health. These include measures for family planning (sex education in schools, information, and provision of contraceptives, availability of safe abortion); prenatal care (adequate nutrition in pregnancy, avoiding smoking, alcohol, and drugs; appropriate birth attendants, screening for phenylketonuria and congenital hypothyroidism); immunization; optimal nutrition (growth monitoring, iron and vitamin A, and iodine supplementation, correction of iron deficiency anaemia, school-based programmes for treating worm infestation); child safety (preventing road traffic accidents and accidental poisoning, use of lead free petrol and paint); and provision of home visits and day care. These components can be integrated in primary care and school based programmes, but many will be more feasible in some countries than in others because of cultural, political, religious, or other considerations.

Cultural issues in service development

Programmes that have given importance to local systems and values are usually more successful than programmes that neglect local realities and concerns (Desjarlais *et al.* 1995). Therefore, it is important to pay attention to local cultures and belief systems. Understanding and working with the local community may also identify local strengths and resources that can be mobilized to support community programmes.

Perceptions may be very different—what outsiders perceive to be risky or neglectful societal behaviour may seem to many communities to be appropriate, adaptive, and beneficial. For example, child labour may be seen as necessary in the path to economic development or even family survival.

Medical anthropological studies in developing countries indicate the importance of greater qualitative understanding of the meaning of disease and illness in a particular culture prior to introducing an intervention (Yach 1992; Yoder 1997). For example, conduct disorders may be seen as disciplinary problems rather than as symptoms requiring medical attention. Similarly, disorders of scholastic skills may not manifest themselves in non-literate communities. Therefore it is necessary to develop and evaluate culture specific assessments and interventions, which are contextualized as far as possible, in their family's and community's structure of meanings, relationships, and language (Tharp 1991). An example of treating children in a culturally appropriate way by designing new culture-specific treatment is quoted by Minde and Nikapota (1993), the so-called 'ceunto therapy' developed by Constantino and colleagues for Peurto Rican and other Spanish speaking children. Traditional folk tales describing troublesome conflicts and suggesting approaches that can modify unpleasant consequences, are read to young children and function as a stimulus to discussion and learning of coping strategies. It was shown that this therapy decreased anxiety in at-risk young schoolchildren more than Western-style therapy and no therapy, and that the effect lasted for at least 12 months.

Many problems can be managed effectively outside the formal healthcare system (Kleinman *et al.* 1978). Even a small shift in the boundary between cases managed within the traditional care system and those cared for by health services could overwhelm the services. Gadit (1996) has stressed the need for therapists to become familiar with ethnoculturally determined methods of treatment and to explore the possibilities of collaboration with traditional agencies of care. However, it would be foolhardy to blindly accept all traditional beliefs and practices as beneficial. Rahman *et al.* (1998) have shown that many such beliefs and practices are stigmatizing and oppressive towards people with mental disorders.

Training issues in service development

In developing countries, the population covered by a single psychiatrist ranges from half a million to 3 million. It is therefore recognized that most child mental health work, in the foreseeable future, will be done not by child psychiatrists but by paediatricians, primary care doctors, and other professionals, such as primary care workers and teachers, working with children. This calls for a change in the role of the specialized child mental health professional, whose focal activity becomes the training and supervision of other health professionals, rather than direct clinical work. The models of service discussed above complement this role.

At the same time efforts should be made to include child mental health training in the curricula of undergraduate medical students and other health workers. Also, post-graduate psychiatric courses in developing countries are geared towards adult mental illnesses, while children constitute a third to half of the population in these countries. These courses may need to be revised to include child mental health. The curricula need to reflect the integrated nature of child health services by having input from psychiatry, psychology, paediatrics, women's health, social sciences, and public health. The knowledge-base and expertise established in developed countries can contribute usefully to this process (Cox 1989). Training can be offered here on child development and psychopathology, diagnosis, and treatment, as well as measurement and research methods. However, trainees who come abroad for training should ensure that they are not alienated from their cultures of origin or feel clinically unprepared to work in a different environment on their return.

Research needs

Health research directly relevant to the needs of the peoples of developing countries is essential for equity in development, as well as for improving health planning and management.

Desjarlais *et al* (1995) advocate a broad base for mental health research in developing countries, recognizing that mental and behavioural health is at once a social, psychological, and biological process inseparable from general health. In outlining the principles of research in ethnoculturally diverse settings, they call for such efforts to be culturally relevant and focused on local problems, perspectives, and realities. They recommend community based research, with local participation and investment in the process. They also emphasize interdisciplinary research, observing that such research approaches are more helpful than those based on a single disciplinary perspective.

The application of these principles can be illustrated by a research project currently being undertaken in rural Pakistan (Rahman *et al.* 2002). Prior studies in these areas have reported high rates of depression in women of child-bearing age. Many of these women suffer from post-natal depression. In the same areas, childhood morbidity and mortality rates are also high, the predominant causes being diarrhoea, malnutrition, and other infections. The continuous care and attention of children is a demanding task, and poor mental health in mothers might be expected to have consequences on their children's health, nutrition, and psychological well-being. This project explores the associations between current maternal depression, and their infants' physical morbidity and nutritional status. It is hypothesized that children of mothers with depression will have higher levels of morbidity from infectious illnesses, and poorer growth compared to children of mothers without the disorder. The project also aims to uncover the potential mechanisms for this association and suggest possible interventions.

There are a number of benefits from this approach. First, it focuses on an important public health problem. It recognizes that malnutrition and infectious diseases not only affect the physical, but also the long-term psychological, cognitive, and intellectual health of children. Conversely, it recognizes the role of maternal bonding and child-care practices in, not only the psychological but also, physical health of the child. It therefore uses a broad-based and holistic approach to child mental health. Second, community members are keen to invest in the health of their children and are able to relate easily to the potential benefits of this study. They have therefore participated enthusiastically in the preliminary phases. Third, by focusing on the relationship between maternal mental health and child health, it highlights the issue of women's mental health in a more culturally and socially acceptable manner. Finally, the interdisciplinary nature of the study has helped in the building of bridges between disciplines in healthcare. Healthcare programmes arising from such holistic approaches are more likely to succeed than narrowly focused ones.

Conclusions

The last three decades have seen significant developments in the field of child and adolescent mental health in developing countries. Because of paucity of resources and trained manpower, innovative approaches have been tried to meet the needs of the populations.

Attempts have been made to plan services in a rational way, keeping in mind the needs of local populations. Many feasible and cost-effective models of service delivery have been suggested to meet these needs. Prominent among these are the primary care, schools-based, and public health approaches. These models are not mutually exclusive and have been successfully integrated into existing primary healthcare programmes. Understanding and working with the local community has helped to identify local strengths and resources that can be mobilised to support community programmes, providing a sustainable and culturally relevant basis for new developments. The knowledge generated from these approaches can benefit all countries as they search for solutions to similar problems in their ethnically diverse communities.

Acknowledgement

This chapter is based on an annotation by the same authors titled: Developing child mental health in developing countries, published in (2000) in the *Journal of Child Psychology and Psychiatry*, **41**, 539–546. We are grateful to Cambridge University Press for permission to reproduce it here.

References

Abiodun, O.A. (1993) Emotional illness in a pediatric population in Nigeria. *Journal of Tropical Pediatrics*, **39**, 49–51.

Armbruster, P., Gerstein, S.H., and Fallon, T. (1997) Bridging the gap between service need and service utilization: A school-based mental health program. *Community Mental Health Journal*, **33**, 199–211.

Bird, H.R. (1996) Epidemiology of childhood disorders in a cross-cultural context. *Journal of Child Psychology and Psychiatry*, **37**, 35–49.

Cederblad, M. (1968) A child psychiatric study on Sudanese Arab children. *Acta Psychiatrica Scandinavica* Supplement, **200**, 1–230.

Comer, J.P. (1980) *School power: Implications of an intervention project*. New York: Free Press.

Cowen, E.L., Trost, M.A., Lorion, R.P., Dorr, D., Izzo, L.D., and Isaacson, R.V. (1975) *New ways in school mental health: Early detection and prevention of school maladaptation*. New York: Human Sciences Press.

Cox, A.D. (1989) Child and adolescent psychiatry. In *Postgraduate training in psychiatry: Options for international collaboration* (ed. G. Edwards and N. Holden), pp. 66–70. Geneva: Division of Mental Health, World Health Organization.

De Jong, J.T.V.M. (1996) A comprehensive public mental health programme in Guinea-Bissau: a useful model for African, Asian and Latin American countries. *Psychological Medicine*, **26**, 97–108.

De Silva, M., Nikapota, A., and Vidyasagara, N.W. (1988) Advocacy and opportunity—planning for child mental health in Sri Lanka. *Health Policy and Planning*, **3**, 302–7.

Desjarlais, R., Eisenberg, L., Good, B., and Kleinman, A. (1995) *World mental health: problems and priorities in low-income countries*, pp. 255–266. Oxford: Oxford University Press.

Duncan, J.G., Brooks-Gunn, J., and Klebanov, P.K. (1994) Economic deprivation and early childhood development. *Child Development*, **65**, 296–318.

Eapen, V., al-Gazali, L., bin-Othman, S., and Abou-Saleh, M. (1998) Mental health problems among school children in United Arab Emirates: Prevalence and risk factors. *Journal of the American Academy of Child and Adolescent Psychiatry*, **37**, 880–6.

Eisenberg, L. (1992) Child mental health in the Americas: a public health approach. *Bulletin of PAHO*, **26**, 230–41.

Eisenberg, L. (1994) Social policy and child health. *Acta Paediatrica*, **394** (Supplement), 7–13.

Gadit, A.A. (1996) Scope of ethnopsychiatry in Pakistan (editorial). *Journal of the Pakistan Medical Association*, **46**, 119.

Garner, P., Torres, T.T., and Alonso, P. (1994) Trial design in developing countries (editorial). *British Medical Journal*, **309**, 825–6.

Giel, R., Bishaw, M., and van Luijk, J.N. (1969). Behaviour disorders in Ethiopian children. *Folia Psychiatrica, Neurologica et Neurochirurgica Nurlandica*, **72**, 395–400.

Giel, R., de Arango, M.V., Climent, C.E., Harding, T.W., Ibrahim, H.H.A., Ladrido-Ignacio, L. *et al.* (1981) Childhood mental disorders in primary healthcare: Results of observations in four developing countries. *Pediatrics*, **68**, 677–83.

Giel, R., and Harding, T. (1971) Psychiatric priorities in developing countries. *British Journal of Psychiatry*, **128**, 513–22.

Graham, P. (1981) Epidemiological approaches to child mental health in developing countries. In *Psychopathology of children and youth: a cross-cultural perspective* (ed. E.F. Purcell), pp. 28–50. New York: Josiah Macy Jr. Foundation.

Grantham-McGregor, S.M. and Fernald L.C. (1997) Nutritional deficiencies and subsequent effects on mental and behavioural development in children. *Southeast Asian Journal of Tropical Medicine and Public Health*, **28**, 50–68.

Guiness, E.A. (1992) Patterns of mental illness in the early stages of urbanization. *British Journal of Psychiatry*, **160**, 4–11.

Gureje, O., Omigbodun O., Gater, R., Acha, R.A., Ikuesan, B.A., and Morris, J. (1994) Psychiatric disorders in primary care clinic. *British Journal of Psychiatry*, **165**, 527–30.

Hackett, R. and Hackett L. (1999) Child psychiatry across cultures. *International Review of Psychiatry*, **11**, 225–35.

Hackett, R.J., Hackett, L., Bhakta, P., and Gowers, S. (1999) The prevalence and associations of psychiatric disorders in children in Kerala, South India. *Journal of Child Psychology and Psychiatry*, **40**, 801–7.

Harrington, R.C., Kerfoot, M., and Verduyn, C. (1999) Developing needs led child and adolescent mental health services: issues and prospects. *European Child and Adolescent Psychiatry*, **8**, 1–10.

Hend...n, R., Birrell Weisen, R., and Orley, J. (1994) *Mental health programmes in schools*. WHO/MNH/PSF/93. 3, First Revision. Division of Mental Health, Geneva: World Health Organization.

Kapur, M. (1997) *Mental health in Indian schools*. New Delhi, Thousand Oaks, and London: Sage Publications.

Kleinman, A., Eisenberg, L.,and Good, B. (1978) Clinical lessons from anthropologic and cross-cultural research. *Annals of Internal Medicine*, **88**, 251–8.

Kroegar, A. (1983) Health interview surveys in developing countries: a review of the methods and results. *International Journal of Epidemiology*, **12**, 465–81.

Meyers, R. (1992) *The twelve who survive*. London and New York: Routledge.

Minde, K.K. (1988) Effect of social change on the behaviour of school-age children. A transcultural perspective. *Pediatrician*, **15**, 170–5.

Minde, K.K. and Nikapota, A.D. (1993) Child psychiatry and the developing world: Recent developments. *Transcultural Psychiatric Research Review*, **30**, 325–46.

Mollica, R.F., Charles, P., Son, L., Murray, C.C., and Tor, S. (1997) Effects of war trauma on Cambodian refugee adolescents' functional health and mental health status. *Journal of the American Academy of Child and Adolescent Psychiatry*, **36**, 1098–106.

Morley, D. (1973) *Paediatric priorities in the developing world*. London: Butterworths.

NHS Health Advisory Service. (1995) Child and adolescent mental health services. *Together we stand*. London: HMSO.

Nikapota, A.D. (1984) Contribution of integrated mental health services to child mental health. *International Journal of Mental Health*, **12**, 77–95.

Nikapota, A.D. (1991) Child psychiatry in developing countries. *British Journal of Psychiatry*, **158**, 743–51.

Pillay, A.L., and Lockhat, M.R. (1997) Developing community mental health services for children in South Africa. *Social Science and Medicine*, **45**, 1493–501.

Pollitt, E. (1994) Poverty and child development: relevance of research in developing countries to the United States. *Child Development*, **65**, 283–95.

Punamaki, R.L. (1989) Mental health aspects of political oppression and violence. III: Children as victims of political repression and violence. *International Journal of Mental Health*, **18**, 3–130.

Rahim, S.I.A. and Cederbled, M. (1984) Effects of rapid urbanisation on child behaviour and health in a part of Khartoum, Sudan. *Journal of Child Psychology and Psychiatry*, **25**, 629–42.

Rahman, A., Mubbashar, M.H., Gater, R., and Goldberg, D. (1998) Randomised trial of impact of school mental-health programme in rural Rawalpindi, Pakistan. *Lancet*, **352**, 1022–5.

Rahman, A., Harrington, R.C., and Bunn, J. (2002) Can maternal depression increase infant risk of illness and growth impairment in developing countries? *Child: Care, Health and Development*, **28**, 51–6.

Richman, N. (1993) Annotation: Children in situations of political violence. *Journal of Child Psychology and Psychiatry*, **34**, 1286–302.

Saeed, K., Wirz, S., Gater, R., Mubbashar, M.H., Tomkins, A., and Sullivan, K. (1999) Detection of disabilities by schoolchildren: a pilot study in rural Pakistan. *Tropical Doctor*, **29** (3), 151–5.

Sartorius, N. and Graham, P. (1984) Child mental health: experience of eight countries. *WHO Chronicle*, **38**, 208–11.

Sartorius, N. and Harding, T.W. (1983) The WHO collaborative study on strategies for extending mental healthcare. I. The genesis of the study. *American Journal of Psychiatry*, **140**, 1470–3.

Tharp, R.G. (1991) Cultural diversity and treatment of children. *Journal of Consulting and Clinical Psychology*, **59**, 799–812.

Tremblay, M.A. (1989) The key informant technique: A non-ethnographic application. In *Field research: a sourcebook and manual* (ed. R.D. Burgess), pp. 98–104. London and New York: Routledge.

UNICEF. (1996) *The state of the world's children 1996*. New York: Oxford University Press.

UNICEF. (1989) *Convention on the rights of the child*. New York: UNICEF.

Wallace, S.A., Crown, J.M., Berger, M., and Cox, A.D. (1997) Child and adolescent mental health. In *Healthcare needs assessment. The epidemiologically based needs assessment reviews* (ed. A. Stevens and J. Raftery), pp. 55–127. Oxford: Radcliffe Medical Press.

Walton, J.R., Nuttall, R.L., and Nuttall, E.V. (1997) The impact of war on the mental health of children: A Salvadoran study. *Child Abuse and Neglect*, **21**, 737–49.

Wig, N.N., Suleiman, M.A., Routledge, R., Srinivasa Murthy R., Ladrido-Ignacio, L., Ibrahim, H.H.A., and Harding, T.W. (1980) Community reactions to mental disorders: A key informant study in three developing countries. *Acta Psychiatrica Scandinavica*, **61**, 111–26.

World Health Organization. (1977) *Child mental health and psychosocial development*. Technical report series 613. Geneva: World Health Organization.

World Health Organization. (1981) *Report from the WHO collaborative study on strategies for extending mental healthcare*. Geneva: World Health Organization.

World Health Organization. (1987) *Children at work: special health risks*. Geneva: World Health Organization.

World Health Organization. (1996) *Public mental health. Guidelines for the elaboration and management of National Mental Health Programmes*. Geneva: World Health Organization.

World Health Organization. (1997) *Promoting health through schools*. Technical report series 870. Geneva: World Health Organization.

Yach, D. (1992) The use and value of qualitative methods in health research in developing countries. *Social Science and Medicine*, **35**, 603–12.

Yoder, P.S. (1997) Negotiating relevance: Belief, knowledge, and practice in international health projects. *Medical Anthropology Quarterly*, **11**, 131–46.

Part 4

Planning, commissioning, and delivering child and adolescent mental health services

Chapter 27

A picture of child and adolescent mental health services in England and Wales at the end of the twentieth century

David Browning

Introduction

In 1998 and 1999, the Audit Commission undertook a major review of the child and adolescent mental health services in England and Wales. The Commission oversees the external audit of local authorities and the National Health Service in both countries and is required by parliament to undertake audits that enable it to comment on the economy, efficiency and effectiveness of services. Its remit is thus very wide, and, over the years, it has undertaken a number of reviews of children's services including hospital services (Audit Commission 1993), health and social services that promote the wellbeing of children (Audit Commission 1994), youth justice (Audit Commission 1996a) and various aspects of education (Audit Commission 1996b, 1999a).

The Audit Commission's audit of child and adolescent mental health services

Child and adolescent mental health services (CAMHS) were selected for audit as part of this wider programme of reviews of children's services across the public sector. The results were published in September 1999 (Audit Commission 1999b). This chapter provides a snapshot of CAMHS as they were at the end of the twentieth century. For this reason, the chapter is written in the past tense. It provides a milestone against which staff should be able to benchmark progress locally and nationally in the interval since 1999.

During the previous reviews of health, social, and youth justice services, the services often mentioned the need for good CAMHS and the difficulties they faced if links were not good. They commented repeatedly on the central importance of CAMHS to the well-being of children and the effectiveness of many other children's services. One central feature of the audit was, therefore, how well CAMHS were working with these other agencies.

What was striking from the start was how little was known about CAMHS. Even the levels of expenditure and numbers of staff employed were not recorded separately—usually because budgets were combined with adult mental health services. A major task of the audit was to establish a baseline of information about the services and how they worked.

At that time, and increasingly since then, CAMHS were being described within the framework of the four tier strategic framework first proposed by the NHS Health Advisory Service

(NHS Health Advisory 1995). This model recognizes that many services are provided at Tier 1 by general practitioners, health visitors, and other primary healthcare staff, teachers, social workers, and voluntary agencies. Specialist CAMHS are provided at Tier 2, Tier 3, and Tier 4. The intent and elements of this strategic framework has been reviewed earlier this book by Richardson (see Chapter 4).

The audit conducted by the Audit Commission primarily covered Tiers 2 and 3, with some reference to Tier 4. It included 60% of the health authorities commissioning Specialist CAMHS in England and Wales, and over 90% of the NHS Trusts providing these specialist services. The main part of the audit was carried out using questionnaires. Nearly 3000 practitioners contributed significantly to the process by completing a diary over a 4-week period, and by recording information on about 30 000 children—with more detail recorded on the presenting problems of about 25 000 of these children.

A number of key messages emerged. They validated and added detail to the earlier findings of the NHS Health Advisory Service, which had reviewed services through four complementary surveys of commissioning provision. The children and young people who were receiving help from specialist CAMHS presented with a wide range of problems, many of which were complex and severe. But the amount and type of specialist service provision available to respond varied widely between areas, with some areas having very little. Many of these services were also poorly linked with other local services, with most having relatively little contact with practitioners providing the Tier 1 functions. Access to specialist services was usually tightly restricted and while commissioning of CAMHS was making progress overall, it still had some way to go in many areas.

The children and young people receiving specialist CAMHS

The children and young people receiving specialist services came from a wide variety of localities across England and Wales from inner-city areas to remote rural areas. Boys outnumbered girls by more than two to one in the younger age bands, but girls outnumbered boys from mid-teens onwards. Just 3% were cared for as in-patients, and most of these were teenage girls between the ages of 15 and 18. The number from ethnic minority backgrounds was at least representative of the wider population as a whole.

The children and young people presented with a range of problems. To describe these, the Audit Commission used the Health of the Nation Outcome Scales for Children and Adolescents (HoNOSCA). For any young person, more than one category of problem could be recorded. Fewer than 5% presented with only one problem, and five was the most frequent number recorded (out of a possible 13 categories used in the audit). The four categories recorded most frequently (in 60–80% of children and young people, and in girls as well as boys) were:

    problems with family life and relationships;

    problems involving emotional and related symptoms, including eating disorders;

    problems with peer relationships; and

    disruptive, anti-social or aggressive behaviour.

Certain groups of children and those living in certain conditions are at greater risk of developing mental health problems than others. Factors known to be associated with children's vulnerability to mental health problems and disorders were recorded, and the audits found that:

    40% were living with only one natural parent compared with 21% of all families with dependent children;

34% were living in families where the main bread winner was unemployed—well above the national average;

27% had some form of learning disability;

19% were living with a parent with mental illness; and

9% were looked after by the local authority compared with 0.5% in the general population.

Thus, the specialist CAMHS were certainly working with children and young people with many complex and challenging problems, and from backgrounds that exacerbated their problems.

Variation in provision

The services available to address these needs varied widely from area to area. About £150 million (at 1999 prices) were spent on Specialist CAMHS in 1998–99 but the level of expenditure per head of population under 18 varied by a factor of seven between different health authorities; that is from under £5 per head to nearly £35 per head. Most of this variation was more readily explained by historical spending patterns than needs. One-third of NHS Trusts did not have a clear picture of what was spent on CAMHS, mainly because the budget was not separated out from that for services for adults.

NHS Trusts also varied substantially in their mix of staff. All of the 124 NHS Trusts that were audited provided community-based Specialist CAMHS. Just under half (57) also provided day and/or in-patient services. Half of the trusts provided community services with fewer than 11 full time staff, and many had just a handful.

A wide mix of professionals worked in Specialist CAMHS, including consultant psychiatrists, other medical staff, psychologists, and psychotherapists, other therapists of various kinds, social workers, nurses, and teachers. But the combinations in individual trusts varied widely in ways that could not be explained by need. It appeared that some NHS Trusts did not have access to the full range of skills regarded as necessary for the satisfactory delivery of Specialist CAMHS. Nearly all trusts employed psychiatrists and clinical psychologists, and two-thirds employed psychiatric nurses and social workers, but all other professionals were much less commonly represented. Almost half of the child psychotherapy posts in England and Wales were in the London region, with very few north of Birmingham. The Audit Commission concluded that this was almost certainly because, for many years, all child psychotherapist training centres were based in North London. It is only recently that training courses have been established in other parts of the Country. The London region also had nearly half the vacancies across England and Wales.

Not surprisingly, given the wide variation in provision, children with similar problems were seen by different professions with different therapeutic methods in different NHS Trusts and not seen at all in those with fewer resources. Only just over a third of trusts (38%) reported having a written operational policy on the roles, professional relationships, and responsibilities of the different professionals involved in CAMHS. The overall result was that provision was very patchy and uneven across England and Wales, with considerable inequity for children and young people who needed these specialist services. Those who gained access were likely to get different treatments, which depended more on where they lived than on what they needed.

The Audit Commission concluded that greater consistency between areas was clearly needed—underpinned by a clear model of what a local CAMHS should consist of, in terms of both services and staff.

Links with other agencies

The four-tier strategic framework requires enhanced volume and capability of Tier 1 services backed by much better provision of support from Specialist CAMHS for staff who deliver non-specialist or Tier 1 services. But the 4-week diaries compiled by 3000 professionals who worked in Specialist CAMHS showed that only 1% of their time was spent giving this support. One NHS Trust estimated that 10% was needed to do the job properly. Following a recommendation in *Together we stand* for development of what it termed Primary Mental Health Work, some NHS Trusts were beginning to employ link workers of various kinds to help provide the necessary support, and were managing to reduce inappropriate referrals and waiting times for specialist services in the process.

In contrast, professionals reported spending 22% of their time on administrative tasks. While good recording is an essential part of professional work, the Audit Commission thought there was probably scope for releasing time for more networking and support by employing clerks and better computer systems.

Referral routes also created barriers to Specialist CAMHS. More than half of all referrals came from GPs, with a further 15% from paediatricians. Only 14% came from social services and education combined, although there were significant variations between trusts. Two-thirds of youth justice managers reported problems gaining access to CAMHS. While tight access criteria helped to avoid time-wasting inappropriate referrals, they also introduced major delays and barriers. Waiting times in some trusts were excessive: 10% could not offer a first appointment for a non-urgent case within 6 months. Some NHS Trusts were developing named lists of professionals who delivered Tier 1 services, who had been given referral rights following discussions and training—possibly using protocols—about who could benefit from a referral. But whatever approach is adopted, the improvement of links with services was clearly needed by many Specialist CAMHS.

Co-ordinating the commissioning of services

Overall the picture that emerged was one of wide variation in the services and resources deployed across England and Wales with little relation to need, and limited links with other agencies. A key priority was for those who commission services to start to get a grip on patterns of provision, resources, and needs, and to work towards a local service that is better co-ordinated, more needs-based and more equitable.

At the time of the audits, health authorities were the lead commissioners as primary care trusts (PCTs) in England and Local Health Boards (LHBs) in Wales had not then been established. In 1995, *Together we stand* reported very little involvement by managers in CAMHS, either as commissioners or service delivery managers. However, by 1998 most health authorities had appointed a member of staff to take the lead and set the strategic direction for services as part of their Health Improvement Programmes (HIPs). Most lead officers were also members of inter-agency groups for commissioning children's services including CAMHS, although the task of getting CAMHS on the agenda for these groups and agreeing a common approach was not reported as an easy one.

Preliminary tasks for those staff who reported that they commissioned CAMHS included agreeing the age range to be covered. Nearly a third (29%) stopped at age 16, which meant that young people of 16 and over received treatment from adult services, which was not considered appropriate by many. A similar number of health authorities (again 29%) stopped at 18, while just under a quarter (22%) was prepared to treat young people into early adulthood. That left a fifth (20%) that were unclear about the age range covered, suggesting, thereby, that it had not been defined. Identifying the appropriate age range for services was, therefore, a key first step for many commissioners.

Assessing needs was then a second step. Two-thirds of commissioners reported mapping areas of deprivation. Most were involving education and social services authorities in assessment of need, but GPs and youth justice services were less commonly involved. Only just over a third (35%) had consulted service users and their families directly. Thus, again, a key priority for many commissioners was to determine with others who they should be targeting, and then to set the agenda for joint working.

Four out of five health authorities also said that they were taking stock of Specialist CAMHS, although their reviews were commonly restricted to identifying unmet needs and the consequent requirements for service developments.

After assessing needs and reviewing services, the challenge facing commissioners was then to work with CAMHS to transcribe needs into service requirements. Here, a major problem was a gap in the knowledge of 'what works'; at that time there was only a limited evidence-base available to commissioners for the efficacy of CAMHS interventions. Such evidence as there was tended to focus on treatments for defined psychiatric conditions, and single conditions without complicating factors. More was known about treatments for younger children and about the shorter rather than the longer-term effects of treatment. Thus the very real issue of complexity of need was identified as a key matter for further work.

This produced a major dilemma. By focusing on what was known to work, commissioners risked providing only a relatively narrow range of specialized interventions. By responding to requests for help from education, social services, and others, they would risk providing support in ways that were less well proven. Clearly, more research was needed to help resolve this dilemma. But the overall message from research was that many interventions that might be made by CAMHS were generally associated with significant improvements, and, even where resolution of problems and disorders was unlikely, relief of symptoms could be significant. Hence, providing interventions in ways that were less well proven appeared to be justified, especially if staff used the opportunity to collect data to increase the evidence base.

Monitoring outcomes systematically was one way of helping to develop a pragmatic evidence base, but information systems were found to be poor. Information was usually limited to administrative rather than clinical material. Many Specialist CAMHS needed better information technology and systems to support their clinical work.

Progress with commissioning overall

Thus, while commissioning of Specialist CAMHS was definitely beginning to make progress, and had developed since it was surveyed in 1994, it still had a way to go. Less than half of all health authorities had a written policy for securing the mental health of children and young people, with a further quarter developing one. Less than half had a commissioning plan for CAMHS although most of the rest were working on one.

To assess progress overall, the Commission developed a set of quality indicators for both commissioners and service providers (NHS Trusts). Both were scored in relation to each indicator and the scores added across all indicators to provide a composite picture. This provided a broad picture of progress.

High-scoring health authorities with evidence of good commissioning practice appeared to have paid specific attention to the interfaces between the four tiers of services. Low-scoring health authorities, in contrast, tended to lack focus, and the lead person often had insufficient authority. They lacked adequate information from local needs assessments or reviews of services. They often excluded non-NHS services from their considerations, and had no evidence of joint inter-agency strategic development. Often, GPs were not involved in the development of any strategy either. But, interestingly, effective commissioning did not appear to depend on the amount spent, as no relationship was found between amount spent per head and overall score.

What distinguished the high-scoring trusts that provided the best services seemed to be clear, informed, imaginative, and understanding management of the service. In contrast, low-scoring trusts appeared to lack any clear sense of purpose. They often lacked specialists who should have been key members of a multidisciplinary team—notably, clinical psychologists, child psychotherapists, and social workers. They reported no special interests in particular services, such as for eating disorders or work with adolescents. Waiting times after referral were long, and referrals were usually restricted to those from GPs. Contacts with social services, education, and youth justice services were usually limited. Limits were often placed on the age ranges seen. They seemed to be more focused on restricting access than providing help.

Interestingly, size did not seem to matter. The overall indicator of quality was not associated with size of the NHS Trust, and many small trusts had high scores.

Conclusion

At the end of the twentieth century, Specialist CAMHS were a very mixed bag. The level of resources available to them and services provided by them varied widely, without any apparent relationship to need. Nevertheless, some were providing good services overall in spite of the difficulties and, usually, because of clear and imaginative direction and a sense of purpose from within the trusts themselves.

Systematic commissioning of services by health authorities, while better than in 1994, was still at an early stage of development. Some authorities had made good progress, but many were clearly struggling. They were not giving CAMHS much priority, and the lead person lacked authority. Joint working with other agencies such as the education, social and youth justice services was poor.

Thus, the agenda facing those staff who are charged with improving CAMHS overall was a large and challenging one. But a base of good commissioning and good services was being established in some places, providing a foundation on which to build.

References

Audit Commission (1993) *Children first.* London: Audit Commission.

Audit Commission (1994) *Seen but not heard.* London: Audit Commission.

Audit Commission (1996a) *Misspent youth.* London: Audit Commission.

Audit Commission (1996b) *Counting to five—education for under-fives.* London: Audit Commission.

Audit Commission (1999a) *Missing out—management of school attendance and exclusion.* London: Audit Commission.

Audit Commission (1999b) *Children in mind.* London: Audit Commission.

NHS Health Advisory Service (1995) *Together we stand.* London: HMSO.

Chapter 28

Mapping specialist child and adolescent mental health services in England

Gyles Glover, Claire Hartley, Richard Dean, and Bob Foster

Introduction

Children in mind, the report of the Audit Commission (1999) on specialist child and adolescent mental health services (Specialist CAMHS) in England and Wales (also see Chapter 27), drew attention to the increasing recognition over the past twenty years of the importance of child and adolescent mental health problems and disorders, and the continuing lack of routinely-collected data about the provision and activity of services for them. The importance of CAMHS was subsequently recognized in a number of governmental funding rounds in England, including the 1999 NHS Modernization Fund (Department of Health 1999) and the child and adolescent mental health service grant (Department of Health 2003). The need for information is being addressed in a number of ways, of which service mapping is one.

Most of the discussion about information requirements in *Children in mind* focused on collection of data about assessing and caring for individual children and young people. Work is under way to address this complex task but, judging from the work involved in developing the adult mental health minimum data set (Glover 2000, Glover and Sinclair Smith 2000), it may be five to ten years before national results are available. However, an equally important area which the Commission tackled in its own data gathering, but about which its report said little, concerns documenting the varied pattern of services and staff provided in different areas of the country and how they change over time. The task of establishing a rolling annual mapping of these features is substantially simpler and has been undertaken annually in adult mental health services in England since the autumn of 2000 (Barnes *et al.* 2001, Glover and Barnes 2002, Glover and Barnes 2003). Building on this experience, and following a pilot study with three mental health services in London, Coventry, and County Durham (Hartley and Glover 2002), the Centre for Public Mental Health in Durham was commissioned by the UK government's Department of Health to undertake an initial mapping round in England in the autumn of 2002. This chapter describes its design and some of its headline findings. We provide further detail in the final report of the first round of CAMHS mapping (Glover *et al.* 2003). Readers who work outside England will be able to draw lessons for similar activities in other jurisdictions from our experience.

Conceptual issues and design

At its simplest level, from a central government perspective, the mapping exercise is required to monitor fulfillment of service provision increases that were set out as part of the Public Service Agreement for 2003-2006 (Department of Health 2003). The Audit Commission's perspective is wider: shared information, put into context by benchmarks for similar places forms a vehicle for partners from different agencies to assess needs, review services, plan local priorities, and monitor implementation, and is the medium in which inter-agency partnerships can be cultured. Three areas of design are involved in this type of exercise: delineation of the geographic and/or organizational areas from which responses will be asked; classification of services that are provided; and the practical arrangements.

The central unit for our mapping was the 'service'. Originally, we had hoped that this would equate roughly to the activities in the purview of former Health Authority 'CAMHS Leads'. This would have provided a multi-agency perspective (health, social services, and education) for defined populations of children and young people in each local area. However, while these posts existed in many areas, the network was not comprehensive. In this circumstance, we attempted to find a head of CAMHS provision in a relevant provider organization in each area who could provide a similar cross-agency perspective. This raised the problem that many services had no neat geographic area of coverage, thereby making analysis of provision in relation to population very difficult.

The most obvious difficulty in classifying the elements of services provided is the lack of any normative blueprint for team or organizational arrangements. Services differ widely both in the patterns of staff they employ and the groupings within which they work. We were keen to identify underlying patterns of teams for the key reason that we wanted to develop a structure that would enable us to merge gathering statistical data with producing the facility of a local service directory. This necessitates a focus on services rather than on individual clinicians. However, despite wide preliminary consultation during and after the pilot work, no neat classification of teams emerged before the start of the main body of our work. Therefore, we asked each CAMHS to provide some details of the service as a whole (including details of total staff and vacancies) and to list the teams that each provided, indicating for each a name, budget, location, and waiting list details. We asked for a description, in free text, of what each team's type was. They were classified post hoc.

In the absence of an adequate typology or coding structure for team types and, hence, the need to develop our own, we had little option but to follow the Audit Commission approach (Audit Commission 1999) and used an additional individual questionnaire for clinical staff to provide some corroboration of our categorization of teams. This included details of their professional group and employment grade, the types of therapy they practised, and for which they had received specialist training, and details of the cases they had seen in the previous month including their treatment duration. It also asked for an estimation of the broad profile of how the employed time of the staff was spent and the availability to them of information technology. We asked, in particular, about which sources were available to help them to answer our questions about their cases.

We did not have the resources available to use agency coding clerks to computerize the large volumes of data. In the pilot work, we experimented with a custom-written database in Microsoft Access. This proved impossible to support adequately on the wide range of hardware and operating system environments that we encountered across services in England. So, for the roll out of the main body of our work, we opted for a mixed solution: we supplied printed forms locally and the data on them were then entered into an internet-based database by a clerk at each site. Extensive checks of the completeness and coherence of the data were built into the web pages and a summary version of the data was produced as a sign-off sheet to be endorsed by the chief executive responsible for each service. The process was not optional, and, at least within the NHS, timeliness and performance in making the submission was the subject of an indicator for the centrally-driven annual round of performance management of providers of services.

Results

Data were collected from 124 services providing Specialist CAMHS in England and relate to the month of September 2002. This number represented 95.4% of the relevant NHS services (later, we became aware of six Specialist CAMHS that had made no return). Inevitably, the boundary is slightly blurred as the threshold of what constitutes providing Specialist CAMHS is also a little blurred. For example, our instructions on scope did not include clinics run by paediatricians (as compared with those delivered by specialists in child and adolescent mental health) providing assessment of the syndromic attention-deficit hyperactivity disorder: an omission that was criticized during the course of our work. Some informants reported on only their own services and not those provided by local partner agencies. Independent-sector organizations (mostly providing Tier 4 services) were not surveyed, and funding used to commission out-of-area placements was not identified. These omissions are probably, proportionately, relatively small in relationship to the activity overall. Where data are reported in relation to population size, the population estimates for 2002 of those child and young people aged 0-17 have been used, derived from the 2001 census of the population. In answer to two general questions: 54% of services indicated that they provide on-call services, while only 35.8% reported special provision for children and young people whose mental illness occurred in the context of a learning disability.

Funding

Data on the spend on Specialist CAMHS were collected only in relation to the teams reported. Thus, we did not get a full picture of commissioners' patterns of spending. In particular, spending on independent sector in-patient care was not covered. However, it was judged to be unrealistic to identify a set of commissioner reporters in the first year of the exercise, particularly as data were collected at the point of greatest period of turmoil following the re-organization of the NHS consequent on the English government's policy on 'Shifting the Balance of Power' (Department of Health 2001). The total spend that we identified was £241.3 m; that is, roughly, £21.70 per child or young person aged 0-17. Of this, £185.8 m (77%) was spent locally on specialist teams. The range between regions for local and wider teams was from £17.70 to £28.20 per child or young person. The national figure for annual spend could be reasonably comparable with the Audit Commission's finding had they provided a national average figure (Audit Commission 1999). From that Commission's graphs, it appears to have been about £12 per child or young person under 18 in the period between 1997 and 1999. The Commission's report was of Health Authority commissioned spend and, unlike our data, would have included inpatient care commissioned from the independent sector. The range the Commission cites (£7 to £31 per child under 18) was for smaller administrative areas (Health Authorities) and, as is to be expected, it shows a wider fluctuation than the range for the Regions that we are able to show.

Teams

The specialist clinical services delivered were grouped into teams. There was considerable organizational variation in how local services identified teams (e.g. by target population, area served, and composition). Seven hundred and thirty-two (732) teams were reported on, although, judging by the descriptions given, eight had no clinical function and are removed from most analyses. Teams were initially classified by their broad function and catchment area (Table 28.1). The classification of team type was undertaken by one of us (GG) from free text responses about the name and type of teams. Services were informed how their teams had been

Table 28.1 Numbers of teams reported categorised by broad type and catchment areas showing numbers with no individual staff data returns and average number of professional groups represented in the others.

Team type	Local	Wide	National	Missing staff data	No of prof groups
Generic locality					
Generic/locality	229	0	0	9 (3.9%)	4.3
Tier 2/3	74	1	0	7 (9.3%)	4.1
Community	26	1	0	1 (3.7%)	3.7
Tier 1/2	16	2	0	1 (5.6%)	1.9
Adolescent	21	4	0	0	3.3
Psychiatry Department	7	2	0	0	2.6
Special client groups					
Child & Family Therapy	36	3	0	6 (15.4%)	3.9
Social Services/Looked After Children	15	0	1	1 (6.3%)	2.2
Paediatric liaison	14	1	0	2 (13.3%)	2.2
Youth Offending Team	22	2	0	6 (25.%)	1.2
Education	5	1	0	0	1.8
Learning disabilities	12	0	0	0	2.2
Specialist team	36	17	13	14 (21.2%)	2.4
Specialist T4 or day					
Day service	15	1	0	2 (12.5%)	3.6
Tier 4/In-patient	7	46	15	3 (4.4%)	4.3
Other					
Psychologists	49	3	1	4 (7.5%)	1.3
Psychiatrists	2	0	1	2 (66.7%)	1.0
Unclassifiable and other	21	0	2	4 (17.4%)	1.9
Non clinical					
Not clinical	4	0	4	5 (62.5%)	1.0

classified and asked to indicate if they felt that any of the other emerging classes would be more appropriate. Three hundred and eighty-three (383) of the teams reported on (52.9% of 724) were classified as generic local teams. The phrases used to describe these included 'community', generic', 'locality', 'Tier 2/3', 'Tier 1/2', 'adolescent', or 'psychiatry'. Twelve (12) teams were described as 'psychiatry' and their staffing returns indicated that nine of these were generic local teams. Essentially, these are teams that provide the first line of specialist care for all types of problem or disorder and, usually, from a local catchment area. One hundred and seventy-eight (178) teams (24.4%) provided care for children and young people with specific types of problem. Eighty-four (84) teams (11.6%) provided intensive day or in-patient support for clients with particularly challenging problems. A further 56 teams (7.6%) were described with words suggesting single discipline teams, and 48 of them comprised child clinical psychologists. The latter teams accounted for roughly one fifth of clinical psychologists who appear to be less well integrated than other professional groups in multi-disciplinary teams and working. Twenty-three (23) teams were unclassifiable.

Staff

Overall staff data from the service questionnaires were reported in seven categories. The total workforce of 7339.9 whole time equivalents (WTE) comprised 5982.5 professional care staff, 1226.4 administrators, and 131 managers. Of the professional practitioners, 92.5 (15.4%) were doctors, 2292.8 (38.3%) nurses, 879.6 (14.7%) clinical psychologists, 1152.6 (19.3%) other clinical staff, 501.4 (8.4%) social services staff, and 233.4 (8.4%) education staff. As the two latter categories were mainly employed by agencies that are outside the NHS, it seems likely to us that the counts of them may have been less complete.

Staff figures show a striking variation in numbers per unit population of children and young people. London showed substantially greater availability of all but nursing staff. This was largely attributable to the presence of many specialist units in the national centres that are located there. While many of these units were identified as national centres, there must be some question as to the actual availability of these staff to children and young people outside the south-east of England except in in-patient settings. The large number of nursing staff in the North East was partly, though not wholly explained by one in-patient unit that specializes in caring for mentally ill children and young people with a coincident or co-morbid learning disability.

In addition to the wide overall range in staff provision, there were also notable differences in the profile of staffing and the level of staff vacancies. Clinical psychologists made up 20.4% of the professional staff in the West Midlands, 17.6% in London, 15.4% in the East Midlands, 15.3% in the North West, 14.2% in the South West, 12.3% in Northern and Yorkshire, 12.2% in the South East, and 9.9% in the Eastern region.

More detailed data about staff roles were available from the individual staff questionnaires, though these were clearly less complete. Overall, 5722 responses were received, comprising a total of roughly 4296.7 WTE staff, suggesting a response rate of 71.8%. The inexactness here arises because WTEs were calculated from weekly working hours reported by staff. Many reported figures well in excess of what is normally contracted, so numbers were expressed as a proportion of 36, (the most commonly occuring figure) rounded to a maximum of one.

Overall, 73% of professional staff worked in local teams. For nurses, this figure was much lower (54.1%) reflecting the disproportionate staffing needs of in-patient units which usually cover wide catchment areas. Seventy-eight point six per cent (78.6%) of doctors, 89.9% of

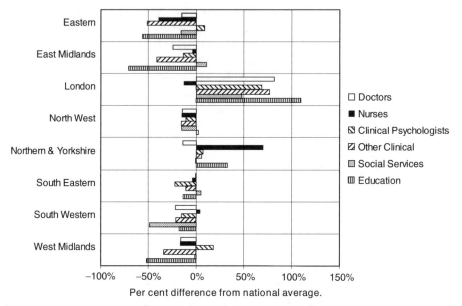

Fig. 28.1 Variations in care staff per 100k population aged 0-17 (figures expressed as a percentage of national average by region and broad staff group).

clinical psychologists, 87.4% of psychotherapists, and 91.2% of social workers were based in local teams.

Six hundred and ninety (690) staff (442.1 WTE) described themselves as psychotherapists and 50 (41.6 WTE) as primary mental health workers. Both figures underestimate the total number performing these roles, as informants were asked to identify themselves initially on the basis of their main qualification, thus many of these will have described themselves as psychologists, social workers, doctors, or nurses. We have a contemporary estimate of the extent of this for primary mental health workers, a new role recommended by the NHS Health Advisory Service (HAS) in *Together we stand* and noted to be growing in the Audit Commission's report. As the mapping was taking place, more than 200 individuals, identifying themselves as primary mental health workers, applied to attend a conference on their work.

Cases seen, waiting times, and waiting-lists

Information about cases seen was collected through the staff returns. Hence this should be seen as an underestimate of the national picture, although probably by less than the rate of staff non-response as it is likely that a proportion of this was due to staff holidays, long-term leave, or sickness implying a level of genuine inactivity during the period surveyed. The data covered children and young people who were seen within the month of September 2002. Caseload data were only analysed from the 5415 staff (4063.8 WTE) who reported that they had a direct clinical caseload. To allow for the cases being seen by more than one therapist, we asked staff to report the total number of children and young people that they had seen, and the number of them for which they were the sole clinician. On the assumption that others would be seen by pairs of therapists, we calculated 'case equivalents' as the number seen alone plus half the difference between this figure and the total. In order to calculate patterns of referral sources and presenting problems, each clinician's data were weighted by the ratio of their case-equivalent number to their total cases.

Table 28.2 sets out the overall patterns of case numbers and their ages, treatment duration, and most common conditions for the different types of team. Eight point six per cent (8.6%) of cases were currently being 'looked after' by their local authority. The figure of 80,598.0 case equivalents represents the reported prevalent cases for one month; that is 725.2 per 100k of children and young people who are aged 0 to 17. The range between regions was from 528.8 in the North West to 882.6 in London. The overall figure comprises 237 with emotional disorders, 105 with conduct disorder, 90 with ADHD, 46 with deliberate self-harm, 43 with autistic spectrum disorders, 25 with a learning disability, 21 with developmental disorder, 21 with psychosis, 16 with a habit disorder, 6 with substance misuse, and 82 for whom it was impossible to identify a principal problem. Probably, we think, all of these figures represent an underestimation of between 15% and 25% because of the incompleteness of staff returns. Individual staff caseloads averaged 19.4 per WTE and were highest for doctors (28.6), clinical psychologists (23.0), and social workers (21.0). The average caseloads of nurses were similar (21.7) for those staff who work in ordinary clinical settings, but are predictably smaller (7.1) for those who work in in-patient or day-patient settings.

Striking regional variations in staff caseloads were seen. Doctors' caseloads ranged from 40 in the East Midlands to 22.3 in the North West, clinical psychologists' from 29.2 in the South West to 19.7 in Eastern, and Social Workers' from 28.4 in the South East to 18.4 in the East Midlands. Caseloads for nurses who work outside in-patient and day units ranged from 27.6 in the South East to 19.2 in London.

Analysis of referral sources is complicated by the fact that 17.5% of cases were referred to the individual seeing them from somewhere within the same NHS Trust. Excluding these, nationally more than half the referrals (54.7%) came from primary health services, 15% came from child health services, 11.6% from social services, and 8% from education departments and schools. This pattern was broadly similar for all regions except London where 8% of referrals came from other NHS Trusts, 15.4% from social services, and 14.3% from education sources with primary care referrals making up only 37%.

Different types of teams had different referral patterns that, we think, reflect obvious associations. There was also wide variation in the types of clinical problems seen by different CAMH professionals. Doctors' caseloads had a disproportionately large share of cases with ADHD; psychotherapists, counsellors, and creative therapists had many cases of emotional disorders; and primary mental health workers had many cases with conduct disorders.

Nationally, 191.9 children and young people per 100k population were on a waiting list with 38.1 having waited in excess of six months. This varied substantially between regions with 252.1 per 100k children and young people in total waiting in the South Eastern region and 134.7 in the Eastern. Numbers waiting more than six months ranged from 62.4 in the South Eastern to 10.8 in London. However, contrary to some popular opinion, nationally, only one in five children and young people on the waiting list had waited six months or more and this figure exceeded one in four only in two regions and then only slightly (maximum 26.2% - North Western region). On average, staff reported that they spent just under half (48.2%) of their time in direct clinical work, 21.8% on administrative and managerial tasks, 11.5% in consultation and liaison about clinical cases, 8% in training and education, and 4.1% in research and evaluation. While there were some predictable exceptions, apart from the more junior or less qualified grades of nurse, (mostly employed in in-patient units and spending 70% to 80% of their time in direct clinical contact), this pattern was remarkably consistent.

Table 28.2 Staff and staff caseload details by type of care team

Team type	WTE staff	Case equivalents	Age 0 to 10 (%)	In treatment 6 months plus (%)	Emotional disorder (%)	Conduct disorder (%)	ADHD (%)	Autistic spectrum (%)
Generic local teams								
Adolescent	146.5	2319.0	4.8	35.6	36.1	11.4	3.5	2.3
Community	115.5	2733.0	46.7	42.3	37.7	16.8	14.6	3.9
Generic/locality	1565.1	39959.0	40.2	38.5	34.2	14.7	14.7	6.1
Tier 1/2	57.7	1023.0	54.4	10.6	33.1	19.3	6.0	2.7
Tier 2/3	423.0	10689.5	42.0	36.5	35.8	16.9	13.2	5.2
Special client group teams								
Child & Family Therapy	225.1	4379.5	41.3	43.6	40.4	17.7	9.8	4.3
Education	10.5	180.0	50.1	38.1	36.4	32.8	8.5	2.3
Learning disabilities	36.8	639.5	51.2	52.8	5.7	3.2	7.8	21.1
Paediatric liaison	35.1	968.5	42.3	38.7	29.8	7.2	15.4	9.3
Social Services/Looked After Children	46.4	661.5	39.9	43.6	35.2	14.3	1.2	0.8
Specialist team	134.7	1982.5	40.4	37.5	23.6	9.0	13.7	10.1
Youth Offending Team	26.1	512.0	1.8	12.6	25.6	34.5	2.6	1.0
Specialist Tier 4 or Day								
Day Service	83.5	1214.5	63.6	37.9	25.9	20.6	18.2	6.8
Tier 4/In-patient	909.2	7273.0	12.5	25.5	23.0	4.5	6.0	5.6
Other								
Psychiatry	49.8	1075.5	36.9	33.4	25.4	13.2	23.1	8.7
Psychology	155.0	3964.0	57.4	33.8	28.3	22.7	4.8	7.1
Unclassifiable and Other	44.0	1015.0	40.3	33.3	32.1	10.3	10.8	16.0
Total	4063.8	80589.0	38.4	36.7	32.8	14.5	12.4	6.0

Staff were asked about the types of treatment that they provide. This showed some predictable patterns. Psychologists used CBT, psychotherapists practiced psychotherapy, and doctors and nurses used drug treatments. However, they also indicated that most CAMH professionals saw themselves as practising an eclectic model of care: other treatment approaches considered included family therapy, creative therapies, parent training, counselling, and 'other'. Excluding the final category, the overall average number of approaches used per staff member (weighted for WTEs worked) was 3.2, with doctors indicating they used on average 3.9 approaches, nurses 3.4, social workers 3.2, and clinical psychologists 3.1.

Day and in-patient services

A total of 628 in-patient beds (42.2 per 100k of the population aged 0 to 17) and 9,039 day places (608.9 per 100k) provided by the NHS were identified. Independent sector provision was not covered. The total in-patient bed figure agrees closely with the figure of 632 NHS beds in England identified by detailed analysis from the NICAPS study (David Daniel, personal communication, 2004 and O'Herlihy *et al.* 2003). Both varied substantially by region, with in-patient beds ranging from 8.2 in London to 3.5 per 100k in the Eastern region and day places from 104.9 in the South Eastern to 49.3 in the Eastern regions.

Local data sources for answering the questions

Both local heads of service, who answered questions on services levels and staff who answered the individuals staff questions were asked about the availability of IT support to help them to answer our mapping questions. Just over two thirds of service heads (69.1%) reported at least some contribution, though this was described as major by only two (1.6%). However, 58% of clinical staff reported either using their memory plus notes (26.7%), which must have been time consuming, or memory alone (31.3%), which must have been unreliable. In addition to providing an indication of the reliability of the data supplied, these observations provide an indication of the poverty of data support available generally in services for clinical audit.

Concluding comments

The exercise that we report here must be seen as the first of its kind. In our experience, data collections of this type do not settle down until year three. There were successes and failures. Data showed signs of being erratic. In one place, it seemed that more information than was appropriate was entered about caring for children and young people with learning disabilities. In two others, whole services reported each staff member as a distinct team. This may reflect true differences in the service pattern or it may reflect failure to communicate the intended approach. For many NHS Trusts, collecting some of the information proved extremely difficult. This was especially the case when they attempted to allocate the costs to teams and determine the overall costs of services. We asked staff to report the ethnic mix of their clients. However, these data were too incomplete for meaningful reporting.

The service and team data were interesting, but it was a bad error not to link the reporting of overall staff numbers by service heads to the teams in which they work. The retrospective coding of team types was unavoidable, but extremely time consuming and, in an important number of cases, difficult or impossible from the information given. It is not realistic to expect 100% coverage of staff data returns; hence, while the data obtained from these questionnaires can be illuminating about patterns of work, caseloads, and activities for different staff groups, data collected through this route cannot be relied upon to give precise details about individual teams as findings will always be suceptible to distortion. One or two missed staff returns may constitute a substantial fraction of a team's work.

Many data items were collected because of the lack of patient-based data sources about what the services do. A patient-based data set would clearly be better suited to collecting information on presenting problems, sources of referral, age, sex and ethnic profiles, durations of involvement, interventions provided, and outcomes.

However with these provisos, a start has been made and some baselines have been drawn. Perhaps most usefully for the task of mapping, greater clarity has been achieved about classifying types of CAMHS teams. This should allow us to place far less reliance on individual staff questionnaires in future and, possibly, to drop them altogether.

References

Audit Commission (1999) *Children in mind.* London: Audit Commission.

Barnes, D., Dyer, W., and Glover, G. (2001) *Mental health service provision for working age adults in England 2000.* Durham: Centre for Public Mental Health, Durham University.

David Daniel, personal communication, Head of Mental Health Statistics, Department of Health (2004) CAMHS bed provision in England 1999 – 2003, based on the NICAPS 1999 findings reported by Anne O'Herlihy and Hannah Farr.

Department of Health (1999) HSC 1999/126 : LAC (99) 22 NHS *Moderni\ation fund and mental health grant for child and adolescent mental health services 1999/2002.* London: Department of Health.

Department of Health (2001) *Shifting the balance of power. Securing delivery.* London: Department of Health.

Department of Health (2002) *Improvement, expansion and reform: the next 3 years—priorities and planning framework 2003–2006.* London: Department of Health.

Department of Health (2003) HSC 2003/003: LAC (2003) 2 *Child and adolescent mental health service (CAMHS) grant guidance 2003/04.* London: Department of Health.

Glover, G. (2000) A comprehensive clinical database for mental health care in England. *Social Psychiatry and Psychiatric Epidemiology,* **35**, 523–9.

Glover, G. and Barnes, C. (2002) *Mental health service provision for working age adults in England, 2001.* Durham: Centre for Public Mental Health, Durham University.

Glover, G. and Barnes, C. (2003) *Mental health service provision for working age adults in England, 2002.* Leeds: National Institute of Mental Health in England.

Glover, G. and Sinclair-Smith, H. (2000) Computerised information systems in English Mental Health Care Providers. *Social Psychiatry and Psychiatric Epidemiology,* **35**, 518–22.

Glover, G., Dean, R., Hartley, C., and Foster, B. (2003) *National Child and Adolescent Mental Health Service Mapping Exercise.* London: Department of Health.

Hartley, C. and Glover, G. (2002) *Final report on the feasibility of a national child and adolescent mental health service mapping exercise.* London: Unpublished report to the Department of Health.

NHS Health Advisory Service (1995) *Together we stand—the commissioning, role and management of child and adolescent mental health services.* London: HMSO.

O'Herlihy, A., Worrall, A., Lelliot, P., Jaffa, T., Hill, P. and Banerjee, S. (2003) Distribution and characteristics of in-patient child and adolescent mental health services in England and Wales. *British Journal of Psychiatry,* **183**, 547–51.

University of Durham (2003) *National CAMH service mapping exercise 2002.* Available on *http://www.dur.ac.uk/service.mapping/CAMH.*

Chapter 29

Assessing need, mapping services, and setting priorities

Zarrina Kurtz

Introduction

During the last five years of the twentieth century, child and adolescent mental health services (CAMHS) became widely recognised as a significant field of service provision in England and Wales, heralded by the publication of two highly influential reports in 1995: *Together we stand* (NHS Health Advisory Service [HAS] 1995) and *A handbook on child and adolescent mental health* (Department of Health and Department of Education 1995). Surveys carried out over this period showed that there was great variation in the level and type of provision in different parts of the country (Kurtz *et al.* 1994; Audit Commission 1999), and that child and adolescent mental health services were rarely actively commissioned (Vanstraelen and Cottrell 1994). The amount spent on specialist child and adolescent mental health services per head of child population (aged up to 18), was found to vary by a factor of seven, with health authority funding accounting for a very small proportion (an average of around 5%) of local NHS mental health budgets (Audit Commission 1999). However, from 1999/2000, largely in response to increasing national and political appreciation of the mental health needs of young people, the Department of Health has made available, year-on-year, specifically designated funds for development across the full range of services for the mental health of children, adolescents and their families (NHS 1999; DoH 2003a). The Emerging Findings from England's National Service Framework for Children includes the expectation that a comprehensive CAMHS will be available in all areas by 2006 (DoH 2003b, c). In addition, a number of major government initiatives, such as Sure Start (Hall 2000), are targeting reduction in risk factors, such as family and child poverty, which are significantly associated with child and adolescent mental health problems (Meltzer *et al.* 2000).

The 1994 national survey (Kurtz *et al.* 1994) showed that the distribution of resources in local CAMHS provision was not linked to any indication of local population needs, and that even in those health authority areas where services had, to some extent, been commissioned, commissioning had rarely been carried out on the basis of an assessment of local needs. Five years later, among approximately 60% of health authorities in England and Wales reviewed by the Audit Commission, although some assessment of needs had been carried out, this had rarely been used to inform commissioning of services. This situation is notable in that the assessment of population needs had been established as a pre-requisite for commissioning local services, and as a key role for purchasers, in the internal market set up in 1990 under the NHS Reorganisation Act.

In 1991, guidance was issued to district health authorities in England on the assessment of needs, and this had three main elements (NHS ME):

1. Epidemiological and expert professional evidence about the level and types of mental health problems in the population of children and young people, and about factors that are known to increase risks.

2. Review of the treatment and management strategies available and their known efficacy and cost-effectiveness, again based on research evidence and on expert opinion; the performance of local services to be assessed in these terms.

3. The views of local people, both users of services and the general public, on what services they regard as important and on their accessibility and acceptability. Direct consultation with the public, particularly with people who have used the services and their carers, is necessary, but relevant non-statutory organizations and community health councils can act as representatives of user and carer views.

This guidance recognized the complexity in conducting a full assessment of needs, and the importance of incorporating the experience, views, and opinions of those who know most about the particular needs and services under consideration, i.e. local people, users, and service providers in the field. More recently, a series of six articles on health needs assessment in the *British Medical Journal* (Stephens and Gillam 1998) covers the topic in considerable detail, pointing out that, technically, needs for healthcare imply that there is the ability to benefit from service provision, that the critical examination of local service provision as an integral part of needs assessment, and reinforcing its pivotal role in planning (Williams and Wright 1998):

> The epidemiological approach to health needs assessment is the traditional public
> health approach to describing need in relation to specific health problems using estimates
> of the incidence and prevalence, and other surrogates of health impact derived from studies
> carried out locally or elsewhere. This approach has been extended to the consideration,
> alongside these measures, of the ways in which existing services are delivered and the
> effectiveness and cost effectiveness of interventions intended to meet the needs thus
> described. This is a logical extension as there is little point in estimating the burden
> of ill health (except for determining priorities for future research) if nothing can be
> done about it.

In the field of CAMHS, the 1991 health service model for the assessment of needs and matching review of local services has limitations, which are usually regarded as being due to its having been developed on a traditional medical model. Child and adolescent mental health needs frequently present in ways that do not conform to strict medical diagnoses, and similarly, these needs may often be met by a range of professional disciplines and non-health service agencies, most notably education and social services. Services from these agencies were included as part of comprehensive CAMHS provision for the first time in the 1994 survey (Kurtz *et al.*). This survey also mapped for the first time, the extent of voluntary sector provision for child and adolescent mental health.

This chapter describes how, for the purposes of planning, commissioning, and delivering child and adolescent mental health services, needs can be assessed and services mapped, i.e. what is involved in gathering the information required to identify the changes necessary to improve the health of the population and to set priorities.

Assessing needs

Epidemiology

Defining mental health problems and disorders

The usual starting point for assessing needs for CAMHS, is to gather epidemiological information about the mental health disorders that may benefit from service provision. As with other
medical conditions, child and adolescent mental health disorders are described according to
the standard taxonomies of the World Health Organization's International Classification of
Diseases (ICD) or the American Psychiatric Association's diagnostic and statistical manual
(DSM). Both classifications are multi-axial and based upon patterns of symptomatology. They
take into account research findings and consensus on aetiology, psychosocial risk factors, and
prognosis. These classification systems are revised regularly (ICD-10 most recently in 1992 and
DSM-IV in 1994) and are now more directly comparable with each other than were previous
versions (Fonagy *et al.* 2002).

The remit of the relatively new field of child and adolescent psychiatry is, essentially, the
diagnosis and treatment of the disorders included in the child and adolescent sections of these
disease classifications. Not only have these sections greatly expanded in recent editions, indicating a growing and increasingly defined field, but many of the conditions now included, e.g.
child abuse and substance misuse, imply the need for more diverse specialist diagnostic and
treatment knowledge and skills. Within clinical practice, disorders (such as post-traumatic
stress disorder and disorders of attachment) are also becoming increasingly recognized that
are, as yet, categorized incompletely and differently in the standard clssifications.

However, a mental health need cannot be equated with a case of a disorder, as it can in many
medical conditions. Mental disorders in children and adolescents manifest in their behaviour
and in the way they feel; the way the disorder is defined and its seriousness depends also upon
the extent to which it interferes with the child's functioning and normal processes of development. Interference with a child's capacity to make progress academically and to make friends at
school may, for example, be an integral part of an anxiety disorder (Fonagy *et al.* 2002), although
the time sequence of manifestation may suggest that these are precursor or precipitating
factors, or arise as a consequence of a more tightly defined mental health disorder.

A useful definition of psychiatric disorder was given by Rutter and Graham (1968) as:

> An abnormality of emotion, behaviour or relationships which is developmentally inappropriate
> and of sufficient duration and severity to cause persistent suffering or handicap to the child
> and/or distress or disturbance to the family or community.

More recent classifications of mental health problems distinguish between problems, defined
as 'a disturbance of function in one area of relationships, mood, behaviour, or development of
sufficient severity to require professional intervention', and disorders, defined as 'either a severe
problem (commonly persistent), or the co-occurrence of a number of problems, usually in the
presence of a number of risk factors' (Wallace *et al.* 1997). The NHS Health Advisory Service
(1995) defined and distinguished mental health problems, mental disorders and mental
illnesses. Problems and disorders can be either quantitatively or qualitatively different from
normal. Tantrums or stealing would be regarded as quantitatively different while autism or
psychotic symptoms are examples of qualitative differences.

The 'diagnosis' depends upon what the child, the parent/carer, teacher, and others report, and
the clinician observes; there are no diagnostic tests. It has been shown that the recognition of

mental health needs, and the way in which they are conceptualized and described are different among parents, communities, and professionals from different backgrounds (Evans and Brown 1993). In defining needs in minority ethnic communities in Britain, for example, there are well-rehearsed but poorly resolved difficulties because the boundary between what is seen as disease or dysfunction on one hand, and mental health on the other, is strongly influenced by cultural factors (Sashidharan and Commander 1998).

Along with the growth in the number of conditions officially recognized as child and adolescent mental health disorders, studies have shown that they frequently present in atypical ways, and that significant disturbance in a child may not fit a medical diagnostic classification. A child's need for a service is often recognized by parents, by teachers, or by the social services as primarily a disciplinary, educational, or protection matter, with little or no appreciation of the mental health component, let alone the role that mental health expertise could play in helping with the problem. Understandable reluctance to label a child as having 'mental health' problems is part of the explanation. However, all those who work with children increasingly acknowledge that mental health makes up a significant proportion of their work, although difficulties arise in the use of single operational definitions by all agencies. In addition, mental health needs may go unrecognized because children present problems that are labelled according to the particular setting, such as non-attendance or low achievement in school, and persistent offending in the youth justice system. In primary care, between 2 and 5% of children attend with mental health problems as the primary complaint but about a quarter of children consulting have been shown to have psychiatric disorders (Garralda and Bailey 1986a, b, 1989).

Perception of the need for services has been shown to differ between parents and their general practitioner (GP), unrelated to the presence of a psychiatric disorder diagnosed on the basis of a standardized questionnaire (Evans and Brown 1993). The GPs thought that a lower number than those with an assessed psychiatric disorder needed specialist mental health services, while the parents of a much higher number of children thought that their children would benefit, although a high proportion of these children did not have a psychiatric diagnosis on assessment.

Risk groups

Mental health problems tend to occur more frequently in a number of well established risk situations—with the likelihood increasing as the number of risk factors increases—and these indicate particular service needs. Knowledge about the risk factors for child and adolescent mental health problems is growing fast, and estimates of risks in numerical terms are given by Wallace and colleagues (1997). In local needs assessment and service development, the most important consideration is not the estimation of actual numbers but the identification of the children and young people at high risk and where they are to be found, and the understanding of their needs. The prevalence of conditions is higher in adolescents than in younger children, and where children and their families live in poverty or disadvantaged circumstances (Meltzer *et al.* 2000). These and other groups of young people in whom particular risks for mental health problems have been established are listed in the *Handbook on child and adolescent mental health* (DoH/DoE 1995) as follows:

young offenders and children from a criminal background;

children who are being looked after by local authorities or who have recently ended a period of public care;

children with learning difficulties;

children with emotional and behavioural difficulties;

children who have been sexually, physically, or emotionally abused;

children with a chronic physical illness;

children with a physical disability;

children with sensory impairments;

children of parents with mental illness;

children of parents with a substance abuse problem;

children who have experienced or witnessed sudden and extreme trauma;

children who are refugees.

Special studies have identified the profile of mental health needs among some of these high-risk groups, such as children in the looked-after system (McCann et al. 1996; Meltzer et al. 2004), which indicates the kinds of intervention and service models that are likely to be effective. But we still lack comprehensive evidence of the holistic needs of children as they present in real life.

Thus, the assessment of needs must encompass assessment of population risks for child and adolescent mental health problems. Information should be collected on local socio-economic conditions, such as unemployment, homelessness, and eligibility for free school meals, with the population prevalence distribution according to these characteristics. It can be helpful to locate housing estates and school pyramids where particular needs are concentrated. Although the figures for many indicators of socio-economic deprivation depend upon political and service definitions, the location of risk groups is an important element in needs assessment, particularly for the provision of preventive and targeted services. Similarly, the particular needs of children excluded from school, in minority ethnic communities, in special schools, children's homes, secure accommodation, and out-of-borough placements must be identified and their location mapped.

Population and risk-group information can be obtained from a number of sources, including: the Director of Public Health's Annual Reports; the health improvement programme (HImP); population profiles compiled by primary care organizations; the Children's Services Plan; Quality Protects Management Action Plan; the Behaviour Support Plan; Connexions; Youth Offending Team; Early Years Plan; Sure Start Proposals; and local special studies.

Resilience and protective factors

In recent times, attention has been directed to understanding why it is that many children who suffer adverse circumstances and a combination of risk factors do not develop problems or a disorder. Three key groups of factors appear to be protective (p. 25, HAS 1995):

self-esteem, sociability, and autonomy;

family compassion, warmth, and absence of parental discord;

social support systems that encourage personal effort and coping.

Services that promote these characteristics and situations for children and families serve to promote child and adolescent mental health, and the need for these services should be included in local assessment. The need for services such as parenting programmes, parent support groups, and nurture clubs in primary schools is particularly acute among children and families known to be vulnerable with respect to mental health problems.

Using the numbers

Local population needs are rarely directly assessed by local studies that, in effect, aggregate standardized assessments of the needs of individual children in non-referred populations. These studies are not practicable because of the considerable resources and time they require.

Usually, local estimates of prevalence are based on national, international and special studies, with the figures derived from children with disorders defined strictly in research terms, although these may differ in different studies, carried out in populations with differing charac- teristics. However, in Great Britain, local estimates for the prevalence of mental health disorder can now be made on the basis of a nationally representative study of psychiatric morbidity in children aged 5–15 years, carried out by the Office for National Statistics (ONS) (Meltzer 2000).

Even so, the findings do not readily translate into figures for caseloads and casemix as they present in real life, notably because a high proportion (up to 60%) of children are found to have a variable mix of psychiatric diagnoses, problems and risk factors (Fonagy *et al.* 2002). Morbidity profiles are largely derived from studies of service users: 92 (of 124 participating) trusts recorded a problem profile for children presenting to the Specialist CAMHS in the national Audit Commission project (Audit Commission 1999), all using the Health of the Nation Outcome Scales for Children and Adolescents (HoNOSCA) (Gowers *et al.* 1999). Fewer than 5% of children presented to these services with only one problem and the most frequent number of problems presented was five. Holistic profiles of the local population of children and families, whether known to CAMHS or not, represent the ideal for needs assessment, but are rarely put together.

However, a recent study has described the mental health needs of children in a deprived area of inner London, encompassing risk factors as well as manifest problems (Davis *et al.* 2000). Based on home interviews with mothers and children, nearly 72% of the children were found to have at least one moderate-to-severe problem, and nearly 37% had three or more. Along with defined mental health problems, associated difficulties were described as: disruptive behaviour, tantrums, and eating problems in the 0–4-year-olds; anxiety, persistent lying, depressed mood, temper control, and defiance in the 5–10s; temper control, depressed mood, defiance, food faddiness/eating problems, and father-relationship problems in the 11–13s; and crime, school discipline problems, multiple sexual relationships, lying, high smoking/alcohol use, truancy, somatic anxiety, sleep problems, mood swings, temper control, and drug use in the 14–16s. Over 85% of the sample had at least one risk factor for child mental health prob- lems, and over 51% had three or more. The most common risk factors included maternal and paternal mental health problems; environmental problems in relation to housing and neigh- bours; social isolation; chronic physical health problems in the parents; and trouble with the police. The number of problems per child was significantly correlated with the number of risk factors. In the light of these findings, Davis and colleagues (2000) suggested five levels of sever- ity and complexity of problems with an appropriate service response at each level. The follow- ing percentages of the sample were apportioned to each level: 5.2% with the least severe problems; 19.5% at the next level; 19.0% at the next level; 25.7% requiring a multidisciplinary CAMH team approach; and 2.4% requiring a highly specialist service.

In a study in four districts, Kurtz and colleagues (1995) estimated, on the basis of a number of research studies, population percentages requiring services at Tier 1 as 15%; at Tier 2 as 7%; at Tier 3 as 1.85%; and at Tier 4, as 0.075%.

The discrepancies between diagnosable child and adolescent mental health disorders from research-based figures and from the ways in which young people present to services, described above, highlight the limitations inherent in a purely numerical approach to assessing local needs in this field—except for comparison with national or regional averages, which may identify a par- ticular local problem. But a summary of a needs assessment, carried out in North and Mid-Hants Health Authority, given in the Audit Commission report (p. 61, 1999) shows what can be learnt.

Service effectiveness

It is here that one should begin to consider needs from the perspective of the ability to benefit from service provision. The evidence on the effectiveness of service provision in meeting defined needs in the field of CAMH is limited and largely confined to studies of treatment efficacy for definable psychiatric conditions in children (Kurtz 1996). Each psychiatric disorder has a range of therapeutic approaches that have been shown to be effective, although in most cases, there is little agreement about which is the most effective. The overall message from research on psychotherapeutic treatments is that, across the range, they are generally associated with significant improvements. But there is little research on problems as they present in clinical practice or in the school. Much more is known about the treatment of single conditions that are not associated with others, and which do not have the complication of serious educational and social problems. Partly for these reasons, more is known about the efficacy of treatments in younger children than in adolescents. More is also known about the shorter rather than the longer term effects of interventions. And greater treatment effects have been measured in terms of psychiatric symptoms than in terms of adjustment or achievement.

Intervention appears to be justified at all developmental stages, but the generally poor long-term prognosis of even early childhood disorder suggests that intervention should be as early as possible, and that preventive strategies are highly important. These should target children, adolescents, and families known to be at high risk, and the effectiveness of a number of approaches has been established, especially when linked to universal services (Cox 1993; Fonagy 1998). The need for preventive services is also clearly indicated because the specialist services, as currently provided, do not, in the main, fulfil the requirements for treatment efficacy in individual conditions as indicated by the studies (Weisz *et al.* 1995). And for many reasons (including staff shortages, lack of appropriate skills) they fail to address the problems presented by children in ways that the research on effectiveness would indicate.

A number of recent summaries of the evidence for the effectiveness of interventions in child and adolescent mental health are readily available (Kurtz 1996; Target and Fonagy 1996; Wallace *et al.* 1997; Harrington *et al.* 1999). An exhaustive systematic review of the literature on the effectiveness of interventions in child and adolescent mental health has also been published (Fonagy *et al.* 2002).

The home background and parental involvement are crucial to the way in which work with children can be carried out and to its effectiveness. Special efforts may be needed to engage the family in treatment, which may actually be delivered by parents who may themselves, in turn, need treatment or support (Kazdin *et al.* 1990). Treatment may accelerate improvement in the child or help to reduce risk of recurrence, and provide other benefits such as improved family functioning.

In maintaining supervision over the course of chronic disorders, difficulties can be expected at particular times, such as when a child changes school or a parent leaves home. These sorts of events may also trigger the first manifestation of problems. For these reasons, a legitimate aim of treatment can be the maintenance of normal developmental processes in a child who, without treatment, might suffer setbacks because of an emotional or behavioural disorder.

The effect of psychiatric and psychological intervention may be nullified if education and social services are not concurrently supporting the child and the family. Particular attention to optimizing the education of a child with a mental health disorder, and work with his or her family, are likely to improve psychological symptoms and functioning. Equally, psychological treatments may show most impact in terms of improved educational and social skills and function. These effects may not become apparent until years after treatment or preventive management has been carried out, but may be those most valued by the young person and the family. Thus assessment of the individual child's needs must take into account what is going on in other domains of his or her life.

Similarly, assessment of population needs for mental health services must take account of health, education and social services, and may well include housing, play and local amenities, and the voluntary sector, as well as certain services for adults. It is also clearly important to retain a range of specialized therapeutic approaches so that children of widely differing ages and social contexts can all be offered effective help for their particular problems or disorders. An effective service will have the capacity to combine these in the most effective way for each individual child. As in the case of individual children, multi-pronged approaches to the promotion of mental health in communities of children have shown encouraging results. Almost all the evidence comes from the United States (Bickman *et al.* 1992), although evaluation of such approaches has started in the United Kingdom (Kurtz and James 2004).

Some of the most telling evidence is for the link between effectiveness and the style of therapeutic approach and service delivery (Bickman 1996; Davies and Spurr 1998). Particularly in prevention, a didactic approach has been demonstrated to be less successful than one focused on relationship building, treating the mother as the person with responsibility to promote the development of her child (Attride-Stirling *et al.* 2001).

Mapping services

A full description of the currently available service provision is an integral part of the local assessment of needs—above all, to identify unmet needs—and in order to plan, commission, and deliver improved services. The extent and type of local provision should be mapped, covering the promotion of child and adolescent mental health, prevention of problems, identification and early intervention, treatment and management interventions, follow-up and longer term care. In any local area, it will be found that these functions are provided, in one way or another, by a great variety of services, projects and agencies.

To start with, it is helpful to compile a local service 'map' according to the tiered strategic framework, described in *Together we stand* (HAS 1995), although a number of services will probably not fit neatly into the way the service tiers are described. In this framework, the types of service that can contribute to the mental health of children and young people, what they do and how they work, have been conceptually organized into four tiers, each of which addresses a different type of problem, the level of severity and complexity increasing from Tier 1 to Tier 4.

Although the tiers are defined slightly differently in Wales as compared with England, Box 29.1 provides examples of what this over-arching 'map' of services may look like in any one area. It is based on a detailed study carried out in four district health authorities (Kurtz *et al.* 1995). This local map will identify all the stakeholders, and often for the first time, faces them with a comprehensive picture of the resources available locally, albeit under labels that do not include the words 'mental health' or even 'emotional and behavioural difficulties'.

Box 29.1 Example of services that may be available for the mental health of children and adolescents in a typical district

NB Increasingly, at all tiers, work is carried out jointly by staff from at least two agencies

Tier 1

Health or health-led

Primary healthcare, with general support by GPs, health visitors, midwives.

Health visitor advice to individual families on child development, feeding, sleep, anti-social behaviour.

Post-natal depression screening by health visitors.

Specialist health visitor clinic for enuresis; joint clinic with community paediatrician for encopresis.

School nurse drop-in counselling service.

Community paediatrician/school nurse behaviour management sessions in schools.

Paediatric community nurse support for children with chronic illness, e.g. cystic fibrosis, diabetes, sickle cell disorder.

Social services or SS-led

Child protection.

Family support and family centres; parenting programmes.

Learning disability team, including respite care.

Young carers project.

Looked-after children service; foster carers; children's homes.

Education or education-led

Early years service; portage; nurture groups in primary schools.

All teachers.

School pastoral system.

PSHE curriculum.

Healthy schools initiative.

Anti-bullying programme.

Special needs co-ordinators.

Youth service.

Connexions.

Voluntary sector

Relate.

CRUSE bereavement service.

NCH action for children creche, playschool, and family resource centre.

Home start.

Barnardo's leaving care project.

Children's society teenage drop-in and counselling centre.

Young people's housing project.

Special projects

Sure Start.

Children's fund nurture groups in primary schools; Saturday clubs to promote racial identity and community integration with minority ethnic communities.

Tier 2

Health or health-led

Individual health members of the specialist multidisciplinary CAMHS working alone.

Primary mental health worker covering a particularly deprived locality.

Children's clinical psychology service; sessions in health centres and to SS child disability team.

Consultant paediatrician clinics in general practice for ADHD, chronic fatigue syndrome.

Paediatrician with a special interest in learning disability session in respite care unit.

RMN working with young people who are clients of the youth offending team.

Social services or SS-led

Individual social workers offering family therapy in family centres.

Therapy-trained social worker-run post-abuse therapy group.

Education or education-led

Educational psychology service

Behaviour support service.

Educational welfare service.

Pupil referral unit.

Home tuition service.

Secondary school outreach, e.g. offering counselling for parents and anger management.

School for the deaf.

Voluntary sector

Drugs and alcohol youth worker.

Autistic society school for children with autistic spectrum disorder.

Tier 3

Health or health-led

Multidisciplinary specialist child and adolescent mental health teams, with child and adolescent psychiatrists, clinical psychologists, nurse specialists, family therapists, occupational therapists; includes social workers.

Specialist CAMHS adolescent team.

Box 29.1 (continued) Example of services that may be available for the mental health of children and adolescents in a typical district

Education or education-led

EBD special school.

Tier 4

Health or health-led

Contract for child and adolescent psychiatry inpatient care with NHS provider.

Extra-contractual referrals to specialist eating disorder unit out-of-district.

Extra-contractual referrals to national catchment adolescent forensic unit.

Social services or SS-led

Out-of-county placements in therapeutic communities and secure units.

Education or education-led

Hospital teaching service.

Out-of-county placements in specialist residential schools.

Once as full a description as possible of this range of local provision has been assembled, an attempt should be made to map the actual location of each service linked to the population distribution; and for each service, the characteristics of the client group served (e.g. age group, type of problem) and the expertise and interventions offered by the service. In this way, assessment can be made of the local child population's 'ability to benefit' from currently available services. A useful framework for this is given by the seven dimensions of good quality, first described for healthcare provision by Maxwell (1984). Services should be:

equitable

accessible

acceptable

appropriate

effective

ethical

efficient.

These dimensions are inter-related, in that equitable provision is, to a greater or lesser extent, dependent upon matters of accessibility and acceptability. It cannot be seen as equitable if a service exists but it is known to be poorly acceptable to the population that it serves.

The information required to map services may need to be put together from a number of different sources, many of which will be the same as those with information about needs; for example, the Children's Services Plan. Details about the Specialist CAMHS should be available from trust business plans and monitoring information. It is remarkable, however, how little reliable information is available at present, in most parts of the country, regarding the full problem and risk profile of children that are seen, even by the Specialist CAMHS, the interventions they receive, and the outcomes achieved (Audit Commission 1999 and Chapter 27). Most of this information must be obtained from service providers (clinicians and managers) themselves (see section on stakeholders below). A national mapping exercise of Specialist CAMHS now reports a core data set annually on http://www.dur.ac.uk/service.mapping/ CAMH/index.php. (see Chapter 28.)

A full service map should—for the Specialist CAMHS—describe the case load case mix (presenting problems, co-morbidity, severity, basic child characteristics such as age, ethnic group, place of residence); the source of referral; staff numbers and disciplines, with skill mix; interventions delivered; clinical process such as joint working; waiting times and non-attendance rates; and outcomes, including user and carer satisfaction. Details of the ways in which services are offered should be covered, such as the location and timing of outreach clinics; consultation, supervision, liaison and training activity; key duties such as 24-hour and emergency cover arrangements; and special services such as an adolescent team, a service for looked after children, work with the child disability team, and so on.

As full information as possible, along the same lines, should be obtained for Tier 1 services, such as health visitor enuresis clinics, parenting sessions and paediatric ADHD clinics, and relevant services provided by non-NHS agencies, such as family centres, foster care, and special schools. The way in which these services provide for child and adolescent mental health and the working relationships between them and the Specialist CAMHS should be described, with indications of their accessibilty, acceptability and other elements of good practice.

Involving stakeholders

Much of the most useful information about the mental health needs of children and adolescents—which is sensitive to local circumstances—will be obtained from service providers. The staff who work hands-on with children, young people and families will also hold the information necessary to build a full picture of what local services actually provide, and will have informed views on unmet needs, the reasons for gaps in service provision and their consequences, as well as on service strengths. Thus, in assessing needs and mapping services, information should be sought from as full a range as possible, of clinicians and managers of services, such as those set out in Box 29.1. This is a time-consuming exercise but is a crucial part of the process, bringing together the multiplicity of experience and opinion that is necessary to understand the complexity of children's needs in the field of mental health. Without the benefit of these wide-ranging views, it may well be impossible to find ways to improve the provision of services. The process allows all providers to feel involved in the decisions that will be taken as a result of assessment of needs. In addition, it will often uncover unanticipated strengths and possibilities for development that would not be revealed solely by documented or official descriptions of services.

User and community participation

Users of services and those with needs who do not obtain the help they require are the primary stakeholders. Thus, the assessment of needs should be informed by the views of the communities that are served by local providers, and by users of local services.

Members of local communities, more particularly families with children and young people, can inform needs assessment on four aspects: whether they know of the existence of the services that are available to meet their needs, and how accurate and complete is their knowledge; what kinds of services they feel most comfortable using; whether they have ready access to appropriate sources of information to guide them when they want help; and what are the assumptions, beliefs and specific areas of knowledge that need to be addressed in information giving and in tailoring services to meet expectations. In addition, consultation itself can act to provide information and bring about more realistic expectations of services. Findings from consultation regarding services other than child and adolescent mental health services, such as leaving care services, are often highly relevant. A number of research studies also provide information that can be applied to the local situation.

As an example, the Mental Health Foundation published the results of a qualitative study undertaken by The Centre for the Child and Society at Glasgow University, which explored the perceptions and attitudes of 169 Scottish young people aged 12–14 years (Laws 1998). This found that young people use a different language to describe mental health, that medical and professional terminology is regarded as stigmatizing and off-putting, and that these differences inhibit communication and form a barrier between young people and mental health professionals. The report concluded that the roles of mental health professionals and the services they offer are not well understood by young people, but they value counselling and helplines. Young people who have direct experience of services, either personally or through another family member or friend, develop a better understanding of mental health issues and make competent decisions and choices about care and treatment. And the support of family and friends emerges as important in the needs of young people with mental health problems, and of those caring for others with mental health problems.

User-consultation projects conducted by the Reach Out Group in Whitley Bay, and a Young People's Project in Cornwall called *Hear our voice* both concluded that statutory services were failing to meet the needs of young people whose lives were in chaos, and that informal approaches in community settings were the most successful ways of reaching the most needy young people (Laws 1998).

These findings are a guide to what to look for in defining unmet needs for appropriate and acceptable provision. It is important, in addition, to seek locally specific information, which must include the views and experience of users of the Specialist CAMHS. Gathering this type of information should be a regular component of CAMHS audit, and an integral part of the service map on quality and effectiveness. An excellent guide that covers all aspects of consultation and participation in child and adolescent mental health services, including the avoidance of tokenism, has been produced by Save the Children for the NHS Executive Trent Region (Hedges and McKeown 2000).

Setting priorities

Unmet need

There is no one way in which a comprehensive service should be provided and in different areas, different functions will be delivered by different services in different ways. Examining the local service map in the light of the assessed local needs will identify the strengths and weaknesses in current provision, and highlight unmet needs as the basis for setting priorities for service development.

Unmet need can occur because:

some children are not recognized as having a helpable problem;

the full range of services do not cover all the local population geographically or/and by age group;

children do not reach an appropriate service in time for effective intervention, or do not, for one reason or another, derive full benefit from the services on offer;

services do not offer the necessary range of skills, expertise and interventions;

there are too few resources effectively to meet the mental health needs of the local child and adolescent population.

Whenever research findings on the prevalence of mental health problems are applied to local populations of children, the resulting numbers of expected 'cases' are alarmingly high, running to between 7 and 10 times the number known to the Specialist CAMHS. However, these numbers are misleading and should not be given undue importance as indicating unmet needs. They are derived for children with disorders studied in strictly defined research terms which do not translate helpfully into case-load and case-mix as they present in real life, particularly for the many children who present with more than one condition.

Another difficulty with using these figures arises because, overall, estimated numbers are usually matched against the case-load of the local Specialist CAMHS, while an unknown proportion of children may well be known to other local services, and may well expect to receive effective treatment from them. In a study to assess needs and unmet needs in four districts (Kurtz et al. 1995), the prevalence of disorders of different severities was matched against the number of children known to services at the appropriate tiers and it was found that very many fewer children were known to the services than would be expected, except at Tier 4. And even in this special study—let alone what might be available from routinely collected information—the data from Tier 1 were very incomplete; it was often difficult to analyse separately data for Tiers 2 and 3; and particularly for Tier 4, it was almost impossible to tell whether the specialist services were dealing with the appropriate children, let alone all of those who might derive benefit.

With the present state of the epidemiological information and local information systems, what can be learned by applying prevalence figures to local populations in commissioning is limited. It can be assumed, in line with the recent national morbidity study (Meltzer et al. 2000), that over 10% of young people in any local area in Great Britain have significant mental health needs that would benefit from service provision. That these needs cover the spectrum of mental health problems and disorders, and will have serious and costly long term impact if neglected, should be used to raise awareness locally and to make the case for an appropriate allocation of resources.

Comparing the full range of local services against the local picture of needs for child and adolescent mental health will almost certainly reveal a lack of provision for some groups of children—according to age group (such as those over the age of 16); type of problem (such as autistic spectrum disorder); or risk group (such as children in the looked after system). Certain types of service may be patchily or poorly developed, such as youth counselling services or early intervention at Tier 1. Some specialisms may not be available, such as the psychiatry of learning disability for young people or forensic adolescent psychiatry. And there may be evidence that access to services is poor for people residing in some geographical parts of the local area, or services may not be used because they are poorly acceptable. Service strengths will also

Box 29.2 Distribution of the costs of conduct disorder in children

19% National Health Service

7.6% Social Services

36% Local Education Authority

0.4% Voluntary Sector

37% Families

be identified, such as specialist resources in the voluntary sector and mental health promoting initiatives in the education sector.

In setting local service development priorities, both the prevalence of child and adolescent mental health problems, their impact on child and family life and the known likelihood of their having serious mental health and other consequences in later life, should be taken into account.

Mental health problems in children increase demands on personal social services, education, health and juvenile justice services, and are costly for families. In a study of conduct disorder, the figures shown in Box 29.2 for the yearly costs emerged (Knapp *et al.* 1999).

Preliminary findings from this study of the lifetime costs of conduct disorder up to age 28, found that those individuals who had had conduct disorder at age 10 cost over £100 000 more in services used than those without conduct disorder (Knapp *et al.* 1999). In a presentation to an inquiry carried out by the Mental Health Foundation, one of the authors was able to make a strong case for the cost-effectiveness of early interventions. He argued that if conduct disorders affecting 15% of the childhood population and costing approximately £100 000 until the young person was 26 could be reduced to those of problems affecting 10% of the childhood population and costing 'only' £70 000 per child, a saving of £30 000 could be made for each child initially experiencing conduct disorder. Thus the cost-benefit of early intervention is large, even if the treatment effect is moderate.

Depending upon the local profile of unmet needs, priorities may also include the development of a multi-agency adolescent service—perhaps a Specialist CAMHS with explicit expertise in assessing and managing the mix of problems with which adolescents commonly present, including early psychosis and substance misuse-related problems, or a non-stigmatizing user-friendly centre for young people, which offers skilled counselling and ready access to specialist mental health expertise.

However, it is unlikely that the identification of the main areas of unmet need in a local area will automatically dictate the priorities for strategic development. A proper and open process of debate about prioritization—once again involving all the relevant stakeholders (who should be as informed as possible regarding the local assessed needs, unmet needs and service strengths and weaknesses)—is needed if implementation of strategic priorities is to succeed (Meslin *et al.* 1994).

Klein (1993) has made the case for the proper process in setting priorities, thus:

> To invoke the concept of rationing implies rationality, i.e. the use of reason, in determining the allocation of resources: the sense that, if these resources are limited, the way in which they are

distributed to individuals should not be arbitrary but justifiable by appeal to some principles. There are two main—albeit 'ideal-type'—models for taking decisions about rationing. The first may be called the technological model. Here, the assumption is that, given more information about outcomes, effectiveness and so on, it will be possible to devise priorities almost automatically from the data. The information will speak for itself provided the computer is properly programmed. It is a model that would allow top-down decision-making for purchasing authorities. In the second model, the assumption is that information will always be incomplete and there will always be different views about the criteria to be used in evaluating it. It is a model which sees priorities emerging from a process of argument. The first model depends on technological rationality and puts emphasis on more research and the development of better expertise. The second is based on process rationality and puts emphasis on improving access to the network of those engaged in debate. The conditions for the first model do not yet exist. Clearly, in operating the second model, the ethical and moral dimensions of the issues are highlighted.

There is no question that responsibility for priority setting must be taken by a multidiscipli-nary group of people of sufficient seniority to take decisions and commit funds. Indeed, such a group is required to carry out a meaningful assessment of needs for child and adolescent mental health services and to initiate and facilitate a service review. The group should include commissioners, specialist clinicians, and managers, practitioners and managers from universal children's services (primary care and education) and those working with known high risk and hard-to-reach groups. This working group needs to integrate the functions of assessing needs, mapping services, identifying unmet needs, prioritizing, commissioning, evaluating, and adjusting further service development according to changes in needs and what is learnt from service evaluation. Members of the group should agree working definitions for mental health needs and the ways in which these can be met locally, and they should become increasingly well-informed about child and adolescent mental health. From agency-specific information a multifaceted picture of the local mental health needs will be built up, and will also contribute to the corporate knowledge about approaches that work in a variety of environments. Although well recognized difficulties are inherent in the process of setting priorities among a multidisci-plinary multi-agency group (Stronks *et al.* 1997), the work of such a group is fundamentally important for service development to meet the mental health needs of children and adolescents.

This group should also be responsible for co-ordinating and commissioning, where neces-sary, specific studies to gain understanding of particular needs (such as may arise because there is a school for deaf children in the local area, or a secure unit) and the evaluation of new serv-ice responses to identified needs. The group should also take the responsibility for developing a strategy for user and community participation in child and adolescent mental health services.

Concluding remarks

In conclusion, when assessing needs and setting priorities, it is crucial to bear in mind that services for the mental health of children and adolescents should work as a service system; the way needs are met in one component of the system will have implications for how other com-ponents should work.

It is essential that a collective overview of the system is maintained and that priorites for service development can be adjusted in response to an iterative needs assessment process and service evaluation. Although it is necessary to keep up-to-date, year on year assessment of how services are meeting needs can be carried out in less detail, using rapid appraisal methods (Annett and Ritkin 1995; Murray Scott 1999).

References

Annett, H. and Ritkin, S.B. (1995) *Guidelines for rapid participatory appraisal to assess community health needs.* Geneva: World Health Organization.

Attride-Stirling, J., Davis, H., Markless, G., Sclare, I., and Day, C. (2001) 'Someone to Talk to Who'll Listen': Addressing the psychosocial needs of children and families. *Journal of Community & Applied Social Psychology*, 11, 179–91.

Audit Commission (1999) *Children in mind: child and adolescent mental health services.* London: Audit Commission.

Bickman, L., Heflinger, C., Pio, G., and Behar, L. (1992) Evaluation planning for an innovative children's mental health system. *Clinical Psychology Review*, 12, 853–65.

Bickman, L. (1996) A continuum of care: more is not always better. *American Psychologist*, 51, 689–701.

Cox, A.D. (1993) Preventive aspects of child psychiatry. *Archives of Disease in Childhood*, 68, 691–701.

Davis, H., Day, C., Cox, A., and Cutler, L. (2000) Child and adolescent mental health needs: assessment and service implications in an inner city area. *Clinical Child Psychology and Psychiatry*, 5, 169–88.

Davis, H. and Spurr, P. (1998) Parent counselling: an evaluation of a community child mental health service. *Journal of Child Psychology and Psychiatry*, 39(3), 365–76.

Department of Health and Department for Education (1995) *A handbook on child and adolescent mental health.* Manchester: HMSO.

Department of Health (2003a) HSC 2003/003: LAC(2003)2. *Child and adolescent mental health service (camhs) grant guidance 2003/04.* London: Department of Health.

Department of Health (2003b) *Getting the right start: the National Service framework for children, young people and maternity services—emerging findings.* London: Department of Health.

Department of Health (2003c) *Improvement, expansion and reform: the next three years priorities and planning framework 2003–2006.* London: Department of Health.

Evans, S. and Brown, R. (1993) Perception of need for child psychiatric services among parents and GPs. *Health Trends*, 25, 11.

Fonagy, P. (1998) Prevention, the appropriate target of infant psychotherapy. *Infant Mental Health Journal*, 19 (2), 124–50.

Fonagy, P., Target, M., Cottrell, D., Phillips, J., and Kurtz, Z. (2002) *What works for whom? A critical review of treatments for children and adolescents.* New York: Guilford Press.

Garralda, M.E. and Bailey, D. (1986a) Children with psychiatric disorders in primary care. *Journal of Child Psychology and Psychiatry*, 27, 611–24.

Garralda, M.E. and Bailey, D. (1986b) Psychological deviance in children attending general practice. *Psychological Medicine*, 16, 423–9.

Garralda, M.E. and Bailey, D. (1989) Psychiatric disorders in general paediatric referrals. *Archives of Disease in Childhood*, 64, 1727–33.

Gowers, S.G., Harrington, R.C., Whitton, A., Lelliott, P., Beevor, A., Wing, J., *et al.* (1999) Brief scale for measuring the outcomes of emotional and behavioural disorders in children: Health of the Nation Outcome Scales for Children and Adolescents (HoNOSCA). *British Journal of Psychiatry*, 174, 413–6.

Hall, D.M.B. (2000) What is Sure Start? *Archives of Disease in Childhood*, 82, 435–7.

Harrington, R.C., Kerfoot, M., and Verduyn, C. (1999) Developing needs led child and adolescent mental health services: issues and prospects. *European Child and Adolescent Psychiatry*, 8, 1–10.

Hedges, C. and McKeown, C. (2000) *Give us a voice: consultation and participation in child and adolescent mental health services within the Trent region.* NHS Executive Trent and Save the Children.

Kazdin, A.E. (1990) Premature Termination from Treatment among Children Referred for Antisocial Behavior. *Journal of Child Psychology and Psychiatry*, **31** (3), 415–25.

Klein, R. (1993) Rationality and rationing: diffused or concentrated decision-making? In *Rationing of healthcare in medicine* (ed. M. Tunbridge), pp.73–81. London: Royal College of Physicians.

Knapp, M.R.J., Scott, S., and Davies, J. (1999) The cost of antisocial behaviour in younger children: a pilot study of economic and family impact. *Clinical Child Psychology and Psychiatry*, **4**, 457–73.

Kurtz, Z., Thornes, R., and Wolkind, S. (1994) *Services for the mental health of children and young people in England: a national review.* London: Department of Health.

Kurtz, Z., Thornes, R., Wolkind, S. (1995) *Services for the mental health of children and young people in England: assessment of needs and unmet need.* London: Department of Health.

Kurtz, Z. (1996) *Treating children well. A guide to using the evidence base in commissioning and managing services for the mental health of children and young people.* London: The Mental Health Foundation.

Kurtz, Z. and James, C. (2003) *What's new: learning from the CAMHS innovation projects.* London: Department of Health.

Laws, S. (1998) *Hear me! consulting with young people on mental health issues.* London: The Mental Health Foundation.

Maxwell, R.J. (1984) Quality assessment in health. *British Medical Journal*, **288**, 1470–2.

McCann, J.B., James, A., Wilson, S., and Dunn, G. (1996) Prevalence of psychiatric disorders in young people in the care system. *British Medical Journal*, **313**, 1529–30.

Meltzer, H., Gatward, R., Goodman, R., and Ford, T. (2000) *Mental health of children and adolescents in Great Britain. A survey carried out in 1999 by the Social Survey Division of ONS.* London: TSO.

Meltzer, H., Gatward, R., Corbin, T., Goodman, R., and Ford, T. (2003) *The mental health of young people looked after by local authorities in England. The report of a survey carried out in 2002 by Social Survey Division of the Office for National Statistics on behalf of the Department of Health.* London: TSO.

Meslin, E.M., Lemieux-Charles, L., and Wortley, J.Y. (1994) *Teaching clinician-managers how to address ethical issues in resource allocation decisions.* Resource Package. Technical Report No. 16. Toronto: Hospital Management Research Unit, Department of Health Administration, University of Toronto, Canada.

Murray Scott, A. (1999) Experiences with 'rapid appraisal' in primary care; involving the public in assessing health needs, orienting staff and educating medical students. *British Medical Journal*, **318**, 440–4.

NHS Health Advisory Service (1995) *Together we stand. Thematic review on the commissioning, role and and management of child and adolescent mental health services.* London: HMSO.

NHS Management Executive (1991) *Assessing healthcare needs. DHA project discussion paper.* Leeds: NHSME.

NHS (1999) *Modernization Fund and Mental Health Grant for Child and Adolescent Mental Health Services 1999/2002.* Health Service Circular HSC 1999/126, Local Authority Circular LAC(99)22. London: Department of Health.

Rutter, M. and Graham, P. (1968) The reliability and validity of the psychiatric assessment of the child. *British Journal of Psychiatry*, **114**, 563–79.

Sashidharan, S.P. and Commander, M.J. (1998) Mental health. In *Assessing health needs of people from minority ethnic groups* (ed. S. Rawaf and V. Bahl), pp. 281–290. London: Royal College of Physicians and Faculty of Public Health Medicine.

Stephens, A. and Gillam, S. (1998) Needs assessment: from theory to practice. *British Medical Journal*, **316**, 1448–52.

Stronks, K., Strijbis, A-M., Wendte, J.F., and Gunning-Schepers, L.J. (1997) Who should decide? Qualitative analysis of panel data from public, patients, healthcare professionals, and insurers on priorities in healthcare. *British Medical Journal*, **315**, 92–6.

Target, M. and Fonagy, P. (1996) The psychological treatment of child and adolescent psychiatric disorders. In *What works for whom: a review of the effectiveness of the psychotherapies* (ed. A. Roth, and P. Fonagy). pp. 263–300. New York: Guilford Press.

Vanstraelen, M. and Cottrell, D. (1994) Child and adolescent mental health services: purchasers' knowledge and plans. *British Medical Journal*, **309**, 259–61.

Wallace, S.A., Crown, J.M., Berger, M., and Cox, A.D. (1997) Child and Adolescent Mental Health. In *Healthcare needs assessment—the epidemiologically based needs assessment reviews. Second series.* (ed. A. Stevens and J. Raftery), pp. 55–128. Oxford and New York: Radcliffe Medical Press.

Weisz, J.R., Donenberg, G.R., Han, S.S., and Kauneckis, D. (1995) Child and adolescent psychotherapy outcomes in experiments versus clinics: Why the disparity? *Journal of Abnormal Child Psychology*, **23** (1), 83–106.

Williams, R. and Wright, J. (1998) Epidemiological issues in health needs assessment. *British Medical Journal*, **316**, 1379–82.

Chapter 30

Developing Tier 1 services

Peter Bower and Wendy Macdonald

Defining Tier 1

The NHS Health Advisory Service (HAS) proposed a four-tier model of child and adolescent mental health services (CAMHS) (NHS Health Advisory Service 1995). Tier 1 was defined as 'agencies that offer first line services to the public and with whom they make direct contact' (p. 135). Included in this definition are general practitioners (GPs) and health visitors (HVs), teachers, school nurses, and school medical officers, social workers, and other workers from the statutory and voluntary agencies.

Primary healthcare is a key exemplar of Tier 1 services. Primary care services provide first-contact access, but additionally are defined as providing longitudinal care; access to comprehensive health and social care; co-ordination of individual patient care; family-centred provision of care; and a local community orientation (Starfield 1992; Appleton 2000).

As Appleton (2000) has noted, other services such as schools, may meet some aspects of this definition. They also have other advantages over health services, such as the fact that children access school routinely, and teachers have specialized knowledge of childrens' normal development. The voluntary sector also has a role at primary care level, providing access to services such as counselling, as well as facilities for self-referrals (Wallace *et al.* 1997).

The authors of this chapter work at the National Primary Care Research and Development Centre (NPCRDC) at the University of Manchester, a Department of Health funded policy research unit. NPCRDC was funded to conduct a study of current provision of CAMHS in primary care, which was focused on general practice-based services. The study involved surveys of GPs and provider trusts, a systematic review, and detailed case study evaluation of services. This chapter will thus use general practice and primary care to illustrate issues in the development of Tier 1 services.

Strategy in Tier 1 services—the relevance of primary care trusts and local health boards

Williams (2000) defined strategy in terms of two key dimensions:

   agreement on what services are intended to achieve (their intent);

   the way in which they are to develop (their direction).

Harrington *et al.* (1999) lamented the lack of planning associated with CAMHS in specialist settings. However, the emphasis on strategy within primary care has traditionally been even more limited, partly because of the lack of a unified approach to primary care provision. However, the development of primary care groups and trusts (PCTs) may increase the degree to which primary care is engaged in strategic approaches to provision, given their budgetary control, responsibility for commissioning, and the requirement that they develop health improvement programmes (HIMPs) in conjunction with health authorities. 'The central challenges of health improvement facing [PCTs] are to adopt a public health perspective, make strategic needs-led plans to improve population health and devise deliverable action plans involving agencies across and outside the NHS' (Abbott and Gillam 2001, p. 47).

Experience from NPCRDC's longitudinal survey of the development of PCTs (Wilkin *et al.* 1999) indicates that PCTs have a number of features that may encourage a more strategic approach to commissioning and providing services. PCTs provide a unified organization for primary care, and differ from fundholding in that they may encourage greater consideration of issues such as equity of access to services within a PCT (as opposed to the focus on the availability of services within individual practices). In addition, the development of PCTs has advantages for liaison with specialist services, because specialist services will only liase with a few PCTs, which will facilitate setting joint priorities (Kramer and Garralda 2000). Information gathered from our qualitative case study evaluation of CAMHS provision in England suggests that health authorities have had some success in implementing change when they have devolved strategic responsibility for CAMHS to locality managers with representation on PCT boards. These managers have knowledge of local needs and are already working with people who are, and will be, involved in the organization of CAMH services now and in the future.

However, PCTs are new and developing organizations, attempting to undertake an ambitious programme of development in primary care with limited managerial resources (Wilkin *et al.* 1999). Priority may be given to meeting the national targets set by documents such as the National Plan—for example, joint commissioning between health and social services (which is of particular relevance to CAMHS) may prioritize services for older people (although there is evidence that a minority of PCTs are engaged in joint commissioning around children and family services). PCTs are also controlled largely by generalist primary care professionals, and the focus of their work may naturally reflect generalist concerns and aspirations. There is a danger that CAMHS will not receive significant attention in the early years of PCT development without specific guidance from central government (a National Service Framework for CAMHS for example) or may be dependent on the presence of a 'local champion' to facilitate changes in service delivery.

What are Tier 1 services supposed to achieve?

According to the HAS report (1995), the purpose of Tier 1 CAMHS are as follows:

1. Working to prevent more serious mental health problems by early intervention.
2. Enabling families, especially those with young children, to function in a manner that is sensitive and responsive to both positive and negative behavioural cues.
3. Enabling families to address difficulties at as early a stage as possible.
4. Enabling families to resolve parenting difficulties effectively.
5. Enabling children, young people and families to feel that they are effective partners in the intervention process.
6. Providing expertise through staff who have mental health responsibilities legitimately incorporated in their work.

The Audit Commission (1999) provided a more succinct description of the role of non-specialist primary care professionals:

1. Identifying mental health problems early in their development.

2. Offering general advice and treatment for less severe mental health problems.

3. Pursuing opportunities for mental health promotion and problem prevention.

In part these roles reflect the 'gatekeeping' function of primary care, and the influence of the 'filters to care' model (Goldberg and Huxley 1980, 1992), which highlighted the key role of the GP in the identification of problems and thus access to appropriate management within primary and secondary care. The focus on prevention is another key facet of primary care.

However, it is important to keep in mind that intent is bounded to some degree by current evidence of effectiveness—the methods of achieving some goals (e.g. primary prevention of problems) may not currently be available, and those goals may remain aspirational. Harrington *et al.* (1999) point out that previous reviews of CAMHS have tended to underplay the role of the evidence-base in planning, highlighting principles such as easy access and a multidisciplinary approach.

Given this broad understanding of intent, it is necessary to have an understanding of the current starting point i.e. current need and demand, the nature of existing service provision and the key problems facing services. These are the subjects of the following sections.

What is the need and demand for Tier 1 CAMHS?

Generally, the prevalence of child and adolescent mental health problems is thought to be around 20% (Target and Fonagy 1996). Bernard and Garralda (1995) reviewed findings from a number of countries and reported that between 20 and 25% of children and adolescents who attended primary care practitioners have a psychiatric disorder. However, it is the presenting complaint in only a small percentage of cases. Thirty-eight per cent of adolescents presenting in primary care met DSM-IIIR criteria for psychiatric disorder during the preceding year (Kramer and Garralda 1998).

It was reported that only 10% of children with a diagnosis causing impairment were in contact with mental health services (Rutter *et al.* 1970). However, service utilization says little about reasons for poor uptake of services or factors that could improve utilization. For example, parents of children with a diagnosed disorder did not always see their child as in need of treatment (Rutter *et al.* 1970). There is low agreement between need as defined by objective measures of disorder, need as defined by parents, demand and actual supply of services (Evans and Brown 1993).

What is current provision in Tier 1?

There is a real dearth of information available on current CAMHS provision in Tier 1. Although 50% of GPs have an adult psychiatric placement during their vocational training (Gask and Croft 2000), many feel that the training is not highly relevant to general practice and its relevance to child and adolescent disorders must be even more limited.

We recently conducted a postal survey of current provision in general practice, which showed relatively low levels of provision of relevant services, such as GPs with training and interest in the subject, clinics for adolescents or post-natal depression, or paediatricians working on-site within practices (Bower *et al.* 2003). However, a minority of practices did report working more closely with specialist services (e.g. specialists working in primary care, or liasing with GPs and other primary care staff). A small proportion of practices also reported access to primary child and adolescent mental health workers (NHS Health Advisory Service 1995). These developments in interface working will be considered in more detail below.

What are the current problems with management of child and adolescent mental health disorders at Tier 1?

Again, there is a real lack of data on problems faced by GPs and other primary care staff in managing child and adolescent mental health problems. Most surveys of GPs' views of the accessibility and effectiveness of specialist services have demonstrated relatively low levels of satisfaction with services, with waiting times and lack of information on referred patients key perceived problems (Mutale 1995; Weeramanthri and Keaney 2000). Management of patients during the long wait for specialist intervention may also cause difficulty. Weeramanthri and Keaney (2000) found low levels of training in child and adolescent mental health, and that training was also perceived as a low priority by GPs. Rawlinson and Williams (2000) also noted the lack of knowledge among primary care staff about specialist services.

There is little information on perceived problems from the perspective of parents and children. Turner (1998) reported the results of two focus groups that suggested that parents did not consider GPs or HVs to be an obvious source of help for an emotionally disturbed schoolchild, although they appreciated the care received for pre-school children and would appreciate similar, if low key, service for schoolchildren.

Developing CAMHS in primary care—models of working

Based on work in adult psychiatry on the interface between primary care and specialist services (Pincus 1987; Gask et al. 1997), there are three main approaches to CAMHS provision in primary care in the UK. Each has different implications for the two key dimensions of quality of health services: (a) access to care and (b) the effectiveness of care (Campbell et al. 2000).

Management by primary healthcare teams

Although identified as a potentially cost-effective method of treatment and prevention, little is known about the effectiveness of management by GPs and HVs. As generalists, primary care professionals vary widely in their attitudes to mental health work. Even those who are willing to increase their role in this area may not have received adequate training for such work, and thus may lack the necessary skills and confidence (Hewitt et al. 1990).

There are two key types of training for primary care professionals (Appleton 2000). The first is for those who intend to remain generalists, but wish to improve skills in basic detection and management. A relevant example is the study by Bernard et al. (1999) who provided a single structured teaching session (using either vignettes or video) and demonstrated some changes in attitudes and recognition behaviour in volunteer GPs. Because of the first-contact role of the GP, this model should impact most on access to care.

The second type is for those who plan to devote a specific proportion of their time to child and adolescent mental health and thus provide a clinical service under Tier 2 supervision. An example of this is the parent advisor training provided to HVs and CMOs to allow them to develop 'a respectful partnership with parents as a way of supporting them and enhancing their self-esteem' (Davis et al. 1997; Davis and Spurr 1998).

Management by specialist mental health services

Fundholding, and the related changes in the financial arrangements in primary care led to an expansion in the use of specialist out-patient clinics, where psychiatrists work alongside the primary care team, taking responsibility for identified mental health cases (Subotsky and Brown 1997). This may increase patient access to care (reducing travel distances, or reducing the stigma associated with attending specialist units). There is also the potential to increase liaison and communication with primary care staff. Although this model is fairly widespread in adult psychiatry (Strathdee and Williams 1984), there are only a few examples of such use in CAMHS (Senior 1994; Subotsky and Brown 1997; Daws 1999).

Consultation-liaison models

The exact definition of 'consultation-liaison' varies between health settings and countries (Bower and Sibbald 2000). In UK primary care, it refers to arrangements whereby specialists are located in primary care, but act to support and assist management by the primary health-care team rather than take responsibility for individual patients themselves (Gask *et al.* 1997). Patients are only referred to secondary care after discussion with the liaison specialist. The potential benefits of such a model of working are increased appropriateness of referral to specialist clinicians; improved communication between primary care and specialist clinicians; and improvements over time in the ability of primary care clinicians to effectively manage a significant proportion of problems without specialist involvement.

Appleton (2000) describes a number of different types of consultation:

informal *ad hoc* consultation initiated by primary care;

client-centred consultation via regular meetings;

consultee-centred consultation via regular meetings;

consultation about organizational change;

mediation by Tier 2 between primary care professionals regarding co-ordination of care.

Primary mental health workers

The HAS report (1995) supported the proposition that direct provision of services by Specialist CAMHS professionals may be a less efficient use of their skills than consultation-liaison approaches. They proposed the creation of a specific new role, the primary mental health workers (PMHWs), to implement this model. The role of PMHWs is as follows:

consolidating the skills of existing primary care workers;

helping primary care workers to develop new skills and build their confidence through training and education;

aiding recognition of child and adolescent mental health disorders and their referral to more specialist tiers, if appropriate;

assessing and treating some individuals with mental health problems who are considered appropriate for management in Tier 1 services.

Thus PMHWs can work as specialists in primary care providing direct clinical intervention, as well as the preferred consultation-liaison role. The exact mix will depend on the skills of the particular clinicians involved and other local circumstances (Macdonald *et al.* 2004).

Advantages and disadvantages of the different models of working

It has long been suggested in adult psychiatry that training the GP and other primary care staff would be the most cost-effective way of improving mental healthcare for the population, given that almost all patients with mental health problems present to primary care staff. A similar argument could be made in child and adolescent mental health, and such a model could potentially meet the three aims of Tier 1 CAMHS—identification, management, and prevention. However, despite the attractions of such a model, resources are not always available for training, validated training packages have not always been produced, and the motivation of generalist Tier 1 staff for training is not always high (Weeramanthri and Keaney 2000).

Moving specialists into primary care has the advantage that access to specialist care may be increased for patients. Having a specialist on-site as an accessible resource may also raise the profile of child and adolescent mental health and lead to increases in recognition and referrals (Thompson and Place 1995). There is also the possibility of beneficial spin-offs in terms of increased interaction between specialist and generalist. However, there are time costs to the specialist, and research has indicated that locating specialists in primary care does not always lead to significant interaction with primary care staff (Reeves *et al.* 2000).

Consultation–liaison may be the most attractive model, in that it involves aspects of both previous models (i.e. locating specialists in primary care and an explicit focus on improving the skills of the primary care team). However, evidence for the effectiveness of consultation–liaison is limited (see below), and it may be as dependent as the first model (management by primary care staff) on the willingness of Tier 1 professionals to take on additional roles and responsibilities. Experience in adult services suggests that direct provision of services by mental health professionals is the preferred model from the perspective of GPs (Gask and Croft 2000).

Access to child and adolescent mental health interventions in primary care

Some studies have examined the usefulness of screening in primary care for mental health problems. Donovan and McCarthy (1988) invited 16–17-year-olds registered with a practice to attend to discuss 'any medical or general problem'. A single letter achieved 50% response, and depression was a commonly reported problem. Westman and Garralda (1996) attempted to use the context of a health-promotion clinic to explore adolescents' mental and physical health concerns. Attendance was low, but half of those attending did have a probable psychiatric disorder. However, most had already attended the GP that year, so it was unclear whether the use of health-promotion clinics in this way would be cost-effective compared to improving the skills of the GP.

Effectiveness of child and adolescent mental health interventions in primary care

The gold-standard for issues of effectiveness is the randomized controlled trial (RCT). However, there are significant complexities associated with the use of RCTs within the child mental health field (Roth and Fonagy 1996) *and* primary care (Ward *et al.* 1995). Nevertheless, an increasing number of studies and reviews have examined the evidence for the effectiveness of interventions such as CBT in childhood depression (Harrington *et al.* 1998).

However, the populations on which these reviews are based are rarely primary care populations: rather, they represent patients referred to specialist services. If access to care for patients presenting in primary care increases, it is likely that the types of problems receiving care will change significantly, e.g. increased access may lead to a lowering of the severity 'threshold' for referral. Although generalizing results from specialist data is a reasonable option in the absence of primary care data, there is always the possibility that the estimates may not be valid.

A systematic review

We conducted a systematic review to examine the education and training of primary care professionals in child and adolescent mental health, the effectiveness of interventions provided by primary care staff (such as GPs and health visitors), the effectiveness of interventions by specialists working in primary care, and consultation-liaison (Bower *et al.* 2001). Because of the lack of available literature, a range of study designs were included, such as RCTs, non-randomized studies with control groups, and simple before and after studies without controls. Generally, the available literature was very limited in quantity, scope and quality. The broad results of the review are summarised in Table 30.1.

Although policy has highlighted the role of the primary care team in the further development of CAMHS, at present such developments cannot depend on a reliable base of evidence on which to make decisions. This leaves commissioners with two choices. The first is to make decisions based on generalizing research from other contexts. The problems with this approach have been outlined above. Alternatively, decisions may have to be based on criteria other than effectiveness. However, if the promise of evidence-based policy making and service development is to be realized, a significant research effort may have to be initiated soon, given the methodological complexities of work in this area and the need for long term follow-ups of the effects of interventions with children.

Table 30.1 Summary of the results of the systematic review (Bower *et al.* 2001)

Type of intervention	Studies Included	Summary of results
Educational interventions for primary care staff.	Bowler 1984; Appleton *et al.* 1988; Stevenson *et al.* 1988; Weir *et al.* 1988; Hewitt *et al.* 1989; Seeley *et al.* 1996; Davis *et al.* 1997; Bernard *et al.* 1999	Parent advisor training has preliminary support from a controlled study, but studies of the effects of training nurses in behavioural management failed to demonstrate effects on child outcomes. Other evidence restricted to uncontrolled studies and limited outcomes (e.g. self-reported attitudes and knowledge).
Treatment by primary care staff.	Cullen 1976; Crawford *et al.* 1989; Scott and Richards 1990; Hewitt 1991; Galbraith *et al.* 1993; Cullen and Cullen 1996; Oliansky *et al.* 1997	Little evidence that treatment by primary care and community staff is effective, although the number of included studies is small.
Treatment by specialists working in primary care.	Graves and Hastrup 1981; Blakey 1986; Benson and Turk 1988; Martin 1988; Finney *et al.* 1989; Nicol *et al.* 1993; Coverley *et al.* 1995; Cooper and Murray 1997; Davis and Spurr 1998	Studies generally suggest that such approaches are superior to routine primary care, but most were uncontrolled and thus the evidence is only suggestive at best.
Consultation-liaison methods.	Neira-Munoz and Ward 1999	Preliminary evidence from a single study that consultation-liaison approaches may influence the referral behaviour of primary care staff.

New developments in providing CAMHS

Primary mental health workers

As stated above, the HAS proposed the introduction of this new role. A recent study by Lacey (1999) found that 22 of 98 trusts responding to her postal survey employed such a worker. Disciplines involved were a combination of specialist nurses, child psychologists, and social workers sharing the role (50%), specialist nurses working alone (40%), child psychologists alone (5%), and social workers alone (5%). In terms of their work, the median proportion of time spent in primary care was 35%. The median time in consultation was 30%, training 18%, joint assessment 10%, and direct work 20%. Some services were involved in 100% direct work.

Neira-Munoz and Ward (1998) conducted an evaluation of PMHWs (described briefly in Table 30.1). The workers assessed referrals, ran liaison clinics with primary care staff, and acted as solo clinicians. The presence of the worker was associated with a marked reduction in referrals from the intervention practices, as compared to a much more modest reduction in the control practices (although no significance tests were reported). More referrals to specialist services from the intervention practices were rated as 'appropriate', and fewer had to be redirected to other agencies. The new service was rated highly by GPs and HVs, although it is of interest that only one-third of doctors thought that the liaison clinics increased their knowledge and skills in this area, which is supposedly one of the main benefits of consultation-liaison. Lacey (1999) also asked respondents about the effects of PMHWs on referral rates to specialist services. Half the services had not evaluated the effect on referral rates, 22% could demonstrate a reduction, but 18% reported an increase, which is often a by-product of bringing specialist mental health staff into the primary care setting. There were no differences in waiting times for services with and without PMHWs. This issue has also been part of our qualitative case-study evaluation. One site also reported that a PMHW reduced referrals to Tier 3 CAMHS by 75%. However, there are a number of factors that have contributed to this success, such as the skill and experience of the workers, and the existence of a well-developed and clearly defined support structure provided by the Tier 3 team.

The HAS PMHWs are Tier 2 workers who liaise with primary care. In contrast, the NHS Plan (2000) promised the deployment of 1000 additional graduate primary care mental health workers (PMHWs) who were to assist GPs to manage common mental health problems in adults *and* children. Although the exact role of these workers remains to be decided, the new PMHWs also differ from the HAS workers in that they are expected to be Tier 1 based, rather than Tier 2 staff working in Tier 1. Given that these new posts are expected to be filled with graduate psychologists, it is not clear what role they will be able to take up in relation to children, especially given the limited evidence-base uncovered by the systematic review concerning effective interventions that are both brief and simple to use.

Flintshire theory-based model

This comprehensive model (Appleton and Hammond-Rowley 2000) of CAMHS provision is based in a single urban community, and involves engaging with that community through needs assessment and interviews with professionals. The aims of the service were (a) to reduce psychological morbidity in young school-age children and (b) to increase parenting confidence in families with young school-age children.

Interventions were based on universal school-based programmes, parenting skills interventions, consultation–liaison services for primary and community care, and a referral-based family consultation service. Primary child and adolescent mental health specialists are attached to each of the primary schools and general practices. Thus this model involves aspects of two models described above—specialists working in primary care, and consultation–liaison.

This service is being evaluated both for its effects on behaviour problems and parenting confidence, but also for the overall cost-effectiveness of the model.

Community child and family mental health services

Davis *et al.* (1997) describe an alternative Tier 2 service, with significant interface with primary care services. A key aspect of the model is the training of local HVs and paediatric community medical officers in the skills of parent counselling, parenting and child behaviour management. These workers function on a home-visiting basis. Also, a specialist early intervention service is based in GP surgeries. Child mental health specialists spend half a day a week in each of the practices running clinics for parents and children of all ages. These services also provide consultation–liaison and are involved with a number of voluntary organizations. They are also conducting a study looking at HVs working in a promotional model, beginning before birth, with the principles of the parent advisor.

School-based interventions include parent advisor training with school nurses and a clinical psychologist working in a primary school to see if child mental health services can be made as accessible in schools as they are in GP settings. Work involved direct work, groups, health promotion to classes, and regular consultation with teaching staff. This model thus involves the use of primary care staff (in a specialist capacity), specialists working in primary care, and consultation-liaison.

Ways of supporting and developing Tier 1 services

Primary care professionals are faced with multiple demands on their time and an increasingly time-consuming agenda concerned with improving quality of care in several areas, including adult mental health. They require clear advice and assistance on ways of implementing improvements in primary care services so as to meet the aspirations of documents such as the National Service Frameworks (Gask *et al.* 2000).

Key barriers to development include the availability of funding, the low priority afforded to CAMHS in primary care, variability in the attitudes and enthusiasm of GPs and other primary care staff, and the rapid pace of change in primary care associated with the development of PCTs and the new clinical governance agenda.

Gask and Croft (2000) describe some of the key barriers associated with setting up a consultation–liaison service, which may have more general relevance for facilitating change in primary care. Important issues include:

What are the agendas and expectations of the key players? Is the change driven by GPs, dissatisfied by specialist services, or are the concerns of specialist services (e.g. concerning workload) driving the agenda? Differing agendas were noted as a key problem in NPCRDC's evaluation of total purchasing pilots and their attempts to deliver change in adult mental health services (Lee *et al.* 1999).

What is the history of co-operation? The development of relationships takes time without a significant history of co-operation over previous projects.

What resources and expertise are available now?

What is the level of motivation for change? Again, the total purchasing evaluation noted the importance of key individuals leading change (Lee *et al.* 1999).

Gask and Croft (2000) also described the key steps in achieving change in primary care.

1. Identification of the evidence base. As noted above, the research literature in child and adolescent mental health in primary care is very limited. However, this can be augmented by local needs assessments, experience from other successful projects, and national guidelines.

2. Bringing together the key players at a local level. This was one of the forms of consultation identified by Appleton (2000). Mildred *et al.* (1999) demonstrated how both sides at the interface could benefit from greater understanding of the context of their work and the problems that they face.

3. Local needs assessment. Experience in total purchasing projects in adult mental health indicated that needs assessments are sometimes based on professionals' conceptions of need, which may not always provide a full or accurate picture (Lee *et al.* 1999).

4. Involvement of service users. This is a significant challenge in relation to CAMHS. Although local involvement is to be preferred, some national publications have examined this issue and may be of use (Laws *et al.* 1999; Armstrong *et al.* 2001).

These authors caution that change may well be slow and should proceed in a stepwise fashion, sensitive to the barriers identified and available resources.

Conclusions

It has been noted that many health experts begin their description of how best to improve services in their particular discipline with the statement that 'the GP is ideally placed...' (Balint 1993). There is a significant gap between the potential of primary care services in child and adolescent mental health and the current ability of those services to improve access and effectiveness in this area, when there are so many competing priorities. Significant advances have been made, and the results of ongoing research studies should further highlight effective methods of organising services in the future. However, the task for clinicians, managers and researchers remains significant.

References

Abbott, S. and Gillam, S. (2001) Health Improvement. In *The national tracker survey of primary care groups and trusts* (ed. D. Wilkin, S. Gillam, B. Leese), pp. 47–50. Manchester: NPCRDC.

Appleton, P. (2000) Tier 2 CAMHS and its interface with primary care. *Advances in Psychiatric Treatment*, **6**, 388–96.

Appleton, P. and Hammond-Rowley, S. (2000) Addressing the population burden of child and adolescent mental health problems: a primary care model. *Child Psychology and Psychiatry Review*, **5**, 9–16.

Appleton, P., Pritchard, P., and Pritchard, A. (1988) *Evaluation of a 12 month in-service course for health visitors in behavioural intervention methods with infants and pre-school children.* Unpublished manuscript.

Armstrong, C., Hill, M., and Secker, J. (2001) *Listening to children.* London: Mental Health Foundation.

Audit Commission (1999) *Children in mind: child and adolescent mental health services.* Portsmouth: Audit Commission.

Balint, E., Courtenay, M., Elder, A., Hull, S., and Julian, P. (1993) *The Doctor, the Patient and the Group: Balint revisited.* London: Routledge.

Benson, P. and Turk, T. (1988) Group therapy in a general practice setting for frequent attenders: a controlled study of mothers with pre-school children. *Journal of the Royal College of General Practitioners*, **38**, 539–41.

Bernard, P. and Garralda, E. (1995) Child and adolescent mental health practice in primary care. *Current Opinion in Psychiatry*, **8**, 206–9.

Bernard, P., Garralda, E., Hughes, T., and Tylee, A. (1999) Evaluation of a teaching package in adolescent psychiatry for general practitioner registrars. *Education for General Practice*, **10**, 21–8.

Blakey, R. (1986) Psychological treatment in general practice: its effect on patients and their families. *Journal of the Royal College of General Practitioners*, **36**, 209–11.

Bower, P. and Sibbald, B. (2000) Do consultation-liaison services change the behaviour of primary care providers? A review. *General Hospital Psychiatry*, **22**, 84–96.

Bower, P., Garralda, E., Kramer, T., Harrington, R., and Sibbald, B. (2001) The treatment of child and adolescent mental health problems in primary care: a systematic review. *Family Practice*, **18**, 373–82.

Bower, P., Macdonald, W., Sibbald, B., Garralda, E., Kramer, T., Bradley, S., *et al.* (2003) Postal survey of services for child and adolescent mental health problems in general practice in England. *Primary Care Mental Health*, **1**, 17–26.

Bowler, J. and Watson, P. (1984) A child behaviour workshop. *Health Visitor*, **57**, 302–3.

Campbell, S., Roland, M., and Buetow, S. (2000) Defining quality of care. *Social Science and Medicine*, **51**, 1611–25.

Cooper, P. and Murray, L. (1997) The impact of psychological treatments of postpartum depression on maternal mood and infant development. In *Postpartum depression and child development* (ed. L. Murray, P. Cooper), pp. 201–20. New York: The Guilford Press.

Coverley, C., Garralda, M., and Bowman, F. (1995) Psychiatric intervention in primary care for mothers whose schoolchildren have psychiatric disorder. *British Journal of General Practice*, **45**, 235–7.

Crawford, W., Bennet, R., and Hewitt, K. (1989) Sleep problems in pre-school children. *Health Visitor*, **62**, 79–81.

Cullen, K. (1976) A six year controlled trial of prevention of children's behaviour disorders. *Journal of Pediatrics*, **88**, 662–6.

Cullen, K. and Cullen, A. (1996) Long-term follow up of the Busselton six year controlled trial of prevention of children's behaviour disorders. *Journal of Pediatrics*, **129**, 136–9.

Davis, H. and Spurr, P. (1998) Parent counselling: an evaluation of a community child mental health service. *Journal of Child Psychology and Psychiatry*, **39**, 365–76.

Davis, H., Spurr, P., Cox, A., Lynch, M., Von Roenne, A., and Hahn, K. (1997) A description and evaluation of a community child mental health service. *Clinical Child Psychology and Psychiatry*, **2**, 221–38.

Daws, D. (1999) Child psychotherapy in the baby clinic of a general practice. *Clinical Child Psychology and Psychiatry*, **4**, 9–22.

Donovan, C. and McCarthy, S. (1988) Is there a place for adolescent screening in general practice? *Health Trends*, **20**, 64–6.

Evans, S. and Brown, R. (1993) Perception of need for child psychiatry services among parents and general practitioners. *Health Trends*, **25**, 53–6.

Finney, J., Lemanek, K., Cataldo, M., Katz, H., and Fuqua, R. (1989) Pediatric psychology in primary healthcare: brief targeted therapy for recurrent abdominal pain. *Behaviour Therapy*, **20**, 283–91.

Finney, J., Riley, A., and Cataldo, M. (1991) Psychology in primary healthcare: effects of brief targeted therapy on children's medical care utilisation. *Journal of Pediatric Psychology*, **16**, 447–61.

Galbraith, L., Hewitt, K., and Pritchard, L., (1993) Behavioural treatment for sleep disturbance. *Health Visitor*, **66**, 169–71.

Gask, L. and Croft, J. (2000) Methods of working with primary care. *Advances in Psychiatric Treatment*, **6**, 442–9.

Gask, L., Sibbald, B., and Creed, F. (1997) Evaluating models of working at the interface between mental health services and primary care. *British Journal of Psychiatry*, **170**, 6–11.

Gask, L., Rogers, A., Roland, M., Morris, D. (2000) *Improving quality in primary care: a practical guide to the National Service Framework for Mental Health*. Manchester: University of Manchester, NPCRDC.

Goldberg, D. and Huxley, P. (1980). *Mental illness in the community: the pathway to psychiatric care*. London: Tavistock.

Goldberg, D. and Huxley, P. (1992) *Common mental disorders: a biosocial model*. London: Routledge.

Graves, R. and Hastrup, J. (1981) Psychological intervention and medical utilisation in children and adolescents of low-income families. *Professional Psychology*, **12**, 426–33.

Harrington, R., Whittaker, J., Shoebridge, P., and Campbell, F. (1998) Systematic review of efficacy of cognitive-behaviour therapies in childhood and adolescent depressive disorder. *British Medical Journal*, **316**, 1559–63.

Harrington, R., Kerfoot, M., and Verduyn, C. (1999) Developing needs led child and adolescent mental health services: issues and prospects. *European Child and Adolescent Psychiatry*, **8**, 1–10.

Hewitt, K. (1991) Parent education in preventing behaviour problems. *Health Visitor*, **64**, 415.

Hewitt, K., Hobday, A., and Crawford, A. (1989) What do health visitors gain from behavioural workshops? *Child: Care, Health and Development*, **15**, 265–75.

Hewitt, K., Appleton, P., Douglas, J., Fundudis, T., and Stevenson, J. (1990) Health visitor based services for pre-school children with behaviour problems. *Health Visitor*, **63**, 160–2.

Kramer, T. and Garralda, E. (1998) Psychiatric disorders in adolescents in primary care. *British Journal of Psychiatry*, **173**, 508–13.

Kramer, T. and Garralda, E. (2000) Child and adolescent mental health problems in primary care. *Advances in Psychiatric Treatment*, **6**, 287–94.

Lacey, I. (1999) The role of the child primary mental health worker. *Journal of Advanced Nursing*, **30**, 220–8.

Laws, S., Armitt, D., Metzendorf, W., Percival, P., and Reisel, J. *Time to listen: young peoples' experiences of mental health services*. London: Save the Children, 1999.

Lee, J., Gask, L., Roland, M., and Donnan, S. (1999) *National evaluation of total purchasing pilots: total purchasing and extended fundholding of mental health services*. London: King's Fund.

Macdonald, W., Bradley, S., Bower, P., Kramer, T., Sibbald, B., Garralda, E., *et al.* (2004) Primary mental health workers in child and adolescent mental health. *Journal of Advanced Nursing*, **46**, 78–87.

Martin, S.L. (1988) *The effectiveness of a multidisciplinary primary healthcare model in the prevention of children's mental health problems*. Unpublished PhD thesis. University of North Carolina at Chapel Hill.

Mildred, H., Brann, P., Luk, E., and Fisher, S. (1999) Collaboration between general practitioners and a child and adolescent mental health service. *Australian Family Physician*, **29**, 177–81.

Mutale, T. (1995) Fundholders and child mental health services. *Psychiatric Bulletin*, **19**, 417–20.

Neira-Munoz, E. and Ward, D. (1998) Side by side. *Health Service Journal*, **108**, 26–7.

NHS Health Advisory Service (1995) *Child and adolescent mental health services: together we stand*. London: HMSO.

Nicol, R., Stretch, D., and Fundudis, T. (1993) *Preschool children in troubled families*. Chichester: John Wiley and Sons.

Oliansky, D., Wildenhaus, K., Manlove, K., Arnold, T., and Schoener, E. (1997) Effectiveness of brief interventions in reducing substance use among at-risk primary care patients in three community-based clinics. *Substance Abuse*, **18**, 95–103.

Pincus, H. (1987) Patient-oriented models for linking primary care and mental healthcare. *General Hospital Psychiatry*, **9**, 95–101.

Rawlinson, S. and Williams, R. (2000) The primary-secondary care interface in child and adolescent mental health services, the relevance of burden. *Current Opinion in Psychiatry*, **13**, 389–95.

Reeves, D., Alborz, A., Hickson, F., Bamford, J., and Gosden, T. (2000) Community provision of hearing aids and related audiology services. *Health Technology Assessment*, **4** (4).

Roth, A. and Fonagy, P. (1996) *What works for whom? A critical review of psychotherapy research*. London: Guilford Press.

Rutter, M., Tizard, J., and Whitmore, K. (1970) *Education, health and behaviour*. London: Longmans.

Scott, G. and Richards, P. (1990) Night waking in infants: effects of providing advice and support for parents. *Journal of Child Psychology and Psychiatry*, **31**, 551–67.

Secretary of State for Health (2000) *The NHS Plan*. London: HMSO.

Seeley, S., Murray, L., and Cooper, P. (1996) The outcomes for mothers and babies of health visitor intervention. *Health Visitor*, **69**, 135–8.

Senior, R. (1994) Family therapy in general practice: 'we have a clinic here on Friday afternoon…'. *Journal of Family Therapy*, **16**, 313–27.

Starfield, B. (1992) *Primary care: concept, evaluation and policy*. New York: Oxford University Press.

Stevenson, J., Bailey, V., and Simpson, J. (1988) Feasible intervention in families with parenting difficulties: a primary preventive perspective on child abuse. In *Early prediction and prevention of child abuse* (ed. K. Browne, C. Davies, and P. Stratton), pp. 121–38. Chichester: John Wiley and Sons.

Strathdee, G. and Williams, P. (1984) A survey of psychiatrists in primary care: the silent growth of a new service. *Journal of the Royal College of General Practitioners*, **34**, 615–8.

Subotsky, F. and Brown, R. (1997) Working alongside the general practitioner: a child psychiatric clinic in the general practice setting. *Child: Care, Health and Development*, **16**, 189–96.

Target, M. and Fonagy, P. (1996) The psychological treatment of child and adolescent psychiatric disorders. In *What works for whom? A critical review of psychotherapy research* (ed. A. Roth and P. Fonagy), pp. 263–320. New York: Guilford Press.

Thompson, A. and Place, M. (1995) What influences general practitioners' use of child psychiatry services? *Psychiatric Bulletin*, **19**, 10–12.

Turner, S. (1998) Parents do not see GPs as source of help for emotionally disturbed schoolchildren [letter]. *British Medical Journal*, **317**, 212.

Wallace, S., Crown, J., Berger, M., and Cox, A. (1997) Child and Adolescent Mental Health. In *Healthcare needs assessment: the epidemiologically based needs assessment reviews* (ed. A. Stevens and J. Raftery), pp. 55–128. Oxford: Radcliffe Medical Press.

Ward, E., King, M., Lloyd, M., Bower, P., and Friedli, K. (1999) Conducting randomized trials in general practice: methodological and practical issues. *British Journal of General Practice*, **49**, 919–22.

Weeramanthri, T. and Keaney, F. (2000) What do inner city general practitioners want from a child and adolescent mental health service? *Psychiatric Bulletin*, **24**, 258–60.

Westman, A. and Garralda, E. (1996) Mental health promotion for young adolescents in primary care: a feasibility study [letter]. *British Journal of General Practice*, **46**, 317.

Weir, I. and Dinnick, S. (1988) Behaviour modification in the treatment of sleep problems occurring in young children: a controlled trial using health visitors as therapists. *Child: Care, Health and Development*, **14**, 355–67.

Wilkin, D., Gillam, S., and Leese, B. (1999) *The national tracker survey of primary care groups and trusts: progress and challenges 1999/2000*. Manchester: University of Manchester, NPCRDC.

Williams, R. (2000) A cunning plan, the role of research evidence in translating policy into effective child and adolescent mental health services. *Current Opinion in Psychiatry*, **13**, 361–8.

Chapter 31

Case study: the primary mental health team—Leicester, Leicestershire, and Rutland CAMHS

Fiona Gale and Panos Vostanis

Background

The HAS four-tier model of service provision suggested the development of the primary mental health worker (PMHW) role at the interface between Tier 1 (primary care professionals) and Tiers 2/3 (Specialist CAMHS). These recommendations were also affirmed by reports from the House of Commons Health Committee (DoH 1997), The Mental Health Foundation (1999), and the Audit Commission (2000), which emphasized the need to develop more effective inter-agency collaboration in the provision of CAMHS, through the development of appropriate liaison between primary care and Specialist CAMHS. These policies have led to the development and expansion of PMHW post in CAMHS on a national basis.

In the mid-1990s, Leicestershire CAMHS were faced with an increasing number of referrals, lengthy waiting-lists, and limited ability to liaise with, or support, potential referrers in primary care. In response, a joint strategy for child and adolescent mental health services was developed between the health authority, three local authorities, and the voluntary sector. Within this strategy, the need for development of the PMHW role was identified and after successful bids, funding has been awarded for 13 PMHW posts.

The team: philosophy and objectives

The philosophy of the team is to strengthen and support the provision of CAMHS at Tier 1. The active promotion of mental health in children and their families is achieved by offering a needs-led service, through work with the professionals who are more likely to see children on a day-to-day basis. The objective is to increase knowledge of, and accessibility to, services appropriate to meet the mental health needs of children, thus reducing stigma. Through the promotion of the principle of joint working and planning with other agencies and services, primary care professionals can be empowered to develop their existing skills in recognizing and managing child mental health. This consequently enables different CAMHS components to maximize their efficiency by targeting clients and problems appropriate to their skills and expertise.

The team thus advocates the concept of 'universal CAMHS', in which the responsibility for children's mental health is integral to all professionals who work with them.

Team description

Located within Tier 2/3 CAMHS, the primary mental health team currently consists of 13 PMHWs, seven of whom work to specific target areas in the community, three with the youth offending teams (YOTs) and two for looked-after children (LACs). Leadership, development, and co-ordination of the team are provided by the senior PMHW. The team works closely with a CAMHS multi-agency training co-ordinator, a training post for primary care staff (Sebuliba and Vostanis 2001) and multi-agency child behaviour intervention initiatives (CBIIs) based in the community.

Background and experience

The PMHWs are employed on a specifically designed PMHW pay scale, which is aligned to nursing and midwives grade 'H' salary. The professionals undertaking the PMHW roles are from a variety of professional backgrounds and experience, namely mental health nursing and social work. Their experience includes, recent work in child and adolescent mental health, health visiting, adolescent forensic psychiatry, social services teams, and the voluntary sector. This range of skills and experience has proved invaluable in establishing a rich resource and team are able to consult and advise on a wide range of issues that may influence children's mental health.

Clinical supervision

The senior PMHW provides supervision relating to the components of the role; supervision of direct intervention is provided by the multidisciplinary CAMH team and the PMHWs also have regular peer supervision, which is significant in utilising experience and knowledge from the different disciplines within the team.

Target populations

The Leicestershire cover inner-city, semi-urban, and rural areas of a general population of approximately 900 000 across three local authorities (Leicester, Leicestershire, and Rutland). There are approximately 200 000 young people under the age of 17 years. According to epidemiological research (Mental Health Foundation 1999), more than 15% (around 30 000) will be experiencing significant mental health problems at any one time. The community PMHWs operate within identified target localities of approximately 50 000–60 000 population (or 11 000 children).

Being allocated to a locality enables the PMHW to become involved in detailed negotiation with professionals in that community, developing a needs-led service (Gale and Vostanis, in press). As funding was gradually obtained, target areas were prioritized through local data of rates of child mental health need, referrals to Specialist CAMHS, child protection registrations, and use of educational resources for behavioural, emotional, and learning difficulties. It is envisaged, however, that all areas of the target population will eventually be covered by PMHWs. The PMHWs for young offenders and children looked-after work across the whole CAMHS population, in relation to these vulnerable groups (Callaghan et al. 2002).

The Leicester model of primary mental health work

The model has been developed from previous research regarding the PMHW role (Gale 1999), from mental health consultation and liaison models in adult psychiatry and mental health nursing (Caplan 1970; Roberts 1997; Tunmore 1997). An integrative approach proposed by Regel and Davies (1995) has been applied in liaison mental health nursing. This is based on biological, psychological, and sociological theories, which complement the range of backgrounds from which PMHWs are drawn.

The PMHW model is viewed as a process, with three levels of intervention. Each level can precipitate a move to the next level, and there can be an interface with other agencies or Specialist CAMHS at any stage, dependant on the determined level of need. The process starts in all instances with consultation and may progress to joint working with the referring professional or an identified professional deemed more appropriate to meet the child's needs, liaison with other agencies or, in some instances, direct intervention with children and families.

First, the PMHW actively filters referrals to the CAMHS community teams, through their referral meeting and, second, work is determined through direct requests for consultation by primary care professionals. Using this model helps both the PMHW and primary care professionals to define the level of support and intervention. This approach is necessary to achieve the common goals; i.e. managing the child's mental health needs successfully in primary care or ensuring access to the service appropriate to the determined level of need. This includes identifying those children presenting with more severe mental health difficulties or disorders requiring Specialist CAMHS intervention (Arcelus *et al.* 2001).

Components of the primary mental health worker role

First-level intervention: consultation, supervision, and training

Consultation

Within the Leicester model, the consultant (PMHW) works indirectly on a problem with the consultee (primary care professional), where the consultee is defined as a competent autonomous practitioner who may accept or reject advice (Caplan 1970; Tunmore 1997). The aim is to define the child's mental health needs and to consider the most appropriate ways of meeting them. Consultation within the PMHW role is viewed as being on a continuum ranging from telephone advice and support to advanced face-to-face consultation, where the PMHW and the primary care professional meet regularly to agree goals and review work.

Supervision

Within the role, supervision is defined as the development of skills and knowledge regarding the assessment and management of children's mental health problems, enabling the primary care professional to learn and practice new management techniques (Regel and Davies 1995). It differs from previous levels of consultation described, as it is primarily educative. The aim is to improve the ability of the professional to manage a problem more effectively by increasing their skill-base and enabling practice. Other than taking place on a case-by-case basis, supervision can also be used with groups of professionals. For example, in Leicester, PMHWs have been involved in a project to train health visitors in solution focused brief therapy (Evan *et al.* 1999) and to provide them with specific supervision to enable them to use it in their practice.

Training

Training offered to primary care professionals should enable them to develop an understanding of children's mental health issues and should consolidate their existing knowledge through experiential learning (Sebuliba and Vostanis 2001). It should not seek to turn front-line staff into specialists in children's mental health, but rather enable them to recognize and manage child mental health problems at an early stage. This can be achieved by providing them with a broad knowledge-base and a theoretical framework to make informed choices on the best care approach for each child (Dogra *et al.* 2001).

The PMHWs are involved in designing and delivering a 2-day introduction to children's mental health in their areas, which feeds into a phased multi-agency training programme in child mental health. They also co-ordinate regular multi-agency training and case discussion mental health forums in their localities.

Second-level intervention: liaison and joint working

Liaison

The liaison component of the role is defined as 'collaboration between agencies to work towards defining the best approach to meet the child's needs'. This is based on work by Lipowski (1968) who advocated a 'team approach', in which psychiatrists were complemented by colleagues from other agencies to create a core team to meet the needs of the individual. The model includes notions of networking and collaboration between agencies and professionals (Baird and Praty 1989; Roberts 1997).

Liaison with primary care professionals at an early stage following referral to CAMHS, can also take place using various approaches. These include direct liaison from PMHW to the referrer to discuss which services may be more appropriate to meet a child's needs, liaison with potential services, or organization of multi-agency meetings to agree plan of care.

Joint work with primary care professionals

Joint work between primary care professionals and PMHWs is agreed and negotiated through the process of consultation. Examples of this include:

joint assessment with a practitioner already involved in a case, for the purpose of understanding the child's or the family's needs in relation to mental health;

support for the practitioner in the work they are already undertaking, assisting them in developing choices for intervention;

education and support about the assessment process or a specific management technique; and

development of jointly facilitated groups in the community for young people and parents.

The joint-working process should be a two-way learning activity, in that both professionals set agreed aims and objectives for a piece of work. Once the joint-working process has ended, it is important that supportive, consultative, or supervisory plans are put into place for the Tier 1 professional who continues the work with the case, thus enabling ongoing communication and management.

Third-level intervention: direct intervention with children and families

At any stage of the model it may be necessary for the PMHW to undertake a mental health assessment and/or direct intervention with the child and their family. This approach would be implemented when it is apparent that the child's difficulties are not responding to methods and interventions tried by the primary care professional, or when it is established that the primary care professional has concerns regarding the child's mental health needs, which cannot be supported through the consultation/joint-working process. Cases selected for this approach are usually not considered appropriate for a more specialist intervention from CAMHS or another agency. The child must also be suitable for management by primary care professionals, once the intervention is complete (Davis *et al.* 1997). In such cases, the PMHW will offer a brief focused intervention, followed by a formal review with the child, the family and, where possible, primary care professionals involved. The intervention is tailored to meet the needs of the child and family, i.e. parenting training, cognitive-behavioural therapy, solution-focused brief therapy, and anger management. Each child and family should be seen for an assessment session, to ensure detection of mental health problems, which may require intervention form Specialist CAMHS.

Lessons so far: the challenges in implementing the PMHW role

There are many challenges in the successful implementation of their role including:

A new way of working. As a new role for most professionals, there may be have some resultant training and supervision implications.

Clinical supervision. With professionals from different backgrounds it is difficult to find a Supervisor with all necessary skills. Supervision protocols need to reflect the needs of the team and the service.

Interface/proximity to CAMHS. This varies around the country. In Leicester it was felt necessary to have the PMHW based within Specialist CAMHS, to enable children presenting with more severe mental health needs to gain a timely response.

Primary care perceptions: consultation vs. direct work. This can be viewed as a controversial approach in meeting the mental health needs of children, and can challenge professionals' preconceptions on who should provide for children's mental health needs. There is sometimes pressure to see cases directly rather than work through consultation. One solution was the development of the PMHW model and philosophy, which is explained to professionals to help them understand the role. The challenge of engaging professionals in collaborative working still stands as they continue to make often unnecessary referrals to CAMHS, and thus perceive the PMHW role as 'gate keeping'.

Training for PMHWs. The PMHW role calls for senior, experienced CAMHS professionals. As more posts are developed, the range of professionals able to undertake the role is becoming depleted. It is therefore necessary to develop training and development programmes for PMHWs, so CAMHS can start to 'grow their own' workforce.

Fluidity between the tiers. It has become apparent that there is the increasing need for fluidity between CAMHS tiers. The PMHW is in a prime position to manage the interface between Tier 1 and Specialist CAMHS in both directions, i.e. referrals to Specialist CAMHS, as well as children who have received a specialist intervention being managed at Tier 1.

Access to CAMHS for minority ethnic groups/vulnerable groups. The PMHW needs to be proactive in working with professionals and community leaders representing these groups to establish the most appropriate ways of providing a service. Just because PMHWs are more available does not always mean these groups will have more access by default.

References

Arcelus, J., Gale, F., and Vostanis, P. (2001) Characteristics of children and parents attending a primary mental health service. *European Child and Adolescent Psychiatry Newsletter*, Mar; **10** (1), 91–5.

Audit Commission (2000) *With children in mind: child and adolescent mental health services.* Oxford: Audit Commission Publications.

Baird, S.B. and Praty, M.P. (1989) Administratively enhancing CNS contributions. In *The clinical nurse specialist in theory and practice* (2nd edn) (ed. A.B. Hamric and J.A. Spross). Philadelphia: W.B. Saunders.

Callaghan, J., Young, B., and Vostanis, P. (2002) *Primary mental health workers within youth offending teams: evaluation of a new service model.* Leicester: University of Leicester.

Caplan, G. (1970) *The theory and practice of mental health consultation.* London: Tavistock.

Davis, H., Spurr, P., Cox, A., Lynchm M., Von Roenne, A., and Hahn, K. (1997) A description and evaluation of a community child mental health service. *Clinical Child Psychology and Psychiatry,* **2**, 221–38.

Department of Health (1997) *Developing partnerships in mental health.* London: HMSO.

Dogra, N., Parkin, A., Gale, F., and Frake, C. (2001) *A multi-disciplinary handbook of child and adolescent mental health for front-line professionals.* London: Jessica Kingsley Publishers.

Evan, G., Iverson, C., and Ratner, H. (1999) *Problem to solution: brief therapy with individuals and families* (revised and expanded edition). London: Brief Therapy Practice.

Gale, F.J. (1999) *When tiers are not enough: an evaluation of the perceptions and experiences amongst primary care professionals of the primary mental health worker role within CAMHS.* Birmingham, University of Central England: Unpublished MA Thesis in Research Methodology.

Gale, F. and Vostanis, P. (2003) Developing the primary mental health worker role within child and adolescent mental health services. *Clinical Child Psychology and Psychiatry,* **8**, 227–40.

Lipowski, Z.J. (1968) Review of consultation psychiatry and psychosomatic medicine III: thematic issues. *Psychosomatic medicine,* **33**, 395–422.

Mental Health Foundation (1999) *Bright futures; promoting children and young people's mental health.* London: Mental Health Foundation.

Regel, S. and Davies, J. (1995) The future of mental health nurses in liaison psychiatry. *British Journal of Nursing,* **4** (18), 1052–6.

Roberts, D. (1997) Liaison mental health nursing: origins, definition and prospects. *Journal of Advanced Nursing,* **25**, 101–8.

Sebuliba, D. and Vostanis, P. (2001) Child and adolescent mental health training from primary care staff. *Clinical Child Psychology and Psychiatry,* **6**, 191–204.

Tunmore, R. (1997) Mental Health Liaison and Consultation. *Nursing Standard,* **11**, 46–51.

Chapter 32

Demand for and use of public sector child and adolescent mental health services

Richard Williams, Sarah Rawlinson, Owen Davies, and Wendy Barber

Introduction

This chapter explores the rising demand on specialist child and adolescent mental health services (CAMHS) that has been reported recurrently over the last two decades in the UK and elsewhere.

Many agencies have endeavoured to cope with the imbalance between supply and demand by directing variable amounts of additional resource to them or by altering how services respond within the same resource envelope. Inevitably, policymakers, strategic and operational managers, and practitioners discover that there is a substantial time-lag built into resolving many workforce challenges as an answer to increasing demand. In particular, there are recruitment and retention challenges, and the shortage of professionals in the UK and many parts of the world is all too apparent. There are also challenges arising from the increasing expectations that parallel increased abilities to deliver modern and effective services. Consequently, most specialist services are developing policies and practices to better manage the demands on them and all of these matters have considerable implications for training.

In this chapter, we examine the reasons for the expanding demand, the processes of referral that are common in public sector Specialist CAMHS, the impact of waiting on the efficacy and effectiveness of existing services, and we survey the responses that have been put in place and researched in a number of countries. Interestingly, although we quote many UK sources, the research we summarize provides evidence of similar imbalances between demand and supply impacting on delivery of CAMHS across the world.

At the end, we commend a more fundamental approach that requires examination of the functions required of Specialist CAMHS and re-design of services, alongside allocation of more staff and other resources. The challenges include those of: defining the client group; more effective determination of the functions desired of each tier of service; judicious application of the evidence about effective service interventions; and balancing stakeholder opinions on the services they require with innovative ways of using the professional workforce in the context of the clinical realities.

The context—rising demand and increasing recognition of complexity

Barton *et al.* (2002) provide a background summary of the epidemiology of mental health problems and disorders and some service delivery research that focuses, mainly, on the UK.

In 1999, Knapp and Henderson provided an overview from a health economic perspective. In this context there are widely held beliefs in the UK and elsewhere in the world that Specialist CAMHS have come under increasing pressure from rising demand and that this has been particularly the case in the last two decades. In the UK, there was little effective action taken to adjust resources to adequately meet this demand, until the last decade of the 20th century. As we write, most of the new revenue recently announced in England has yet to reach the frontline of service delivery. There also appears to be a general consensus that the pressure on services is not related solely to problems in recruiting and retaining professional staff.

Now that there is an evident imbalance between the volume of services that can be delivered, and the volume and changing nature of the demand on them, there is considerable pressure to examine ways in which to better manage the interfaces between specialist services and those who would use them or refer others to them. The implication of failing to take a strategic approach to the problem is that of perpetuating ineffective and/or sub-optimal service delivery and of not tackling one of the most potent factors that have stood in the way of better inter-disciplinary and cross-agency collaboration.

Rising volume of demand

There is evidence of a true increase in the prevalence of disorders (Rutter *et al.* 1970; Rutter and Smith 1995). Nonetheless, at first glance, the Audit Commission report of 1999 appears to throw doubt on the reality of a widely held belief that the volume of referrals to Specialist CAMHS across England and Wales has risen partially as a consequence of the increased incidence and prevalence of diagnosable disorder. It said:

> Many Trusts told Auditors of pressure from rising numbers of referrals with no adjustment in resources to meet this demand. However, one-third of the Trust Auditors could not produce figures to back this claim.

Examination of the summary data that 85 Trusts could provide, revealed that increases in workload in some counter-balanced decreases in referrals received by others.

What was not in doubt, endorsed by the Audit Commission report, was a common perception held by the staff of the Specialist CAMHS of them being under increasing pressure of demand. The Audit Commission offered three explanations:

> trusts with good data systems were also the ones that have developed links with referrers to relieve demand;

> complexity of referred cases was rising causing a perception of increased demand on services though not necessarily, as a consequence of an increasing number of cases; and

> high staff vacancy rates were placing greater strain on the fewer remaining staff.

Several years later, the National CAMHS Mapping Exercise in England provides support for several of these views (Glover *et al.* 2003 and Chapter 28). It showed that an average of 10% of some 6000 professional posts in Specialist CAMHS were vacant in 2002 (medical posts: 15%; psychology posts: 13%; nursing posts: 9%). Also, although 67% of 123 NHS Trusts reported that they were able to rely on IT systems to make some contribution to responding to the survey, only 2 (1.6%) could draw all the data required from IT and 31% said that IT systems did not help them at all to respond to the survey. Furthermore, our experience suggests that, in many places, it is likely that extended waiting times lead to reduced referrals through frustration experienced by referrers. If so, then a crude form of homeostatic device is a feature of current referral systems, even where there is no demand management *per se* in operation.

Our review of the wider literature suggests that the reason why demand has increased in many services is complex. By way of illustration, we have grouped examples of the contributory factors.

Prevalence and recognition factors:

increasing prevalence of child and adolescent mental disorder (Rutter *et al.* 1970; Rutter and Smith 1995);

increased and better recognition of disorder (Bowman and Garralda 1993);

reduction of the stigma attached to psychiatric referral.

Service effectiveness factors:

the capability of professionals in Specialist CAMHS has increased rapidly in the last 20 years;

there is growing evidence to support the effectiveness of a number of interventions and continuing research in the field showing the long-term health economic advantages of intervening with problems in childhood (see Chapter 8).

Service change factors:

the demise of child guidance clinics with restriction or the loss of the previous roles and/or numbers of certain professions from Specialist CAMHS;

narrowing of the focus of agencies that had previously invested more in CAMHS arising from pressure from other work (e.g. pressures on social services arising from child protection and other statutory duties and restriction of the role of education psychologists through their greater commitment to statutory (e.g. 'Statementing') procedures.

Client group definition factors:

there has been a noticeable tendency for all sectors see diagnosis as casting the lead role to the health sector for increasing numbers of children and adolescents with problems with their mental health;

paradoxically, we have received much anecdotal evidence that education authorities, for example, in the UK are increasingly requiring medical diagnoses to establish eligibility for special education and education support services and the finance for them—this leads to pressure being put on Specialist CAMHS from families for doctors to see patients to make diagnoses and reduced satisfaction when none are offered or are inappropriate.

Service planning and resource factors:

impediments to timely and effective service delivery arising from increasing numbers of referrals and slowing response times (a circular process, as we shall see);

difficulties in recruiting and retaining specialist professionals;

increasing demands on pressured professionals to spend a greater proportion of their time away from direct and indirect client-related activities.

One opinion that is frequently expressed in conversation with professionals is that unplanned re-distribution of referrals across the agencies has occurred and resulted in increased pressure on Specialist CAMHS. This reflects failures in inter-agency collaboration in a circular way, i.e. both as cause and effect. In 1995, the NHS Health Advisory Service (HAS) reported that nowhere in England or Wales could it find an example in which the four major groups of agencies (local education authorities, local authority social services departments, the NHS, and the voluntary sector) were in effective partnership (Williams and Richardson 1995). Arguably, these agencies should contribute to well-coordinated networks. Experience and research

(Williams and Salmon 2002) shows that lack of collaboration between agencies leads to:

lack of shared definitions, tasks, roles, and vision;

inappropriate assumptions about the roles of others;

gaps in communications;

single agencies defining problems as lying in the zone of responsibility of another agency when this is neither negotiated with, nor accepted by the receiving agency; and

over-tasking of staff of current services resulting in individual agencies resorting to defining their own priorities unilaterally.

Our experience is that these sorts of events are much more likely to arise when there is a substantial mismatch between supply and demand and poor relationships between the contributing agencies.

These factors operate in a situation in which services are far from 'saturation' level (i.e. most are only able to respond effectively and in a timely way to a fraction of the potential demand that could be thrown up by society) (Rutter and Smith 1995; Stallard and Potter 1999; Meltzer *et al.* 2000; Zwaanswijk *et al.* 2003). Put in another way, there is evidence that the volume of services in the UK falls far short of parity with what is required to respond effectively to the levels of need arising from mental disorder in the population. This conclusion appears to have been at least obliquely endorsed by the Secretary for State for Health in England when the government made a Public Service Agreement, as a result of which much greater financial resource will be made available to achieve targets for increased access to CAMHS (Target 7 in Department of Health 2002). But, while new finance is available in England, the same cannot be said elsewhere in the UK where, at best, the resources remain uncertain to support services, to take on additional volumes or complexity of work, despite the growing evidence-base about the importance of doing so (National Assembly for Wales 2002).

In addition, these opinions and our other findings appear to us to support our contentions that:

it is necessary to better understand the local and national circumstances to guide significant investment; and

present information systems are still too poor in many places, and the premises upon which services operate too poorly understood, to enable the necessary analysis.

We hope that this chapter will assist readers to find the way forward.

Complexity and co-morbidity

Not only is there evidence of increasing volume of demand on specialist services but, as we have said, it is apparent that there have also been changes in the complexity of demand that has been placed upon specialist services (Williams 2002). Chapter 27 reports on the Audit Commission's findings which indicated that, in 1998–99, the most frequent number of problems experienced by children and young people attending Specialist CAMHS was five (fewer than 5% had one problem) but that the commissioning and delivery of services did not necessarily match this finding. The CAMHS mapping exercise showed that in 2002, 65% of young people seen by Specialist CAMHS had multiple problems. In part, this situation may reflect a real increase in complexity, but we think it has also arisen from better recognition of the range of needs or 'wants' of families. It also arises from better awareness and recognition of co-morbidity of mental health problems and disorders with other physical health, education, social/welfare, and substance misuse conditions.

Many of these co-morbid conditions interact to increase risk. Finding high levels of co-morbidity is not surprising, as mental health problems and mental disorders co-occur with lower use of services, and education and social problems. All these problems share overlapping risk and resilience factors (Williams *et al.* 2004).

Viewed from the client perspective, co-morbidity is a professional conception that describes situations in which single syndromes or diagnoses do not adequately describe the common experiences and needs of the population at risk, thereby making more than one diagnosis, or a multi-axial formulation, essential to adequately describe the problems they face. Patients/clients service users and their carers do not see or experience their problems in this, apparently, disjointed way. The significance of co-morbidity to professional practice and to service re-design is that it emphasizes the importance of viewing people's needs from a broad perspective in which their own voices are heard. Furthermore, there is some evidence that services are more likely to be effective if they intervene with more than one problem and with the background risk factors. This supports the contention that our services should become broader and better articulated to respond to the real and inter-connected needs of the public. Similarly, much work in general practice has shown the importance of narrative-based approaches to understanding the dilemmas of the clients of our services.

In the UK, these contentions have been growing noticeably in prominence in the last decade. They add fuel to the need to understand complexity of need but also result in increased demands being made from one agency to another. Inter-agency work is demanding of time and skill if true collaboration is to be produced and cost-shifting, the inevitable alternative, is to be avoided.

Another contemporary and particular example of the impact of this shift in approach to the needs of the population comes from study of the impact of the Youth Justice Board. Created in 1998, the Board has made rapid advances in improving the responsiveness of the youth justice system. Its challenges to public sector services have reached out well beyond its core remit to include endeavours to reduce juvenile crime by attention to the risk factors (also shared with social exclusion and mental disorder) and the consequences of criminality. The result is greatly increased demands on Specialist CAMHS.

Similarly, CAMHS are being challenged to change their response styles by many agencies. The HAS, Audit Commission, and governmental policy all encourage the development of the capability of primary care services to intervene (preventatively and therapeutically) earlier and more effectively with children, young people, and families who have mental health problems. The specialist services are being actively encouraged to provide greater support to that endeavour. However, there is some evidence that doing so re-directs the work of the specialist services. While some demand may be re-channeled by making primary-level services more effective, re-directing professional time away from direct work with clients also poses parallel challenges, that is until the availability of suitably trained staff can be increased.

Summary

Our exploration, so far, suggests that there is:

increasing demand framed by requests for increasing volumes of services and better responses to complex problems;

increasing apprehension of the real complexity of people's problems; and

changing patterns of demand and expectation arising from wider shifts in the philosophy of public sector services and demand on them.

Referral processes

What is a referral?

A referral consists of a number of explicit and/or implicit decisions made by a variety of people. Zwaanswijk *et al.* (2003) describe five levels or stages, each separated by a filter. These authors summarize 47 recent empirical studies on parental and adolescent problem recognition and help-seeking, and problem recognition by general practitioners in order to better understand 'the discrepancy between rates of child and adolescent psychopathology and rates of mental health service use'. In our opinion, their paper is more influential for its collation of the literature than for its depth and breadth of analysis. Leff and Bennett (1998) have provided a commentary on referral pathways and Laitinen-Krispijn *et al.* (1999) have used a record linkage study to predict adolescent mental health service use.

Our approach is illustrated by Fig. 32.1, which shows aspects of that decision process in respect of referrals from GPs. We have included this figure, not because we think that referrals from GPs should be the norm, but because the Audit Commission showed that more than 50% do come by this route (see Chapter 27).

In reality, Little and Bullock from the Dartington Social Research Unit have drawn attention to five 'prominent career routes' taken by children in trouble and how they depend more on the 'life route' decisions made by their families and 'process' decisions made by the agencies, than they do on need (Little and Bullock 2004; Williams 2004). As we show, there is a distinct resonance between their findings and the effects of the concepts of burden and impact on deciding who goes to which agency.

Whatever, the circumstances relating to how referrals are distributed across originating agencies, we have found that, usually, the mechanism for referring cases between agencies and professionals to Specialist CAMHS is, in the UK, akin to that used by GPs in the NHS. Thus, it is similar to the outline in Fig. 32.1. Perhaps, in part, this reflects the increased prominence of the NHS in CAMHS of the last two decades.

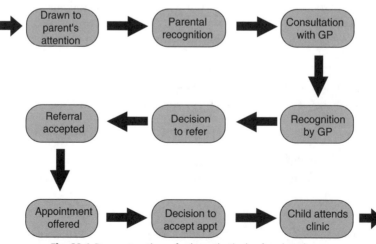

Fig. 32.1 Deconstruction of a hypothetical referral pathway.

More generally, the pathway from children and families to Specialist CAMHS can be modelled as a series of steps that represent decision points (Wolpert and Fredman 1996). Commonly, in our view, the steps in that pathway that can be identified by the process of deconstruction are:

Step 1: A parent or other adult recognizes that a child has problems and that they have failed to respond to informal interventions at home, school, or elsewhere (relatively rarely in the UK, a child or young person recognizes their own problems and takes action for themselves).

Step 2: The parent or other adult decides to seek help from a professional agency.

Step 3: Adult and/or the child or young person consults with a non-specialist service.

Step 4: The staff of the non-specialist service recognize that a child or young person has problems.

Step 5: A practitioner decides whether to offer intervention within that non-specialist service or to refer the child or young person (who is now conventionally a 'client' or 'patient') elsewhere.

Step 6: The practitioner refers the child, young person or family to Specialist CAMHS.

Step 7: The Specialist CAMHS decides whether or not to accept the referral and, if so, prioritizes the 'case'.

Step 8: A practitioner(s) from the Specialist CAMHS offers an appointment to the child, young person and/or family.

Step 9: The family receives the appointment and someone, usually an adult, decides to attend the Specialist CAMHS or otherwise.

Another way of construing this pathway is as a sequential set of filters in which default at any level results in failure of progression or selection of an alternative route. There is some research relating to each of four steps that has been carried out in more than one country and in more than one continent. This may imply that there are similar issues and concerns about the dynamics of the relationship between CAMHS and their clientele. In the past in the UK, many Specialist CAMHS accepted 'self-referrals' and, in some countries, direct contact between families and specialist services is usual. Although the number of decision-makers in the pathway is reduced in such circumstances, the general scenario that we outline here holds good.

We have already quoted evidence indicating that only a proportion of young people in need are referred. In England, the CAMHS mapping exercise recorded that 9822 cases were seen in the previous month (Glover *et al.* 2003; Centre for Public Health 2003). If this is taken as an average, the approximate figure for cases referred and surviving the process we describe here to be seen is in the order of 120 000 per annum. A crude estimation, based on the ONS survey of 1999 (Meltzer *et al.* 2000) suggests that this is at best around 10% of the population in serious need. Stallard and Potter showed that their service saw 1.9% compared with a predicted 8.9% of the population during their three-month audit (1999). Kurtz (Chapter 29) suggests that 'expected' cases run at 7 to 10 times the number known to Specialist CAMHS. Whatever the inevitable inaccuracy of these estimates, they show that there is a much larger potential pool of referees than assessment and treatment opportunities in Specialist CAMHS presently.

Referrability is defined as the frequency with which a child's problem is reported as a presenting complaint compared to the frequency of the problem in the general population (Weisz and Weiss 1991). This concept covers not only manifestations of a child's problem but also their carer's response, their ability to cope, and the tolerance of the culture for the symptoms the child expresses, at least in so far as referral might signify someone's opinion that assistance is required from other than directly accessible sources of help to which a referral is not required.

The notion of referrability provokes questions about why it is that some people are referred while others, with similar problems, are not. While we cannot answer this question with confidence, there are clues. For example, Vostanis *et al.* (2003) have carried out further work on the study conducted by Meltzer *et al.* (2000) in 1999 of the mental disorders experienced by children and young people in Great Britain. They have found that 'children with conduct disorders had significantly higher lifetime rates of using social and education services than children with other psychiatric disorders. Contact with primary health, specialist health, and educational services was significantly associated with comorbid physical and psychiatric disorders. In contrast, contact with social services was associated with family discord and social sector tenancy.'

In the next five sections we deconstruct the referral pathway to provide a partially evidence-based commentary on some of the key steps. Readers might like to consider the paper by Rawlinson and Williams for a fuller summary of the literature as at 2000.

Recognition by parents or carers and deciding to seek help

Angold *et al.* showed that parents' perceptions of need were related to the use of CAMHS (1998). They defined burden as 'the presence of problems, difficulties or adverse life events which affect the life (lives) of the psychiatric patients and others'. Their conception of burden is dynamic, as it encompasses the manifestation of children's problems and their parents' ability to cope. Research has shown that the burden is much less associated with use of services to which young people may refer themselves and that the impact of a problem on the individual experiencing it appears to be more significant to self-recognition and opinion-seeking. Significantly, children who are depressed or anxious are experienced by their carers as less burdensome then those with other problems, particular, problems relating to conduct. Research supports anecdotal experience of parent-initiated service contact being more likely in the case of disruptive disorders, whereas depression and anxiety are more related to children's perceptions of their need (Wu *et al.* 1999).

Zwaanswijk *et al.* (2003) conclude that:

> … although the presence of child psychopathology does not automatically lead to parental problem recognition, the chance of concern about, and help seeking … was confirmed to increase with comorbidity, and with increasing severity and persistence of problems. Adolescents' experience of psychological distress and functional impairment was confirmed to increase their help-seeking.

Age, the presence of medical and school-related problems, informal help-seeking, past treatment of parents or relatives, family size and type of maltreatment were also shown to influence help-seeking. On the other hand, they report studies from several countries that show a 'negative association between ethic minority status and parental and adolescent help seeking though this association disappeared when socio-economic variables were controlled'.

Evidence also supports the contention that parents' recognition of their children's psychological problems and making the decision to seek help are influenced, not only by their perceptions of the needs of their child, but also by their own needs (Garralda and Bailey 1988). Parents with their own pre-existing mental health problems, for example, experience more burden than those who do not. It appears that this is particularly the case for children who have hyperactivity and conduct disorder (MacLeod *et al.* 1999). Gasquet *et al.* (1999) have shown that use of specialist mental health services is associated with having: multiple problems; functional physical disorder; family problems; separated parents; multiple contacts with other doctors; and having confided in teachers or other youth advisers.

In 2003, Meltzer *et al.* published the results of a 3-year follow-up study conducted by the Office for National Statistics relating to the survey of the mental health of children and adolescents in Great Britain carried out in 1999. It found that the onset and persistence of mental disorders were linked to child, family, household, and social characteristics.

> Persistence of emotional disorders was particularly linked with mothers' poor mental health, whereas the persistence of conduct disorders was associated with the child having special educational needs, being shouted at frequently and mothers' poor mental health.
> About two-thirds of parents who had children with a persistent disorder or of those who had developed a disorder had sought help or advice from a professional in the year prior to the follow up survey, and around a quarter overall, used specialist health services.

A subset of parents was selected for a telephone interview, if they had used specialist, education, or primary care services in the year prior to follow-up, or if their child had significant problems when surveyed in 1999 and at follow-up. Twenty per cent of children participating in the telephone survey had been in contact with Specialist CAMHS during the previous year. However, 'the most common reasons parents gave for not contacting any services were:

they felt they would be branded a failure or blamed (29%);

they didn't know where to go for help for mental health problems (17%); or

they thought that intervention either would not be helpful or might actually make things worse (12%).'

Recognition by primary-level or non-specialist services

Generally, research has shown low levels of recognition of mental disorder by primary level professionals in primary care (Bowman and Garralda 1993). Kramer and Garralda (1998) found a rate of psychiatric disorder of 38% in a group of adolescents who had attended their GPs more than three times in the past year. They reported that the GPs recognized around 20% of the psychiatric disorder in this group. Lavigne *et al.* (1998) found that mental health service use was associated with being older, having greater impairment, and having a family that was in conflict.

Angold *et al.* (1999) showed that impairment was a stronger predictor of mental health service use than diagnosis, and Goodman (1999) found that impact scores on his Strengths and Difficulties Questionnaire were better predictors than symptom scores and discriminated between population and clinic samples. Thus, there appear to be similar sorts of burden-related processes in operation at this step of the referral pathway as at the parental or adult recognition stage.

Zwaanswijk *et al.* (2003), summarizing recent studies, found that GPs recognized problems more frequently in boys, older children, and children of single parents. They found evidence that life events, severity of psychopathology, past treatment for psychosocial problems, academic problems, length of visit to the primary care physician, and acquaintance with the child have been cited as influencing GPs' recognition of mental health problems and disorders. But, overall, they concluded that 'this aspect of the help-seeking pathway remains relatively uncharted ...'.

Referral from primary to secondary healthcare services

The concepts of referrability and burden are inter-related. Bailey and Garralda (1989) found in their research that the overt expectations of referrers to Specialist CAMHS are similar to those for other specialist services. They seek specialist opinions, advice, treatment provision, and advice for families. This suggests that in arenas well outside children's mental health, decisions about referral are also based on experience of burden and are not simply related to impact on the children who are the subject of consideration.

Social factors such as parental unemployment, financial problems, and lack of support from extended families, also appear to influence decisions about referral, as does parental distress and their own psychiatric history (Garralda and Bailey 1988). Bailey and Garralda described GPs as reacting to parents' anxiety and requests for referral to Specialist CAMHS. In 1998, the *Psychiatric Bulletin* carried an article reporting interviews of 47 GPs on their views about prioritizing children's' mental health problem (Jones and Bhadrinath 1998). The GPs were reported as highly motivated by the desire to share anxiety and responsibility with the specialists, even though mental health services were not necessarily seen as the most appropriate lead agency. In other words, the notion of 'treatability' did not appear to be the sole, or even, in many cases, the most significant matter impacting on deciding to refer. Other audits have shown that most children who are referred have long-standing, multiple, and complex problems (Stallard and Potter 1999).

The reactions of Specialist CAMHS to receiving referrals

It is becoming more apparent now that services vary in the way in which they respond to receiving referrals. Even within services, different teams adopt different stances in respect of how they respond to the demands placed upon them. The volume of published material in this regard is small. So, we reach into our experience covering the last 30 years in a variety of different services to suggest that, not only do practices vary within and between services, but there are indications of a historical shift in the responsiveness of Specialist CAMHS over time.

When the first author started work in CAMH in the mid-1970s, a common statement made by, what are now known as Specialist CAMHS (often, in those days, a non-systematic and historically derived mixture of child guidance clinics, hospital-based child psychiatry departments, adolescent psychiatric services, and slender academic departments), was that their policy was to take all referrals and to offer appointments to all children and/or families that were referred. In effect, many practitioners prided themselves on, not only offering specialist services but also, on offering primary levels of mental health service through their direct accessibility to the public and their overt encouragement of what were described as 'self-referrals'. The vast majority of these self-referrals were not made by young people but were made by family adults who sought advice from a specialist service rather than, or in addition to, attending other primary level or directly accessible services. In other words, usually they reflected burden on adults rather than or in addition to impact on younger people. Many specialist services offered appointments on the basis of reacting to the chronological order of receipt of the referrals or by endeavouring to prioritize referrals using the material contained in a referral letter or gleaned from a telephone call made by a family adult. There is little published material to illustrate how successful were these processes.

In more recent times, and in response to perceptions of demand increasing more rapidly than capacity and capability of specialist services, many have reviewed their policies on accepting referrals. In some, it was spurred by the report of the NHS Health Advisory Service (HAS) report *Together we stand*, which led to a much greater awareness of limitations of the training and the ability to provide first-line responses to children who may have problems with their mental health of primary level or direct access services (also see Buston 2002). Realizing that re-distribution of scarce services was not feasible, and that considerable development of primary level services was required, the HAS recommended that roles of primary mental health workers be developed, as, at least, a partial response.

A number of themes are identifiable. First, many services have reconsidered whether or not they should encourage and accept 'self-referrals'. Many have also reviewed what might otherwise be termed their eligibility criteria for referral. Some services have identified what they regard as their core business and have stratified the work they do into three layers. The first of these is work that is regarded as essential, the second layer is work that is desirable, resources permitting, and the third is work that may be required by the population but in which the Specialist CAMHS might only be one of a number of local agencies that might be legitimately regarded as providing responses. A good example of this latter category includes the provision of parent training services that could legitimately be seen as the province of social services departments, education authorities, the NHS and the voluntary sector.

Other services have endeavoured to manage demand through either issuing or agreeing protocols in conjunction with their referrers or instituting scoring systems or adapting the duration and quantity of contact that they offer to families in response to increasing demand.

Our continuing contact with practice shows that commissioning agencies are not clear about why some groups of young people are afforded accelerated attention within Specialist CAMHS, while others are put on to a waiting-list of variable length. Anecdotal conversation with NHS staff in the UK suggests a reasonable coherence of view among specialist practitioners about the types of case and the sorts of circumstances affecting young people that constitute reasons for urgency. By contrast, there is a diversity of opinion in the specialist services about their client group overall (HAS 1995; Goodman 1997). Levels of agreement between referrers, those people referred, and staff of specialist services, concerning what problems constitute a legitimate demand on Specialist CAMHS, are precarious (Evans and Brown 1993). Further support for this contention comes from a recent study of the opinions expressed by professional staff in a Specialist CAMHS about 170 consecutive letters of referral received in 1999 by that service (Sparrow, Barber and Williams personal communication). Deliberately, specialist practitioners were asked a highly subjective question in this audit about whether they considered each referral to be 'appropriate' or otherwise. The results are summarized in Table 32.1.

If, for a moment, readers take the view that all referrers saw at least some advantage accruing to the referred individual and/or their family from their being sent to the Specialist CAMHS, then Table 32.1 does suggest a substantial mismatch between the views of the referrers and those of the staff of the specialist service about its role. Our experience of conducting this audit also supports the opinion that assigning priorities on the basis of the contents of the letters written by referrers is

Table 32.1 Opinions of staff in a Specialist CAMHS about the 'appropriateness' of the referrals they received

Opinion of Tier 2 staff teams about the congruence between each referral and the core business of the specialist service	Number	Percentage
Referral considered likely to be appropriate	79	46.5
Referral considered to be inappropriate	65	38.2
No opinion as to appropriateness possible	26	15.3
Totals	170	100

far from easy and/or satisfactory. In our view, there are distinct limitations as to the value of spending lengthy periods in allocation meetings on the basis of the content of many referral letters.

At much the same time that we conducted this audit within a specialist service, we also established communications with a number of GP referrers in different parts of the UK to begin to learn from them why it is that they had or had not made referrals. In common with recent literature, the subjective opinion most often provided by this process indicated that many GPs are very unclear about what they might expect from Specialist CAMHS. Overall, their opinion was that their own knowledge and skills in this arena is insufficient for them to take on children's mental health problems (Buston 2002). Another view expressed frequently was they felt very uncertain about how best to get help for some families, particularly for those who recurrently seek help for a wide array of social and educational problems. A substantial proportion of the GPs with whom we talked saw referral to Specialist CAMHS as an avenue for action though they volunteered that they were unsure at best about the appropriateness of the resource to which they were referring young people.

Our sense from conducting this pilot phase of a substantial qualitative research study is that GPs see many young people with a wide array of different types of problems over a considerable range of severity as potential candidates for referral to Specialist CAMHS. On the other hand, despite the thin literature in this arena, our sense is that many specialist practitioners have a reasonable measure of agreement between them as to what they see as constituting reasons for urgency. Thus, we find from published and unpublished material (some of which is available on the World Wide Web) suggestions that many services identify their core business often by diagnostic categories or problems for which they see themselves as primarily responsible rather than on the basis of need or level of impairment.

If our tentative observations are accurate, they support observations made a decade ago by Wilkin and Rowland (1993) who highlighted the need for reliable up-to-date information, together with meaningful ways of measuring performance, in order to better manage the situation. They urged greater communication, especially between consultants and their referrers, not just about waiting times but about referral objectives and patient follow-up.

Deciding to attend a specialist service

Much of the literature in this arena relates to non-attendance or, as children and young people are described impersonally in many services, DNAs (did not attend). Initially, it may be surprising to unfamiliar readers that, having survived so many filtering processes before being offered an appointment, families might, then, decide not to attend.

Attendance at Specialist CAMHS has been perceived by some observers as poor when compared with other specialist services. In fact, anecdotal evidence and local audits suggest that non-attendance rates are not especially low in many Specialist CAMHS. It may be that the time offered to families at their initial attendance makes their non-appearance much more visible than a similar circumstance at, say, an orthopaedic surgery clinic. Initial non-attendance rates have been shown to be as low as 14% (Cottrell et al. 1988) or as high as 38% (Piacentini et al. 1995; McKay et al. 1996). One study compared attendance at a child psychiatric clinic with that of paediatric ENT and general paediatric clinics (El-Bhadri and McCardle 1998). Although the samples cited were small, the investigators found no significant differences in initial attendance rates between each of these clinics.

In their audits, Stallard and Potter (1999) found that nearly 1 in 5 of those referred did not attend their initial appointment, but that, in nearly half of these instances, someone had contacted the clinic to rearrange the appointment. As a result, only 11% of their appointments identified for initial attenders were unfilled. However, on the basis of the information derived from the original referral letter, the clinic staff was unable to predict accurately who would attend and who would fail to do so.

No consistent differences between non-attenders and attenders have been found relating to the age and sex of the child, family status, nature of symptoms, referral source, area of residence, having problems with transport, having problems with language, having multiple social problems, parental separation, and/or there being a history of previous failed attendance (Cottrell *et al.* 1988).

CAMHS also vary in how accessible they are to children and young people. In some situations, access can be gained easily; in others it is poor (Audit Commission 1999). But there is recent evidence from a randomized trial that the location of clinics is not necessarily the most material factor in families' perceptions of acceptability (Harrington *et al.* 2000). Factors that have been shown to be more important as regards attendance include parental understanding of, and agreement to, the referral and the duration of wait since referral (Lefebre *et al.* 1983; Cottrell *et al.* 1988; Jaffa and Griffin 1990). We conclude that it is temporal proximity rather more than geographical proximity that determines families' perceptions of accessibility.

There is strong evidence that poor attendance rates at Specialist CAMHS are closely associated with longer waiting-lists (Lefebre *et al.* 1983; Jaffa and Griffin 1990; Munjal *et al.* 1994; Stern and Brown 1994). Figure 32.2 summarizes the relationship between referral rates, waiting times, and rates of families that do not attend without previously notifying the specialist service that they could not or would not come.

Le Febvre *et al.* showed that for over 50% of non-attenders, long waiting times was the single most important factor that influenced their choice of non-attending. There is evidence that there may be a cut-off point in waiting time that is significant in this decision, which may be as short as 2 weeks before the effects summarized in Fig. 32.2 begin to operate (Jaffa and Griffin 1990). Long waiting times are a significant cause for complaint for some of those who do eventually attend (Subotsky and Berelowitz 1990).

We conclude that parents who understand why their child has been referred, who agree with the referral, and who wait less long, are more likely to bring their children to appointments.

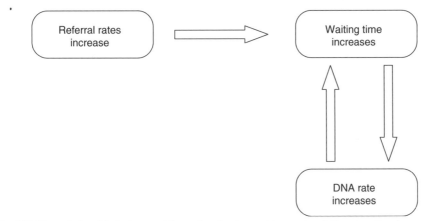

Fig. 32.2 The relationship between rising referral rates and increasing failure to attend appointments.

Research supports interventions to improve engagement with referred families. Nonetheless, one study showed that prior telephone contact reduced DNA rates, whereas a similar study has shown no effect.

Waiting-lists and times

The functions of waiting-lists

Any waiting-list identifies a portion of the demand made for services. Waiting-lists also restrict access to services for a selection of people with certain conditions. The presence and length of lists and waiting times throughout the NHS causes concern to service users, providers, commissioners, and policymakers (Health Services Management Centre 1998). Arguably, waiting-lists represent improvements in health waiting to be given (Gudex *et al.* 1990).

We observe that waiting-lists may provide, often inadvertently, one or a combination of the following functions:

regulation of demand placed on services that are insufficient to meet that demand, by creating a buffer of referrals held in suspense or a barrier to their onward progression;

an estimate of the uplift in services required to more adequately meet demand;

legitimatization of contrary opinion about the need for particular types of service;

a way to manage a volume of cases or conditions about which clinicians find decision-making difficult, or those that consume large amounts of resource;

regulation of demand represented by those conditions clinicians believe may respond poorly to current interventions (e.g. conduct disorders);

a reservoir in case- and cost-shifting between agencies.

Reducing waiting-lists and waiting times has been at the top of successive governments' health priorities. Their centrality in health policy remains, despite strong arguments about why we should not concentrate policy so substantially on waiting-lists in a setting of continuing increases in the numbers and complexity of cases with which services deal.

There is a range of concerns. One is that concentrating on waiting-lists and times fails to recognize the recent rapid rises in public sector throughput. As long ago as 1989, Frankel noted that the number of patients on in-patient waiting-lists constituted 1% of the population of England and Wales, but that this represented only 14% of the in-patient throughput of the NHS. Our concern is that the waiting approach to resourcing and tasking the NHS appears to be based on a false premise of there being a finite amount of morbidity in all areas of ill health. On the contrary, a common observation in the NHS, as in other demand-sensitive systems, is that increasing the volume and responsiveness of services stimulates demand and fuels expectations. In other words, increasing turnover reduces waiting-lists temporarily only for them to re-emerge. Thus, there are indications from a number of the waiting-list initiatives that they do not make fundamental impacts on the performance on the whole of the health-care system.

Behind these matters is another rather more grave concern. It is that deflecting resources towards reducing waiting-lists risks moving health service investment away from certain specialisms and, in particular, away from conditions that require longer-term care. Concentrating on waiting-lists risks moving resource-allocation processes away from mechanisms that reflect a realistic balance with the true nature of the health needs of the population and the evidence of effectiveness. This situation describes a schism within clinical governance created by tensions between differing political and professional values, pressures and evidence.

Waiting for Specialist CAMHS

Most published work on waiting-lists has concentrated on in-patient services, though, more recently, increasing attention is being paid to out-patients. Although experience suggests that many of the circumstances that we have considered in general terms here may apply to CAMHS, the literature relating to waiting-lists, waiting times, and related initiatives, is relatively thin. So, it is difficult for us to document the history of waiting-lists in CAMHS and we rely on what published work there is, and our own and others' experiences.

These sources suggest that out-patient waiting-lists for Specialist CAMHS have developed particularly in the last 10–20 years. It is apparent from our survey of the plans of the many statutory agencies in the UK for Specialist CAMHS published on the World Wide Web, that concerns about waiting times and waiting-lists in CAMHS are ubiquitous. There is also evidence that opinion about problems has engendered increased attention being given to Specialist CAMHS by the responsible authorities (Community Care 1998), those involved in waiting, the media (Turner 1998) and providers of services.

In the past, the existence of a waiting-list has been seen as endorsing the need for particular services and as an indicator of unmet need. Often, missing from such examinations is whether the needs of the populations served are being appropriately targeted; nonetheless, waiting-lists are frequently cited as supporting evidence for uplifting the volume or capacity of a service or as a reason for re-engineering it.

Some legitimacy is afforded this claim by the centrality of increases in accessibility within the Public Service Agreement of 2002 between the Department of Health in England and the Government in the UK (Target 7 in Department of Health 2002). On this basis, we contend that growing waiting-lists is one of the factors that have propelled concern about Specialist CAMHS at professional, health authority, local authority, and government levels. When demand for CAMHS did not so demonstrably outstrip supply, there was less pressure to examine the situation.

An indication of the level of the problem in the UK can be gained from the findings of the Audit Commission, which reported in 1999 that 10% of NHS trusts could not offer an initial appointment for non-urgent cases within 6 months (Chapter 27). The CAMHS mapping exercise conducted in England in 2002 showed, as stated previously, that 9822 cases were recorded as being 'seen' by Specialist CAMHS in the previous month: 24% had waited 3 weeks or less, another 61% between 4 and 25 weeks, and 15% longer than this. In the same period, 21 329 more cases were waiting (51% had waited less than 12 weeks and 20% had waited more than 26 weeks). The cases seen represented 99 per 100 000 population and those waiting 215 per 100 000—another indicator of the excess of demand over supply.

Responding to waiting-lists

Stallard and Sayers (1998) opine that there are several reasons why it is important to reduce waiting times for first appointments. They say:

> … from a clinician's perspective it is important to respond swiftly to referrals in order to assess the urgency and severity of the difficulties and prevent problems escalating or becoming more firmly established …. An ability to respond quickly is an important criteria adopted by many refers in

evaluating child and adolescent mental health services. From a service management perspective there is need to ensure that limited resources are used effectively and that the number of failed appointments remains low .... Finally, it is important to provide service users with an accessible and responsive service. Delays may result in clients becoming dispirited or less motivated and leaving them feeling dissatisfied with the service they eventually receive.

Typically, there has been a number of ways in which Specialist CAMHS have endeavoured to tackle their waiting-lists. The intervention most commonly recommended to tackle the problem is an increase of resources (i.e. uplift in the volume of service available aimed at bringing the volume of supply closer to the volume of demand) (Pope 1993). Recently, the UK government has allocated very substantial new finance to CAMHS to fund a very substantial uplift in service accessibility in England. The focus of Target 7 of the Public Service Agreement on accessibility plainly indicates that the present initiatives being taken by the Department of Health fall broadly into this first category of response.

However, previously and now, in jurisdictions other than England, increases in resource have been much less systematic and much more modest. Also, the current problems in recruiting, training, and retaining sufficient professional staff, for even the current levels of service in the UK, should not be underestimated. In these circumstances, the staff of present specialist services have responded in a variety of innovating ways with the intention of using existing or slowly expanding resources to greater effect. These innovations can be grouped into a number of categories. They are schemes to:

improve the quality of referrals made;

more explicitly prioritize or select from the referrals received;

improve the involvement, motivation, and compliance of families with appointments; and

change responses provided by existing services.

Readers will see that these innovations operate at different points in the referral process. We begin by summarizing a number of initiatives that endeavour to improve use of specialist services by streamlining the relationships between the non-specialist services and Specialist CAMHS, and better selecting referees for prioritized waiting-lists.

Raising the quality of referrals

Listing eligible referrers Many services have moved from having, so-called, 'open' referral systems to stipulating more restricted lists of professionals from whom the specialist services are prepared to take referrals. Often, the intention is to raise the quality of referrals received but also to recruit certain practitioners to act as preliminary gatekeepers. We have found no formal evaluation of these schemes.

Standardising referral formats In other instances, specialist services have endeavoured to standardize the referrals they receive by publishing lists of the information they require in referral letters or by asking referrers to fill in standard referral forms. Again, we have found no formal evaluations.

Prioritizing referrals

Restricting the types of patient' problems that are accepted Typically, services that adopt this approach seek to narrow the gateway of referral by stipulating what types of problem that they accept. In our experience, these categories are often stated in diagnostic terms, though, as we have seen, this creates a schism with many referrers, as they tend not to use the same criteria. There is little written about schemes of this type, but we believe, from anecdotal report, that they are very commonly used and particularly when services are hard pressed.

Referral filtering In other instances, specialist services endeavour to filter referrals before or immediately after their receipt. Often, this also involves sign-posting unsuccessful referers to other agencies. It may build on the first category by the staff of the receiving agency communicating prospectively to potential referrers that they cannot prioritize certain types of problem. Another way in which filtering processes are used is to offer an alternative service in which the potential patient may not be taken on directly by a specialist. Good examples of this include provision of: mental health consultations to referrers (in which the patient/client is not seen); support, training, and advice to would-be referrers (so that they can continue to work more effectively with the young people); and joint working (in which specialists may offer occasional contacts for a referred person jointly with the potential referrer in order to augment the practice of the would-be referrer). Very often, these latter roles have been taken on by primary mental health workers and elsewhere, this book reviews their roles and impacts (see Chapters 30, 31 and 33). In some services, primary mental health workers have taken on an explicit role as gatekeeper and some Specialist CAMHS do not accept referrals unless they have been either discussed with, or routed through, a primary mental health worker.

Formal referral as confirmation of negotiation The previous methods of filtering and prioritizing referrals may either be imposed by the specialist services upon their referrers or be negotiated between potential referrers and the specialist services.

Other methods involve putting the amount of time that might be expended in resisting or prioritizing referrals after their receipt into explicit negotiation beforehand, with the intention to create a two-stage referral process. In schemes of this kind, specialist services do not take referrals unless there has been some negotiation prior to them being dispatched. Thus, referral letters do not come 'out of the blue' but are expected as a summary or confirmation of telephone or face-to-face contacts between specialist practitioners and referrers. We are aware of a number of schemes in which the specialist services publish the availability of their staff by telephone at certain times in the week, so that potential referrers can contact them within a ring-fenced time to discuss their concerns, the options, and the kinds of information required if a referral is the agreed course. Other services offer regular meetings between specialist practitioners and referrers at which face-to-face negotiations can take place.

Two-tier waiting-lists Very many Specialist CAMHS have, either explicitly or implicitly, broken their waiting-lists into a number of levels. These services may categorize the referrals they receive into those that they think require very urgent responses (immediately or within days), those that require rapid responses (an appointment as soon as one can be provided), and those cases that might listed for non-accelerated responses.

However, our experience has shown that there are problems of two main types with operating schemes of this kind. First, it is often very difficult to make decisions on priority on the basis of the information provided in referral letters. Second, many services have found that the number of patients to whom they give prioritized appointments absorbs most, if not all, of their capacity, which leaves the remaining, non-prioritized cases, on slow moving, static, or lengthening waiting-lists. Therefore, schemes of this kind have often been supplemented by referral scoring or prioritization against explicit criteria in order to improve their efficiency and fairness.

A variety of these schemes has been reported from across the world. They endeavour to struggle with the dual challenges of allocating insufficient resources and doing so in ways that are fair, though limitations remain. In the case of the Western Canada Waiting-list Project (WCWL), its creators elected to adopt a set of criteria incorporating indicators of each patient's severity of illness, family and social factors, and estimates of the likely outcomes associated with intervention by Specialist CAMHS (Smith and Hadorn 2002). The evaluation of this scheme recognized that its approach was essentially a diagnosis and not a needs-led one, which does not fully take into account representations from families or their advocates, and that it did little to address the issue of low-scoring patients who might never reach the top of the list. The success of schemes of this kind plainly depends on the quality of information provided by referrers.

One of the problems with all of the schemes that we have covered so far is that the initiative for them has most usually come from a specialist service, which is endeavouring to offer its slender resources equitably through rational and overt gatekeeping processes. We think that, without other changes, there can be little motivation for referrers to share that gatekeeping task because, as we have shown early in this chapter, there is some evidence that what referrers want from specialist services may differ from the roles that the specialists see for themselves.

The WCWL initiative showed that the specialists tended to prioritize young people with internalized problems and better prospects of benefiting from the interventions available. Nonetheless, the concept of burden indicates that non-specialists and families are more likely to recognize and seek specialist intervention for young people who have externalizing problems. Again, the language used by referrers and specialists may differ with the latter preferring a greater accent on diagnostic categories, while families tend to articulate their needs in more ordinary terms. Primary level practitioners appear to sit between the two. Often, they believe that they lack the expertise to make the necessary assessments and this encourages them to adopt the position of their patients/clients. Inevitably, unless the innovations described in our first two categories are negotiated between the specialist and non-specialist services, a variety of tensions will remain between them.

Next, we turn to two categories of innovation in which specialist practitioners have endeavoured to use their slender resources differently.

Improving the involvement and compliance of families

A variety of techniques has been used to ensure that appointments go to families who will take them up with a view to reducing the number of DNAs and, thereby, promote more prompt responses.

Telephone prompts The first method has been to employ telephone prompts. There have been several studies of interventions to reduce non-attendance rates through introductory telephone calls made by practitioners or administrative staff of the specialist service before the initial interview. McKay et al. (1996) found that families who received telephone calls aimed at engaging them were more likely to attend or to call in advance and rearrange their first appointment (72.7% versus 45.3%). Mathai and Markantonakis (1990) found that a telephone call before the appointment significantly increased attendance rates. However, earlier, Burgoyne et al. (1983) found that telephone prompting had little or no effect on attendance, and that telephone ownership was a marker for socio-economic status. In summary, the evidence for the effectiveness of telephone prompts remains unresolved and, like the other measures in this category, it is difficult to free interventions of this kind from markers of socio-economic status.

Opt-in systems Traditionally, specialist practitioners offer appointments then wait to see if their clients attend on the day. Recently, specialist services have reported use of schemes in which families are asked to declare whether or not they wish to have, and will take up, an appointment before it is offered or prior to its confirmation. In opt-in systems, if a client does not confirm in advance, an appointment is not offered.

In our experience, the systems used are of two types. In the first, upon receipt of a referral, the specialist clinic sends a letter to the potential clients asking them to get back in touch to confirm that they wish the referral to proceed to an appointment. In the second, a letter is sent but its wording assumes that the family will wish to receive an appointment by asking a representative to make a telephone call to the clinic to speak personally to a secretary to arrange their own appointment at a time that is mutually convenient. A third and particular variant of opt-in schemes is contacting longer term waiters to ask if they still wish to be seen with a view to removing those who say no, or do not respond, from waiting-lists (Henderson 1998).

Studies evaluating these schemes have shown mixed impacts on appointment failures. Again, the problems might lie in implicit socio-economic matters hidden in systems of this kind. For example, most of the systems that we have looked at depend on written communications from the clinic to the client and this must, therefore, presume sufficient levels of literacy. However, claims made in the UK in recent years are that adult functional illiteracy may be as high as 20%. If so, approaches based on letters may not be universally effective, and may disadvantage certain people who are more at risk of mental disorder.

Changes in specialist clinic responses

This category presumes that a specialist practitioner is prepared to offer an appointment and that the family is prepared to attend. Traditionally, appointments are sent to first-attenders with a presumption that an assessment is made by a practitioner who then arranges for management of each case to be continued in a way that is appropriate to the outcome of the assessment. In other words, the presumption is of a full assessment and that such clinic resources as there are will be made available subsequently. In a number of reported projects, clinics have varied this traditional pattern of response.

Triage and brief assessment clinics Some services have set up clinics to offer brief assessment only (i.e. briefer than would be offered to fully evaluate the case) with the intention of selecting from a number of subsequent courses. Jones *et al.* (2000), for example, have reported what they call a 'triage style assessment' in which they endeavour to allocate cases into the categories of:

immediate action;

further assessment;

priority waiting-list;

routine waiting-list; and

closure.

They directed a sample of new referral and waiting-list cases into their triage system. A multi-disciplinary group assembled, before families were seen, to review the referrals, generate hypotheses, and consider the assessment and action plans to be made. They set aside two triage days each month and a standardized letter was sent to each family prior to their appointment, together with Goodman's Strength and Difficulties Questionnaire and a self-styled questionnaire. Appointments were not conditional upon families returning questionnaires but parents were asked to confirm their intention to attend. If no confirmation was received, the administrative staff at the clinic contacted a parent by telephone to elicit his/her wishes. At the triage session, each family was offered an hour-long assessment, including a semi-structured interview, to gain an overview of the presenting problem. After the multidisciplinary team agreed the outcome later in the day, the referrer and family were informed of its decision.

Jones *et al.* (2000) report on a total 155 patients who had passed through their scheme. They say that 'an unusually high percentage of patients attended the first appointment (81.3%)'. On the basis of the other evidence we have reviewed, we think that finding may result from the reduced waiting times and the several mechanisms built in to gain commitment. As a result of the triage process, 43 cases (27.7%) were closed because they did not require a further appointment, were referred on to a more appropriate service, or did not attend; 25% were considered to require immediate allocation and a similar number was placed on the routine waiting-list; 10% were put on the priority waiting-list. The authors say that they have now adopted this initiative as standard practice.

Brief interventions Our final category is of initiatives that have limited the clinical time allocated to individual cases. A common approach reported is of employing the '2 plus 1' model that was developed initially for adult mental health problems by Barkham and Shapero (1989). Brief interventions are not new in CAMHS, as there are publications showing that high percentages of referrals are seen three times or fewer (Beer 1992; Hoare *et al.* 1996). This could be taken to suggest that moving towards briefer interventions would be a legitimate approach but it might also suggest that, if a majority of cases are seen briefly already, the impact of doing so may turn out to be relatively restricted.

Conclusions

This chapter has surveyed the relationships of Specialist CAMHS with potential and actual clients of those services and with professionals in the wider array of services that may have an impact on children's mental health and which may wish to refer clients/patients to specialists. We have looked at the imbalance between demand and supply, and the slender research on aspects of referral pathways with the intention of laying before readers a survey of what is known about performance of services from the literature and anecdotal information. We have surveyed initiatives taken by the specialist services to manage demand, which include gatekeeping, prioritizing referrals, and endeavours to respond more efficiently and more equitably. In our view, each of these has its place in managed healthcare systems but also limitations.

While constructing this review, we have come to a number of over-riding conclusions, which are:

1. There is need to improve input made by young people and their families to the processes by which services decide what they do and how they operate.

2. There is need for greater clarity at national, regional, and local levels about the realistic role of each of the services that comprise comprehensive CAMHS.

3. When planning services, we must recognize that some people are not motivated to attend statutory services that are provided in traditional ways but that they still have needs.

4. There is a requirement for diversity rather than single types of response but we need to conduct much more research orientated to show how best to apply and co-ordinate them effectively.

5. We should recognize that all health, education, social and non-statutory services have finite capacities and capabilities and avoid wishing unrealistic demands onto them.

6. Vertical and horizontal integration between the services that, together, make up CAMHS need to be improved in order to ensure that children and young people are offered access to the most appropriate services in the most appropriate settings.

7. There is a need to achieve better integration between specialist services and those services to which young people (often those with internalized problems for which there is an improving evidence-base for the effectiveness of interventions) may prefer to go.

8. Further work is needed in many areas to clarify agreements between general services and Specialist CAMHS about indicators for urgent or high priority responses.

9. Local services need clarity about how they corporately provide advice to children, young people and families when their problems, needs, and dilemmas do not appear to fit the system.

   In order to achieve these aims we should:

   use explicit plans and protocols for demand management that take account of the views of all appropriate stakeholders;

   re-organize some of our services so that they respond to need and are not solely lead by diagnostic category;

   consider how the needs of clients/patients for information can be met in ways that are not predicated on presumptions of literacy;

   recognize the concepts of burden and impact and, in particular, recognize that referrability and burden are closely aligned and that young people with internalized problems and high impact may receive, inadvertently, a lower profile of response from traditional referral mechanisms;

   recognize that the notions of complexity and co-morbidity indicate that many children, young people, and families have multiple problems and/or needs and many may require input from a variety of services at one or the same time or in an ordered sequence;

   recognize that better matching is required between 'wants', need, evidence of service effectiveness, and available expertise and skill; and

   design information systems that are truly supportive of the real needs of young people and families and the work of CAMHS.

All of these matters could be seen as reasons for us to review the adequacy of traditional letter-based referral systems in favour of clearer and more focused negotiations on the basis of need, capacity, and capability,

   Milton in 'On his blindness' said, 'They also serve who stand and wait'. We have found that studying the children, young people, families, and referrers who are waiting for specialist services contributes rewardingly to designing future CAMHS. So, we conclude that much more research is required into the lessons to be gleaned from knowing how our services actually work, followed by active responses to those findings if we are to turn children's waiting into better services.

References

Angold, A., Messer, S., Stangl, D., Farmer, E.M.Z., Costello, E.J., and Burns, B.J. (1998) Perceived parental burden and service use for child and adolescent psychiatric disorders. *Am J Public Health*, **88**, 75–80.

Angold, A., Costello, E., Farmer, E., Burns, B.J., and Erkanli, A. (1999) Impaired but undiagnosed. *J Am Acad Child Adolesc Psychiatry*, **8**, 129–37.

Audit Commission (1999) *Children in mind—child and adolescent mental health services.* London: Audit Commission.

Bailey, D. and Garralda, M.E. (1989) Referral to child psychiatry: parent and doctor motives and expectations. *J Child Psychol Psychiatry*, **33**, 449–58.

Barkham, M. and Shapiro, D.A. (1989) Towards resolving the problem of waiting-lists: psychotherapy in two plus one sessions. *Clinical Psychology Forum*, **23**, 15–8.

Barton, H., Davey, I., Street, E., and Williams, R. (2002) *Mental health in childhood, children and young people who have mental health problems and mental disorders and mental health services for young people.* Health and Social Services Committee of the National Assembly for Wales. Internet: http://www.wales.gov.uk/assemblydata/3CBED339000BCF0700003BC400000000.rtf

Beer, R. (1992) A preschool child psychiatric service: predictors of post-assessment default. *Child: Care, Health and Assessment*, **18**, 1–13.

Bowman, F. and Garralda, M.E. (1993) Psychiatric morbidity among children who are frequent attenders in general practice. *British Journal of General Practice*, **43**, 6–9.

Burgoyne, R., Acosta, F., and Yamamoto, J. (1983) Telephone prompting to increase attendance at a psychiatric out-patient clinic. *Am J Psychiatry*, **140**, 345–7.

Buston, K. (2002) Adolescents with mental health problems: what do they say about health services? *Journal of Adolescence*, **25**, 231–42.

Centre for Public Mental Health, University of Durham (for Department of Health) 2003 *National Child and Adolescent Mental Health Service Mapping Exercise.* http://www.dur.ac.uk/service. mapping/CAMH

Community Care (1998) Children with mental health problems failed by services. *Community Care*, 27th August, p. 6.

Cottrell, D., Hill, P., Walk, D., Dearnaley, J., and Lerotheron, A. (1988) Factors influencing non-attendance at child psychiatry out-patient appointments. *Br J Psychiatry*, **152**, 201–4.

Department of Health (2002) *Technical note for the spending review 2002—public service agreement.* http://www.doh.gov.uk/psa/psa02.htm

El-Bhadri, S.M. and McCardle, P. (1998) Attendance at child psychiatric clinics ± comparison with attendance at child medical and surgical clinics. *Psychiatr Bull*, **22**, 554–6.

Evans, S. and Brown, R. (1993) Perception of need for child psychiatric services among parents and GPs. *Health Trends*, **25**, 11.

Frankel, S. (1989) The natural history of waiting-lists—some wider explanations for an unnecessary problem. *Health Trends*, **21**, 56–8.

Garralda, M.E. and Bailey, D. (1988) Child and family factors associated with referral to child psychiatrists. *Br J Psychiatry*, **153**, 81–9.

Gasquet, I., Ledoux, S., Chavance, M., and Choquet, M. (1999) Consultation of mental health professionals by French adolescents with probable psychiatric problems. *Acta Psychiatr Scand*, **99**, 126–34.

Glover, G., Dean, R., Hartley, C., and Foster, B. (2003) *National child and adolescent mental health service mapping exercise.* London: Department of Health.

Goodman, R. (1997) *Child and adolescent mental health services: reasoned advice to commissioners and providers. Maudsley discussion paper no. 4.* London: Institute of Psychiatry.

Goodman, R. (1999) The extended version of the strengths and difficulties questionnaire as a guide to child psychiatric caseness and consequent burden. *Child Psychol Psychiatry*, **40**, 791–9.

Gudex, C., Williams, A., Jourdan, M., Mason, R., Maynard, Y., O'Flynn, R., *et al.* (1990) Prioritizing waiting-lists. *Health Trends*, **3**, 103–8.

Harrington, R., Peters, S., Green, J., Byford, S., Woods, J., and McGowan, R. (2000) Randomised comparison of the effectiveness and costs of community and hospital based mental health services for children with behaviour disorders. *British Medical Journal*, **321**, 1047–50.

Health Services Management Centre (1998) *Examining some of England's longest waiting-lists. Half year report. Inter-authority comparisons and consultancy.* Birmingham: University of Birmingham.

Henderson, J. (1998) 'Reply-paid letters gave our service users a choice and us a break' letter. *Health Service Journal*, 13 August.

Hoare, P., Norton, B., Chisolm, D., and Parry-Jones, W. (1996) An audit of 7000 successive child and adolescent psychiatry referrals in Scotland. *Clinical Child Psychology and Psychiatry*, **1**, 229–49.

Jaffa, T. and Griffin, S. (1990) Does a shorter wait for a first appointment improve the attendance rate in child psychiatry? *Assoc Child Psychol Psychiatr Rev Newslett*, **12**, 9–11.

Jones, E., Lucey, C., and Wadland, L. (2000) Triage: a waiting-list initiative in a child mental health service. *Psychiatric Bulletin* **24**, 57–9.

Jones, S.M. and Bhadrinath, B.R. (1998) GPs views on prioritization of child and adolescent mental health problems. *Psychiatr Bull*, **22**, 484–6.

Knapp, M. and Henderson, J. (1999) Health economics perspectives and evaluation of child and adolescent mental health services. *Current Opinion in Psychiatry*, **12**, 393–7.

Kramer, T. and Garralda, M.E. (1998) Psychiatric disorders in adolescents in primary care. *Br J Psychiatry*, **173**, 508–14.

Laitinen-Krispijn, S., Van der Ende, J., Wierdsma, A., and Verhulst, F. (1999) Predicting adolescent mental health service use in a prospective record linkage study. *J Am Acad Child Adolesc Psychiatry*, **38**, 1073–80.

Lavigne, J., Arend, R., Rosenbaum, D., Binns, H.J., Christoffel, K.K., Burns, A., *et al.* (1998) Mental health service use among young children receiving pediatric primary care. *J Am Acad Child Adolesc Psychiatry*, **37**, 1175–83.

Lefebvre, A., Sommerauer, J., Cohen, N., Waldron, S., and Perry, I. (1983) Where did all the 'no-shows' go? *Can J Psychiatry*, **28**, 387–90.

Leff, S. and Bennett, J. (1998) Developing guidelines for community child health staff and examining the referral pathways and outcomes of care in the support of emotionally and behaviourally disturbed children. *Public Health*, **112**, 237–41.

Little, M. and Bullock, R. (2004) Administrative frameworks and services for very difficult adolescents in England. In *Forensic adolescent psychiatry* (ed. S. Bailey and M. Dolan), Chapter 24. London: Arnold.

MacLeod, R., McNamee, J., Boyle, M., Offord, D.R., and Friedrich, M. (1999) Identification of childhood psychiatric disorder by informant: comparisons of clinic and community samples. *Can J Psychiatry*, **44**, 144–50.

Mathai, M. and Markantonakis, A. (1990) Improving initial attendance to a child and family psychiatric clinic. *Psychiatr Bull*, **14**, 151–2.

McKay, M., McCadam, K., and Gonzales, J. (1996) Addressing the barriers to mental health services for inner city children and their caretakers. *Community Ment Health J*, **32**, 353–61.

Meltzer, H., Gatward, R., Goodman, R., and Ford, T. (2000) *Mental health of children and adolescents in Great Britain.* London: The Stationery Office.

Meltzer, H., Gatward, R., Corbin, T., Goodman, R., and Ford, T. (2003) *Persistence, onset, risk factors and outcomes of childhood mental disorders.* London: The Stationery Office.

Munjal, A., Latimer, M., and McCune, N. (1994) Attendance at child psychiatry new patient clinics. *Irish J Psychol Med*, 11, 182–4.

National Assembly for Wales (2002) Too serious a thing—the Carlile Review March 2002. Cardiff: National Assembly for Wales.

Newton, N., Henderson, J., and Goldacre, M. (1995) Waiting-list Dynamics and the Impact of Earmarked Funding. *British Medical Journal*, 311, 783–5.

NHS Health Advisory Service (HAS) (1995) *Together we stand*. London: HMSO.

Parliamentary Under Secretary of State for Health, speaking on 2 February (1999) *Developing effective child and adolescent mental health services, current initiatives and innovations.*

Piacentini, J., Rotherham-Borus, M., Gillis, J., Graae, F., Trautman, P., Garcia-Leeds, C., *et al.* (1995) Demographic predictors of treatment attendance among adolescent suicide attempters. *J Consult Clin Psychol*, 63, 469–74.

Pope, C. (1993) Waiting times for out-patient appointments. *British Medical Journal*, 306, 408–9.

Radical Statistics Health Group (1995) NHS 'Indicators of success': what do they tell us? *British Medical Journal*, 310, 1045–50.

Rawlinson, S. and Williams, R. (2000) The primary-secondary care interface in CAMHS—burden as a defining feature. *Current Opinion in Psychiatry*, 13, 389–95.

Richards, H. (1990) What do they do at the child guidance? *Assoc Child Psychol Psychiatr Rev Newslett*, 12, 13–7.

Rutter, M., Tizard, J., and Whitmore, K. (ed.) (1970) *Education, health and behaviour*. London: Longman.

Rutter, M. and Smith, D.J. (1995) *Psychosocial disorders in young people*. Chichester: Wiley.

Smith, D.H. and Hadorn, D.C. (The Steering Committee of the Western Canada Waiting-list Project) (2002) Lining up for children's mental health services: a tool for prioritizing waiting-lists. *J Am Acad Child Adolesc Psychiatry*, 41, 367–77.

Stallard, P. and Potter, R. (1999) Making sense of child and adolescent mental health services. *Psychiatr Bull*, 23, 217–21.

Stallard, P. and Sayers, J. (1998) An opt-in appointment system and brief therapy: perspectives on a waiting-list initiative. *Clinical Child Psychology and Psychiatry*, 3, 199–212.

Stern, G. and Brown, R. (1994) The effect of a waiting-list on attendance at initial appointments in a child and family clinic. *Child: Care, Health and Development*, 20, 219–30.

Subotsky, F. and Berelowitz, G. (1990) Consumer views at a community child guidance clinic. *Assoc Child Psychol Psychiatr Rev Newslett*, 12, 8–12.

Turner, P. (1998) 350 city youngsters on psychiatric waiting-list. *South Wales Evening Post*, 7 August.

Vostanis, P., Meltzer, H., Goodman, R., and Ford, T. (2003) Service utilisation by children with conduct disorders—findings from the GB national study. *European Child and Adolescent Psychiatry*, 12, 231–8.

Weisz, J.R. and Weiss, B. (1991) Studying the Referrability of Child Clinical Problems. *Journal of Consulting and Clinical Psychology*, 59, 266–73.

Wilkin, D. and Roland, M. (1993) *Waiting times for first out-patient appointment in the NHS*. Manchester: Centre for Primary Care Research, University of Manchester.

Williams, R. (2002) Complexity, uncertainty and decision-making in an evidence-based world. *Current Opinion in Psychiatry*, 15, 343–7.

Williams, R. and Richardson, G. (ed.) (1995) *Together we stand*. London: HMSO.

Williams, R. and Salmon, G. (2002) Collaboration in commissioning and delivering child and adolescent mental health services. *Current Opinion in Psychiatry*, 15, 349–53.

Williams, R., Gilvarry, E., and Christian, J. (2004) Models of service delivery. In *Young people and substance misuse*. London: Gaskell.

Williams, R. A strategic approach to commissioning and delivering forensic child and adolescent mental health services. In *Forensic adolescent psychiatry* (ed. S. Bailey and M. Dolan), Chapter 23. London: Arnold, in press.

Wolpert, M. and Fredman, G. (1996) Child characteristics influencing referral to mental health services. *Child Psychol Psychiatry Rev*, 1, 98–103.

Wu, P., Hoven, C., Bird, H., Moore, R.E., Cohen, P., Alegria, M., *et al.* (1999) Depressive and disruptive disorders and mental health service utilization in children and adolescents. *J Am Acad Child Adolesc Psychiatry*, 38, 1081–90.

Zwaanswijk, M., Verhaak, P., Bensing, J., van der Ende, J., and Velhulst, F.C. (2003). Help seeking for emotional and behavioural problems in children and adolescents—a review of recent literature. *European Child and Adolescent Psychiatry*, 12, 153–61.

Chapter 33

Consultation: more than talking about talking?

Anna Brazier and Fiona Gale

Introduction

Consultation has been offered as part of childrens' mental health services at least from the time of the child guidance movement. Robin Skynner commented on the value of offering consultative services in his address to a London Child Guidance Inter-Clinic conference in 1967 (Skynner 1967): 'Through consultation—we increase the capacity of others to carry a share of the treatment load' and to 'illuminate the social, psychological and psychiatric aspects of problems they [front line staff] meet in the course of their own work' (p. 50). His vivid descriptions of consultancy emphasize its personal impact and multidisciplinary concerns; practitioner issues that are as relevant to us now as they were 30 years ago.

This chapter explores the nature of consultation processes in the context of children's services and looks at the range of theoretical ideas that may inform the practice of consultation today. This chapter offers a rapid introduction to the area. We recommend supplementary sources in each section to aid readers to explore particular areas in more depth.

Definitions

Definitions of consultation and consultancy vary according to context, and references to consultation practices can be found in the literature relating to many professions. In the health literature, consultation usually refers to a medical consultation where a client/patient is seeking a medical opinion, or to professionals seeking to consult with each other about specialist matters. We find an important distinction between *consultation* and *supervision* in the counseling and psychotherapy literature. Hawkins and Shohet (1989, 2000) suggest that supervision and consultation in the helping professions may involve different combinations of 'normative, supportive, and formative' elements.

Definitions also need to take account of service contexts. For health practitioners working in the UK today, services are more and more likely to be organized within the strategic framework provided by *Together we stand* (NHS Health Advisory Service 1995). Those providing Tier 2 functioning are increasingly required to offer training support, consultation, and training to professional colleagues at Tier 1. Thus, there has been, and will be, a demand for more expertise in areas of work other than direct assessment of, and therapy with, children and their families. In this context, we identify the following features of consultation:

a consultant offers specialist expertise;

a consultation is a meeting during which a consultant sets a frame that invites a consultee to set out their dilemma or concern;

a consultation is a collaborative exercise where professional responsibility remains with the consultee within their own professional guidelines (this aspect is explored further under elements of an initial consultation which examines contract setting).

A request to participate in a training initiative involving a new team of primary mental health workers in the area in which one of us works, prompted the first author to think about, and articulate more clearly, the different theoretical frameworks that influence practice as a consultant. The request challenged those involved in the training to think about different practices and to consider how we might go about offering some of these ideas to others. These ideas and frameworks are offered in the next section under the following headings:

current developments in the UK;

key elements of an initial consultation;

reconsidering the helping relationship;

a micro-skills approach to consultation: intentional interviewing;

stages of change: motivational interviewing;

models of supervision;

systemic ideas and consultation;

the application of solution-focused approaches.

Towards the end we provide thoughts on elements of practice, service contexts, and implications for service design.

Current developments in the UK

In order to meet the demands from primary care for services, many Specialist CAMHS have developed liaison schemes in which a child and adolescent psychiatrist, clinical psychologist, or community psychiatric nurse offer advice and consultation to potential referrers. Following on from the HAS report, many CAMHS have recently enhanced their support and liaison provisions for professionals in primary care by introducing the role of primary mental health worker (PMHW).

Primary mental health workers are professionals who are based within and are part of Specialist CAMHS: they work at the interface between primary care and Specialist CAMHS. They may come from a range of backgrounds, i.e. nursing, social work, clinical psychology, or psychiatry, and should have knowledge and expertise in working with children and adolescents with a range of mental health problems and disorders. Their function is to strengthen and support child and adolescent mental health provision within primary care.

The role can include providing consultation and advice on issues relating to: emotional well-being; training on children's mental health issues; supervision and joint working with professionals in the primary care services; joint assessment; and direct work with children and families.

Primary mental health work is continuing to be developed around the UK, with consultation being a main feature of the role in all cases (Arcelus *et al.* 2001). A national survey of CAMHS, undertaken in 1998, showed that 25% of NHS Trusts were developing the role and 40% were examining the possibility of developing the role (Lacey 1999). The developments fall into a number of styles, including services in which the role is provided by professionals as a part of their wider professionals role within Specialist CAMHS or through full-time posts, or as small-scale community initiatives. In Warwickshire, the clinical nurse specialist provides defined times for telephone and face-to-face consultation on a part-time basis in Specialist CAMHS

(Lacey 1998); and in Portsmouth, specialist mental health workers provide consultation, support, and advice to GP practices (Neira-Munoz and Ward 1998) and, now, schools. In Coventry (Gale 1999) and Birmingham, full-time posts have been developed; and, in Norfolk, small community-based multi-agency teams have been introduced, which accept and respond to referrals. Multi-agency teams provide a combination of consultation, training, and some locality-based initiatives for parents and professionals in Gwent in South Wales. In Leicester, Leicestershire, and Rutland, a team of 12 work with professionals in providing care services within defined localities; with professionals working with looked-after children; and in the youth offending teams.

Consultation has been developed as part of the role of primary mental health workers in a variety of formats, which may be on a continuum from one-off telephone and face-to-face consultations, to regular consultation/supervision groups and training for practitioners. Most commonly, the service offered is by telephone and face-to-face consultation. Regular consultation groups are also run in many areas with health visitors, school nurses, and also within staff in GP surgeries. The specialist worker acts mainly as facilitator for discussion and also provides advice, where necessary. It can also be useful for them to work closely with professional community forums and voluntary agencies (e.g. parenting networks, home-start, special needs forums, volunteer groups, local voluntary action forums and domestic violence forums), with a view to providing education and information on children's mental health issues. These activities can strengthen these professionals' confidence in recognizing and intervening with young people who have problems with their mental health or disorders.

The aims and activities of these initiatives can be summarized as follows:

Aims:

> to increase appropriate referral to and use of scarce specialist services;

> to increase speed of identification of mental disorders and provision of appropriate responses to children in need;

> to reduce anxiety in the system and facilitate thoughtful and planned responses;

> to increase general understanding of all staff who come into contact with children and young people about how to promote children's well-being.

Key activities:

> provision of accurate and up-to-date information about local services;

> provision of high-quality information in accessible form about common childhood problems;

> provision of easy access for front-line staff to a 'thinking space' in a range of formats;

> provision of high-quality training in response to assessed need;

> provision of one-off joint consultations with front-line staff and families; and

> provision of information about need and demand service strategists planners and commissioners.

Therefore, consultation must take place within a wider framework of service arrangements, objectives, and plans. This requires that it should be well resourced in respect of administration and IT. Consultants require access to up-to-date and accurate information about clinical problems and local services in a format (e.g. leaflets, books, videos, CDs, etc.) that can be shard easily with other professionals. Consultation services also require collaborative relationships with the specialist services, so that recommendations for referral can be made confidently, where necessary.

Consultants require a range of skills. The main elements or tasks of a consultation are outlined below. This outline provides the frame of reference for the overview of theoretical models to come, and also the skills analysis required, against which to appoint and train consultants.

Key elements of an initial consultation

Setting the frame at the start of a consultation requires good listening skills and the capacity not to offer advice prematurely. This is described by Ivey (2002) as 'the basic listening sequence'. His intentional interviewing model is outlined in the next section. The key elements of an initial meeting are introduced here as stages:

The first stage is to make a contract. This requires abilities to set appropriate boundaries and to attend to any mismatch of expectations. The stages of change model, presented later in this chapter, provide a framework for considering this aspect of a consultation. In some settings, a written contract outlining accountability will be important. In the model outlined here, practitioners/consultees remain responsible for decision-making and action.

The next stage requires consultants to widen the frame of the concern or dilemma presented by the consultee. This could relate to the context of the concern, details of the problem, or the nature of the dilemma. To do this, a consultant needs a theoretical framework to guide their enquiry. The supervision models presented later in this chapter taken together with the sections on solution focused and systemic consultation provide an introduction to this area.

Throughout a consultation, a consultant should assess the nature of the concern. They require a sufficient knowledge to collaborate with a consultee about appropriate action. This implies an ability to pick up signs of problems that require immediate attention (e.g. child protection matters, risk of self-harm, possible serious psychiatric disorder) and sufficient experience, training, and support to contain the anxieties of others about serious concerns. This experience and knowledge is the foundation of the expertise offered by specialist practitioners in child and family work. These abilities plainly set consultation as advanced, in terms of the skills required, and indicate that this kind of work should only be taken on by experienced and well-trained and supervised practitioners.

A consultant should also monitor and review the progress and process of the meeting throughout, so that the focus can be renegotiated if needed. Where the agreement for consultation over a number of meetings is continuing, consultants should able to establish a relationship in which the process of practice can be explored and challenged. We believe that Hawkins and Shohet's process model of supervision presented later can facilitate this kind of enquiry.

At the end of a meeting, consultants should to be able to close at an agreed time, and to summarize and record appropriately.

Reconsidering the helping relationship

Taking on a consultative role means that staff have to make a fundamental shift in their understanding of the nature of helping. A consulting relationship usually requires a shift in thinking for both consultant and consultee. For the consultant who is used to offering answers, or used to 'doing for', the challenge is to make the shift towards listening and asking questions. For a consultee who is used to waiting to be told, or have the problem 'taken out of my hands', the challenge is to take responsibility, to work with the consultant, to be ready to think again, and to take a new perspective.

In order to understand what kinds of shifts may be required of us (in either role), we believe that it is appropriate to explore what expectations we bring from our personal and professional lives. The following questions could form the beginning of such a process of enquiry that can be done individually or as part of team building:

Do I have experience of being consulted and asking for consultation?

In which role do I feel most at ease, and what barriers are there to me having experience of each role?

Which aspects of my professional training are most/least helpful in the two roles?

What personal habits and interactional style will help or hinder me in these roles?

What are the similarities and differences between a therapeutic and consulting role?

New consultants and consultees require opportunities to think and talk about changing roles. We regard this as part of both the initial training and continuing supervision. To this end, any new projects must include funding and time set aside for adequate training and supervision.

The following sections explore the range of theoretical frameworks that may inform a consultation process. In this case, the 'what' of the consultation is a knowledge-base in child and family development, and its possible associated problems and remedies. This is the expertise assumed of practitioners who deliver functions that fall into Tiers 2, 3, and 4. Information about child and family problems and disorders, which may be helpful to those who work in primary care, is well summarized in Spender *et al.* (2000).

A micro-skills approach to consultation: intentional interviewing

Ivey (2002) offers a way of breaking down interpersonal skills so that they can be practiced in isolation and built up again in different combinations, depending on the intention of the interview. Hence the name of the approach: intentional interviewing. Self-observation and the capacity to choose from a range of responses are the key skills that Ivey's model is designed to establish. The foundation skills make up the 'basic listening sequence', which is relevant in therapy and in consultation. These skills are:

attending, culturally appropriate eye contact, body language, vocal qualities, and verbal tracking skills;

using open and closed questions;

observation;

encouraging, paraphrasing, and summarizing; and

reflection of feeling.

During consultation, the combination of skills used should maximize respect for the professional skills of the consultee and maximize the potential for empowerment and problem-solving. For example, too much ill-timed reflection of feeling during a consultation may inflame a consultee who is seeking information. One of the strengths of this model is that it provides a framework for offering detailed feedback from recorded sessions (consultation about consultation), and/or for requesting direct feedback from consultees about the balance of skill use.

Stages of change: motivational interviewing

Miller and Rollnick (2002) offer a framework for thinking about change that has been used extensively in a range of mental health service settings. They believe that, if staff fail to understand clients' position in relation to contemplating change, it is likely that there will be a mismatch between the clients' positions and the interventions offered by the staff. This kind of mismatch increases the potential for resistance. In this model, resistance to change is understood as relational and not as residing within a 'difficult' client (or consultee), and as a result of interactional processes between client and staff members. This motivational model presents helpful questions to ask at different stages of work, and encourages the staff member to think about their contribution to a client's position with regard to contemplating change.

The model suggests the following stages: pre-contemplation, in which the client is not yet thinking about change; contemplation, in which the client is considering the pros and cons of change; action, in which changes are being made; maintenance, in which changes are being sustained; and relapse, in which client has returned to former behaviour.

This approach suggests that consultants should assess their consultees' positions with regard to change (e.g. their approach or way of thinking about each client) and enable their consultees to think about their clients' positions in regard to this also.

Models of supervision

We take it as basic standards for services of acceptable quality that all staff should be provided with coherent and effective supervision. Yet, we are aware that the rollout of supervisors in Specialist CAMHS is presently incomplete. In addition, some staff who work at primary care level may have, or wish to acquire and sustain, more specialist therapy skills and may ask for specialist consultation for particular pieces of work. Clinical supervision models are, therefore, important and of great significance to our approach to consultation. These models tend to be either generic or therapy model-specific. In therapy-specific models, consultants tend to model the therapy in the consultation.

In the examples that follow, we provide a flavour of the many approaches that flourish in CAMHS.

A consultant working from a cognitive-behavioural perspective might well model the therapy skill of agenda-setting, eliciting automatic thoughts, and opportunities to give clear feedback. In a children's service, they would focus on the ways in which a staff member translates these ideas, so that there is a fit with the developmental stage of each child, and with the understanding of the adults involved.

Analytic and psychodynamic consultants might model boundary setting and regularity of place and time. In this way, they set a frame that would allow material relating to the processes of transference to emerge and be available for comment and consideration. There would be a greater focus on the internal world of each child, and on the feeling responses in adult carers and in the staff.

Attachment theorists would be particularly interested in how meetings and partings are dealt with, in the context of continuity and change in relationships. Again, this reflects on how these themes relate to the families and staff, as they negotiate transitions in life and in consulting relationships.

Consultants using a systemic model invite their consultees to consider multiple perspectives, to wonder about how they came to understand things as they do, and to think about what would have to change in order for them to think differently. Systemic consultants are interested in the ways in which beliefs have grown up between people, and how these beliefs affect behaviour and feelings. Thus, systemic consultations usually offer consultees opportunities to widen their frame of reference, to reconsider ideas they may have rejected along the way, and to look at why they may have become very attached to one way of describing things. They are interested in the relationship between staff and clients. However, once the work has began, they will be even more interested in how relationships are changing in the wider network, and what different kinds of conversations can be had, both in the consulting room and beyond. The usefulness of this model in consultation practice is discussed in more detail later in this chapter, together with a section on solution-focused approaches.

Generic supervision models offer a framework for thinking about consultation processes, irrespective of the model of approach to change and/or therapy that is adopted. Stoltenberg's developmental model, described in Watkins (1997), concentrates on adapting supervisory environments to suit the learning stage of each supervisee. It is suggested that less experienced practitioners (here experience relates to the familiarity of the dilemma to the consultee, not their experience as a whole) require more structure and direction. The environment in supervision is, therefore, tuned to this developmental process. While, the model is presented in the context of training and supervising therapists, we argue here that there are elements in the model that can help us to think about consultation. These elements are:

awareness;

motivation;

autonomy (here meaning felt autonomy or confidence as we are not referring to trainees);

consultation environment.

An inexperienced practitioner may be high in motivation, low in awareness, and low in felt autonomy. This pattern may be evident in enthusiastic but unaware consultees, who are seeking direction. More experienced staff may face reduction of motivation as they become more aware of complexity. This pattern may emerge in consultants who are aware but seen to be overwhelmed and also embarrassed by their need to consult. We think that it is important that consultants do not ascribe these elements to the person who comes for consultation but rather look towards how the particular dilemma has generated the different responses in the consultees. To summarize, in this model, the consultation environment, that is the balance of structure and support, and the extent of direction and challenge, should be adjusted to meet the needs of each consultee and the dilemmas each bring.

By contrast, Hawkin and Shohet's (2000) model offers what they describe as a 'holistic and integrative model which draws upon psychodynamic, humanistic, cognitive, behavioural and systemic approaches to therapeutic work' (p. xvii). Their framework encourages supervisors/consultants to think in different ways with the trainees/consultees about particular areas of concern. These are described as supervisor modes. Within each mode, certain questions promote different kinds of discussion. The modes focus on:

the content of each session (i.e. on detailed description without 'premature' understanding);

intervention (what as been tried, what could be tried);

relationships (between consultees and consultants, and between clients and staff, in terms of understanding of the psychodynamic, transference, and counter-transference issues); and

wider organizational contexts.

In summary, we believe that a thorough understanding of supervision models, together with supervised practice, offers 'would be' consultants the widest range of potential interventions.

In the next section, two related consultation frameworks, systemic and solution-focused, are offered. These models share a stance that does not pathologize problems and places emphasis on empowerment and feedback. This makes them particularly suited to the aims and key activities that we outlined at the beginning of this chapter.

Systemic ideas and consultation

The ideas presented here have evolved and continue to evolve from the 'Milan' school of family therapy. Many practitioners now tend to describe themselves as 'Post-Milan Systemic Psychotherapists', a title that, although rather clumsy, reflects the changes in the approach over the last 20 years. The approach is now applied in wider contexts than families and post-modern ideas, e.g. social constructionism, are having major impacts. In the outline below, we summarize some of the central ideas and techniques. Rivett and Street (2003) provide an up-to-date critical analysis of the field.

Key ideas in systemic work

Systems focus. Problems do not arise solely from individuals, but in the relationships that develop between people.

Deconstruction. Problems and difficulties are socially constructed through language and interaction. In order to deconstruct a problem, questions are asked in the areas of beliefs, behaviour, and relationships.

Circularity and reciprocity. Causation is not seen as linear but reciprocal and transactional.

Hypothesizing guides areas of enquiry. Hypotheses are seen as more or less useful in terms of the questions and subsequent conversations they generate.

Narrative and story telling are seen as important. Stories are understood to be the threads we use to make sense of our experiences.

Neutrality and multiple engagement. The stance of therapists is a central consideration. Therapists are encouraged to engage with as many perspectives as are presented and to invite more. The idea of neutrality has promoted much discussion in the literature. We understand this concept to mean remaining non-judgmental and involved, while at the same time using questions to challenge the unacceptable.

Remaining curious requires staff to remain in a position of not quite understanding. In this way, staff may prevent themselves from staying with one formulation or hypothesis when it is no longer useful.

Self-reflexivity. Therapists are required to consider the beliefs and behaviours they bring to their work so that they can use themselves in their work effectively and thoughtfully

Feedback from the client is central to assessing usefulness of hypotheses and questions.

Key techniques in systemic work

Introducing difference is a key task carried out through asking certain kinds of questions and offering reflections.

Circular questions are questions asked of everyone in turn about beliefs, behaviour, and changing relationships.

Reflecting teams offer conversations in the presence of, and, conversations structured in such a way as to introduce difference

Observation offers opportunities for additional perspectives and feedback.

Live and video supervision help staff to stay curious and this facilitates awareness of relationships between clients and staff.

Systemic consultation in practice

Using these ideas as a consultant, requires the basic skills that we outlined earlier. These are: setting the frame; using the basic listening sequence; and using a relevant and up-to-date knowledge-base. In addition, a consultant using a systemic framework asks particular kinds of questions, which are based on the ideas that we have just outlined. We present examples of these questions in the hope that they will give those readers who are unfamiliar with this way of working a clearer picture of the approach.

Questions about the context of the request for consultation

Who is aware that you are contacting us/whose idea was it that we talk?

Who, in the system, might be surprised/relieved/upset to hear that you have contacted us?

What might they hope will/will not happen?

Is there anything we might come up with today that would disappoint/anger etc. X?

Can you tell me what you imagine A and X might be talking to each other about in relation to this?

Questions about the behaviour (and beliefs about the behaviour) that is causing concern

What do you think X would say about how come things have got like this?

Who do you think might be surprised by B's description of C's behaviour, and would anyone else describe it in that way, and who might describe it differently?

If D thought XXX, what difference do you think that would make to her handling of him?

What ideas do you have about why E does that?

How have those ideas helped/hindered her/you in tackling the difficulties?

If things carry on like this, what do people/you think will happen ... what are they/you afraid of?

Who, of the people involved, do we know least about (have we heard least from)?

How has F's description of the difficulty changed over time, what was happening around that change in description?

Questions that re-visit the process of the consultation

As we have been talking, what has struck you most about our conversation?

Which of the ideas we have discussed do you think has been most/least useful?

Which ideas/hypotheses would be hardest to give up at this point?

How similar or different is this conversation from ones you have had already about this and in which ways?

Ideas to use in teams

Exploring core beliefs about behaviour and helping that staff bring to their work.

Noticing pattern and language, how are problems discussed in the team, how can the team ensure that discussions stay open and curious?

Using team structures to promote reflection.

The application of solution-focused approaches

Solution-focused brief therapy was developed in the early 1980s by Steve de Shazer, Insoo Kim Berg and their team at the Brief Therapy Centre in Milwaukee. Initially, it was created as a model for therapy that uses concepts of solution-focused thinking. However, there are a variety of wider contexts in which the precepts can be applied, which include consultation and supervision, team building, coaching, and corporate thinking.

The central premise of solution focused brief therapy is that, during conversations, there should be a shift from problem-domination to solution-orientation, thus enabling development in the client or professional. When applied to consultation, the approach has a number of basic assumptions and these are:

Attempts to understand the origins or causes of problems are not necessarily a step towards their resolution. Indeed, in some instances, discussing problems can become unhelpful in developing useful solutions;

Successful work depends on knowing what the consultee wants to achieve. Once this has been established, the aim of the approach is to find the quickest and most effective way of achieving the defined goals;

Even if a problem seems not to have a resolution, there are always times when the consultee is actually finding ways to solve it, efficient use of time is establishing 'what works' and building upon it;

In most consultations, the consultee should be able to ascertain when a problem has been resolved. Sometimes, small changes that are identified within consultation sessions can set in motion a solution to the problems or lead the system to change in other areas.

As in most consultative relationships, the consultee retains responsibility for taking action, where necessary, after a meeting. Therefore, it is important for both parties (consultee and consultant) to come to an agreement or, in a different language, to have a contract about how consultations will be run. It is the duty of the consultee to assess whether, in retrospect, the consultation has been useful.

Consultation relationships should be reciprocal. Therefore, when approached for a solution-focused consultation, the consultant will assume that the consultee has access to the necessary resources to resolve the problems s/he is bringing. The consultant offers their expertise in setting the frame and in facilitating the process of finding a solution.

When using this approach, the consultant does not attempt to be directive or attempt to solve the problems for the consultee. A consultation session enables consultees to examine for themselves new possibilities and directions in tackling their work. To facilitate this process consultants use questions that elicit strengths and highlight resources. In this way, consultees are supported to begin to believe that there is potential for change to take place.

Elements of practice

The elements, which form the basis of practice in consultation, include the following.

Establishing a context for collaboration

Consultation is a collaborative enterprise to which the consultee will bring their own knowledge and expertise. It is, therefore, important to pay attention to what has been useful in the past and how both parties will know when the process is working and what is the preferred approach for the consultee.

Identifying a preferred future

Goal-setting is central to the process. It is paramount for goals to be described and explored in detail as the consultant has no separate goal for the work other than those agreed with the consultee.

Professional development

The key consideration when deciding on a preferred future is for the consultee to define the circumstances in which they will believe that their work is progressing

Case-related

The initial focus should include agreements about how the consultee will know that a session has been useful. Ways of achieving this include asking the consultee to identify what it would take to convince them that the encounter had been useful or by asking, what would be different? Sometimes, it is useful to ask the consultee about 'third-person perspectives' (i.e. what would your client see happening if this work has been successful)? It is also important help the consultee to notice or identify when small changes are being made sufficient to indicate the case is moving forward.

Establishing what is working

Our approach to consultation includes identifying what is causing forward movement, either for the consultee or the client of the consultee. Rather than focusing on what elements the consultee should be changing, it is vital to encourage consultees to identify what more they could be doing. This involves discussing indicators of progress.

Scaling questions

Scaling questions can be useful in enabling a consultee to develop a clear focus on how far they have progressed toward meeting their goals. They also enable to positively integrate into their work differences in perspective between the client, consultee, consultant, and agency. As examples, the following types of questions can be useful:

On a scale of 1 to 10, 10 representing the achievement of your goals where 1 is no progress, where do you feel you are?

What tells you things are at … and not at 1?

What tells you things have moved to that point?

Scaling questions are particularly helpful in assisting consultees to consider less concrete matters such as confidence and progress.

Identifying resources and determining a context of competence

The context of competence focuses consultees on determining what is available to them to assist them to achieve goals. It is also important to identify the qualities that consultees bring to their work, thereby developing a context of resourcefulness and openness to change (George *et al.* 2001).

Constructive feedback

The effects of consultative conversations can be amplified by giving feedback on the qualities of the consultee and the useful aspects of the process that are identified during a session. At the end of the session it is useful to see if a consultee wants to follow up on the conversation or whether they are satisfied with the current outcomes.

Organizational and service contexts

Throughout this chapter, we have made reference to the wider organizational context in which the work of consultants and consultees takes place. Consultants may encourage in consultees greater awareness of the complexity of cases or dilemmas at the peril of fostering a sense in consultees of them being overwhelmed. It is one thing to foster openness and a willingness to consult within one's own agency, but another to attempt to facilitate different ways of working across agencies. Yet, if specialist mental health staff from various backgrounds are hoping to offer something new and helpful to those staff who work in primary care, they must aim to promote a positive climate for learning. This is a culture in which we think that everyone in a particular locale, whatever their role, feel supported in their work with children and families.

The Centre for Parent and Child Support (CPCS) aims to promote psychosocial well-being through consultation, training, and research. Its well-researched interventions highlight the impact that tailored training followed by structured supervision can have on the work of health visitors and community doctors (Hilton Davis and Crispin Day). Information about its projects is available on the web site, http://www.cpcs.org.uk/default.asp. All the projects involve innovative interventions in which evaluated training and consultation have been shown to make high impact on management of young people and families by staff of primary services.

Peter Birleson (1999) has written about turning CAMHS into learning organizations. He argues that:

> 'A learning organisation works to identify and remove blocks to learning, and build structural and cultural support for continuous learning, adaptation and improvement in order to meet organisational objectives and the needs and aspirations of those involved.

He suggests that, in working towards these aims, they have developed an organization in which 'we can admit what we do not know, collaborate in developing our knowledge, and be more committed and more eclectic in trying to improve work practices and enhance consumer outcome'. It requires commitment and inspiration from planners at every level and across agencies to enable such a culture to emerge. However, establishing good relationships that enable more staff to ask for consultation across agencies does begin to build a network of professionals. As a result, they can begin to feel cared for and become part of Skynner's (1967) sufficient network of care for troubled children and families, in which there is increased understanding and a sharing of the load through effective communication and consultation.

An example: training in consultation

An invitation made to the first author to provide training to a new primary healthcare consultation team was the impetus for us to begin gathering together the ideas presented in this chapter. Naturally, in any training plan, the balance of contributions from the different theoretical frameworks depends on the skill mix of the 'trainees'. The training package offered in one area of Gwent comprised of an initial three days followed by more days on chosen topics. The aim of the initial package was to enable team members to get to know each other and to begin to identify the skills they had already within the team and also their future training needs relating to others, which they anticipated that they might require. Team members came from different backgrounds, including those of social work, health visiting, educational psychology and nursing. The initial three days:

Day one

Introductions—to each other and the project, coupled with invitations to share personal and professional background.

Children and mental health—refresher training and discussions of themes relevant to the project.

What is consultation? Introduction of the main elements of consultation and their implications for helping relationships.

A skills exchange exercise—a facilitated discussion to explore skill mix

Day two

Role play consultations—working in threes to practice giving feedback, using the Ivey micro-skills model recognizing existing skills.

A strategic overview of CAMHS in Wales.

Day three

Systemic ideas and consultation.

Practice using a micro-skills model.

Working in a team, organizational issues, and a role-play of a team referral meeting.

Predictions of future training needs.

The training days were evaluated by using rating scales and interviews. The recorded interviews were analysed using a grounded theory approach. The themes from the interviews were found to fall into two core categories, which were: evaluation of training and team issues. The future training needs that were identified included mental health and team issues. The sub-categories under the theme of team issues highlighted the importance of recognizing the process aspects of team formation right from the start. These were identified as: the impact of relationships and beliefs on teamwork; the nature of future decision-making in the team; identifying roles and functions within the team and in respect of other agencies; skill mix; and recognizing individual's personal emotional responses to anticipated future demands.

Evaluating the roles of the primary mental health workers

Gale (1999) explored primary care professionals' perceptions of the primary mental health worker role using a survey questionnaire and semi-structured interviews ($n = 116$). The findings indicated that certain facets of the role were more important to those interviewed. Professionals who worked in primary care valued a combination of consultation, training, and supervision, followed by joint working and liaison. Seventy nine per cent ($n = 92$) of these professionals indicated that consultation was of most value to them. Forty six per cent of them felt they had been able to tackle children's mental health problems as a result of working with a primary mental health worker. In the semi-structured interviews, one professional said of consultation '… it's knowing that I am going in the right direction and having somebody to discuss it with is very valuable for me, the PMHWs do that …'. Another said, '… for like the very depressed child… sometimes I think I would really like discussion, just plan. I think sometimes a thing can be quite complicated and they involve various people. And I think again it's the clarification is most important …'.

In this chapter we have sought to introduce readers to the concept of consultation and to highlight a range of theoretical frameworks that can inform the process. The importance of service contexts has been emphasized and we have offered brief illustrations of projects that have been run in two different areas in the UK. The last section summarizes the key ideas that we commend to planners and managers of services who seek to enhance provision of the consultation in their area.

Imperatives for future service design and delivery

Sufficient seniority must be given to potential coordinators of consultation services. This acknowledges both the complexity of the consultation task and the level of skills needed to train others. It also ensures the credibility of services within these complex professional networks.

Training and continuing supervision should be offered to both consultants and consultees. This means that appropriate and clear line management and supervision arrangements must be made for all disciplines involved. The time for supervision must be adequately costed, and should be seen as an essential part of the work.

Information and management systems must be constructed that do not mitigate against promoting a learning culture within services and across agencies. These systems should not unintentionally devalue time spent in consultation and training. A common problem is for information systems to focus too heavily on 'head counts' or direct contacts with clients.

The experience of most schemes is that good primary level provision does not necessarily reduce the demand for specialist services.

Potentially good schemes can get into difficulty if existing formal and informal arrangements and relationships have not been taken into account when planning, implementing and evaluating them.

Many new schemes have underestimated the time needed to make links and establish new habits within the networks of existing services. This must be recognized when setting targets.

Talking about talking: a final word

It can be easy for those not trained in consultation and supervision to see talking about talking as little more than tea and sympathy. Without an understanding of the theoretical frameworks that underpin this way of working, it can be difficult to understand the nature of these activities and easy to underestimate their importance to the success of developing CAMHS. Not only do managers need to understand and support these activities, they also need to integrate this understanding into protocols for staff development and appraisal and service monitoring. This is essential if we are to work towards establishing services which can provide high quality, sufficient networks of care, for all of our children and young people.

References

Arcelus, J., Gale, F., and Vostanis, P. (2001) Child mental health problems in primary care. In *Promoting collaborative primary mental health care* (ed. F. Badger and P. Nolan). London: Nelson Thornes.

Birleson, P. (1999) Turning child and adolescent mental-health services into learning organizations. *Clinical Child Psychology*, **4**, 265–74.

De Shazer, S. (1985) *Keys to solution in brief therapy*. New York: Norton Press.

Gale, F. (1999) *When Tiers are not enough; an evaluation of the perceptions and experiences amongst primary care professionals of the primary mental health worker role within child and adolescent mental health*. Unpublished Thesis. MA in Research Methodology, University of Central England, Birmingham.

George, E., Iveson, C., and Ratner, H. (2001) *Supervision and consultation: a solution focused approach*. London: BT Press.

Hawkins, D. and Shohet, R. (1989, 2000) *Supervision in the helping professions*. Buckingham: Open University Press.

Ivey, A.E. (2002) *Intentional interviewing and counseling*. London: Wadsworth.

Lacey, I. (1998) The role of the child primary mental health worker. *Journal of Advanced Nursing* **30** (1), 220–8.

Miller, M.R. and Rollrick, S. (2002) *Motivational interviewing: preparing people for change* (2nd edn). New York: Guilford Press.

Neira-Munoz, E. and Ward, D. (1998) Side by side. *Health Service Journal*, 13 August, 26–7.

NHS Health Advisory Service (HAS) (1995) *Together we stand. The commissioning, role and management of child and adolescent mental health services*. London: HMSO.

Rivett, R. and Street, E. (2003) *Family therapy in focus*. London: Sage.

Scaife, J. (2001) *Supervision in the mental health professions: a practitioner's guide*. Hove: Bruner-Routledge.

Skynner, R. (1967) *Child Guidance from within: Reactions to new pressures*. Paper given at the 23rd Child Guidance Inter-Clinic Conference, London: NAMH Publications.

Spender, Q., Salt, N., Dawkins, J., Kendrick, T., and Hill, P. (2001) *Child mental health in primary care*. Oxford: Radcliffe Medical Press.

Watkins C.E. (ed.) (1997) *Handbook of psychotherapy supervision*. New York: Wiley.

Chapter 34

Child and adolescent mental health services—roles, functions, and management in an era of change

Mike Shooter and Alison Lagier

Introduction

To understand the complexity of the changes that CAMHS are going through in their structure and function, and to appreciate the problems of managing CAMHS through those changes, we need a model. It is difficult to think of a better model than that which CAMHS practitioners so often use for those in their care—child development. What are the tasks facing the developing child and what style of parenting is needed for healthy development to take place?

The good enough parent, in its broadest Winnicottian sense, is one who provides a secure envelope within which a child can experiment with acceptable risks; one who patrols the boundaries within which the child is free to establish its own identity—attitudes to self, family, peer group, and community; how those attitudes are expressed; and to what lengths it is permissible to follow them in social relationships.

Just so, the good enough manager is one who is neither so domineering that other members of the team are never allowed to think for themselves, nor so *laissez-faire* that individual members have to find a premature adulthood in the absence of leadership. And just so with this chapter. It does not aim to lay down a prescription for the structure, function, and management of every CAMHS; nor is it an argument for free experiment. Rather, it outlines the broad principles within which debate can take place and services can find their own solutions. In the process, it identifies the fault lines in poorly working services, the imperatives for change that impinge on those fault lines, and the proper management of such change.

Faltering services

Let us begin by describing a typical CAMHS of a decade or more ago—no service in particular, but every service in general. Like so many services, it has grown 'like topsy' over the years, cobbling together whole-time, part-time, and bits of jobs from many different disciplines, as the opportunity arose. Some are managed and paid for wholly within the health budget; some work partly within the health trust but are paid for and managed from an outside agency, such as the local authority. It is unclear what particular roles and responsibility each job holder has.

The service has a general, egalitarian ethos with individual practitioners having a good deal of case autonomy; but there is no formal protocol for this. Practice differs from one consultant team to another and referral agents, such as general practitioners, have no guide to referral pathways and responsibilities. The service has been dominated in the past by a succession of parental figures in psychiatry and nursing but this has begun to fragment as new consultants develop different ways of working and a personal understanding with agencies in their area.

The out-patient service has followed 'patch' lines without the geographical boundaries ever being made clear. They have changed many times. General practitioners often ignore them in favour of the consultant with whom they get on best, and there is an increasing traffic of disaffected families across the borders. Many referrers in primary care, paediatrics, schools, and social services say that they find difficulty working out who to refer and end up doing the work themselves. Some of the CAMHS team say that they spend far too much time doing non-specialist, day-to-day work with families in whom primary care seems to have lost interest once they have been referred.

Although the consultants spend most of their time in the out-patient clinics, they have access to day-patient and in-patient facilities covering the whole service. The consultants have managed these facilities sometimes in a shared capacity, sometimes by taking turns. In effect, the units are under the control of senior nursing staff for whom there is little rotation across the different theatres of work. There is no doubt that a good deal of effective work is done on the units in individual and group therapies, but little is written down other than in the daily nursing records. The units are increasingly stretched by the demands of long-term work with behaviourally disturbed adolescents from chaotic backgrounds. Emergency referrals of seriously ill adolescents have begun to find their way onto the adult wards at weekends—to the shock of carers and anger of ward staff.

The service is said to be doing 'as well as it has always done' but there are growing signs of unrest. Waiting-lists are getting longer. Several recent complaints have come in from families but the protocol for investigating them has been unclear. It is getting more difficult to recruit permanent staff and the number of agency staff and locums is increasing. The service is not as popular as it once was with trainees. The consultants meet less and less often, citing pressures of work. The psychologists seem to be developing a separate service of their own, with no clear demarcation between it and CAMHS. It has been impossible to answer commissioners' questions because no detailed figures have ever been kept by which to audit service progress.

In reality, of-course, this is a service that has lost its way. It is reminiscent of so many that were assessed by the Health Advisory Service in the preparation of its report, *Together we stand*, on the commissioning, role, and management of CAMHS so many years ago (NHS Health Advisory Service 1996) but regretfully still familiar today (Carlile Review 2002) This is by no means an exhaustive list, but it would not be difficult to pinpoint ten principles of good practice being flouted here. No hierarchy is implied and all are inter-dependent (Box 34.1).

Ten points of poor practice

1. Vague service aims

Arguments rage about the value of mission statements, which are meaningless without a clear idea of how they might be translated into practice. But a service needs a general statement of what it is setting out to achieve and what its place is, therefore, amongst the matrix of services involved with children, adolescents, and their families. The above service has inherited a vague

Box 34.1 Ten points of poor practice

1. Vague service aims.
2. Lack of management.
3. Confused roles and responsibilities.
4. Weak internal communication.
5. Poor record keeping.
6. Idiosyncractic clinical practice.
7. Indecisive service remit.
8. Unclear referral pathways.
9. Audit aversion.
10. Precarious commissioning.

set of values and traditions from the past. There is no agreed idea of what they imply and whether they are still the most effective way to go about delivering a CAMHS in a modern business world.

2. Lack of management

As a result, this service cannot be said to be 'managed', though it is 'led' in many different and often conflicting ways. The ethos of the service has been enshrined in the past within the person of senior figures who acted as dictators of what should be done, with varying degrees of benevolence. Now individual consultants are developing their own sub-services within their own geographical patch, alongside other agencies in their own areas. Not surprisingly, the fault lines show up most where collaboration is important, as in the day and in-patient units with the plethora of tasks the staff are asked to perform (Royal College of Psychiatrists Council Report CR76 1999). Thus, with no central management, no service protocols can be laid down and the scene is set for fragmentation.

3. Confusion of roles and responsibilities

CAMHS are nothing if not multidisciplinary, but multidisciplinary teams need agreed roles and lines of responsibility. This service has grown up on the premise that all are equal and roles can be diffused across different disciplines with a great deal of individual autonomy. In reality, there was always a power battle within such services, between different disciplines and their management structures and between different individuals with varying degrees of interest, training and expertise—'a systems dilemma' (Reder 2003). When crises came, this often descended into mutual recrimination in which staff retreated into a psychiatric, nursing, or social work identity and a senior figure (usually the consultant) was chosen to carry the can as 'responsible medical officer', as if that phrase had any validity outside the Mental Health Act. If different members do not have a clear idea of what particular role they bring to the team, it will be confusing to them, to outside agencies who do not know who is in charge of their referral, and to patients and carers, who do not know where to turn to in any situation. If they do have a clear idea of their role, the staff members can take a proper responsibility for what they do, on both a clinical and legal level (Carlile Review 2002).

4. Weak internal communication

Despite such dangers, small-scale traditional CAMHS often compensated for their lack of structure with frequent internal communication. Staff sat down and discussed what was happening in individual teams and cross-service groups, and close relationships were developed on a basis of familiarity and respect. As services fragment, such face-to-face meetings become practically impossible or emotionally avoided—as with the consultant group here. Weakening lines of internal communications between staff are likely to be reflected downwards, in relationships with patients and carers, and upwards, in relationships with other agencies. It is just such a situation that is identified over and over again in inquiry reports as one of the key elements in clinical case disaster (Department of Health 2002).

5. Poor record keeping

Ironically, frequent personal contact often meant that things were never written down. Some disciplines, like nursing, had their own protocol for record keeping and stuck to it, independently of everyone else. But medical consultants rarely recorded the content of their regular contact with patients, for example, on a day or in-patient unit. Their knowledge of their patients and their families and their circumstances might have been an intimate one, but it could not easily be passed on or drawn upon when the consultant was not around. At the very least, this did not make for good case management; at its worst, it led to consultants being pilloried in court when lawyers looked with contempt at sets of notes with months between entries. More comprehensive sets of notes were kept of out-patient appointments but to no consistent formula. They were often recorded in files kept in conjunction with paediatrics, with all the lack of confidentiality that implied. While we would never equate good communication entirely with written records, it is difficult to achieve without them (Working Together to Safeguard Children 1999).

6. Idiosyncratic clinical practice

In such circumstances, free from any protocols, individual consultants and their teams became idiosyncratic in attitudes and practice. The advent of CPD and yearly appraisal meant that there was some monitoring of overall performance, but this still allowed clinicians to follow different sets of criteria for referral and treatment in their own areas. To some extent, of-course, that could be seen as healthy. Patients and their carers often say that they do not want a homogeneous consultant mass who fear all innovation lest breaking the guidelines will lead to the steps of the court house or the GMC. What they want is choice—between different teams with different approaches, each practising to the same high standard. But where services have no overall approach to a particularly demanding illness, such as ADHD, the result can seem like postcode anarchy, and leave disaffected families and their referrers to play off one part of a service against another. The key to good, consistent practice and informed patient choice lies in the evidence that is freely available but often difficult to find one's way around (Scott *et al.* 2001).

7. Indecisive service remit

Clarity of remit is made impossible by such idiosyncrasy. At any moment in time, there are over 10 million under 18-year-olds in the United Kingdom. All are vulnerable without the proper, health promoting, preventative inputs. One-fifth of these, 2 million, will already have problems sufficient to interfere with the normal enjoyment of childhood and adolescence. Half of these, 1 million, will be suffering with classifiable psychiatric diagnoses. Even the top 3% of these—the most severely disordered children (psychotic, dangerously disturbed, suicidally depressed or on the edge of anorexic, metabolic collapse)—will present terrifying figures when extrapolated to a local service level. In the face of them, the well-functioning CAMHS must decide what level of need it can satisfy with the resources available to it—and communicate that clearly in protocols agreed with commissioners and referral agents (Wallace *et al.* 1997). But different consultants, unmanaged by agreed protocols, may have very different ideas about where to draw the line around an appropriate referral. This leaves everyone confused, not least the patients, who may find themselves rejected by one team and accepted by another.

8. Unclear referral pathways

With a shaky internal structure, and poor external liaison with other agencies, a CAMHS is unlikely to have a clear pathway for referrals once made. This means that there can be no tiered pyramid of broadbased primary care, narrowing through increasingly specialized secondary, tertiary, and quaternary facilities. There will be no clear criteria for how patients are passed up and down through those levels of care, and no sense of whose job it is to do what to the patients at each stage of that journey. Still less will there be any plan between agencies to provide a package of care, to which many agencies will offer an input simultaneously, and the balance of which may shift over time as the patient's disorder gets better or worse. The result will be the sort of complaints in the service described, that primary carers are doing specialist jobs and vice versa. As ever, the lack of agreed pathways is likely to be shown up most keenly in the emergency situation, with potentially dangerous consequences. And safety must come first; once safety 'as a fundamental pre-requisite has been addressed, attention must turn to the pursuit of quality' (Learning from Bristol 2001).

9. Audit aversion

It is possible that the mystique of such services, of working with difficult children and adolescents in idiosyncratic ways and in a culture alien to most of medicine (including adult psychiatry), may have 'protected' CAMHS from too close an inquiry into their clinical and cost-effectiveness. That mystique may even have been encouraged by some consultants for just such machiavellian reasons. If you haven't got any figures, you can't be held to account. Others, on a matter of principle, may have been reluctant to do anything so 'demeaning' to a patient's distress as to label it with a diagnostic classification, even if an appropriate one could be found. What that has done, of-course, is to make impossible any audit of the effectiveness of treatments in general and of individual consultants or their services in particular. At the very best, this is a waste of the precious resources available to CAMHS teams and is selling the patients short (NICAPS 2003).

10. Precarious commissioning

At its worst, however, this lack of audit, together with all the other vagaries of the poorly functioning CAMHS, prevents the writing of a business case with which to persuade commissioners that existing resources, or increased funding, would be well spent. In the modern NHS, commissioners look for a service that is being well-managed with a clear remit in mind, a clear structure to fit that remit, agreed protocols, and regular audit along relevant outcome measures (Kurtz 1996). Without such evidence of good management, the commissioners may well turn elsewhere. The traditional, fragmenting service we started off with, 'fragile and vulnerable

Box 34.2 Ten pressures for change

1. Increasing demand.
2. Changes in allied services.
3. Political imperatives.
4. Reassessing service roles and values.
5. Empowering users and their carers.
6. Incidents, complaints, and investigations.
7. External reviews.
8. Trust reconfigurations.
9. Risk management.
10. Patterns of commissioning.

to the financial and political tensions that exist between statutory authorities' (Mental Health Foundation 1999), may have had its day in every sense.

In such a precarious state, a service is ill-equipped to withstand the rigours of change without the fault lines we have talked about becoming unbridgeable cracks. The pressures for change within the NHS as a whole, within psychiatry in particular, and within child and adolescent work especially, are huge. Again this is not a complete list of discrete factors, but ten imperatives for change are clearly identifiable (Box 34.2).

Ten pressures for change

1. Increasing demand

The balance has shifted between resources (static at best) and demand (increasing year by year), such that CAMHS and their staff struggle to cope, individuals become demoralized and leave, recruitment is poor, the workforce is reduced to unsafe levels, and the vicious cycle keeps turning. For services, this means a complex transition from deciding between vertical priorities of disorders to horizontal levels of seriousness. In the past, we have made decisions between competing disorders—the looked-after children from local authorities, the ADHD disorders from the school classroom, the psychosomatic problems that bedevil paediatric clinics, or the conduct disorders that are the bane of parent and GP alike and cost the country enormous sums of money every year (Knapp *et al.* 1999). In the future, to make best use of their expertise, CAMHS may have to confine their direct intervention to high levels of severity across all disorders, and find ways of supporting primary care agencies in dealing better with other children and adolescents in their care. In the meantime, individual practitioners struggle to maintain quality over quantity; to establish what they can safely and effectively achieve, and put back the responsibility for waiting-lists to where it really belongs, commissioners.

2. Changes in allied services

Other services within the care of children, adolescents, and families have their own problems and their own ways of dealing with them. Local authority social services have been swamped by the consequences of physical, sexual, emotional abuse, and neglect and the statutory crises they engender. They have little time left for the day-to-day family work they once saw as the bread and butter of their job. School success, for teachers as much as their pupils, is now measured in academic achievement. There is less room for an holistic approach to the 'strugglers' and disadvantaged children may rapidly find themselves excluded. Psychologists and community paediatricians, on the other hand, may seem to be moving into territory once thought to be the exclusive domain of CAMHS, on the back of developmental problems, ADHD, and the like. Looked at positively, differences between services in conceptual approach, models of care, priorities, and points of intervention, can lead to a rich diversity of approach. But the 'lack of a common language' (Everybody's Business 2001) can equally lead to tension between agencies and problem children passed like a relay-baton from one waiting-list to another. At the very least, just as in families, no-one can change their own role without the roles of everyone else being affected too.

3. Political imperatives

And then, of-course, there are the political imperatives for change. Some CAMHS may have fought for these, often in the teeth of disinterest or hostility. Thus it was difficult to get child and adolescent mental health into the National Service Framework for children in England, but having done so it seemed to unlock a great deal of new money, in theory at least, through health and local authority budgets. In Wales, a National Strategy for CAMHS (Everybody's Business 2001) was achieved with little difficulty and politicians expressed themselves committed to it, but with no money attached, even in theory. However welcome these plans may have been, and however clear the evidence base for them, they will all involve change for services and practitioners, often with very new roles and responsibilities attached. Other political solutions have been thrust at clinicians with no evidence-base whatsoever and at a speed that suggests that change itself has become the rationale rather than any reasonable outcome; 'constant change is the enemy of continuity' (Carlile Review 2002).

4. Reassessing roles and values

But not all change is externally driven. Many of the disciplines involved in CAMHS delivery have been reassessing the values they hold most dear and which underpin their perception of their proper role. Nurses, weighed down by everyday patient care, have sought higher skills and management qualifications. Psychiatrists, burdened by the bureaucracy of management, have wondered how to get back to what they most enjoy—face-to-face contact with complex clinical situations. As roles change, CAMHS will need to take that into account within the complicated web of relationships and responsibilities in the multidisciplinary teams.

5. Empowering service users and their carers

The empowerment of users and their carers has been one of the most dramatic and long overdue aspects of modern health service change. Much of this has been achieved at a corporate level, through patients' forums and other bodies. This has tended to outstrip their ability to make a real impact on the treatment of their own illness. The resultant frustration has sometimes turned into open hostility to staff or a sense of learned helplessness, where the expectations of the patient are not matched by the ability of the doctor to satisfy them. Children and adolescents, of course, are in a particularly vulnerable situation. They often feel trapped between the power of the therapist and the influence of family carers, who may be part of the problem rather than a source of support. This will be particularly true of disadvantaged children in local authority care or from black and minority ethnic populations. With the growing intervention of children's advocates, however, the voice of patients will have to be heeded by CAMHS and services modified to be more accessible and acceptable to all groups (Richardson and Joughin 2000). This will involve walking a tight rope between what children say they want, what CAMHS may perceive as their real needs, and what the service can realistically provide.

6. Incidents, complaints, and investigation

Nothing inspires change more than an investigation—from relatively minor patient and carer complaints, through to full blown inquires into serious incidents, such as Statutory Part 8 reviews, and the horrors of the lawsuit. In an increasingly litiginous world, where some actions are inspired by the possibility of getting money rather than justice, such change may be a negative one—a retreat into 'tribalism' and defensive practice that is understandable but in the long run will only increase patients' suspicions (Learning from Bristol 2001). Some change will be positive. Even the Secretary of State has been known to admit in Health Select Committee that medicine is not an exact science, doctors are fallible, and provided they learn from their mistakes, investigations should identify patterns to change rather than pillory individuals (Department of Health 2002). After investigations like that into the Bristol Royal Infirmary or Alder Hey Hospital, this is sometimes difficult to believe. Down at grass roots level, however, CAMHS need at least to offer clear complaints procedures, be ready to direct patients to a second opinion and heed the consequences. Employers should remember that 'staff have rights too'—to appropriate support and a fair hearing (Carlile Review 2002).

7. External reviews

On top of all this, services will be subject to a plethora of external reviews—from Royal College training scheme accreditation visits to regular governmental inspections by agencies such as the Commission for Health Audit and Inspection (CHAI). A clear distinction needs to be maintained between appraisal of the individual doctor's performance and clinical governance—the assessment of services, whose shortcomings may be due to lack of resources rather than any clinical failing. If CAMHS practitioners play the game right, such inspections can put pressure on commissioners to provide more resources and in this the clinicians and users of services may be on the same side. But it can often seem a risky way of bringing about change and one for which CAMHS staff may not feel themselves well trained.

8. Trust reconfigurations

The configuration of trusts has sometimes changed so rapidly that CAMHS within them have not known in what 'bed' they are going to wake up from one year to the next. Such instability undermines any long-term service planning. Where choice has been possible, CAMHS have sometimes opted to work within mental health trusts, along with their adult psychiatry colleagues, sometimes within child health trusts, along with paediatricians, and sometimes within community trusts, along with many other agencies. The same would apply in terms of directorates within larger trusts. The quality of the experience seems to depend more on relationships between senior personnel and their willingness to collaborate across boundaries than on any particular configuration. CAMHS should be wary of too prescriptive a direction. 'The important issue is not where these (services) are located but how they are able to draw upon or contribute to all relevant expertise to meet the needs of individual children' (Everybody's Business 2001).

9. Risk management

The public prejudice that surrounds mental illness, the fears upon which it is based, the newspaper headlines that fan those fears, and the politicians who pander to them, have so concentrated the minds of clinicians on risk that therapy seems to have taken second place. Of course, CAMHS have a duty to protect children and adolescents from the consequences of their illness and other people from the behaviour in which that illness may be expressed; but risk can never be wholly eliminated. Indeed, creative therapeutic relationships, just like parenting, may well demand an element of risk within which children and adolescents may be helped to find new ways of running their own lives. The pressures, however, are immense for clinicians and services working under the shadow of blame if things should go wrong. CAMHS will need a well-worked out protocol for managing risk, for example, in out-of-hours emergency situations, with agreement for co-operation between agencies. This is particularly so when Mental Health Act changes threaten to drive larger numbers of disturbed adolescents towards CAMHS at a time when in-patient facilities are woefully inadequate (Royal College of Psychiatrists Council Report CR106 2002b).

10. Patterns of commissioning

Finally, the pattern of commissioning of CAMHS is changing rapidly as responsibility passes to Primary Care Trusts or Local Health Groups. There are grave anxieties about whether such organizations will have the motivation, the skills, or the breadth of horizon successfully to commission specialized services, but it may also be an opportunity for creative thinking (Everybody's Business 2001). If joint working between different agencies in health, education, and social services is essential to the proper handling of child and family needs, why not jointly commission them to do the job? If those needs are the responsibility of all of us to satisfy, why not pool our resources too, including the budget? Experiments in commissioning abound and CAMHS should treat them as opportunities rather than threats (Davey and Littlewood 1996). Anything has to be better than haphazard bidding for pots of money that appear on a Friday and demand a business case by the following week. We owe both patients and staff a better plan than that.

How then is change to be managed, given that eight years after the HAS report, a member of the Welsh Assembly, when discussing the Carlile Report, could still be amazed that 'so few clinicians who deal with children have any expertise in children's services' (Melding 2002). Because of the complexity involved, the administration of the NHS is turning increasingly to professional 'change managers' to facilitate its agenda. Most CAMHS will not have the luxury of such an appointment. At the opposite end of the scale, however, it cannot be assumed that senior clinicians will pick up the art of management for change by some process of osmosis in their training; they will not. This applies just as much to child psychiatric staff, who ought to know something about change management through their systems therapy and family therapy skills. 'Buggins turn' amongst the consultants—'I've done my whack, now it's your turn to take us through the next phase'—can only lead to dispute and disaster. A manager, even one appointed from within, must be chosen on merit. 'Clinicians should not be required or expected to hold managerial roles on bases other than competence for the job' (Learning from Bristol 2001). The person most qualified may come from any discipline, including an administrative,

---

Box 34.3 Ten processes for managing change

1. Listening to staff.
2. Agreeing a rationale.
3. Laying down of a strategic plan.
4. Assessing need.
5. Assessing the resources required.
6. Reforming structures and protocols.
7. Monitoring staff feelings.
8. Working round resistance.
9. Helping casualties.
10. Auditing outcomes.

---

non-clinical one. Coping with the tensions this may set up with senior staff not used to being managed will be part of the skills involved. Once again, without it being a finite list, we might offer a ten-point process in a strategy for change (Box 34.3).

Ten processes for managing change

The first three stages of that process are aimed at establishing the 'ownership' of change by the service staff. Much of the resentment amongst staff within the NHS has been caused by their feeling that change has been imposed upon them by a government that has assumed that all professionals are Luddites dedicated to the status quo, rather than creative thinkers who might be excited by the prospect of doing things differently and better. The agents of that imposition are often seen as management that interferes with clinical work rather than freeing 'the hands of those whose real abilities lie in caring for patients' (Bell 2003). The good CAMHS manager must dispel that perception.

1. Listening to staff

Thus the ideas and opinions of staff need first to be listened to. It is tempting for a hard-pressed trust executive to look for a quick-fix expert who will spot the problems after minimal consultation and inflict solutions, in a take-it-or-leave-it manner. Any changes thus achieved are likely to be grudgingly accepted, if at all, by staff who will have good reasons for fearing change and will be driven back into their corner if their fears are not appreciated. The most successful change comes from within the organization; surprisingly, the more staff are allowed to contribute ideas about changes, the more they want to be involved in them (Sturt 1995).

2. Agreeing a rationale

Out of this discussion, agreement on the rationale for change may emerge. In other words, staff may have shifted from seeing themselves as the victims of change to feeling that they are the architects of change in their own service. This may need to be achieved with key, senior staff across all disciplines initially, and then with the wider staff in a cascading system. But the ultimate aim is a move away from the stultifying bureaucracy and tribal professionalism that inhibits innovation to a learning culture in which staff can come together around a common goal.

3. Laying down a strategic plan

A strategic plan, including a timetable, can be laid down to meet this goal. Such a timetable is important if the process of change is to have a sense of purpose. As in behaviour therapy with their patients, CAMHS staff will need the overall goal to be broken down into a series of smaller, achievable, more immediate targets—with regular review of where each has got to.

In essence, all this involves putting three huge questions to the CAMHS involved, which together make up an 'organizational diagnosis': 'Where are we?' (in terms of the delivery of services at present); 'Where do we want to get to?' (in terms of future services); and 'How do we best get there?' (in terms of the process of service change) (Sturt 1995). Answering those questions means putting some practical flesh on the theoretical discussions, in a further three stage process.

4. Assessing need

A thorough assessment must be carried out of the needs in the child and adolescent population served by the CAMHS (Harrington *et al.* 1999). This can be done with reference to national statistics for the prevalence of child and adolescent disorder in any population (Meltzer *et al.* 2000) and the local profile of needs built up from such indices as perinatal mortality rates, under sixteen pregnancy rates, the proportion of lone-parent families, the numbers of children on the child protection register or looked after by the local authority, the numbers with a statement of special educational need, children and adolescents absent from school without authority or excluded, children from refugee groups, those with chronic physical illnesses and other vulnerable conditions, those involved with the law in all its forms, unemployment, and substance misuse rates, and so on (Finch *et al.* 2000).

5. Assessing the resources required

Having established the need, a parallel assessment of available resources should follow. This should not be restricted to staff and facilities within CAMHS itself. That service should be seen as an integral part of the network of all agencies dealing with children, adolescents, and their families in the catchment area, including voluntary as well as professional organizations, working collaboratively together in a spectrum of care (Wallace *et al.* 1997). Needless to say, such a concept can only be based on consensus agreements across all those agencies. The strategy for change is a strategy for everyone, not just CAMHS (Finch *et al.* 2001).

6. Reforming structures and protocols

On the basis of these two assessments, practical protocols can be worked out for the handling of problems within a tiered hierarchy of CAMHS services, what particular disorders are appropriate to direct work within that structure, what disorders are the prime responsibility of other agencies with support from CAMHS staff, and what problems are the socio-economic responsibility of politicians. Distressing though it may be, and tempting though it may be for CAMHS staff to become involved with it, re-framing social deprivation as mental illness is to accept responsibility for it without the power to make it better.

However well all this process is carried out, change will be painful for service staff. Just like the children of families in their care, staff will not agree to change unless the pain of it is less than the pain of what they have got, and unless they are offered a different way of doing things that would bring some relief. The next three stages of the process, therefore, are directed at helping with the emotional repercussions of change.

7. Monitoring staff feelings

Staff feelings need to be monitored regularly, through group forums and individual access for staff to the manager. It is one of the functions of a service manager to offer such supports, though the service might consider the employment of an outside facilitator at times of particular difficulty. The manager will need to ensure that adequate supervision is available for all staff. It should include 'scrutinizing and evaluating the work carried out, assessing the strengths and weaknesses of the practitioner and providing coaching development and pastoral support' (Working Together to Safeguard Children 1999).

8. Working round resistance

There is no defence that our patients may erect against the pain of change that staff are not capable of erecting too. Indeed, it has repeatedly been shown that the feelings of patients and staff closely reflect each other—the 'care-giver's plight'. It would hardly be surprising if they found the same ways of dealing with the stress of those feelings. Some may lapse into a mutual learned helplessness in the face of forces apparently beyond their control; some will fight change with a continual, dogged resistance or guerilla, hit and run tactics at key points; some will get stuck in the process of planning for change without ever being able to move on to effect it: 'If we just had one more meeting...'. Such defences will need to be identified and worked around with the same sensitivity the staff would use in individual or family therapy with CAMHS patients. In the cool logic of management theory, this has been talked about as 'force-field analysis', plotting defences and resistances along the path of change and the often surprising sources of power for and against it (Lewin 1972). More empathic CAMHS managers appreciate that changes for some staff might be more like bereavement. We should never underestimate the sense of loss in giving up long-held roles and practices, and the life-style that has grown around them. But as with all bereavement, this is an opportunity for greater fulfilment too.

9. Helping casualties

Inevitably, however, there will be casualties. We know the sort of situations that render both patients and their doctors most vulnerable (Royal College of Psychiatrists Council Report CR101 2002a)—the inexperience of junior doctors and egotism of seniors, the burden of unrealistic expectations, unresolved personal issues and rigid personalities, confusion of roles and conflicts of values, and isolation. It is such pressures that so often lead to inappropriate practice and GMC censure. But the pressure may also lead to frank psychiatric illness. CAMHS staff are no more immune to mental health problems than their patients and it has been shown how many staff are already developing serious levels of distress on general health questionnaires issued to them (Littlewood *et al.* 2003). Such levels of distress demand local and national schemes for mentoring and support, but every service will need clear protocols for how to direct those who need it into active psychiatric treatment. It does not help staff to collude with the fear of stigma, understandable though it may be in those 'in the trade' and fearful of their jobs. Such collusion may in the long run lead to tragedy.

The role of management in an era of change is therefore a complex one demanding many skills. It calls for basic management training for all and advanced level training for key people charged with the task of overall leadership—and, of-course, protected time to perform that task (Everybody's Business 2001) And it is not a one-off exercise. Just as the children, adolescents and families in our care are developing over time, so CAMHS will continue to develop with changing needs.

10. Auditing outcomes

Part of that process must be a built-in monitoring of agreed outcome measures, based on both objective and narrative evidence. Are the service and the staff working more effectively with their patients and are they feeling better in the process? Regular record keeping will facilitate audit of individual elements of the service. All needs to be open to further adjustment in the light of such audit, the closing of the audit loop, in a continuous cycle.

Thus we come back to where this chapter started—with the model of the good enough parent and the good enough manager, shepherding those in their charge through the phases of healthy development. Such a manager can be seen to 'engage' the fledgling CAMHS in the excitement, as well as the difficulty, of change and help it 'work through' those difficulties as staff take a more and more responsible role in the process themselves. Ultimately, of-course, the test of the manager's role is whether 'separation' can be successful too. Has the service matured to the level at which any individual manager is expedient? Can the manager leave without the service collapsing in its parent's wake?

References

Bell, A. (2003) The measurement of management. *British Journal of Health Care Management*, **9**, 115.

Carlile Review (2002) *Too serious a thing*. Cardiff: National Assembly for Wales.

Davey, R. and Littlewood, S. (1996) You pays your money and you takes your choice. Helping purchasers to commission an appropriate CAMHS. *Psychiatric Bulletin*, **20**, 272–4.

Department of Health (2002) *Learning from past experience—a review of serious case reviews*. London: Department of Health.

Everybody's Business (2001) *Child and adolescent mental health services strategy document*. Cardiff: The National Assembly for Wales.

Finch, J., Hill, P., and Clegg, C. (2001) *Standards for CAMHS*. Brighton: HAS/Pavilion Publishing.

Harrington, R., Kerfoot, M., Verluyn, C. *et al.* (1999) Developing needs-led childhood and adolescent mental health services: issues and prospects. *European Child and Adolescent Psychiatry*, **8**, 1–10.

Knapp, M., Scott, S., and Davies, J. (1999) The cost of anti-social behaviour in young children: a pilot study of economic and family impact. *Clinical Child Psychology and Psychiatry*, **4**, 457–73.

Kurtz, Z. (1996) *Treating children well: a guide to using the evidence base in commissioning and managing services for the mental health of children and young people*. London: The Mental Health Foundation.

Learning from Bristol (2001) *The report of the public inquiry into children's heart surgery at the Bristol Royal Infirmary 1984–95*. London: HMSO.

Lewin, K. (1972) Quasi–stationary social equilibria and the problem of permanent change. In *Organizational development: values, process and technology* (ed. N. Margulies and A. Raia), pp. 65–70. New York: McGraw Hill.

Littlewood, S., Case, P., Gaber, R., and Lindsey, C. (2003) Recruitment, retention, satisfaction and stress in consultant child and adolescent psychiatrists. *Psychiatric Bulletin*, 27, 61–8.

Melding, D. (2002) *Plenary session 23rd April on government's response to the Carlile Report*. Cardiff: National Assembly for Wales.

Meltzer, H., Gatward, R., Goodman, R., and Ford T. (2000) *Mental health of children and adolescents in Great Britain*. London: HMSO.

Mental Health Foundation (1999) *Bright futures. Promoting children and young people's mental health*. London.

NHS Health Advisory Service (1996) *Together we stand. Thematic review on the commissioning, role and management of CAMHS*. London: HMSO.

O'Herlihy, A., Worrall, A., Bannerjee, S., Jaffa, T., Hill, P., Mears, A., *et al*. (2001) *National in-patient child and adolescent psychiatry study (NICAPS)*. Final report to the Department of Health. London: Royal College of Psychiatrists Research Unit.

Reder, P. (2003) Consultant responsibilities in CAMHS: a systems dilemma. *Psychiatric Bulletin*, 27, 68–71.

Richardson, J. and Joughin, C. (2000) *The mental health needs of looked after children*. London: Gaskell Publications, Royal College of Psychiatrists.

Royal College of Psychiatrists (1999) *Guidance on staffing of child and adolescent in-patient units*. Council Report CR76. London: Royal College of Psychiatrists.

Royal College of Psychiatrists (2002) *Vulnerable patients, vulnerable doctors. good practice in our clinical relationships*. Council Report CR101. London: Royal College of Psychiatrists.

Royal College of Psychiatrists (2002) *Acute in-patient care for young people with severe mental illness*. Council Report CR106. London: Royal College of Psychiatrists.

Scott, A., Shaw, M., and Joughin, C. (2001) *Finding the evidence. A gateway to the literature in CAMHS*. London: Gaskell Publications, Royal College of Psychiatrists.

Sturt, J. (1995) Managing Change. In *Management for psychiatrists* (2nd edn) (ed. D. Bhugra and A. Burns), pp. 188–99. London: Gaskell Publications, Royal College of Psychiatrists.

Wallace, S., Crown, J., Cox, A., and Berger, M. (1997) Child and adolescent mental health. Health Care needs assessment. In *Epidemiologically base needs assessment reviews* (ed. A. Stevens and S. Rafferty). Oxford: Radcliffe Medical Press.

Working Together to Safeguard Children (1999) Department of Health/Home Office/Department for Education. London: HMSO.

Chapter 35

Teams, team-working, and clinical leadership

Michael Kerfoot and Dave Pottage

Introduction

In this chapter we believe it is important to help commissioners to gain a clear picture of the service's personnel operating within a CAMHS structure and of the configurations of staff that are likely to produce the most effective and efficient models of working. Historically, the CAMHS team comprised a psychiatrist (who was normally the team leader), a psychiatric social worker, and a psychologist. In LEA child guidance clinics this would normally be an educational psychologist and in NHS settings, a clinical psychologist. These personnel formed the core of the 'team' and each had a clearly prescribed (and proscribed) role and function. The psychiatrist was the administrative conduit by which the referral came to the service and was managed, and had the main responsibility for diagnosing the child's illness or problems and for treating the child. The psychiatric social worker was usually the first point of contact for families referred to the service and normally would undertake an exploratory home visit to compile a 'social history' on the case. This document would often form the backbone of the case file, since it provided a detailed developmental history of the child's life, and also of the family members. In the diagnostic phase, the psychiatric social worker would very much represent the social dimension, and in the treatment phase, would take responsibility for undertaking work with parents and other significant adults, and for liasing with community-based services.

The psychologist's main role was in 'testing' the child in order to assess IQ, educational progress, and potential. If involved in treatment, the psychologist would traditionally focus on behavioural programmes. In the past 20 years or so this care configuration has changed in form and content, so that currently both roles have, to some extent, become interchangeable and functions have become more diverse. For example, many CAMHS teams now have CPNs working with them, as well as play therapists, child psychotherapists, and family therapists. The services of a clinical psychologist are now frequently seconded to the team from a separate clinical psychology department, which takes its own referrals, so that CAMHS work is now only one of a number of services offered. Psychiatric social work has, in general, diminished mainly because of the need for departments to staff the heavy child protection agenda that has developed in recent years. Psychiatric social workers, like psychologists, are contracted into the services from a parent department and do not, as a rule, undertake many home visits to families.

Specialist CAMHS is now largely clinic-based with a team of mixed professionals undertaking both separate and joint functions. Teams and team working these days seem to be a 'given', at least in most public services—'team' is commonly used as the basic commodity for service delivery—and as such, incorporated into public service planning and strategic development without the feasibility of the notion itself being questioned in terms of its suitability of purpose.

The notion of team is only one model for achieving an organizational purpose—there are others, mainly built around clarifying superior/subordinate relationships, prescribing functions, and locating purpose within individual contributions. What we wish to stress is that people can work within a role, achieve a purpose, and make a valid contribution, working alongside others within a common location or space, and work for a common organization, but in themselves these features do not constitute a team or teamwork (many academic depts for example).

Our starting point is, therefore, to consider the CAMHS system in terms of whether the notion of 'team' and 'teamwork' seems appropriate to it, as opposed to other ways of organizing the service. In recent years the world of organizational and staff development has become so heavily influenced by the study of human relationships that it is assumed that they form the foundation of every successful organization—to the point where there is now a plethora of activities, methodologies, and literature in the training and development field based on the premise that organizational success flows from meaningful colleague relationships.

It is now possible to become involved in 'team development', 'team building', and 'management development'—programmes that take no account of the purpose, content, and actual experience of participants working reality, preferring instead to foster individual insights through the use of games and exercises, and to produce insights that are then assumed to be influential in changing working behaviour. The important point is that these activities are context-free and their promoters do not, apparently, see any contradiction in this.

We make no such assumption, preferring instead to regard sound working relationships as an outcome of sound working practices that in turn reflect clarity of purpose. Frankly, in our opinion, an over-emphasis on personal relationships as the basis for organizational stability can come to represent another contradiction, in that the organization is dependent for its success upon factors that may be largely out of its control.

The need to work continually on clarity of purpose (as a feature of work itself, as opposed to an adjunct to it), in the light of changing circumstances, is one of the key factors that determine the use of the 'team' as the appropriate organizational approach. This is distinct from the situation where the organizational purpose is achieved through skilful but fixed repetition of a pre-determined task. In this context, the team model is not required and can be achieved through purposeful clear bureaucratic structure, procedure, and accountability.

As we shall clarify, the team model is expensive and risky but necessary in service contexts that are required to present to outside collaborators and commissioners a clarity, permanence, and continuity, while internally requiring high levels of flexibility in responding to fluid situations. It is effective teamwork that works with this tension creatively.

What we are proposing is that any service sector that has the aim of being effective, needs to consider the appropriate model for how it conducts its internal business. What is always counter-productive is when radical change in the nature of service is introduced without due consideration of the internal organizational approach. For example, it is invariably disastrous when a bureaucratic regulatory model is used in situations that can only be effective through a team approach (an increasing reality in local government-based services). Teams can often be self-regulating and will function without the need for external regulation, once it is acknowledged that self-regulation provides the means for internal quality assurance as distinct from the self-defeating passivity that frequently stems from externally imposed regulation.

Why CAMHS require a teamwork approach

CAMHS is a clinical service, and while consisting of a range of specialist contributions, the fact that their purpose is to respond to the needs of their individual patients requires that everyone on the team accepts personal responsibility for the whole teams effort. Accepting responsibility, whilst a requirement, is meaningless without authority.

The team needs clinical leadership, but not to the extent that such leadership interferes with the professional judgment of a professional in the team acting within their particular role and sphere of expertise. That becomes authoritarianism, which undermines collective responsibility.

In the clinical context, which requires many different permutations of resources and responses, the leadership role is not simply to take decisions and issue commands, but to identify and co-ordinate the leadership and decision-making function within a whole range of short-term task-based arrangements. In other words, the clinical team requires an overall leader, but within any sphere of activity, specific leadership and authority is invested in various colleagues according to the logic of the work.

What defines the team is that every individual is responsible for the entire team rather than only for his or her own work. The team, rather than the individual, is the unit of service. What the unit has to do in order to satisfy those that commission their service is not based on a fixed menu of responses, but assumes that, as an overall collective resource, they have the capacity to be effective.

> Team members need not know each other well to perform as a team. But they do need to know each others function and potential contribution 'rapport', 'empathy', 'interpersonal relations' are not needed. Mutual understanding of each others job and common understanding of the task are however essential. (Drucker 1977).

We have outlined why a team approach is appropriate to delivering a CAMHS service, but we need to suggest briefly what constitutes a service. We have spoken earlier about the importance of giving a message of clarity of purpose and consistency to external commissioners and collaborators, and simultaneously achieving maximum internal flexibility in responding to patient need. It is the individual contribution to the team's collective purpose that defines CAMHS as services. A collection of experts, acting as individuals, giving of their best but doing so outside of the connection with the contribution of their colleagues, is a collection of individuals not a service. Individually, they may be highly regarded in their own sphere of expertise but they are not contributing to a service.

Similarly, if the work of the team is not co-ordinated well in terms of, for example, the prioritizing of referrals and the best rationing of the team resource, or if intakes are manipulated to over-reflect the clinical or research interests of any of its members, this also undermines their status as a service.

In the present climate, services must be needs-led so that patients/clients come to feel that their distress has been listened to in *their* terms and responded to in a way that conveys to them the belief that their 'treatment' is tailored to their specific difficulties and individual family characteristics. Too often teams deliver a way or style of working that evidences its own view of itself but which has little external meaning for service users.

Some implications

Services that operate on a team approach create difficulties for the wider organization. In the team 'the whole group must work constantly on explaining both to itself and to managers throughout the organization what it is trying to do, what it is working on and what it has accomplished' (Drucker).

However, in spite of this tension the team, in order to be a team, must retain its flexibility and fluidity, and not solidify around tried and tested approaches, either for its own comfort or that of the wider organization. Teams that become static cease to be teams and lose their capacity for effectiveness. Conversely they can become so fluid and permissive as to lose their sense of internal discipline, a feature essential for flexible working.

How teams manage this conflict will determine the extent to which the team will become a responsive, efficient, and effective working unit. There are several points that may be of use here. First, the issue of clinical leadership must be addressed, agreed, and settled as soon as possible. Traditionally, psychiatrists were always afforded this role, since GPs would only refer to another doctor and would be asking for a 'medical' opinion. The comments of other team members would be incorporated into the correspondence but direct contact between, say, a psychiatric social worker and the GP would have been unusual. The position in today's CAMHS is little different, although the etiquette of doctor–doctor contacts is now more relaxed.

We would suggest that to resolve satisfactorily the issue of clinical leadership the team should decide what the role of 'leader' will be. This means that power is given rather than taken and decisions are reached through consensus rather than conflict. Where issues of clinical leadership have not been addressed openly and directly, then much of the team's activity may be diverted into petty skirmishing, or other activities that can ultimately undermine the team's integrity and undermine its core business.

A second point is that the activities of the team are about work and not personalities. The needs of the particular patient or child determine the decisions made, not the need for a particular team member to be right. It is self-evident, therefore, that the team becomes a forum for regular discussion and review of patient material. Its function is to clarify complex or complicated situations, so that decisions can be taken about assessment, treatment, and management. It also has the function of supporting the team members and promoting their continued professional development. It does this, however, through a careful and detailed consideration of pieces of direct work with patients. The team member is viewed through the work they undertake, rather than alongside it. It is an integral relationship, not a parallel one, and the work with patients must always be at the core of team activity.

Finally, the team must also review its functioning from time to time, so that structures do not become so fixed that their flexibility and responsiveness is reduced. A team is not created to become some kind of organizational or administrative unit for regulating clinical activity.

Interconnectedness, effectiveness and efficiency

We have emphasised in this chapter the two main themes of CAMHS as 'service' and the notion of 'team' as the most appropriate organizational model for offering service. Developing CAMHS in the future along these lines best reflects the increasing realisation of the interconnection of factors in understanding childhood social and emotional development, and problem behaviour. We agree with other writers that planning and evaluation of prevention research might be more effective if:

> ...classification systems were modified in accordance with recent advances in the field of developmental psychopathology, emphasising patterns of adaptation which focus upon social relationships rather than isolated deviant behaviours or traits. (Garber 1984).

It is the attention given to the interconnectedness of psychopathological factors, and the recognition of unifying influences between and within factors that offers the best hope for understanding and responding to disturbance in children and adolescents (Sroufe and Rutter 1984; Maguire and Earls 1991). The position is summarised particularly well by Rutter (1989) when he says:

> Just as we have learned not to polarise nature and nurture as if they were mutually exclusive, alternative explanations, so also we need to get away from the unduly simplified question of whether a person's behaviour is the result of past or present experiences. Not only will behaviour be shaped by the biological substrate, genetically and non-genntically determined, as well as by psychosocial influences, but equally both the past and the present are likely to have effects. Most crucially, however, they are not independent of one another.....it is important to search for unifying principles in the mechanisms underlying the diversity of pathways from childhood to adult life, but in so doing we must consider the pathways in personal terms and in the context of possible person/environment interactions

If 'interconnectedness' is becoming increasingly the vehicle that helps to take forward our understanding of the nature of human psychological and social development and functioning, it seems logical that interconnectedness should increasingly underpin our strategy in taking forward the development of CAMHS. It also explains why the notion of having a team delivering a service is also important, because it is an exemplar of how modernising influences can permeate and modify successfully services that have well-established, traditional ways of working.

The point of a service perspective is that effectiveness and credibility comes from demonstrating in working practices that individual, specialist and expert contributions are determined in relation to each other and the whole, when responding to a child's situation. It means that those who commission the service, those that collaborate with it, and those that receive it experience the service as a sensible process rather than as a series of disjointed events and encounters. In this context, the present Government's emphasis on 'evidence-based practice' may, potentially, have a detrimental effect on the development of CAMHS as a service. Through the implication that the quality of a service should be measured primarily via individual treatment methods the message is conveyed that the organisational and operational context is merely the place where treatment happens. At worst, context is somehow perceived as neutral or, at best, as separate.

We have placed such emphasis on the notion of 'interconnectedness' in order to offer a strong reminder that in the search for credibility, to isolate one factor for analysis can and will result in a serious distortion both of clinical evidence, and the future development of the service. The history of service and practice development in the UK is littered with failed inititatives that were introduced in isolation from the context and culture central to their success. Some of these mistakes were a consequence of the patchy and uneven development in CAMHS nationally, but were also a consequence of the persistent under-funding of this specialty in relation to others.

Earlier we decided that the team organisational model was the most relevant for CAMHS because it seemed the most appropriate model for better incorporating the broadening range of expert and specialist contributions represented there. These in turn reflected the important theoretical developments, and changes in practice which have improved the quality of care, influenced by wider social, educational and paediatric developments (Parry-Jones 1989). However, we have also said that the team model is expensive as a working model in that effectiveness in performance requires significant time and attention to be devoted to the maintenance of the team itself as a working unit (Etzioni 1971). All teams have a built in tendency to become static around familiar working practices, particularly those that have previously demonstrated their effectiveness. When work becomes based upon mere habit it is invariably ineffective. Working patterns and purpose become distorted to fit the comfort and convenience of team members, with effectiveness becoming a secondary consideration.

We believe that team effectiveness stems from the capacity to learn continuously, and to develop and adjust from the analysis of the knowledge located within individual and collective experience (Pottage and Evans 1994). As Parry-Jones (1989) has pointed out:

> ....the specialty has not been spared a recurrent tendency to oversimplify causal explanations and to apply uniform systems of ideas and actions somewhat indiscriminately .... good ideas can be transformed into certainties, and aetiology and treatment can be enveloped in all-embracing credos.

Building reflective practice, learning, appraisal and development into the service as one of its features helps to ensure that working practices remain part of strategic thinking rather than mere habit.

We acknowledge that when approached from a strict efficiency perspective the 'good' team is seen as one that devotes maximum time and effort to delivering the service, and building up an impressive number of patient contacts. From an effectiveness perspective what is important is the optimum use of clinical time. Similarly, we suggest that efficiency measures such as the number of patients seen, service throughput etc., are less valuable than evaluating the features of a working unit that manages its business in such a way as to give confidence to those that commission it. It sends the message that the team has the means to be effective, not simply the intention to be so.

Working on effectiveness and development simultaneously can be looked at as involving a number of interrelated spheres of activity:

- Working on individual and collective clarity of purpose that is continually refined and redefined in the light of internal and external changing circumstances to ensure accurate targeting, equitable prioritising, and the most effective and economical use of specialist resources.

- Gaining access to, and utilising the knowledge located in day to day experience, both clinical and organisational, through regular, detailed individual and collective case monitoring and debriefing.

We have found that incorporating an organisational practice dimension into the clinical audit helps both to emphasise the interrelation between clinical and organisational practice, and to open up the valuable reservoir of knowledge and learning located in day to day working behaviours. This notion is supported by Goodman (1997), who states:

> The desirability of clinical audit is now generally accepted. There is often considerable educational value in reviewing randomly chosen and 'poor outcome' cases at regular audit meetings. The value of these meetings could be increased by inviting 'guest auditors' from outside CAMHS e.g. from Education, Social Services, General Practice, Paediatrics and Public Health.

There is always much debate and speculation about the feasibility of both incorporating research findings within CAMHS and also of the research potential of CAMHS teams, but the research dimension is one that has to be addressed if a team (and service) is genuine in its wish to develop. Parents seeking help for their children need accessible and comprehensive child mental health services. They also have a right to expect that systematic steps have been taken to assess the merits and demerits of the treatments on offer. Unless such steps are taken, there is a danger that parents will have easy access to treatments that are either ineffective or perhaps even harmful. Not only is progress being made in establishing which treatments are effective in, for example, behaviour disorders and depressive disorders, but evidence is also accumulating about treatments that are mostly ineffective (Harrington et al 1999). However, as Goodman (1997) points out:

> It would be a mistake to think that a Mental Health Service could operate solely on the basis of published treatment trials and protocols, for example .... the young person's or family cirumstances and preferences may make standard protocols unthinkable.

In such circumstances, accurate observation using a combination of quantitative and qualitative research methods would be necessary, particularly where the nature or substance of the therapeutic encounter does not lend itself to quantitative ratings alone. The additional point is that research in CAMHS is not something that can or should be left entirely to academic departments. Team members within CAMHS routinely collect data from a variety of sources in order to further their diagnostic and therapeutic work, and the procedures used are often highly structured, disciplined and objective. Team members do not always recognise that the information they generate contributes not only to individual case planning but also to service development by providing direct evidence to test out models of causation, diagnosis and treatment. Their practice gives an authenticity to the notion of research that is often unavailable in research centres that are detached from day to day clinical practice.

Earlier we remarked upon the importance of interconnectedness as a notion that not only takes forward our understanding of the complex nature of human psychological and social development and functioning, but also as a notion that should increasingly underpin our strategy in taking forward the development of child and adolescent mental health services. This also explains our emphasis in this chapter on CAMHS as a service operating on team principles, to show clearly that the modern CAMHS reflects and is congruent with modern understanding. This is presumably what 'best organisational value' is about, and is a solid platform upon which to base future developments.

References

Drucker, P. (1979) *Management: tasks – responsibilities – practices.* (Abridged and revised version). London: Pan Books.

Etzioni, A. (1960) Two approaches to organisational analysis: a critique and suggestion. In *The sociology of organizations* (ed. O. Grusky and G.A. Miller), pp. 103–6. New York: The Free Press.

Garber, J. (1984) Classification of childhood psychopathology: a developmental perspective. *Child Development,* **55**, 30–48.

Goodman, R. (1997) *Child and adolescent mental health services: Reasoned advice to commissioners and providers.* Maudsley Discussion Paper No.4. London: Institute of Psychiatry.

Harrington, R., Kerfoot, M., and Verduyn, C. (1999) Developing needs-led child and adolescent mental health services: issues and prospects. *European Child and Adolescent Psychiatry,* **8**, 1–10.

McGuire, J. and Earls, F. (1991) Prevention of psychiatric disorders in early childhood. *Journal of Child Psychology and Psychiatry,* **32**(1), 129–54.

Parry-Jones, W. (1989) The history of child and adolescent psychiatry: its present day relevance. *Journal of Child Psychology and Psychiatry,* **30**(1), 3–11.

Pottage, D. and Evans, M. (1994) *The competent workplace – the view from within.* London: National Institute of Social Work.

Rutter, M. (1989) Pathways from childhood to adult life. *Journal of Child Psychology and Psychiatry,* **30**(1), 23–51.

Sroufe, L.A. and Rutter, M. (1984) The domain of developmental psychology. *Child Development,* **55**, 17–29.

Chapter 36

Measuring quality in CAMHS: policy, frameworks, and evidence for practice and commissioning

Carol Joughin

Introduction

The drive to ensure quality in mental health service provision began in the UK in the 1960s following a series of hospital scandals. Increasing workloads, limited resources, the development of new treatment approaches, and raising expectations from the public have fuelled the need to demonstrate high-quality service provision. Demonstrating the quality of health service provision is complex and there is still ambivalence over its meaning and the best framework to ensure that it is delivered. This chapter outlines the development of quality measures, presents the policy that underpins quality improvement in services, and discusses the implications of the quality agenda for the development of CAMHS.

Defining quality

For professionals charged with the responsibility to provide 'high-quality' health care, what does the term 'quality' really mean? The definition of quality is currently imprecise. Defining what constitutes 'quality' is 'exasperatingly complex', to use the words of Donabedian when he was discussing quality in general health services (Pirkis *et al.* 1999). This is even more the case when trying to define 'quality' for CAMHS. Donabedian (1992) suggests that quality incorporates:

  effectiveness (achieving the greatest improvements in health currently achievable by the best care);

  efficiency (the ability to provide appropriate care without diminishing improvements in health);

  optimality (achieving a balance between the cost of care and effects of care on health);

  acceptability (achieving conformity with patient preferences);

  legitimacy (achieving conformity to social preferences and ethical canons); and

  equity (conformity to principles guiding the fair distribution of health care in a population) (Pirkis *et al.* 1999).

Measuring quality: structure, process, or outcome?

The elements in Donabedian's framework for ensuring quality can be evaluated by assessing structure, processes, and outcomes of care. There is, however, a continuing debate over the appropriateness of using structure, process, or outcome measures to assess quality.

The structure of care refers to 'relatively stable characteristics of providers of care, of the tools and resources they have at their disposal, and of the physical and organisational settings in which they work' (Mark *et al.* 1997). It relates to the dimension of equity as used by Donabedian (1992).

The process of care refers to 'a set of activities that go on within and between practitioner and patient' (Mark *et al.* 1997). These 'activities' relate to both technical aspects (such as the number of CBT sessions delivered) and interpersonal aspects, and relate to the dimensions of 'acceptability' and 'legitimacy', as referred to by Donabedian (1992).

Donabedian (1992) describes outcomes of care as 'states or conditions attributable to antecedent health care' and relates to the effectiveness of care provided. He believes that outcomes are the most important criteria of good quality; they remain the ultimate validators of effectiveness and quality of medical care (Fessel and Van Brunt 1972). There is no single way of evaluating effectiveness in CAMHS; outcomes of care may be measured by:

symptom severity (the changes of symptoms on a rating scale);

levels of functioning;

social and psychological well-being (independent of symptoms);

quality of life;

child or parent satisfaction or impressions of improvement;

the prevention of the emergence of co-morbid disorders or conditions.

There is very little research in the mental health field that demonstrates that quality structures and processes do in fact lead to quality outcomes (Pirkis *et al.* 1999). However, some authors propose that process measures 'can be sensitive indicators of the quality of care and have many advantages over outcomes (Crombie and Davies 1998). They are generally readily measured and easily interpreted, unlike some outcome measures, which may require detailed questionnaires and subjective assessments. Process measurements can also directly reveal aspects of care that need improving. It should also be noted that poor outcome does not necessarily imply poor quality of care, and good outcomes do not mean that credit can be given to the healthcare system. As can be seen, the relationship between structure, process, and outcome is currently unclear, and this is reflected by the debate about where the emphasis should lie when assessing quality (Brugha and Lindsay 1996). It seems most likely that an integrated approach is needed; that structures, processes, and outcomes all need to be considered when assessing the quality of services (Mark *et al.* 1997).

Quality assurance systems

Quality assurance systems have been introduced in various healthcare settings in an attempt to ensure that quality is delivered. Various models have emerged from the business environment and have now been adapted for use in health services. Quality assurance is based on standards that define the components of a service and the processes that need to be followed. Regular external inspections are performed to ensure that standards are maintained. The assumption is that if standards are correctly defined and are being adhered to, a high-quality service will follow. However, the use of quality assurance and standards alone does not necessarily guarantee improved quality outcomes; it may even suppress the development of better quality by promoting complacency. There is an additional risk of plateauing standards. Total quality management was developed to take quality assurance a step further. It requires continuous and relentless improvements in the total process that provides care, not simply the improved action of individual professionals. Improvements are based on both process and outcomes, and it has an additional focus on the needs of the 'customer'. Service evaluation (frequently with an emphasis on outcome measures) is one of a number of methods used in quality assurance.

Medical/clinical audit, formally introduced in 1989, represented the first step of applying a quality assurance model to practice in the health service (see Chapter 37, this volume).

There are currently a number of standards frameworks available to assess the quality of care in CAMHS. The Health Advisory Service has developed generic standards for CAMHS (The Health Advisory Service 2000), the Royal College of Psychiatrists' Research Unit has developed standards for in-patient services as part of the National In-Patient Child and Adolescent Study (The Royal College of Psychiatrists' Research Unit 2000) delivered through the Quality Network for Inpatient CAMHS (QNIC) and the Health Quality Service (in collaboration with the National Children's Bureau) has developed CAMHS specific standards (Health Quality Service 2000). Although these frameworks provide a useful method of examining both the structure and process of care as well as incorporating 'users' perspectives, they are not government-endorsed national standards, and it remains to be seen if they will be used widely in CAMHS.

The policy framework for quality improvement

Prior to the health reforms in the 1990s, the success of the health service was assessed by measuring its efficiency. The reforms outlined below demonstrate a clear drive to move from measuring efficiency to the effectiveness of care.

Clinical effectiveness

The clinical effectiveness initiative was introduced in 1993 and a national strategy was presented in *Promoting clinical effectiveness* (Department of Health 1996). The initiative aimed to support evidence-based, outcomes driven decision-making. Clinical effectiveness was described as:

> the extent to which specific clinical interventions, when deployed in the field for a particular patient or population, do what they are intended to do—i.e. maintain and improve health and secure the greatest possible health gain from the available resources.

Clinical effectiveness aimed to improve the outcomes of specific clinical interventions. Prior to the introduction of clinical effectiveness initiatives, such as research and development, the development of information systems, quality programmes, and educational programming were performed in relative isolation within trusts. The launch of clinical effectiveness was the first time that the health service was encouraged to examine existing structures and remove boundaries at a local level.

Health policy required that increased clinical effectiveness would be achieved through:

developing an increased knowledge-base of effectiveness and cost-effectiveness;

the dissemination of that knowledge to decision-makers;

using the knowledge-base to change clinical practice and monitoring the results.

In order to influence decision-making by clinicians, patients, and managers, local strategies were needed to inform that decision-making, to change practice where appropriate, and to monitor the outcomes (Department of Health 1996).

Clinical governance

In December 1997, with a change of government 'The New NHS' was launched and heralded the introduction of clinical governance. Clinical governance provided 'a framework through which NHS organizations are accountable for continuously improving the quality of their services and safeguarding high standards of care by creating an environment in which excellence in clinical care will flourish' (Department of Health 1997). Clinical governance placed expectations on individuals and organizations to develop systems that assure the delivery of high-quality care to patients. 'The New NHS' also recognized the importance of collaborative working across health authorities, local authorities, voluntary organizations, and the private sector. Assessment of performance in CAMHS needs to take into account the contribution made by developing successful partnerships across these sectors. The New NHS promised to concentrate on assessing things that count most to patients and the public—high-quality, cost-effective care that leads to improved health.

Clinical governance has been driven by the need to co-ordinate functions that frequently took place in isolation within trusts. The development of strategies, the incorporation of user views and feedback, the findings from clinical audit, clinical risk management, the use of research evidence, information management, and staff development and workforce initiatives, need to be addressed in a co-ordinated and integrated way. Key to the introduction of clinical governance was that chief executives were made accountable for the quality of services for patients.

A first class service published for consultation in 1998 (Department of Health 1998a) specified 21 components of clinical governance[1] and stated that a 'quality organization' will ensure that:

quality improvement processes are in place and integrated within the quality programme for the organization as a whole;

evidence-based practice is in day-to-day use with the infra-structure to support it; and

the quality of data collected to monitor clinical care is itself of a high standard.

It set out a three-pronged strategy to drive performance improvement by setting clear standards, promoting effective delivery of high-quality services locally, and ensuring that external monitoring systems were in place (see Table 36.1).

The National Framework for Assessing Performance would measure how local services were progressing against their targets. The Framework would address six areas of service delivery:

health improvement;

fair access;

effective delivery of appropriate healthcare;

efficiency;

patient/user experiences;

health outcomes of NHS care.

These elements are clearly linked to those described by Donabedian (1992).

---

[1] The Royal College of Psychiatrists Research Unit has developed a Clinical Governance Support service to help providers of mental health and learning disability services implement the requirements of clinical governance (http://www.rcpsych.ac.uk/cru/qual.htm).

Table 36.1 The NHS strategy for performance improvement

Setting standards:	National Standards would be developed through National Service Frameworks (NSF) and the National Institute for Clinical Excellence (NICE). Each NSF would include: the evidence of clinical and cost effectiveness; national standards; and outcome measures.
Delivering standards:	Clinical governance would ensure that national standards and guidance was reflected at a local level.
Monitoring standards:	Health authorities and Primary Care Groups/Trusts would use the NSFs to assess performance. The Commission for Health Improvement would carry out local reviews to check that systems were in place to monitor and improve clinical quality. The National Framework for Assessing Performance was introduced with new emphasis on standards and outcomes.

The NHS plan (Department of Health 2000) further developed the definition of quality by emphasizing that 'quality will not just be restricted to the clinical aspects of care, but will include quality of life and the entire patient experience'. The plan announced that new efficiency targets would be set, which would not permit a trade-off between cost and quality. This focus on patients'/clients' experiences is also evident in the development of a National Patients Survey Programme led by the Commission for Health Improvement and in the promotion of user-satisfaction surveys in social services (Department of Health 1998b).

In early 2001, the government announced that a Children's National Service Framework (NSF) would be developed and that child and adolescent mental health would be addressed within this framework. National standards and outcome measures would then be set for CAMHS. Delivery of standards would be achieved through the local clinical governance frameworks and performance would be measured through health authorities, primary care groups/ trusts, and the Commission for Health Improvement (the Commission for Healthcare Audit and Inspection, from April 2004). The ability of trusts to meet the performance targets set out in the NHS plan would also need to be addressed, and achievement of these targets, alongside meeting standards in the Children's NSF, will influence the star rating allocated to trusts.

Recent reviews of the progress that mental health trusts have made in implementing clinical governance highlight a number of problems that are currently being encountered by services. Reports from both the Commission for Health Improvement and the Clinical Governance Support Service (based at the Royal College of Psychiatrists) highlight common issues of concern. These include: problems with recruitment and pressures on staffing; fragmented information systems leading to little development in performance management; lack of robust processes to ensure user consultation and involvement; inadequate or no strategies for implementing an evidence-based approach to practice; poor clinician engagement in management; lack of cohesion of services within the trust and with other agencies, such as social care. These issues will all be familiar concerns to CAMHS practitioners and they serve to highlight some of the real obstacles to improving the quality of services for children with mental health problems.

Evidence of effective interventions

It is clear that evidence-based practice was a key component of clinical effectiveness and is a key component of clinical governance and of the delivery of high-quality services. There is general consensus over the effectiveness of some treatments for children with mental health problems but considerable uncertainty still exists regarding best practice for many interventions that are currently used in this field. The research base is growing, and people are becoming increasingly skilled at appraising and interpreting the research. However, until these skills become universal, and the quality and span of the research is improved, we will be left with considerable gaps in our evidence-base for effective interventions.

The evidence for the potential effectiveness of CAMHS interventions has been demonstrated in the most part by randomized controlled trials, in which clinical outcomes tend to be assessed over a single or brief period of time. Guidelines are likely to be developed on the strength of this evidence but currently the evidence-base is insufficiently developed to address many of the complexities of working with children with mental health problems.

There are a number of factors that need to be considered when discussing the evidence-base for CAMHS:

The care of children with mental health problems is delivered and commissioned by different agencies and professional groups who have varying opinions on the validity of the current evidence-base. Until a common language is developed, which is shared by professionals in health, education, and social care, difficulties will continue to arise in the acceptance of research findings.

The conceptualization and description of disorders has changed considerably in the last 30 years, making it difficult to apply the findings from early research to practice today.

The majority of randomized controlled trials have been conducted outside the United Kingdom, leading to concerns about the generalizability of the findings.

Research is frequently conducted in carefully controlled, ideal conditions, using a fairly heterogeneous cohort of subjects. It is difficult to apply the findings of such studies to work in clinic settings with children and adolescents who present with complex problems associated with co-morbid conditions.

However, progress is being made. As the needs for evidence in CAMHS has been highlighted over the last few years, organizations such as the National Institute for Clinical Excellence and the Scottish Intercollegiate Guidelines Network (SIGN) are working to develop guidelines for practice. Evidence-based guidelines are now available for the management of attention deficit hyperactivity disorder (Lord and Paisley 2000; Scottish Intercollegiate Guidelines Network 2001) and are being developed for problems such as depression, eating disorders, and conduct disorder. The Department of Health has commissioned a review of research for CAMHS (Fonagy *et al.* 2002). The FOCUS Project based at the Royal College of Psychiatrist's Research Unit has produced a resource to assist professionals to access research (Scott *et al.* 2001) and the National Electronic Library for Health is currently working to improve the resources available for child health related issues.

Commissioning for quality

Before the introduction of clinical effectiveness, the success of the NHS was measured by its activity. As previously described, a shift has been made from purchasing activity to commissioning effective practice.

Strategic health authorities and primary care trusts are now ultimately responsible for the measurement of quality within services.

Measuring outcomes in CAMHS

It is clear that measuring outcomes will become increasingly important, both to ensure effective practice within services (within the framework of clinical governance) and as measures of performance against nationally set standards.

Outcome evaluations need to identify a positive outcome. 'The evaluation must be designed so that it uncovers an important outcome if one really exists (statistical validity), is able to attribute this effect to the programme and not some irrelevant cause (internal validity), identifies the proper elements of the programme that produced the effect on relevant outcome measures (construct validity), and is able to extend the results to situations other than the ones studies (external validity)' (Bickman 1992). A meaningful assessment of outcomes for children must also take into account the complex interactions between the patient and family, and medical educational and social factors, which may have contributed to the referral (Hunter *et al.* 1996). Decisions about what constitutes a 'good outcome' and how this can be measured, also require careful thought. Professionals, parents, and children tend to have different perspectives on the nature of a good outcome. Identifying and measuring appropriate outcomes of care is clearly a challenge for those with a responsibility for setting the quality agenda in CAMHS, as well as for those who are charged to deliver on it.

While it is widely acknowledged that evidence needs to be provided that shows that CAMHS have a positive effect on the lives of children and their families, actually gathering data on the success (or otherwise) of a treatment is not straightforward. Children and adolescents referred to CAMHS often present with complex problems arising from a combination of inter-related causes. The dynamic social context in which they live means that familial, social, and environmental factors continuously influence the nature of the difficulties they experience. It is extremely difficult to disentangle these factors when trying to measure the impact of input from CAMHS professionals. Some key points to consider when addressing outcome evaluations in CAMHS are shown in Box 36.1

Although the principles of good outcome measurement have been well-described, relatively few child and adolescent mental health services have made outcome measurement routine. Standardized outcome-measurement tools, e.g. the child and adolescent version of the Health of the Nation Outcome Scales HoNOSCA (Gowers *et al.* 1999) and the Paddington Complexity Scale (Yates *et al.* 1999), specifically designed for child and adolescent mental health, are gradually being developed and will certainly assist CAMHS professionals to examine this area. The use of specific outcome measure is covered in Chapter 31.

Because of the complexity of outcomes measurement, and the time and resources required to develop robust evaluations, it is likely that performance indicators will continue to be used to assess quality within services.

Performance indicators

Performance indicators are indirect measures of the quality of care. They are relevant because they may increase or decrease the probability of a good outcome. However they are only valuable as a proxy for outcome, once the elements of structure or process are known to have a clear relationship with the desired changes in outcome (Hunter *et al.* 1996).

Performance indicators have already been introduced to social services departments. The White Paper *Modernising social services* and the consultation paper *A new approach for social services performance* set out proposals for a new performance-assessment system for social

Box 36.1 Outcome evaluations in CAMHS (adapted from Pirkis *et al.* 1999)

Measuring outcomes in CAMHS is highly complex. It is difficult to design measures to capture complex information.

Mental health problems (particularly in children) are long-term in nature. Improvements can be seen as points on a continuum rather than absolute. Appropriate time points for measurement need to be considered.

Different outcomes will be relevant to different stakeholders. Also different stakeholders will have different perspectives on the achievement of the same outcome. A range of perspectives is required.

For some (such as children with pervasive developmental disorders), realistic achievements may be small.

Outcomes should be case-mix adjusted. Otherwise it is impossible to know which differences in outcome are due to patient-based factors or provider-based factors.

Conclusions can be strengthened if comparisons are made with groups who have not received such care, or at least against a benchmark.

Instruments need to be relevant, simple, and easy to use.

Staff require training in the use of instruments in order to ensure consistency of measurement.

Information systems need to be developed to manage this data.

services within the Best Value regimen for all local government services. The Department of Health acknowledged in LAC(99) 27 that, while the performance indicators were the best available using existing or planned-for data, a great deal of work remained to be done to improve the quality and coverage of performance assessment framework indicators, which have been taken forward by the NHS plan. When assessed against these indicators, data quality was found to be a concern, and social services were informed that poor-quality data would in itself be considered an indication of poor performance in the future. These issues are likely to present similar challenges to CAMHS, where limited information systems are currently in place and general administrative support frequently falls well below the ideal.

This chapter has attempted to describe some of the key elements of quality and highlight some of the key policy changes that have led the drive for quality improvement. Much work remains to be done to achieve the elements of quality services first described by Donabedian and taken forward by the NHS plan. The acknowledged aim remains to be to provide equitable services which are accessible to all, regardless of circumstances or location and which are based around the needs of the child and family. There is no doubt that clients of child and adolescent mental health services need to be offered reassurance that the treatments offered to them are likely to lead to improved outcomes. It is also the case that promoting effective practice and evidence-based decision-making will help to reduce the current lack of equity in service provision around the UK. However, this chapter highlights some of the difficulties inherent in both delivering and demonstrating high-quality, effective services in CAMHS. In order to make decisions concerning best treatment, at both a national and a local level, more resources need to be targeted at developing a solid research base (with a particular emphasis on pragmatic research and outcomes from a patient's perspective). Information systems need to be developed to manage data, and staff need training and allocated time to use such information to inform their decision-making. Finally, and crucial to the development of high-quality services, are well-trained and well-supported staff, who work in an environment that allows excellence to flourish, and which is able to recruit and retain its workforce. Without initiatives such as these it will be difficult to assess the quality of care and the quality of life for children and adolescents with mental health problems.

References

Bickman, L. (1992) Designing outcome evaluations for children's mental health services: improving internal validity. *New Directions for Programme Evaluation*, **54** (Summer), 57–69.

Brugha, T.S. and Lindsay, F. (1996) Quality of mental health service care: the forgotten pathway from process to outcome. *Social Psychiatry and Psychiatric Epidemiology*, **31**, 89–98.

Crombie, I.K. and Davies, H.T.O. (1998) Beyond health outcomes: the advantages of measuring process. *Journal of Evaluation in Clinical Practice*, **4**, 31–8.

Department of Health (1996) *Promoting clinical effectiveness. a framework for action in and through the NHS*. London: NHS Executive, HMSO.

Department of Health (1997) *The new NHS; modern, dependable*. A White Paper. London: Department of Health, HMSO.

Department of Health (1998a) *A first class service: quality in the new NHS*. London: Department of Health, HMSO.

Department of Health (1998b) *Modernising social services*. CM4169. London: Department of Health, HMSO.

Department of Health (2000) *The NHS plan. A plan for investment. A plan for reform*. CM 4818-I. London: Department of Health.

Donabedian, A. (1992) The role of outcomes in quality assessment and assurance. *Quality Review Bulletin*, **18**, 356–60.

Fessel, W.S. and Van Brunt, E.E. (1972) Assessing the quality of care from the medical record. *New England Journal of Medicine*, **286**, 134–8.

Fonagy, P., Target, M., Cottrell, D., Phillips, J., and Kurtz, Z. (2002) *What works for whom? A critical review of treatments for children and adolescents*. New York: Guilford Press.

Gowers, S.G., Harrington, R.C., Whitton, A., Lelliott, P., Beevor, A., Wing, J. *et al.* (1999) Brief scale for measuring the outcomes of emotional and behavioural disorders in children: health of the nation outcomes scales for children and adolescents (HoNOSCA). *British Journal of Psychiatry*, **174**, 413–16.

Health Quality Service (2000) *Quality standards framework for child and adolescent mental health services*. London: HQS.

Hunter, J., Higginson, I., and Garralda, E. (1996) Systematic literature review: outcome measures for child and adolescent mental health services. *Journal of Public Health Medicine*, **18** (2), 179–206.

Lord, J. and Paisley, S. (2000) *The clinical effectiveness and cost-effectiveness of methylphenidate for hyperactivity in childhood* (version 2). London: National Institute for Clinical Excellence.

Mark, B.A., Salyer, J., and Geddes, N. (1997) Outcomes research: clues to quality and organisational effectiveness? *Outcomes Measurement and Management*, **32** (3), 589–601.

Pirkis, J., Burgess, P., Dunt, D., and Henry, L. (1999) *Measuring quality in Australian mental health services*. Melbourne: Centre for Health Program Evaluation.

Scott, A., Shaw, M., and Joughin, C. (2001) *Finding the evidence: a gateway to the literature in child and adolescent mental health.* London: Gaskell.

Scottish Intercollegiate Guidelines Network (2001) *Attention deficit and hyperactivity disorders in children and young people: a national clinical guideline.* Edinburgh: SIGN.

The Health Advisory Service (2000) *Standards for child and adolescent mental health services.* Brighton: Pavillion Publishing.

The Royal College of Psychiatrists' Research Unit (2000) *National in-patient child and adolescent standards* (unpublished) http://www.rcpsych.ac.uk/cru/qual.htm

Yates, P., Garralda, M.E., and Higginson, I. (1999) Paddington complexity scale and health of the nation outcome scales for children and adolescents. *British Journal of Psychiatry*, **174**, 417–23.

Chapter 37

Data collection, clinical audit, and measuring outcomes

Miranda Wolpert, Margaret Thompson, and Karen Tingay

Introduction

Any child and adolescent mental health service within the NHS seeking to evaluate outcomes on a routine basis must address the following questions:

What is the aim of routine outcome evaluation?

Whose views of outcome should be taken into account?

What needs to be evaluated?

How should it be evaluated?

How should the results be used?

How should this be resourced?

In this chapter, we explore possible answers to these questions and suggest practical ways forward, drawing on our experiences of establishing routine outcome evaluation in Bedfordshire and Luton CAMHS and Southampton CAMHS, respectively.

We start from the position that none of the questions identified above are amenable to simple or non-controversial answers. Choices and compromises need to be made.

Given the complexity of the task, services will need to make their own choices as to measures and methods. However, we also feel that services should be encouraged to use at least some measures and methods in common to allow for the possibility of comparison in the future (recognizing that any future comparisons can only meaningfully be made where comparable contextual data is also available).

This approach, and the suggestions we make below, are broadly in line with the recommendations made by the CAMHS External Working Group contributing to the development of the Children's NSF (http://www.doh.gov.uk/nsf/children/outcomesubgroupreport.pdf).

The approach is also in line with that adopted by the CAMHS Outcome Research Consortium (CORC), a collaboration between CAMHS who have agreed to adopt common measures and a common protocol in relation to evaluation of outcome in their services. This group is chaired by the first author (for further information email: outcome.project@sbchc-tr.anglox.nhs.uk).

Aim of routine evaluation of outcomes

The key aims of routine evaluation of outcome can be broken down into the following four categories:

1. To provide information for clinicians about individual children and their families. This may usefully be shared with the individual children and families involved (case evaluation).

2. To provide information for clinicians and their managers about outcomes for the range of children and families seen by an individual clinician, in order to allow for monitoring of clinical practice in line with clinical governance (clinician evaluation).

3. To provide information for service providers, commissioners, users, and potential users of services about the outcomes of particular projects or services (service evaluation).

4. To provide information for use in specific research projects or particular audit projects (research and audit use).

Whose view of outcome should be evaluated?

Working with children involves a panoply of interested stakeholders, each of whom may have very different views on what constitutes a good 'outcome' for a given clinical contact. These might include, for example, mother, father, referrer, referred child, teacher, other children in the family, and policy makers, amongst others. We know there is very little agreement between these different groups on initial symptoms or view of outcome. For example, even at the level of symptoms, teachers, mothers, and fathers appear to share little more than 10% of the variance in the child's internalizing symptoms (Achenbach 1995).

Clearly routine collection of outcome data from all the above stakeholders would be an overwhelming undertaking. However, it is also clear that no one view will suffice. It is our suggestion that the perspective of the following groups should be routinely evaluated as a minimum:

referred children aged 11 and over;

parents/carers;[1]

clinicians.

We suggest including the view of all referred children aged 11 and over because we think the view of the referred child is a key perspective. We would have liked to suggest collecting views of those children under 11 but have been unable to identify a suitable tool (Southampton is developing a tool for use for young children to be trialled soon).

Some clinicians suggest routinely evaluating views of all siblings in the family because they do not want to single out the identified child as the bearer of the problem. Services may decide to leave this up to individual clinicians or to make a service policy about this, but it is our suggestion that the minimum standard should involve evaluation from the perspective of the referred child.

In terms of parent/carer view—in order to maximize returns, we would suggest not specifying which parent or carer should give their view, but allowing the family to decide as appropriate, as long as it is logged who responds (e.g. mother, father, mother and father, social worker, foster carer, adoptive parent, step-parent).

Whilst services may be interested in views of other groups, e.g. referrers, teachers, etc., it is likely to be too costly to try and include these as part of routine evaluation of outcome, but services may want to audit the views of other groups (e.g. referrer and teacher) periodically or in relation to particular projects or services.

---

[1] From now on we will use 'parent' to include all carers or others who may be in *loco parentis*.

What should be evaluated?

A wide variety of possible different domains have been suggested in terms of understanding and evaluating outcome of treatment. One influential model is that proposed by Kazdin and Kendall (1998), who suggest that outcome can be divided into five domains: social adaptation (which includes school performance and social relationships in general), symptomatic behaviour, relationship to parents and peers, use of service, and mechanisms of treatment. Each of these domains has pros and cons to its usage (for an extended discussion of the issues outlined below see: Fonagy *et al.* 2002).

The most commonly evaluated domain is that of symptom reduction. It is at this level that current measurement of child mental health outcomes is most sophisticated. However, there are limitations to a purely symptom-based approach to outcome assessment. Longitudinal studies of childhood disorders have shown that long-term outcomes are not well predicted by symptom severity alone (Rutter 1999). For example, multiple social adversities can increase the chances of severe problems in adolescence almost 100-fold (Fergusson and Horwood 1999).

The second level of measurement concerns adaptation to the psychosocial environment. Critical dimensions are likely to include meeting the role demands of home and school, and having adequate pro-social interactions with peers and adults, but the range of possible aspects of this domain that could be measured is huge.

The third level of outcome measurement concerns mechanisms, Kazdin and Kendall (1998) stressed that the future of treatment development and outcomes investigations lies in the specification of the processes and mechanisms through which treatments achieved their effects. Surprisingly, outcome studies measuring change at this level frequently fail to demonstrate that symptomatic change was associated with modifications of underlying mechanisms. For example, cognitive-behavioural therapy is sometimes successful without demonstrable changes in cognitive structures (Jacobson *et al.* 1996).

The fourth level concerns transactional aspects of development. Contextual or transactional measures of outcome could, in principle, involve an almost limitless range of measurement domains. Perhaps of greatest relevance, however, is the child's immediate context (parent and family functioning). This might include psychiatric disorder amongst family members and quality of family relationships. Contextual influences beyond family functioning include a wide range of life circumstances, including social stressors and socioeconomic status.

The final level of outcome identified by Kendall and Kazdin concerns the level and experience of service utilization. Economic evaluations of child and adolescent mental health interventions (Knapp 1997) are clearly important but sometimes service use may be increased by 'successful' interventions. For example, some of the benefits of early home visitation may be mediated by the increased use made of a range of other paediatric medical services (Olds and Kitzman 1993).

In addition to service use, satisfaction with services is a clear priority in much current policy development. However it is important to remember that positive experience of services does not necessarily equate with most positive outcome in other domains and vice versa.

It is clear from the forgoing that multiple levels of measurement are indicated. We would recommend that, as a minimum, services seek to evaluate outcomes in relation to the referred child's symptoms and adaptation, family relationships, and both child and parent's experience of service.

In order to make sense of any changes found, it is crucial to collect a wide range of demographic and other information on age, gender, case complexity, and so forth, in order to be in a position to meaningfully interpret any outcome data collected. The Paddington Complexity Scale is used by some services as a simple measure that clinicians complete at first contact that provides core data about case complexity (Yates *et al.* 1999).

The development or purchase of a database is key to the success of any routine outcome evaluation. The databases in both Southampton and Bedfordshire are home grown. There are now commercial systems on the market, for example 'Maisy' (Thompson 1996). These can be customized for local needs at a cost.

Any database must include (as a minimum) information in relation to the following: the referred child; their family; the reasons for referral; who referred; what services were offered and what received, and information about any clinician(s) who saw them.

In Southampton, the CAMHS database has been developed over many years to provide information for research and audit purposes (Thompson *et al.* 2003). The coding system used is based on the database formulated by an Association of Child Psychologists and Psychiatrists (ACPP) working Party (Berger *et al.* 1993).

Box 37.1 outlines the various databases that inter-relate in the Southampton system to allow interrogation, in order that a combination of different reports can be regularly prepared.

Regular reports can be prepared on stored templates (Box 37.2).

Box 37.1 Databases presently available in Southampton CAMHS

Current details containing current family information.

Referral and discharge details.

Problems.

Appointments database.

Research database young child clinic/medication.

Outcome database.

Box 37.2 Regular reports pertaining to any time span available in Southampton

Age and sex of children referred.

Referrers.

Referral by area sector.

Appointments for each therapist for the month.

Cancellations and did not attends (DNA).

Waiting time for first appointment for each therapist.

Discharge report.

Table 37.1 Key elements of information collected in Luton and Bedfordshire CAMHS

Client information	Referral information	Service provision information
Gender	Date of referral	Date first appointment offered
Date of birth	Referring professional	Date of first appointment
Age at referral	Problem category using ACPP codes (as many as necessary)	Waiting time (weeks)
Ethnicity	Date of referral	Date of last appointment
Family composition	Referring professional	Therapy time (weeks from first to last appointment)
Child protection history		How case closed (e.g. DNA, mutual agreement etc)
Peri-natal history		Number of sessions offered
Nature of difficulties pre- and post-interventions using agreed outcome evaluation measures (clinician, child and parent)—quantitative and qualitative information		Number of sessions attended
Service satisfaction measures (child and parent)		Type of intervention(s) offered Discipline(s) of clinicians involved

In Bedfordshire and Luton the databases developed also allow for regular reporting on different aspects. Table 37.1 outlines some of the key elements of information collected in the Bedfordshire and Luton databases (it would be too lengthy to include all fields).

The challenge for any service developing a database is to balance the wish to capture maximum details with the need to ensure that such data are viable to collect and input on a routine basis in the context of already stretched resources. For a database to be useful it must be flexible and to able to be modified year by year. Southampton is now looking at including routine information, pre- and post-intervention, as to the referred child's drug and alcohol use, number of hours in school, community activities and number of family placements. Bedfordshire and Luton are exploring how best to include routine information about social economic status, deprivation, school attendance, and parental mental health.

For a database to function it needs clinic staff that are willing to fill in information correctly and it needs someone to audit and manage that database. Ideally there should be at least two clinicians who are willing to take responsibility and give a lead in relation to this endeavour (preferably from different disciplines to encourage their colleagues). It is vital that clinicians receive feedback from the database on a regular basis that they can appreciate its use.

How should outcome be evaluated?

Questionnaires are one of the most commonly used methods of assessing service users' views (Stallard 1995). The many advantages of survey research are well-documented

(Thompson *et al.* 2003). However, there is some evidence that responses on questionnaires are likely to be more positively skewed than those elicited by in-depth interviews (Cape 1991; Tozer 2000). Whilst interviews are too time-consuming and resource-intensive to do on a routine basis, we would suggest they might supplement a questionnaire-based routine evaluation of outcome with in-depth qualitative studies on particular groups and issues.

For example, in Bedfordshire in recent years, alongside routine evaluation of outcome by questionnaire, a number of in-depth qualitative studies have been undertaken including: looking at why people did not attend (Brooks *et al.* 2002), exploring children's experience of being diagnosed with ADHD (Harbornne 2001), and investigating siblings' experience of being involved in family therapy (Swann 2001).

In terms of the questionnaires—there are a wide range available and each has their advantages and disadvantages (Fonagy *et al.* 2002; Gledhill and Garralda 2002; Hunter *et al.* 1996; Sperlinger 2002; Wolpert *et al.* 2000).

We suggest the following criteria for selecting measures be applied: measures need to be: valid, reliable, acceptable to users, acceptable to clinicians, inexpensive, easy to complete (less than 10 min and simple language), easy to interpret, widely used, and culturally sensitive.

The following are suggested as an example of a likely set of core measures for many services (with the expectation that services will add more specialist measures as local need dictate):

The perspective of clinicians:

> Health of the Nation Outcome Scales—Child and Adolescent (HoNOSCA)(Gowers *et al.* 1998, 1999); completed by clinicians (also an adolescent version for clients aged 13 years and over). Available at: (www.rcpsych.ac.uk).

> Children's Global Assessment Scale (C-GAS); completed by clinicians for all age groups. Available at: (http://depts.washington.edu/wimirt/Index.htm).

Parents' and children's perspectives:

> Strengths and Difficulties Questionnaire (SDQ) (Goodman 1997); completed by referred children aged 11–16 and parents of children aged 3–16. Available at: (www.sdqinfo.com).

> Service satisfaction survey such as that developed by the Commission for Health Improvement (CHI). Available at: (www.chi.nhs.uk/eng/cgr/mental_health/child_ questionnaire.pdf).

In terms of clinician based measures, the HoNOSCA is the most widely used and researched in the UK (Brann *et al.* 2001; Garralda *et al.* 2000; Gowers *et al.* 1999); there is also a user version for young people aged 13 and over. This 13-item scale rates the child's behaviour in terms of the level of 'problems' in relation to the following domains: anti-social behaviour; over-activity and inattention; non-accidental self-injury; substance abuse; scholastic or language skills; physical illness or disability; hallucinations or delusions; non-organic somatic symptoms; emotional and related symptoms; peer relationships; self-care and independence; family life and relationships; and school attendance. Ratings on each scale can be added together to make a total score.

It is however, recognized there are limitations in this scale: especially for the younger age group (Thompson *et al.* 2003), the training materials could be improved; and there are difficulties in establishing consistency between clinicians. Where the HoNOSCA is not acceptable to clinicians, we suggest use of the Children's Global Assessment Scale (C-GAS).

From a user perspective—the SDQ is already widely used, well standardized, exists in a range of languages, is quick to complete, and is acceptable in a range of settings. It has also been found valid for use with children with learning disabilities (Emerson 2003). Although the SDQ has not been validated for children over the age of 16, it has also been used for 17–18-year-olds in some community surveys. This 25-item questionnaire covers both positive and negative behaviours, and also assesses the impact of the difficulties on the child and family. From it you can generate scores for a child's emotional symptoms, conduct problems, hyperactivity, difficulties in peer relationships, and also their levels of pro-social behaviour. There is also a teachers' version available.

In terms of service satisfaction measures, many services have devised their own, but services may choose the version available from Commission for Health Improvement (CHI), the Experience of Service Questionnaire, the individual items of which were derived from consultation with users.

Table 37.2 summarizes the main measures suggested for use by the different age groups of referred children.

A major problem for any routine evaluation of outcome is getting acceptable return rates at follow-up. Problems with low response rates are one of the chief disadvantages of evaluation by questionnaire. In Bedfordshire, return rates from users to the 'pre-therapy' measures over the first two years of introduction of routine evaluation of outcome, were as follows: 56% of children, 70% of parents, and 71% of clinicians. At case closure, the majority of clinicians (64%) completed the evaluation but only 14% of children and 17% of parents completed post-therapy questionnaires.

In order to attempt to maximize response rates, we suggest that core outcome measures should be implemented by the first appointment and at 6 months following the first appointment, or at termination of treatment if this occurs before 6 months. The rationale for choosing a 6-month time point for follow-up, comes from the fact that most children and adolescents seen in CAMHS will have had their problems attended to and treated in that time; it fits in with a system that is as simple to institute administratively and as cost-effectively as possible.

There is obviously room for flexibility and experimentation in this. For example, Southampton has adopted 6-monthly routine evaluations using some measures, but for service satisfaction is planning to adopt a twice yearly snap-shot of the service. For 2 weeks, in October

Table 37.2 Summary of main measures to be used for different age groups

Age range of child or young person in years	Methods of evaluation
0–5	SDQ (parent completed) HoNOSCA or C-GAS (clinician completed) CHI service satisfaction (parent completed)
6–10	SDQ (parent completed) HoNOSCA or C-GAS (clinician completed) CHI service satisfaction (parent and child aged 9+ versions completed)
11–16	SDQ (parent and child versions completed) HoNOSCA or C-GAS (clinician completed) CHI service satisfaction (parent and child versions completed)
16–21	HoNOSCA or C-GAS (clinician completed) HoNOSCA or SDQ (child/young person version) CHI service satisfaction (parent and child versions completed)

and April, every patient who has had a second or subsequent appointment will be surveyed with questionnaires filled in by the patients at the clinic.

In general we would recommend that any follow-up measures be completed as part of routine contact in the clinic (preferably by administrative staff or research assistants) or over the telephone. Telephone interviews can improve compliance rates up to 80%, although they may bias response (Thompson *et al.* 2003). Where possible, telephone contact or questionnaire administration should be undertaken by someone other than the clinician involved in the work, in order to try to minimize the potential skewing of the data, but we recognize this may not be feasible in all cases. How the questionnaire is completed should be logged in the database.

Table 37.3 summarizes a possible protocol, as adopted by the CAMHS Outcome Research Consortium (CORC).

How should the findings be used?

It is important to constantly reiterate that there are likely to be differences in outcome, as viewed from different perspectives, in relation to different domains. Therefore, it is vital to present any findings in the following terms: outcome in relation to a particular domain (e.g. adaptation, emotional problems, etc.), as measured by a particular instrument (e.g. SDQ), from the perspective of a particular respondent (e.g. child).

There is no generally agreed way of determining when change is 'clinically significant' (cf. Fonagy *et al.* 2002). The method we suggest adopting is the 'Reliable Change Index'. This involves setting a criterion for change in standard deviation units, which exceed chance fluctuations, adjusted for the reliability of the instrument (Jacobson and Truax 1991). This has been used in both Bedfordshire (Wolpert *et al.* 2003) and Southampton (Sonuga-Barke *et al.* 2001).

Jacobson and Truax suggest four categories of outcome: deteriorated, no change, improvement, and clinically significant improvement. In Bedfordshire, we felt it was important to apply the same criteria for clinical significance to those children who had deteriorated, as for those who had improved, therefore we decided to adopt five categories of outcome: clinically significant deterioration, deterioration, no change, improvement, and clinically significant improvement.

Table 37.3 A suggested protocol (as adopted by the CAMHS Outcome Research Consortium (CORC))

Clinic activity	Outcome evaluation activity
Referral processed	Basic patient information in-putted into database (including coding using ACPP data sets).
First appointment letter sent	SDQ to be sent with the first appointment letter to parent and/or child together with covering letter explaining the use of any data and requesting consent.
First appointment	Family members hand in completed questionnaire(s).
After first appointment	Clinician completes HoNOSCA or C-GAS.
After 6 months or on ending contact (whichever comes first):	SDQ and CHI service-satisfaction questionnaire completed by Parent and/or child in clinic or over the phone. HoNOSCA or C-GAS completed by clinician. For those small minoriry of cases seen over a number of years, questionnaires will completed on yearly basis.

Below is presented a brief overview of how we have sought to use of the findings in our respective services, in order to achieve the four aims identified at the outset (client evaluation, clinician evaluation, service evaluation, and to support research and audit projects).

Case evaluation

In Bedfordshire and Luton, outcome data for each closed case is presented in a summary form at case closure and sent to the clinician before being added to the file notes. A 'crib sheet' is provided for all clinicians, to help them understand and interpret the scores. It is stressed that it is not possible to say that any changes, whether clinically significant or not, are caused by the therapy or are merely co-temporaneous with it.

Looking at individual cases in this way, it quickly becomes clear that the outcomes in the different domains do not necessarily neatly tally. For example, one child indicated that she felt things were much better, that her behaviour had improved in most areas, and that she he felt that the service had helped quite a lot, but she also indicated she had not felt understood and that some areas of her behaviour had not improved. Such data can be used in supervision to try to understand the findings in the context of the particular case and as a way of developing future practice.

Clinician evaluation

Collation of individual cases, discussed in supervision, becomes a way for clinicians to reflect on their own practice. Thus, if the clinician of the case above found all the children he saw commented on not feeling understood, this may be something to be addressed as a training need.

The experience in Bedfordshire and Luton has been that clinicians reviewing cases in this way start to identify themes and issues. Clinicians have commented that they have found feedback from families, particularly in relation to what they found more or less useful, illuminating and helpful in the development of their own practice. For example, one clinician who adopted a policy of openness with clients, was pleased to have this commented on positively by many of the families she saw.

Clearly, the low response rates from parents and children affect the strength we can give to these findings in terms of monitoring clinical activity. As discussed above, there is likely to be a positive skew, and until we have larger, more representative response rates, we cannot be too sanguine about the very positive feedback received so far. However, even with a likely positive skew, not all the comments and feedback from families have been positive. We have now developed a system in Bedfordshire and Luton whereby all qualitative comments are regularly collated, in an anonymized form, and passed on to the Chair of our Research and Audit Committee, which oversees the outcome evaluation project. If any of these comments are felt to be a potential cause for concern, then the clinician in question is identified from the database and alerted to this, and the comment is passed to the clinical director. In this way, we hope to facilitate clinical governance and make sure any inappropriate practice is identified quickly. We have only had occasion to use this mechanism once so far.

Information about the service or projects

For reasons of space only one example is offered below from Bedfordshire and Luton as to how outcome data might be used as part of evaluation of services. Other examples can be found in Wolpert *et al.* (2003). The example below highlights the strengths and weaknesses of using the available data to look at service-level issues, in the context of low post-therapy return rates for children and families.

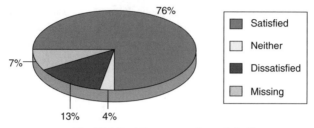

Fig. 37.1 Post-therapy service satisfaction.

The example reported is service satisfaction as measured by a service-specific questionnaire (the services has since starting use the CHI questionnaire) from the parents' perspective.

Of the 415 parents sent post-therapy measures, 71% completed the service satisfaction aspect of the questionnaire (17% return rate). Of these, the majority said they were satisfied with the service they received 76% ($n = 54$), although 13% ($n = 9$) were dissatisfied (see Fig. 37.1).

Qualitative data gave some useful insights into what was liked and disliked. Recurrent positive themes about the service focused on the possibility for family members to talk about difficult issues together. For example, one parent commented:

> The fact that we were talking with the child and not 'behind her back' was useful—it showed us what her problems were and she also heard our side of things.

Children often commented on their feeling of having been listened to. One adolescent wrote that what she had found most useful was:

> Talking as a family where everyone got their points of views heard.

Where users were more negative about their experience, this tended to focus on the length of the wait before being seen following referral. One parent wrote:

> I would have liked an appointment earlier. By the time we had been referred some time had lapsed from my initial visit to the doctor for help.

Another parent felt that they:

> … would (have liked) some background information on what form the meeting would take.

Such information has been used to further develop our service. For example, we re-designed the information leaflet we routinely send to families prior to their first appointment.

In presenting these and other results based on user evaluation, to commissioners, we need to acknowledge the very low response rate and the likely positive skew. However, in the context of fighting for funds for services, with fund holders sceptical about CAMHS having any positive impact, even these results, partial as they are, can be helpful. For some commissioners to discover any children and families value the service can be an eye opener.

This data can also provide information for users and potential users of service. We have developed posters for service users highlighting key findings from our project, such as the one displayed in one of our clinic waiting-rooms reproduced in Fig. 37.2.

Research projects and audits using outcome data

Below are listed a selection of audits and research projects that draw on the databases within the two services, to illustrate some of the ways that data may be used.

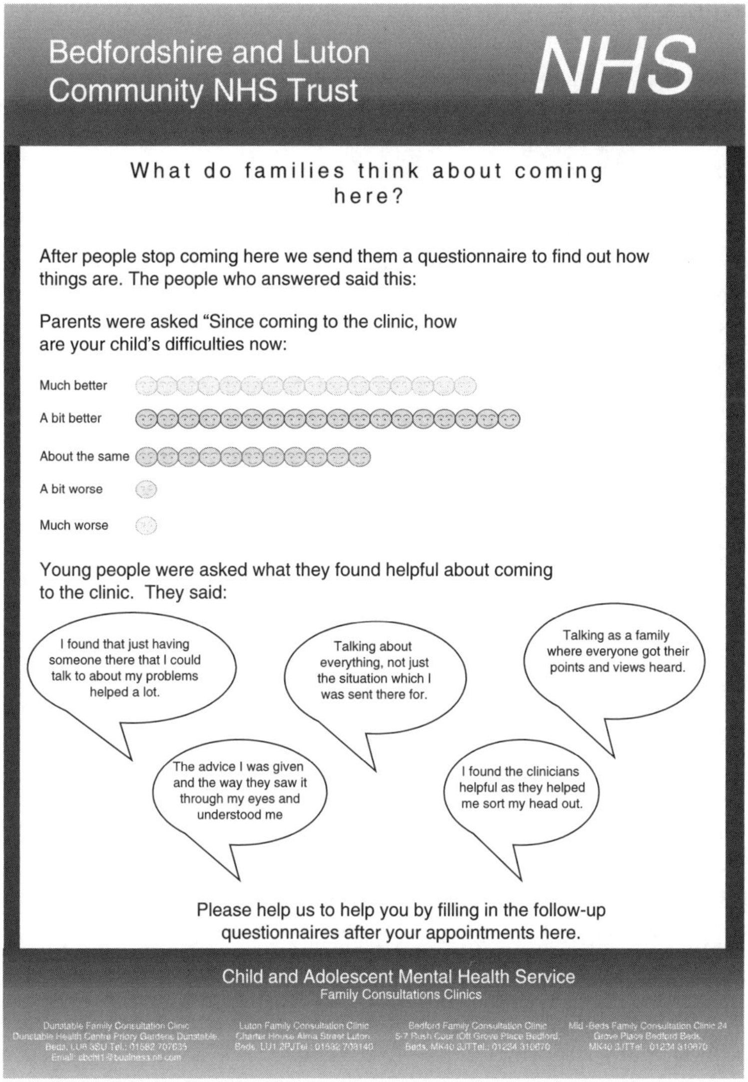

Fig. 37.2 Example of a poster for service users to highlight findings from previous service satisfaction surveys.

Monitoring workload and waiting times

In Southampton and Bedfordshire and Luton, the databases are used to enable clinical staff to monitor workload and for the clinic to monitor referral patterns and to share such information with clinicians themselves, as well as with commissioners and referrers. It is also possible to check how long patients are waiting to be seen, and, by using the priority rating and problem list, it is possible to look at the profile of those waiting for an appointment.

Case-load management and clinical governance

In Southampton each month, the number of appointments each clinician has offered, and the number kept, is printed. A regular printout of open cases is useful for appraisal and supervision sessions, as well as for job plans. The profile of cases can be looked at, with severity codings to look at case weighting. A recent audit of the caseload of all clinicians in the clinic (Laver-Bradbury 2001), indicated that the number of children referred to the clinic with complex problems was increasing and thus the ratio of children who present with less than five problems, compared with those presenting with more than five problems, is going down . This helped the team to understand why everyone was so busy, felt overloaded, and morale was low.

Audit of children in the clinic with attention deficit disorder (ADHD)

A recent audit and research project in Southampton looked at all children in the clinic who were on stimulant medication in July 2000, in order to monitor the protocols we had in place, and to consider whether or not the stimulant medication was appropriate (Thompson *et al.* 2003). The audit indicated that protocols were being used appropriately, and that the mean medication used was about the same as the MTA study; but it highlighted the complexity of children seen at a community AD/HD clinic. The clinic has re-looked at the kind of work offered to the children, especially children with specific speech and communication difficulties, and those with complex families.

Non-attenders and attenders

An appointment database in Southampton allows tracking of all appointments, and our database manager is able to make sure appointments are sent to families and that no appointments are missed. The database also tracks appointments cancelled by clinicians, which is useful for clinical governance issues. The results of a recent audit led the team to conclude that DNAs occurred because of poor briefing by referrers, rather than clinical issues. We have now introduced an opting-in system for first appointments, which has cut our DNA rate to less than 5%.

Register of schedule 2 drugs

Tracking of appointments in Southampton has also enabled us to make sure that all our AD/HD patients on medication have regular monitoring visits. The therapy database enables us to keep a register of all medication prescribed for the young people, which is important, as the stimulant drugs are schedule 2 drugs and a way of monitoring this is essential.

Was the young child clinic cost-effective?

A series of audits was set up to look up at the evaluation of a service for young children with behaviour problems in Southampton. The initial clinic was run with two clinicians but was then re-organized to be run by nurses, and the work sometimes took place in the main clinic but more often in the patient's own locality or at home. Doctors or other therapists were rarely involved and usually only one worker was involved. Costing was cheaper in the second option, although there was no statistical difference in the number of appointments kept (1990–1 mean number of appointments 4.07 SD3.18; 1994–5 mean number of appointments 3.5 SD2.8). This encouraged the team to work even more closely with professionals in primary care, in order for the more simple problems to be dealt with by them. This freed the main clinic to be reserved for more complex cases, where more intensive work was necessary; for example, children with ADHD or complex developmental issues (Thompson *et al.* 2003).

What predicts referral into a child guidance clinic?

The most recent use of the database in Southampton for research purposes was to find children who had been referred into the clinic at some point in the last 8 years, who had been part of a birth cohort of children surveyed with the mothers in 1990–91, when the children were 3 years of age: 77 children had been referred into the clinic. Being a young mother who had had an unhappy childhood predicted referral on multi-regression analysis. On univariate analysis, a hyperactive score, a high score on a behaviour checklist and having a mother who scored highly on the General Health Questionnaire when the child was 3 year of age, was predictive.

An evaluation of the accuracy of the current CAMHS system for prioritizing referrals

A research project is being conducted in Bedfordshire and Luton to compare waiting-list priority codes assigned from the referral letter, with parents' perceptions of the severity of their child's problems, and clinicians perceptions of problem severity at assessment.

Differences in pre-therapy symptom severity, as measured by white British and South Asian parents of children referred to CAMHS

This project is one of a number of cultural research projects carried out by Bedfordshire and Luton. Because of the high ethnic mix found in the county, it is important for the team to consider the cultural needs of the community and to ensure the service meets these needs.

How should routine evaluation be resourced?

It is crucial to have adequate administrative and IT resources to allow outcomes to be evaluated on a routine basis in an ongoing way. Commissioners must take account of this in commissioning services; and include in any costing, the need to build-in appropriate resources to allow for routine outcome evaluation. Our experiences suggests that psychology assistants and administrative staff are crucial in making these systems work. Estimated costs are around £30 000 p.a. but will obviously depending on the size of the service and the resources already in place.

The next step?

Any evaluation of outcome that does not include control groups cannot make claims about cause and effect. However, one future development might be to compare clinical significant change rates for particular types of problem, or groups of children, with those in the research outcome literature. In this way, baselines for good practice may be established, providing, of course, that the relevant contextual factors are taken into account. One way forward might be to employ the notion of 'effective efficacy' as described in Fonagy *et al.* (2002). This refers to 'the proportion of patients encountered in clinical practice who are likely to respond to empirically supported psychosocial interventions'. This involves adjusting predicted efficacy rates from the research literature to allow for a higher degree of co-morbidity in the clinic. These adjusted figures could be used to provide realistic baselines for services to compare their own levels of significant clinical change against.

Conclusion

The work outlined above demonstrates ways of gathering key information that may usefully add to the clinical work. Outcome data from a range of families can help individual clinicians in the evaluation and development of their practice and aid clinical governance. Whilst low post-therapy return rates from users means service evaluation cannot hinge on their responses, service outcomes as measured by the clinicians' evaluations and the responses from those users who do complete the questionnaires, can help inform commissioners, service providers, potential users and researchers alike and aid service development.

References

Achenbach, T. M. (1995) Diagnosis, assessment, and comorbidity in psychosocial treatment research. *Journal of Abnormal Child Psychology*, **23**, 45–64.

Berger, M.H.P., Cottrell, D., Stein, E. *et al.* (1993) *Minimum data base for child psychologists and psychiatrists.* London: ACPP.

Brann. P., Coleman, G., and Luk, E. (2001) Routine outcome measurement in a child and adolescent mental health service: an evaluation of HoNOSCA. *Australian and New Zealand Journal of Psychiatry*, **35**, 370–6.

Brooks, E., Ross, C., Wolpert, M., Christie, D., and Stein, S. (2002) Towards an understanding of did not attend rates in a child and adolescent mental health service. *Clinical Psychology*, **14**, 25–8.

Cape, J. (1991) Quality assurance methods for clinical psychology services. *The Psychologist: Bulletin of the British Psychological Society*, **4**, 499–503.

Emerson, E. (2003) Use of the strengths and difficulties questionnaire to assess the mental health needs of children and adolescents with intellectual disabilities. Personal communication.

Fergusson, D.M. and Horwood, L.J. (1999) Prospective childhood predictors of deviant peer affiliations in adolescence. *Journal of Child Psychology and Psychiatry and Allied Disciplines*, **40**, 581–92.

Fonagy, P., Target, M., Cottrell, D., Phillips, J., and Kurtz, Z. (2002) *What works for whom? A critical review of treatments for children and adolescents.* New York: Guilford Press.

Garralda, M.E., Yates, P., and Higginson, I. (2000) Child and adolescent mental health service use: HoNOSCA as an outcome measure. *British Journal of Psychiatry*, **177**, 52–8.

Gledhill, J. and Garralda, E. (2002) Scales to measure behavioural and emotional adjustment in children and their families. *Psychiatry*, **5**, 32–8.

Goodman, R. (1997) The strengths and difficulties questionnaire: a research note. *Journal of Child Psychology and Psychiatry*, **38**, 581–6.

Goodman, R. (1999) The extended version of the strengths and difficulties questionnaire as a guide to child psychiatric caseness and consequent burden. *Journal of Child Psychology and Psychiatry*, **40**, 791–9.

Gowers, S.G., Harrington, R.C., Whitton, A., Beevor, A., Lelliott, P., Jezzard, R. *et al.* (1998) *Brief report on Health of the Nation Outcome Scales Child and Adolescent Mental Health. (HoNOSCA).* London: CRU.

Gowers, S.G., Harrington, R.C., Whitton, A., Lelliott, P., Beevor, A., Wing, J. *et al.* (1999) Brief scale for measuring the outcomes of emotional and behavioural disorders in children. *British Journal of Psychiatry*, **174**, 413–6.

Harbornne, A. (2001) *Childrens' perceptions of being diagnosed with ADHD and prescribed Ritalin.* Doctoral thesis, University College London.

Hunter, J., Higginson, I., and Garralda, M.E. (1996) Systematic literature review: outcome measures for child and adolescent mental health services. *Journal of Public Health Medicine*, **18**, 197–206.

Jacobson, N.S. and Truax, P. (1991) Clinical significance: a statistical approach to defining meaningful change in psychotherapy research. *Journal of Consulting and Clinical Psychology*, **59**, 12–9.

Jacobson, N.S., Dobson, K.S., Truax, P.A., Addis, M.E., Koerner, K., Gollan, J.K. *et al.* (1996) A component analysis of cognitive-behavioral treatment for depression. *Journal of Consulting and Clinical Psychology*, **64**, 295–304.

Kazdin, A.E. and Kendall, P.C. (1998) Current progress and future plans for developing effective treatments: comments and perspectives. *Journal of Clinical Child Psychology*, **27**, 217–26.

Knapp, M.R.J. (1997) Economic evaluations and interventions for children and adolescents with mental health problems. *Journal of Child Psychology and Psychiatry*, **38**, 3–25.

Laver-Bradbury, C. (2001) *Community child and adolescent mental health long-term case management study*. Unpublished in-depth in practice module as part of Msc, University of Southampton.

Olds, D. and Kitzman, H. (1993) Review of research on home visiting for pregnant women and parents of young children. *Future of Children*, **3**, 53–92.

Rutter, M. (1999) Psychosocial adversity and child psychopathology. *British Journal of Psychiatry*, **174**, 480–93.

Sonuga-Barke, E.J., Daley, D., Thompson, M.J.J., Laver-Bradbury, C., and Weeks, A. (2001) Parent based therapies for attention deficit/hyperactivity disorder: a randomised controlled trial with a community sample. *Journal of American Academy of child and Adolescent Psychiatry*, **40** (4), 1–7.

Sperlinger, D. (2002) *Outcome assessment in routine clinical practice in psychosocial services*. British Psychological Society, Division of Clinical Psychology.

Stallard, P. (1995) Parental satisfaction with intervention: differences between respondents and non-respondents to a postal questionnaire. *British Journal of Clinical Psychology*, **34**, 397–405.

Swann, R. (2001) *Siblings' experiences of family therapy*. Doctoral thesis, University of East London.

Thompson, M.J.J. (1996) Software review: maisy for Windows. *Child Psychology and Psychiatry Review* ;**1** (2).

Thompson, M.J.J., Coll, X., Wilkinson, S., and Utenbroek, D. (2003) The development of an effective mental health service for young children. *Child and Mental Health Review*, **8** (2), 68–78.

Tozer, M. (2000) Learning from the patient experience: evaluating service quality from the perspective of patients and carers. *Clinical Governance Bulletin*, **1**, 3–4.

Wolpert, M., Wilkinson, I., and Fuggle, P. (2000) *Minimum standards for evaluating outcome in clinical practice-position paper of the faculty for children and young people*. Division of Clinical Psychology, British Psychological Society.

Wolpert, M., Stein, S.M., Pakes, K., and Tingay, K. (2003) Establishing routine evaluation of outcome in child and adolescent mental health services: first steps on a thousand mile journey? *Service Practice and Update (March 2003)*. Faculty for Children and Young People of the Division of Clinical Psychology, British Psychological Society.

Yates, P., Garralda, M.E., and Higginson, I. (1999) Paddington Complexity Scale and Health of the Nation Outcome Scales for Children and Adolescents. *British Journal of Psychiatry*, **174**, 417–23.

Chapter 38

Creative practice and innovation in child and adolescent mental health services

Zarrina Kurtz and Cathy James

Effective services to deliver efficacious interventions

Although what is known about the efficacy of treatments for child and adolescent mental health problems is not inconsiderable (Fonagy *et al.* 2002), the effectiveness of child and adolescent mental health services has been much less studied, even in the US and particularly so in the UK. Outcomes achieved in research-based studies of the efficacy of particular treatments show a good deal of discrepancy with the observed effectiveness of these treatments in naturalistic settings such as community clinics, health centres, or homes (Weisz *et al.* 1992; Weisz and Weiss 1993). Based on a systematic review of studies of clinic-based interventions, Weisz and colleagues (Weisz *et al.* 1995a) found that they showed negligible effectiveness. What appears to account for the greater effect sizes in research-based therapy, compared with clinic-based interventions, includes behavioural methods and the use of focused treatment with pre-planning and structure. Children presenting to routine services are known to be likely to have greater severity of problems and levels of co-morbidity than in research settings, with additional problems (associated, for example, with substance misuse or being in the care system), and lower levels of motivation for treatment with high rates of drop-out (Weisz *et al.* 1995b). However, it has been suggested that the organization and structure of a manualized approach may even motivate parents and children to attend sessions with greater enthusiasm than would be the case with less structured approaches.

Even in less controlled situations than the clinic, the effectiveness of interventions has been shown. An example is multi-systemic family intervention, which has achieved remarkable success in a naturalistic setting involving home, school, and community (Borduin *et al.* 1995; Henggeler *et al.* 1995). And parent management training can be more successful in a community setting than in the clinic (Cunningham *et al.* 1995). It is suggested that the central issue might be whether efficacious methods are systematically applied, rather than certain inherent characteristics of the clinical setting (Fonagy *et al.* 2002).

Whole-service evaluation of innovative projects in CAMHS

In England in 1999, a remarkable series of evaluative studies were started on new 3-year projects aimed at delivering innovative services for child and adolescent mental health (Department of Health 1998). These 24 projects were funded by the Department of Health with the explicit aim of stimulating partnership and innovation, and reflecting the government's recognition of the importance of the mental health of children and young people in tackling its social exclusion agenda. Ten of the projects focused on prevention and early intervention, working to reduce known risk factors for child and adolescent mental health problems, and to prevent family breakdown and school exclusion. Nine projects focused on the needs of looked-after children and their parents and carers, and five worked with young people with very severe and complex needs. There was overlap in these two groups in that many young people with complex needs are in the care system. The expectation was that these projects would develop services in areas known to be particularly under-resourced, within what had been shown to be generally unsatisfactory current provision of services to meet well-documented needs (Audit Commission 1999).

Each project was individually evaluated. These studies constitute the first whole-service evaluations of child and adolescent mental health services (CAMHS) in England, and provide considerable information about the process of setting up and running the projects, as well as about outcomes. Outcomes, across the evaluations, were reported in all five domains of the comprehensive model described by Hoagwood et al. (1996): symptoms and diagnoses; child and family functioning; consumer perspectives; the child's environment; and the service system. An over-arching analysis of the collective findings from the individual evaluations enables us to conclude with some confidence what the projects achieved in each of these domains, and what kinds of approaches proved to be effective (Kurtz and James 2004).

Positive outcomes reported by the projects

Before describing and discussing the creative and innovative approaches taken by the projects, we will describe the ways in which they were shown to be effective, ie. the impact of the work they carried out. So far, only short-term outcomes (c.6 months or a year post-intervention) have been reported. Different elements of the projects' work and ways of working led to positive outcomes in different areas, which are described below.

Mental health symptomatology

Unexpectedly high levels of mental health need were found among the children, young people, and parents with whom the projects worked, even those aiming at early intervention. However, many projects were able to show a reduction in the proportion of those with clinically significant problems, and among the most challenging young people, there were reported improvements in conduct problems and disruptive behaviour. Among projects working with looked-after children and those with severe and complex needs, a particular finding was increased self-awareness among the young people and an understanding of their difficulties, as well as their strengths.

Young people's engagement with services

The projects succeeded in carrying out therapeutic work with groups of young people and their families who were well known to have failed to benefit from previous service provision. The young people reported that they were helped, chiefly, in making improvements in their behaviour and their relationships with others, in finding a way through their difficulties, and in accessing other services.

Child and family functioning

Early intervention projects showed a substantial increase in parental understanding of, and confidence in, handling their child's behaviour. Across the board, there was increased engagement with education and a reduction in school exclusion.

Children's environments

Many positive changes in the school environment—leading to positive mental health outcomes for children and more confident and competent school staff—were reported by those projects targeting their work on the education system. Projects working with looked-after children reported that placements were better planned and more stable as a result of their work. There was compelling evidence that the projects had a major effect in improving parenting and carer skills, reducing parents' and carers' stress, and supporting them in a number of therapeutic and practical ways. Both parents and carers reported that the help they had received from the projects enabled them to provide effective help to the children in their care, improved family functioning, and prevented family and placement breakdown.

Service systems

About half the projects reported an impact on the wider local service system for child and adolescent mental health. Some projects were providing extra resources, while others undertook different ways of working to meet previously unmet local needs. The work of the early intervention projects, in particular, usually resulted in a decrease in the waiting time for Specialist CAMHS and where this did not happen, it was thought to be due to the uncovering of previously unmet need. In all instances there was a positive influence on the appropriateness of referrals to Specialist CAMHS. Several projects also influenced the way in which Specialist CAMHS was delivered in the area, with an increased emphasis on the acceptability and accessibility of services.

Projects targeting looked-after children often succeeded in increasing the involvement of Specialist CAMHS in work with this vulnerable group and the understanding of children's mental health needs within social services.

All the projects had a more or less significant effect in increasing inter-agency working; collaborative work with education was regarded as particularly important for successful outcomes.

Approaches employed to achieve positive outcomes

Whole-team reflective learning and re-shaping the service accordingly

The projects based their approaches on currently available evidence indicating the reasons why so many children and young people and their families appear not to derive much benefit from child and adolescent mental health services. Along the way, the projects also gathered new evidence that substantially informed the ways in which their services were shaped. Thus a key and creative aspect of their practice was their continuing efforts to reflect on how things were going, and to modify their therapeutic and organizational approach accordingly, organize appropriate staff training, and perhaps recruit new skills into the team. Some projects were able to attract funding to expand their remit, and several early intervention projects began offering 'top-up' sessions for families after 6 months (or longer), in response to user feedback. One project leader described how important they felt it was to create and sustain a 'learning organization' (Senge 1990).

Tailoring interventions to the assessed needs of families and young people

Projects took time to understand the complex needs of their target group and the particular local context in which they were working, and to include the views of potential service users in this multi-faceted assessment of needs. But they had designated time and resources, which allowed them to tailor services accordingly and to develop the necessary expertise. Projects developed individualized packages for the parent and child, wherever possible, as well as using evidence-based, manualized interventions. Individual packages could address anything from housing and domestic violence issues for the parent, to educational and leisure opportunities for the child:

> It felt like an individualized personal service, listening to us as a family rather than a case [Parent early intervention project].

For young people with complex needs, several projects focused on developing wrap-around packages of care. Again, following a comprehensive assessment of needs, these packages often explicitly included a period of work to engage the young person. Packages included mental health interventions but also focused on physical health, education, and social needs. When difficulties arose, the package was reviewed and enhanced where necessary, rather than the young person being moved on or told that the service was not able to meet their needs. Parents from one project graphically described how their previous experience in seeking help had been to trail from one agency to another, being 'assessed' but with little action resulting. In contrast, they saw this service as one that gathered the necessary resources around the child and their family.

Projects aimed to influence factors in the child's environment, in the family, school, and community. Working with schools meant developing whole school interventions, as well as targeting the problems of particular children; for example, a playground games pack, as well as behaviour strategies for use in the classroom. Projects working with looked-after children were able to influence service systems, such as the training available to residential homes and the availability of leisure facilities, as well as children's individual circumstances.

Recognizing and supporting the needs of parents and carers

Projects recognized the key role they had in supporting and enhancing the skills and confidence of parents in bringing about positive outcomes for children. They aimed to help parents, not only during the period of intervention, but to give them tools that could be used in the future as their child developed. In early intervention, advice and support were offered to some parents without the need for children to be seen. Projects offered evidence-based parenting programmes, as well as individual packages for parents and children. Several projects also worked on improving parents' relationships with other services, such as schools:

> It made me feel stronger inside so when I have to telephone anyone about my son, I can now deal with them better. I can say what I mean now. My confidence has increased enormously [Parent].

With young people looked after and with complex needs, projects worked with parents whenever possible, even when they were no longer the main carer for the young person.

A number of projects identified that the needs of adoptive parents largely went unmet, and offered a specific service for them as well as for foster carers.

The involvement of carers, both foster carers and residential staff, was crucial in the development and success of the projects and in positive outcomes for children. Stable placements and positive relationships with adults are key to children's mental health, and the projects worked on enhancing carers' skills and confidence through training and on-going support. They also recognized the expertise of carers about the children living with them and the need to include carers in the therapeutic process rather than leaving them in the waiting room.

The projects highlighted the need for a culture change, so that seeking help with caring for looked-after children is seen as a strength and not a weakness on the part of carers, and that awareness of children's mental health issues is accepted as an essential pre-requisite for carers and residential staff:

> To admit to needing help may be a huge step for some foster carers but they need the help out there to be able to do it-this service gives that help [Foster carer].

Style of work

Young people and parents in all projects appreciated the open and respectful approach of project staff and reported feeling supported and not judged. Young people valued confidentiality highly, and an approach that built on their strengths, as well as recognizing their difficulties. Parents and professionals welcomed the open approach of the projects and usually felt they were kept well-informed. Projects recognized that they were developing their practice and were open to learning from mistakes. There was an ethos of partnership with both users of the service and with other professionals:

> Well I can't put my finger on it, but… [therapist] just put you at your ease… just made you feel good about yourself and what you were doing [Carer].

Increasing access to services and their acceptability

All the projects aimed to increase accessibility to, and the acceptability of, child mental health expertise for children and families, and for professionals. Some did this by opening up the service to children and families who would not usually meet the threshold for a service. One project was described as providing for 'a level of need previously ignored. Even when a child doesn't fit criteria, they will advise' (education professional).

Projects offered a variety of referral routes (including self-referral) and worked in community venues such as schools and health centres, as well as visiting at home. Home visiting was seen as particularly useful and empowering for families:

> The people [service users] may have to deal with these academic people, you know, who have never lived on a council estate, or dealt with violence or aggression that some of my clients have to deal with, and they're handing out advice which is not practical. It can't work in their lives. My experience with [the project] is that they go in and work with what's possible within the home [Referrer to an inner city early intervention project].

Several project teams included staff who were not CAMHS specialists, such as family support staff and youth workers. They brought an important understanding of the local neighbourhood and the families' ethnicity and culture. In some cases the fact that they shared the same ethnicity as the child or family was a key factor:

> I know English youth workers but in the situation I wouldn't go to them... But she was Bengali....
> she was Asian so it wasn't any different.... It was like one of your sisters [Young man in
> East London].

Parents especially valued a 'hands-on' approach. The parent of a young child described how many professionals had 'advised her' on how to deal with her child's behaviour but the project worker had gone shopping with her and her child, and modelled for her *how* to carry out this advice in practice. These staff both informed, and were guided by specialist members of the CAMH team.

A major consideration for these projects was how to engage with young people, who often felt they already had too much interference from adults in their life. The approach to encouraging engagement took many forms; for example, involving the young person in designing the therapeutic package, providing appealing leisure activities, providing creative therapies, getting young people involved in technology such as video. Many projects offered young people a choice of venues, especially for their first meeting; some young people chose to be seen at home, while others opted for meetings in cafes or parks. Workers required persistence and flexibility, as well as back-up from colleagues. Engagement with the project facilitated young people's present and future engagement with other services that they might benefit from.

Multi-disciplinary and inter-agency working

Multi-agency working was a core activity for all the projects but, in order for services to survive and thrive, they required multi-agency commitment at both strategic and operational levels. In developing early intervention services, some projects worked with a network of providers, from both the voluntary and statutory sectors, to provide choice and flexibility for families and to develop local capacity.

The projects carried out a great deal of collaborative work with staff in day-to-day contact with children and families; for example, in education, social services, and primary care. This collaborative work comprised both formal and informal consultation, training, and joint work. Staff appreciated learning new skills and gaining confidence in using those they already had:

> We all have resources, we just forget we've got them, we forget we know this stuff [Tier 1
> professional].

Several projects used a solution-focused approach, both in working with families, young people, and carers, and in their work with other professionals, and found this useful in developing shared goals.

This wider, inclusive vision of CAMHS was useful in inner city areas where the community was ethnically diverse, but also in rural areas where access to statutory services was limited. It strongly enabled access for families to longer-term support where necessary:

> Because of their flexibility and skills they can share workloads—packages of work with other
> professionals in a variety of venues, home and school. Their service addresses problems straight
> away and helps make speedy improvements. Shared working has improved access to a child and
> adolescent mental health service [School nurse].

The majority of staff welcomed this way of working, as it offered different perspectives on problems and different ways of finding solutions. They learned from colleagues' skills and knowledge, and children and families benefited from having access to a range of professionals whose understanding extended across the education, social services, and health systems. A clear leadership role was vital in the projects, in providing direction for the project and encouraging stability among staff. In turn, project leaders needed support from a robust multi-agency steering group in managing the different expectations of the agencies:

> [The project] is a particularly difficult thing to manage because it is a therapeutic resource but within a social services department. That is tricky because you have got to know about therapy and processes. Then on the other side, you have got the pressure of social services…[Project worker from project for looked-after children].

Discussion: this is what CAMHS practice can look like

The CAMHS innovation projects have convincingly shown the type of work and style of working that result in positive outcomes for children with mental health problems and their families. If methods such as these were developed by all services for children's mental health, the evidence indicates that there would be widespread improvement in outcomes. However, the evidence about the outcomes for children and families attending comparable routine services, and whether these differ from those in the innovation projects, is largely anecdotal and very little researched.

A clear message for all services is that, in order to be effective, they need to assess holistically the needs of children and families and to take considerable care to tailor the interventions offered accordingly. This may take time, and the service needs to be able to respond as needs are revealed or modified during the intervention period. This approach may mitigate against what has been shown to be maximally effective for defined problems in research studies: the delivery of manualized interventions. A service that can respond flexibly and sensitively to individual needs stands the best chance of engaging the young person and the family with the service, building an understanding of, and trust in, the goals and methods of treatment, and maintaining the therapeutic relationship. Engagement is enhanced when the young person's and the family's most urgent practical needs are acknowledged and all possible steps taken to meet them. However, it was shown that children and families appreciate a structured intervention programme and respond very positively to regular monitoring of their progress in the independent and concrete terms that were introduced by the evaluation of the innovation projects. Thus it became clear that the achievement of self-awareness among the young people was often a pre-requisite for making further progress, although it may also indicate specific ongoing needs. Services working with young people with severe and complex needs, in particular, should find ways of marking progress, with the full involvement of the young person themselves. Commissioners of these services would do well to plan for longer term interventions—probably provided by a number of local services working in concert—in order to achieve sustainable progress in positive outcomes for young people and their families.

Even with their explicit, specific, and high profile remit, the CAMHS innovation projects found that a change in attitudes—to the kinds of problem taken on, the goals of treatment, and the ways of working—was necessary among many of their staff. All child and adolescent mental health services should recognize their need to examine critically what they do and how they are doing it. This means that staff should have dedicated time to reflect upon their work, and should acknowledge and be able to act upon their training needs. As an example, all the innovation projects came to recognize that they lacked adequate knowledge, experience, and skills to work effectively with young people from minority ethnic communities. They found that they could gain this expertise by working closely with other local services, such as the youth service, which have longstanding experience and good relationships with community members, as well as directly from community members themselves.

All child and adolescent mental health services need to find ways to reduce the stigma of mental health services and the lack of understanding of their problems by professionals that is often felt by children and families. Some of the ways in which this can be achieved is by involving them in the design of their treatment and its delivery, and the information given to others, as well as in planning service provision. Offering services, as well as a conduit to more specialist help, through universal provision, such as schools, is a vital component in any local service system.

In line with the evidence for effectiveness, work with the index child alone is likely to be the exception rather than the norm. Parents and carers are vital partners and may even be the chief recipients of the professional intervention in support of their child. This is highlighted by the finding in the recent ONS follow-up survey of childhood mental health disorders (Meltzer *et al.* 2003b), that maternal mental health was the most significantly correlated factor in the persistence of emotional disorders in children. In addition, Kazdin (1990), for example, examined differences between children and families referred for anti-social behaviour, who complete treatment versus those who terminated prematurely. Among those who terminated treatment prematurely, children showed more severe conduct disorder symptoms and more delinquent behaviours; mothers reported greater stress from their relations with the child, their own role functioning, and life events; and families were at greater socio-economic disadvantage than those who remained in treatment. In line with approaches shown to be effective in adult psychotherapeutic services, Kazdin suggested that treatment programmes may include components designed specifically to address sources of maternal stress (e.g. marital discord, social isolation), with other approaches to include special orientation and related pre-treatment interviews, various mailings and methods of scheduling appointments, and mone-tary incentives.

Some of the most telling evidence is for the link between effectiveness and the style of thera-peutic approach and service delivery (Bickman 1996; Davis and Spurr 1998). Particularly in prevention, a didactic approach has been demonstrated to be less successful than one focused on relationship-building, treating the mother as the person with responsibility to promote the development of her child (Barnard *et al.* 1985 cited in Fonagy 1998). This approach is the founda-tion of an innovative community child and family mental health service in a part of inner London (Davis *et al.* 2000). Existing staff (mostly health visitors and community paediatricians) have been trained to work as parent advisers, in a style characterized as having 'unconditional regard' for their clients. Evaluation has shown very high satisfaction among those who use the service, but the take-up is disappointingly low (Davis *et al.* 1997). Further development and evaluation of this service focuses on matters related to the engagement of families with the service (Attride-Stirling *et al.* 2001)—an aspect strongly confirmed to be crucial in the 24 projects.

An effective service should have the capacity to offer a highly skilled workforce capable of addressing a whole range of needs, or of setting up joint work with partner services, as neces-sary. This is especially the case for services that expect to work intensively with young people with severe and complex needs, but applies equally for effective practice in preventive and early intervention services. Some of the most successful early intervention projects offered a set number of sessions, but offered them flexibly over a period of time chosen by the family, with good links with other services for wider and longer term support. All services—or service systems—should find ways to define less rigidly the length of a specific intervention and formal discharge, with—again, in order to enhance effective practice—longer periods of skilled support for some children and families and informal continuation of advice and support where this will maintain the family's coping and prevent further help being dependent upon the occurrence of crises.

All CAMHS have a vital role in raising awareness of mental health among all local children's services and in finding every possible opportunity to work with these services to identify children and families at risk and encourage them to obtain the appropriate help. The value of this aspect of practice in CAMHS should be clearly acknowledged. As such, there is little doubt that a comprehensive local CAMHS system should include skilled practice in the prevention of child and adolescent mental health problems, working with universal services such as education but also with young people at high risk in specialist services such as foster care and Youth Offending Teams. It often requires particularly creative approaches to find ways to work with these services and with young people and families in differing local contexts, influenced by differing understandings of mental health in community and service cultures.

Acknowledgement

The authors wish to thank the users, staff and evaluators of the CAMHS Innovation projects for their enthusiasm and commitment. All quotes from service users and staff are taken from project reports and evaluations; these are fully referenced in our Department of Health publication (Kurtz and James 2004).

References

Attride-Stirling, J., Davis, H., Markless, G., Sclare, I., and Day, C. (2001) 'Someone to talk to who'll listen': addressing the psychosocial needs of chilren and families. *Journal of Community and Applied Social Psychology*, **11**, 179–91.

Audit Commission (1999) *Children in mind—child and adolescent mental health services.* London: Audit Commission.

Bickman, L. (1996) A continuum of care: more is not always better. *American Psychologist*, **51**, 689–701.

Borduin, C.M., Mann, B.J., Cone, L.T., Henggeler, S.W., Fucci, B.R., Blaske, D.M., *et al.* (1995) Multisysemic treatment of serious juvenile offenders: long-term prevention of criminality and violence. *Journal of Consulting and Clinical Psychology*, **63**, 569–78.

Cunningham, C.E., Bremner, R., and Boyle, M. (1995) Large group community-based parenting programs for families of pre-schoolers at risk for disruptive behavior disorders: utilization, cost-effectiveness and outcome. *Journal of Child Psychology and Psychiatry*, **36**, 1141–59.

Davis, H. and Spurr, P. (1998) Parent counselling: an evaluation of a community child mental health service. *Journal of Child Psychology and Psychiatry*, **39** (3), 365–76.

Davis, H., Spurr, P., Cox, A., Lynch, M., Von Roenne, A., and Hahn, K. (1997) A description and evaluation of a community child and adolescent mental health service. *Clinical Child Psychology and Psychiatry*, **2**, 221–38.

Davis, H., Day, C., Cox, A., and Cutler, L. (2000) Child and adolescent mental health needs: assessment and service implications in an inner city area. *Clinical Child Psychology and Psychiatry*, **5**, 169–88.

Department of Health (1998) *Specific grant for the development of social care services for people with a mental illness 1998/9: the child and adolescent mental health services (CAMHS fund)* LAC 98(13) HSC1998/008. London: Department of Health.

Fonagy, P. (1998) Prevention, the appropriate target of infant psychotherapy. *Infant Mental Health Journal*, **19** (2), 124–50.

Fonagy, P., Cottrell, D., Target, M., Phillips, J., and Kurtz, Z. (2002) *What works for whom? A critical review of treatments for children and adolescents.* New York and London: The Guilford Press.

Henggeler, S.W., Schoenwald, S.K., and Pickrel, S.G. (1995) Multisystemic therapy: bridging the gap between university and community-based treatment. *Journal of Consulting and Clinical Psychology,* **63**, 709–17.

Hoagwood, K., Jensen, P.S., Petti, T., and Burns, B.J. (1996) Outcomes of mental health care for children and adolescents: I. A comprehensive conceptual model. *Journal of the American Academy of Child and Adolescent Psychiatry,* **35**, 1055–63.

Kazdin, A.E. (1990) Premature termination from treatment among children referred for antisocial behavior. *Journal of Child Psychology and Psychiatry,* **31**(3), 415–25.

Kurtz, Z. and James, C. (2004) *What's new: learning from the CAMHS Innovation projects.* London: Department of Health.

Meltzer, H., Gatward, R., Corbin, T., Goodman, R., and Ford, T. (2003) *The mental health of young people looked after by local authorities in England.* London: The Stationery Office.

Senge, P.M. (1990) *The fifth discipline: the art and practice of the learning organisation.* London: Century.

Weisz, J.R. and Weiss, B. (1993) *Effects of psychotherapy with children and adolescents.* Newbury Park: Sage.

Weisz, J.R., Weiss, B., and Donenberg, G.R. (1992) The lab versus the clinic: effects of child and adolescent psychotherapy. *American Psychologist,* **47**, 1578–85.

Weisz, J.R., Donenberg, G.R., Han, S.S., and Kauneckis, D. (1995a) Child and adolescent psychotherapy outcomes in experiments versus clinics: why the disparity? *Journal of Abnormal Child Psychology,* **23**(1), 83–106.

Weisz, J.R., Weiss, B., Han, S.S., Granger, D.A., and Morton, T. (1995b) Effects of psychotherapy with children and adolescent revisited: a meta-analysis of treatment outcome studies. *Psychological Bulletin,* **117**, 450–68.

Index